MW01614996

CALIFORNIA NURSING PRACTICE ACT

WITH REGULATIONS AND RELATED STATUTES

BOARD OF REGISTERED NURSING

2023

Statutes Include Amendments Through the 2022 Regular Session of the 2021-2022 California Legislature and Regulations Include Amendments Through October 7, 2022 (2022 Register No. 40)

QUESTIONS ABOUT THIS PUBLICATION?

For CUSTOMER SERVICE ASSISTANCE concerning replacement pages, shipments, billing, reprint permission, or other matters,

please contact Customer Support at our self-service portal available 24/7 at *support.lexisnexis.com/print*
or call us at 800-833-9844

For EDITORIAL **content questions** concerning this publication,

please email: *llp.clp@lexisnexis.com*

For **information on other LEXISNEXIS MATTHEW BENDER publications,**

please call us at 877-394-8826
or visit our online bookstore at *www.lexisnexis.com/bookstore*

ISBN: 978-1-66335-700-7

© 2022 Matthew Bender & Company, Inc., a member of the LexisNexis Group.

All rights reserved.

LexisNexis and the Knowledge Burst logo are registered trademarks, and Michie is a trademark of Reed Elsevier Properties Inc., used under license. Matthew Bender is a registered trademark of Matthew Bender Properties Inc.

The California regulations appearing in this publication have been extracted from Barclays Official California Code of Regulations, copyright © 2021, State of California. This material may not be commercially reproduced or sold in printed or electronic form without written permission of Thomson/West, and is subject to the following disclaimer:

THOMSON/WEST MAKES NO WARRANTY OR REPRESENTATION WHATSOEVER, EXPRESS OR IMPLIED, WITH RESPECT TO THE MERCHANTABILITY OR FITNESS FOR ANY PARTICULAR PURPOSE WITH RESPECT TO THE INFORMATION CONTAINED IN THIS PUBLICATION; AND

THOMSON/WEST ASSUMES NO LIABILITY WHATSOEVER WITH RESPECT TO ANY USE OF THIS PUBLICATION OR ANY PORTION THEREOF OR WITH RESPECT TO ANY DAMAGES WHICH MAY RESULT FROM SUCH USE

LexisNexis®

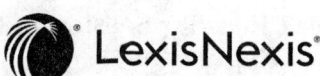

Matthew Bender & Company, Inc.
Editorial Offices
9443 Springboro Pike
Miamisburg, OH 45342
800-833-9844
www.lexisnexis.com

(Pub. 23550)

PREFACE

LexisNexis is pleased to offer to the nursing community the 2023 edition of **California Nursing Practice Act with Regulations and Related Statutes**. This volume is a compilation of selected laws and regulations that affect the nursing industry. It is fully up to date with statutes required by legislative enactments through the 2022 Regular Session of the 2021-2022 California Legislature. Regulations include amendments through October 7, 2022 (2022 Register No. 40).

Included herein is a Table of Sections Affected which may be utilized to facilitate research into recently enacted legislation affecting these Codes. Through the use of state-of-the-art computer software, attorney editors have updated the comprehensive descriptive word index with the enactments of the 2022 legislature.

We are committed to providing legal professionals with the most comprehensive, current and useful publications possible. If you have comments and suggestions, please write to California Codes Editor, LexisNexis, 9443 Springboro Pike, Miamisburg, OH 45342; call us toll-free at 1-800-833-9844; or E-mail us at *llp.clp@lexisnexis.com*. By providing us with your informed comments, you will be assured of having available a working tool which increases in value each year.

Visit the LexisNexis Internet home page at *http://www.lexisnexis.com* for an online bookstore, technical support, customer service, and other company information.

January 2023

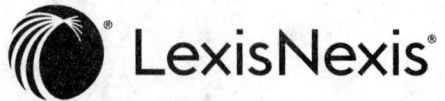

LexisNexis®

NURSING PRACTICE ACT—TABLE OF CONTENTS

Page

NURSING PRACTICE ACT
EXTRACTED FROM
BUSINESS AND PROFESSIONS CODE

DIVISION 2. Healing Arts
CHAPTER 6. Nursing

Article 1. Administration

Section		
2700.	Citation	2
2701.	Board of Registered Nursing; Authority [Repealed effective January 1, 2023]	2
2701.5.	Board subject to review	2
2702.	Membership qualifications	2
2703.	Appointments, terms, vacancies	3
2706.	Removal from office	3
2707.	Elections of officers	4
2708.	Executive officer; Appointment; Duties; Interim executive officer [Repealed effective January 1, 2023]	4
2708.1.	Priority of board; Protection of the public	4
2709.	Regular meetings	4
2709.5.	Mediums of exchange	5
2710.	Special meetings	5
2710.5.	Advisory committees	5
2712.	Quorum	5
2713.	Records	5
2714.	Offices; Venue	5
2715.	Prosecutions; Employment matters; Seal; Rule-making authority	6
2716.	Compensation and expenses	6
2717.	Plan to address nursing shortage	6
2718.	Performance audit of enforcement program [Repealed]	6

Article 2. Scope of Regulation

Section		
2725.	Legislative intent; Practice of nursing defined	7
2725.1.	Dispensation of drugs or devices by registered nurse; Construction	8
2725.2.	Dispensation of self-administered hormonal contraceptives; Injections; Standardized procedure	9
2725.3.	Functions performed by unlicensed personnel	10
2725.4.	Abortion by aspiration techniques; Requirements	11
2725.5.	"Advanced practice registered nurse" defined	12

		Page
2726.	Unauthorized practices	12
2727.	Practices not prohibited	13
2727.5.	Liability for emergency care	13
2728.	Services by attendants and psychiatric technicians; Supervised services of unlicensed graduates of accredited psychiatric technician training programs	13
2728.5.	Utilization of licensed psychiatric technicians and psychiatric technician interim permittees	14
2729.	Services by student nurses	14
2730.	Nurses qualified outside state and engaged to care for patient temporarily in California	15
2731.	Nonprofit religious care	15
2732.	Licensure requirement; Use of "R.N."	15
2732.05.	Verification of current R.N. status	15
2732.1.	Applications; Interim permits; Waiver of examination; Fees	16
2733.	Issuance of temporary license where examination waived	16
2734.	Inactive licenses	17
2736.	Qualifications generally	17
2736.1.	Training in detection and treatment of client abuse, and alcohol and chemical substance dependency	18
2736.5.	Continuing education courses regarding implicit bias	18
2736.6.	Eligibility of vocational nurse to take examination for licensure as registered nurse	19
2737.	Application fee	19
2738.	Holding of examinations	19
2740.	Conduct of examinations; Finality of decisions	19
2741.	Fees with application for reexamination	20
2742.	Issuance of license	20

Article 2.5. Nurse-Midwives

Section		
2746.	Issuance of certificates	20
2746.1.	Compliance with article required	20
2746.2.	Educational prerequisites; Nurse-midwifery committee	21
2746.3.	Renewal of midwife's certificates	21
2746.4.	Practice of midwifery by midwife's certificates	21
2746.5.	Authority conferred by certificate; Required supervision	21
2746.51.	When nurse-midwife may furnish drugs or devices	23
2746.52.	Authority to perform episiotomies and repair lacerations of perineum	26
2746.53.	Furnishing number fees	26
2746.54.	Obtaining informed consent	26
2746.55.	Data collected after transfer to hospital or maternal, fetal, or neonatal death that occurred in the out-of-hospital setting	27
2746.6.	Discipline for performance of abortion	30
2746.7.	Applications and fees	31
2746.8.	Renewal of nurse-midwifery certificates	31

Page

Article 3. Disciplinary Proceedings

Section		Page
2750.	Persons subject to discipline; Conduct of proceedings	32
2751.	Acceptance of surrender of license through stipulated agreement	32
2759.	Scope of discipline	32
2760.	Effect of suspension; Conditions of reinstatement	33
2760.1.	Petition for reinstatement or modification of penalty; Notice to Attorney General; Hearing	33
2761.	Grounds for action	34
2761.1.	Performance of abortion	36
2761.5.	Reporting mechanisms	36
2762.	Drug-related transgressions	37
2764.	Jurisdiction in event license suspended or surrendered	37
2765.	What deemed conviction	38

Article 3.1. Intervention Program

Section		Page
2770.	Legislative intent	38
2770.1.	Definitions	39
2770.2.	Intervention evaluation committees; Composition; Appointments	39
2770.3.	Per diem and expenses of committee members	39
2770.4.	Quorum; Majority vote requirement	40
2770.5.	Election of chairperson and vice chairperson	40
2770.6.	Administration of article	40
2770.7.	Establishment of criteria for acceptance, denial, or termination of registered nurses in program; Investigations; Disciplinary actions	40
2770.8.	Intervention program manager responsibilities; Duties and responsibilities of committees	41
2770.9.	Informing participants of procedures, rights, and responsibilities	41
2770.10.	Authority of committee to convene in closed session	42
2770.11.	Termination of participation for noncompliance with provisions of program	42
2770.12.	Purging of records following intervention program	42
2770.13.	Provision of representation in defamation action resulting from reports or information given to committee	43
2770.14.	Board reports	43

Article 3.5. Nursing Corporations

Section		Page
2775.	Definition	44
2776.	Individual unprofessional conduct	44
2777.	Corporate unprofessional conduct	44
2778.	Name	44
2779.	Shareholders, directors and officers	44

		Page
2780.	Income while shareholder is disqualified	45
2781.	Regulations	45

Article 4. Nursing Schools

Section		
2785.	List of approved schools	45
2785.5.	Board to facilitate efficient transfer agreements between associate degree nursing programs and baccalaureate degree nursing programs	46
2785.6.	Nuring Education and Workforce Advisory Committee	46
2786.	Approval of schools; Implicit bias training requirement	48
2786.1.	Denial or revocation for school not giving credit for military education and experience; Regulations; Review of school's policies and practices regarding credit for military education and experience and posting of information on Web site	50
2786.2.	Private postsecondary school of nursing; Memorandum of understanding;Actively accredited approved schools	50
2786.3.	Nursing programs affected by interruptions due to state of emergency; requests submitted to board of nursing education; approval	52
2786.4.	Payments for student clinical experience placements prohibited	54
2786.5.	Fees	54
2786.6.	Grounds for denial of approval	55
2788.	Inspections; Approval of schools meeting requirements; Notice of defects	55
2789.	Exempt schools	55

Article 5. Penal Provisions

Section		
2795.	Unlawful practice; Misrepresentation of licensee status	56
2796.	Use of "R.N.", etc.	56
2797.	Impersonation of applicants or examinees	56
2798.	Conduct of unapproved school; Unprofessional conduct for registered nurse	57
2799.	Penalty for violations	57
2800.	Applicability of article	57

Article 6. Revenue

Section		
2810.	Board of Registered Nursing Fund	58
2811.	Renewal of licenses; Expiration and reinstatement; Restoration of license in inactive status to active status	58
2811.5.	Continuing education as prerequisite for renewal	59
2811.6.	Availability of continuing education course records for board inspection	60

Page

2812. Reports; Deposit of funds 60
2814. Use of funds 60
2815. Fee schedule for registered nurses 61
2815.1. Increase in license renewal fee 63
2815.5. Fee schedule for nurse-midwives 63
2815.7. Report to the legislature upon proposal or adoption of fee increase 63

Article 6.5. Public Health Nurse Certification

Section
2816. Fee 64
2817. Child abuse and neglect detection training requirement 64
2818. Legislative findings; Use of title "public health nurse" 64
2819. Repeal and adoption of regulations 65
2820. Scope of practice 65

Article 7. Nurse Anesthetists

Section
2825. Citation of article 66
2826. Definitions 66
2827. Anesthesia services; Approval; Permit 67
2828. Nonemployee nurse anesthetists working in acute care facilities 67
2829. Unlawful use of title "nurse anesthetist" 67
2830. Certificate to practice 67
2830.5. Evidence that applicant has met requirements 68
2830.6. Certification 68
2830.7. Fee schedule for nurse anesthetists 68
2831. Written application; Fee 68
2832. Applicant to comply with all provisions of article 69
2833. Renewal of certificate; Reinstatement of expired certificate 69
2833.3. Article not limitation on ability to practice nursing 69
2833.5. Practice not authority to practice medicine or surgery 69
2833.6. Effect of provisions on existing scope of practice 69

Article 8. Nurse Practitioners

Section
2834. Legislative finding of conflicting definitions and usage 70
2835. License requirement 70
2835.5. Requirements for initial qualification or certification as nurse practitioner 70
2835.7. Authorized standardized procedures 71
2836. Establishment of categories and standards 71
2836.1. Furnishing or ordering of drugs or devices by nurse practitioners 71
2836.2. What constitutes furnishing or ordering of drugs or

		Page
	devices	73
2836.3.	Issuance of number to nurse practitioners dispensing drugs or devices	73
2836.4.	Furnishing or ordering buprenorphine	74
2837.	Registered nursing practice not limited	75

Article 8.5. Advanced Practice Registered Nurses

Section		
2837.100.	Legislative intent	75
2837.101.	Definitions	75
2837.102.	Nurse Practitioner Advisory Committee	76
2837.103.	Requirements to perform, in certain settings or organizations, specified functions without standardized procedures	76
2837.103.5.	Conditional authority of nurse practitioner to prescribe, order dispense, procure, and furnish pharmacological agents	78
2837.104.	Requirements to perform, outside of certain settings or organizations, specified functions without standardized procedures	79
2837.105.	Occupational analysis of nurse practitioners performing certain functions	81

Article 9. Clinical Nurse Specialists

Section		
2838.	License required	81
2838.1.	Qualifications and credentials	81
2838.2.	Standards and fees	82
2838.3.	Operative date of article	83
2838.4.	Effect of article	83
	Resolution of Chapter 156	85

CALIFORNIA CODE OF REGULATIONS

TITLE 16. Professional and Vocational Regulations
DIVISION 14. Board of Registered Nursing

Article 1. General Provisions Section

Section		
1402.	Definitions	87
1403.	Delegation of Certain Functions	87
1405.	Authority of Executive Officer	88

Article 2. Registration and Examination

Section		
1409.	Issuance of License	89

		Page
1409.1.	Filing of Names and Addresses	89
1410.	Application	89
1410.1.	Application Processing Times	90
1410.4.	Abandonment of Application	91
1411.5.	Examination Procedure	91
1411.6.	Examination Disclosure	92
1412.	High School Education or the Equivalent	92
1413.	English Comprehension	92
1414.	Interim Permits	92
1414.1.	Foreign Licensees	93
1414.5.	Temporary License	93
1417.	Fees	93
1418.	Eligibility for Licensure of Applicants Who Have Military Education and Experience	96
1419.	Renewal of License	96
1419.1.	Inactive License	97
1419.2.	Renewal Processing Times	97
1419.3.	Reinstatement of Expired License	98
1419.4.	Issuance of Duplicate License	98

Article 3. Prelicensure Nursing Programs

Section		
1420.	Definitions	99
1421.	Application for Approval	100
1422.	Certificate of Approval	101
1423.	Approval Requirements	102
1423.1.	Grounds for Denial or Removal of Board Approval	102
1423.2.	Denial or Revocation of Approval of a Nursing Program	103
1424.	Administration and Organization of the Nursing Program	103
1425.	Faculty—Qualifications and Changes	104
1425.1.	Faculty Responsibilities	106
1426.	Required Curriculum	106
1426.1.	Preceptorship	108
1427.	Clinical Facilities	109
1428.	Student Participation	109
1428.6.	Policies Relating to Establishing Eligibility for Examination	110
1429.	Licensed Vocational Nurses, Thirty (30) Semester or Forty-Five (45) Quarter Unit Option	110
1430.	Previous Education Credit	111
1431.	Licensing Examination Pass Rate Standard	111
1432.	Changes to an Approved Program	111

Article 3.5. Citations and Fines

Section		
1435.	Citations—Content and Service	112
1435.1.	Exceptions	113
1435.15.	Citation Disclosure and Record Purge	113

		Page
1435.2.	Violations and Fines	114
1435.3.	Citations for Unlicensed Individual	114
1435.4.	Criteria to be Considered in Assessing a Fine or Order of Abatement	114
1435.5.	Contested Citations	115
1435.6.	Compliance with Citation/Order of Abatement	115
1435.7.	Notification to Other Boards and Agencies	116

Article 4. Grounds for Discipline, Disciplinary Proceedings and Rehabilitation

Section		
1441.	Unprofessional Conduct	116
1442.	Gross Negligence	117
1443.	Incompetence	117
1443.5.	Standards of Competent Performance	118
1444.	Substantial Relationship Criteria	118
1444.5.	Disciplinary Guidelines	119
1445.	Criteria for Rehabilitation	120
1445.1.	Petition for Reinstatement	121

Article 4.1. Intervention Program Guidelines

Section		
1446.	Definitions	122
1447.	Criteria for Admission	122
1447.1.	Procedure for Review of Applicants	123
1447.2.	Causes for Denial of Admission	123
1448.	Causes for Termination from the Program	123
1448.1.	Notification of Termination	124
1449.	Confidentiality of Records	124

Article 5. Continuing Education

Section		
1450.	Definitions	124
1451.	License Renewal Requirements	125
1451.1.	Expiration of Licenses	126
1451.2.	Continuing Education Courses	126
1452.	Exemption from Continuing Education Requirements	127
1453.	Falsifying Renewal Application	127
1454.	Approved Providers	127
1455.	Continuing Education Hours	128
1456.	Continuing Education Courses	129
1457.	Instructor Qualifications	130
1458.	Course Verification	130
1459.	Advertisement	131
1459.1.	Withdrawal of Approval	131

Page

Article 6. Nurse-Midwives

Section
1460. Qualifications for Certification ... 132
1461. Nurse-Midwifery Committee ... 132
1462. Standards for Nurse-Midwifery Programs ... 132
1463. Scope of Practice ... 134
1463.5. Abortion by Aspiration Techniques ... 134
1466. Renewal of Certificates ... 135

Article 7. Standardized Procedure Guidelines

Section
1470. Purpose ... 135
1471. Definitions ... 136
1472. Standardized Procedure Functions ... 136
1474. Standardized Procedure Guidelines ... 136

Article 8. Standards for Nurse Practitioners

Section
1480. Definitions ... 137
1481. Categories of Nurse Practitioners ... 139
1482. Requirements for Certification As a Nurse Practitioner ... 139
1483. Evaluation of Credentials ... 140
1483.1. Requirements for Nurse Practitioner Education Programs in California ... 141
1483.2. Requirements for Reporting Nurse Practitioner Education Program Changes ... 141
1484. Nurse Practitioner Education ... 142
1485. Scope of Practice ... 145
1485.5. Abortion by Aspiration Techniques ... 145
1486. Requirements for Clinical Practice Experience for Nurse Practitioner Students Enrolled in Non-California based Nurse Practitioner Education Programs ... 146

Article 9. Public Health Nurse

Section
1490. Public Health Nurse Certificate ... 147
1491. Qualifications and Requirements ... 147
1492. Application for Public Health Nurse Certificate ... 149
1493. Issuance of Certificate ... 149

Article 10. Sponsored Free Health Care Events—Requirements for Exemption [Repealed]

Section
1495. Definitions. [Repealed] ... 150
1495.1. Sponsoring Entity Registration and Recordkeeping

		Page
	Requirements. [Repealed]	150
1495.2.	Out-of-State Practitioner Authorization to Participate in Sponsored Event. [Repealed]	150
1495.3.	Termination of Authorization and Appeal. [Repealed]	151
1495.4.	Disclosure Requirements; Name and License Status. [Repealed]	151

BUSINESS & PROFESSIONS CODE

General Provisions

Section		
7.5.	"Conviction"; When action by board following establishment of conviction may be taken; Prohibition against denial of licensure; Application of section	153
12.5.	Violation of regulation adopted pursuant to code provision; Issuance of citation	154
14.1.	Legislative intent	154
22.	"Board"	154
23.	"Department"	154
23.5.	"Director"	154
23.6.	"Appointing power"	155
23.7.	"License"	155
29.5.	Additional qualifications for licensure	155
30.	Provision of federal employer identification number or social security number by licensee	155
31.	Compliance with judgment or order for support upon issuance or renewal of license	158
32.	Legislative findings; AIDS training for health care professionals	159

DIVISION 1. Department of Consumer Affairs
CHAPTER 1. The Department

Section		
100.	Establishment	161
101.	Composition of department	161
101.6.	Purpose	162
103.	Compensation and reimbursement for expenses	163
104.	Display of licenses or registrations	163
105.	Oath of office	163
105.5.	Tenure of members of boards, etc., within department	164
106.	Removal of board members	164
106.5.	Removal of member of licensing board for disclosure of examination information	164
107.	Executive officers	164
107.5.	Official seals	165
108.	Status and powers of boards	165
108.5.	Witness fees and expenses	165
109.	Review of decisions; Investigations	165
110.	Records and property	166

		Page
111.	Commissioners on examination	166
112.	Publication and sale of directories of authorized persons	166
113.	Conferences; Traveling expenses	167
114.	Reinstatement of expired license of licensee serving in military	167
114.3.	Waiver of fees and requirements for active duty members of armed forces and national guard	168
114.5.	Military service; Posting of information on Web site about application of military experience and training towards licensure	169
115.	Applicability of Section 114	169
115.4.	Licensure process expedited for honorably discharged veterans of Armed Forces	169
115.5.	Board required to expedite licensure process for certain applicants; Adoption of regulations [Repealed effective July 1, 2022]	169
115.5.	Board required to expedite licensure process for certain applicants; Adoption of regulations [Operative July 1, 2022]	170
115.6.	Temporary licensure process for spouses of active duty members of Armed Forces [Repealed effective July 1, 2023]	170
115.6.	Temporary licensure process for spouses of active duty members of Armed Forces [Operative July 1, 2023]	172
115.8.	Annual report on military, veteran, and spouse licensure	174
115.9.	Publishing information on licensing options available to military spouses	174
116.	Audit and review of disciplinary proceedings; Report to Legislature	174
118.	Effect of withdrawal of application; Effect of suspension, forfeiture, etc., of license	175
119.	Misdemeanors pertaining to use of licenses	175
121.	Practice during period between renewal and receipt of evidence of renewal	176
122.	Fee for issuance of duplicate certificate	176
123.	Conduct constituting subversion of licensing examination; Penalties and damages	176
123.5.	Enjoining violations	177
124.	Manner of notice	178
125.	Misdemeanor offenses by licensees	178
125.3.	Direction to licensee violating licensing act to pay costs of investigation and enforcement	178
125.5.	Enjoining violations; Restitution orders	179
125.6.	Unlawful discrimination by licensees	180
125.7.	Restraining orders	181
125.8.	Temporary order restraining licensee engaged or about to engage in violation of law	182
125.9.	System for issuance of citations to licensees; Contents; Fines	182
126.	Submission of reports to Governor	184

Page
127. Submission of reports to director ... 184
128. Sale of equipment, supplies, or services for use in violation of licensing requirements ... 184
128.5. Reduction of license fees in event of surplus funds ... 184
129. Handling of complaints; Reports to Legislature ... 185
130. Terms of office of agency members ... 186
131. Maximum number of terms ... 186
132. Requirements for institution or joinder of legal action by state agency against other state or federal agency ... 187
134. Proration of license fees ... 187
135. Reexamination of applicants ... 187
135.4. Refugees, asylees, and special immigrant visa holders; professional licensing; initial licensure process ... 188
135.5. Licensure and citizenship or immigration status ... 188
136. Notification of change of address; Punishment for failure to comply ... 188
137. Regulations requiring inclusion of license numbers in advertising, etc. ... 189
138. Notice that practitioner is licensed; Evaluation of licensing examination ... 189
139. Policy for examination development and validation, and occupational analysis ... 189
139.5. Quarterly internet website posting requirements ... 191
140. Disciplinary action; Licensee's failure to record cash transactions in payment of employee wages ... 191
141. Disciplinary action by foreign jurisdiction; Grounds for disciplinary action by state licensing board ... 191
142. Authority to synchronize renewal dates of licenses; Abandonment date for application; Delinquency fee ... 192
143. Proof of license as condition of bringing action for collection of compensation ... 192
143.5. Provision in agreements to settle certain causes of action prohibited; Adoption of regulations; Exemptions ... 193
144. Requirement of fingerprints for criminal record checks; Applicability ... 193
144.5. Board authority ... 195

CHAPTER 1.5. Unlicensed Activity Enforcement

Section
145. Legislative findings and declarations ... 195
146. Violations of specified authorization statutes as infractions; Punishment ... 195
147. Authority to issue written notice to appear in court ... 197
148. Establishment of administrative citation system ... 197
149. Notice to cease advertising in telephone directory; Contest and hearing; Disconnection of service ... 197

CHAPTER 2. The Director of Consumer Affairs

Section
150.

Page
150150150150Designation 199
151. Appointment and tenure; Salary and traveling expenses 199
152. Departmental organization 199
152.5. Extension of renewal dates 199
152.6. Establishment of license periods and renewal dates 200
153. Investigations 200
154. Matters relating to employees of boards 200
154.5. Legal assistance for experts aiding in investigations of licensees 200
155. Employment of investigators; Inspectors as employees or under contract 201
156.1. Retention of records by providers of services related to treatment of alcohol or drug impairment 201
156.5. Leases for examination or meeting purposes 202
157. Expenses in criminal prosecutions and unprofessional conduct proceedings 202
158. Refunds to applicants 202
159. Administration of oaths 203
159.5. Division of Investigation; Appointments; Health Quality Investigation Unit 203
160. Division of Investigation of the department and Dental Board of California 203
161. Availability of public records at charge sufficient to pay costs 204
162. Evidentiary effect of certificate of records officer as to license, etc. 204
163. Fee for certification of records, etc. 204
164. Form and content of license, certificate, permit, or similar indicia of authority 204
165. Prohibition against submission of fiscal impact analysis relating to pending legislation without prior submission to director for comment 205
166. Development of guidelines for mandatory continuing education programs 205

CHAPTER 3. Funds of the Department

Section

201. Levy for administrative expenses 206
205. Professions and Vocations Fund [Repealed effective July 1, 2022.] 207
205. Professions and Vocations Fund [Operative July 1, 2022.] 207
206. Dishonored check tendered for payment of fine, fee, or penalty 208

CHAPTER 4. Consumer Affairs

Page

Article 3. Powers and Duties

Section
310. Director's powers and duties 209
312. Report to Governor and Legislature 209
313.1. Compliance with section as requirement for effectiveness of specified rules or regulations; Submission of records; Authority for disapproval 210
313.2. Adoption of regulations in conformance with Americans with Disabilities Act 211

Article 3.6. Uniform Standards Regarding Substance-Abusing Healing Arts Licensees

Section
315. Establishment of Substance Abuse Coordination Committee; Members; Duties 212
315.2. Cease practice order 214
315.4. Cease practice order for violation of probation or diversion program 214

Article 4. Representation of Consumers

Section
320. Intervention in administrative or judicial proceedings 215
321. Commencement of legal proceedings 215

Article 5. Consumer Complaints

Section
325. Actionable complaints 215
326. Proceedings on receipt of complaint 216
328. Implementation of Complaint Prioritization Guidelines 216

CHAPTER 6. Public Members

Section
450. Qualifications generally 217
450.2. Avoiding conflict of interest 217
450.3. Conflicting pecuniary interests 218
450.5. Prior industrial and professional pursuits 218
450.6. Age 218
451. Delegation of duties 218
452. "Board" 218
453. Training and orientation program for new board members 219

CHAPTER 7. Licensee

Section
460.

Page
460460460... Powers of local governmental entities 219
461. Asking applicant to reveal arrest record prohibited 220
462. Inactive category of licensure 220
464. Retired category of licensure 221

DIVISION 1.5. Denial, Suspension and Revocation of Licenses

CHAPTER 1. General Provisions

Section
475. Applicability of division 222
476. Exemptions 222
477. “Board”; “License” 223
478. “Application”; “Material” 223

CHAPTER 2. Denial of Licenses

Section
480. Grounds for denial; Effect of obtaining certificate of rehabilitation [Repealed] 224
480. Grounds for denial by board; Effect of obtaining certificate of rehabilitation 224
480.5. Completion of licensure requirements while incarcerated . 227
481. Crime and job-fitness criteria [Repealed] 227
481. Crime and job-fitness criteria 227
482. Rehabilitation criteria [Repealed] 228
482. Rehabilitation criteria 228
484. Attestation to good moral character of applicant 228
485. Procedure upon denial 228
486. Contents of decision or notice 229
487. Hearing; Time 229
488. Hearing request [Repealed] 229
488. Hearing request 229
489. Denial of application without a hearing 230

CHAPTER 3. Suspension and Revocation of Licenses

Section
490. Grounds for suspension or revocation; Discipline for substantially related crimes; Conviction; Legislative findings 231
490.5. Suspension of license for failure to comply with child support order 231
491. Procedure upon suspension or revocation 231
492. Effect of completion of drug diversion program on disciplinary action or denial of license 232
493. Evidentiary effect of record of conviction of crime substantially related to licensee’s qualifications, functions, and duties [Repealed] 232
493. Evidentiary effect of record of conviction of crime

Page

substantially related to licensee's qualifications, functions, and duties 232
494. Interim suspension or restriction order 233
494.5. Agency actions when licensee is on certified list; Definitions; Collection and distribution of certified list information; Timing; Notices; Challenges by applicants and licensees; Release forms; Interagency agreements; Fees; Remedies; Inquiries and disclosure of information; Severability 235
494.6. Suspension under Labor Code Section 244 241

CHAPTER 4. Public Reprovals

Section
495. Public reproval of licentiate or certificate holder for act constituting grounds for suspension or revocation of license or certificate; Proceedings 242

CHAPTER 5. Examination Security

Section
496. Grounds for denial, suspension, or revocation of license 242
498. Fraud, deceit or misrepresentation as grounds for action against license 242
499. Action against license based on licentiate's actions regarding application of another 242

DIVISION 2. Healing Arts
CHAPTER 1. General Provisions

Article 1.5. Advocacy for Appropriate Health Care

Section
510. Protection against retaliation for physicians who "advocate for medically appropriate health care" 243

Article 4. Frauds of Medical Records

Section
580. Sale or barter of degree, certificate, or transcript 245
581. Purchase or fraudulent alteration of diplomas or other writings 245
582. Use of illegally obtained, altered, or counterfeit diploma, certificate, or transcript 246
583. False statements in documents or writings 246
584. Violation of examination security; Impersonation 246
585. Punishment 246

Page

Article 7. Nursing

Section
675. Unaccredited instructional courses 247
676. Applicability of article 247
677. Inspection of records 248
678. Failure to give notice as voiding contract 248
679. Violations 248

Article 7.5. Health Care Practitioners

Section
680. Health care practitioner's disclosure of name and license status 248
681. Securing specimens; Marking containers; Violations; "Locked container" 249
683. Reporting name and license number of licensee prohibited from practicing 250
684. Notice of practice of stem cell therapy not approved by FDA 250
685. Citation of health care practitioner in default of education loan [Repealed] 251
686. Providing services via telehealth 251

Article 10. Federal Personnel and Tribal Health Programs

Section
715. Licenses to practice in state 252
716. Denial of license; Disciplinary action against holder of state license 252
717. Construction of article 253
719. Employment of health care practitioner licensed in another state by tribal health program (First of two) 253
719. Certain persons employed by a tribal health program exempt from licensing requirement (Second of two) 253

Article 10.5. Unprofessional Conduct

Section
726. Commission of act of sexual abuse or misconduct with patient or client 254
730.5. Acupuncture without license 254

Article 11. Professional Reporting

Section
800. Central files of licensees' individual historical records 255
801. Insurers' reports of malpractice settlements or arbitration awards; Insured's written consent to settlement 257
801.01. Report of settlement of arbitration award over a specified

Page

amount in case of alleged negligence, error, or omission in practice or the licensee's rendering of unauthorized professional services; Procedure ... 258
801.1. Report of settlement or arbitration award where state or local government acts as self-insurer in cases of negligence, error, omission in practice, or rendering of unauthorized services resulting in death or personal injury ... 262
802. Reports of malpractice settlements or arbitration awards involving uninsured licensees; Penalties for noncompliance ... 262
803. Report of crime or liability for death or injury on part of specified licensees to licensing agency ... 264
804. Form and content of reports ... 264
806. Statistical reports and recommendations to Legislature ... 265

Article 12. Insurance Fraud

Section
810. Grounds for disciplinary action against health care professional ... 265

Article 12.5. Mental Illness or Physical Illness

Section
820. Examination of licentiate for mental illness or physical illness affecting competency ... 267
821. Effect of licentiate's failure to comply with order for examination ... 267
822. Action by licensing agency ... 268
823. Reinstatement of licentiate ... 268
824. Options open to licensing agency when proceeding against licentiate ... 268
825. "Licensing agency" ... 269
826. Format of proceedings under Sections 821 and 822; Rights and powers ... 269
827. Authority of licensing agency to convene in closed session ... 269
828. Determination of insufficient evidence to bring action against licentiate; Effect on records of proceedings ... 269

CHAPTER 1.5. Exemption from Licensure

Section
900. Requirements for exemption; Immunity from liability ... 270
901. Exemption from licensure requirements for services provided under enumerated circumstances; Prior authorization; Steps necessary for sponsoring entity; Report; List of health care practitioners providing health care services under this section; Compliance [Repealed] .. 271

Page

CHAPTER 3. Clinical Laboratory Technology

Article 3. Application of the Chapter

Section
1242.5. Regulations allowing unlicensed persons to withdraw blood and perform blood tests 271
1242.6. Withdrawal of blood by registered or licensed vocational nurse or respiratory care practitioner 271
1243. When student authorized to perform arterial puncture, etc. 272
1245. Authority to perform blood gas analysis; Application to certified respiratory care practitioner 272
1246. Authority for unlicensed person to perform venipuncture or skin puncture 273

Article 3.5. Hemodialysis Training

Section
1247.3. Treatment by technician; Administration of medications and anesthetics 276

CHAPTER 5. Medicine

Article 18. Corporations

Section
2406. Medical or podiatry corporation defined 277
2406.5. Disclosure statement for physical therapy referral 277

CHAPTER 6.6. Psychologists

Article 1. General Provisions

Section
2908. Exemption of other professions 278

Article 9. Psychological Corporations

Section
2995. Psychological corporation 279

CHAPTER 9. Pharmacy

Article 4. Requirements for Prescriptions

Section
4072. Oral or electronic transmission of prescription by nurse or other healing arts licentiate at health care facility 280

Page

CHAPTER 15. Telephone Medical Advice Services

Section

4999. "Telephone medical advice service" ... 280
4999.1. Application for registration [Repealed] ... 281
4999.2. Compliance with professional requirements; Recordkeeping and retention; Response and notice to department ... 281
4999.3. Discipline and denial of application [Repealed] ... 282
4999.4. Expiration and renewal of registration [Repealed] ... 282
4999.5. Enforcement ... 282
4999.6. Rules and regulations [Repealed] ... 282
4999.7. Effect on other practices and provisions ... 282

DIVISION 7. General Business Regulations
PART 3. Representations to the Public

CHAPTER 1. Advertising

Article 1. False Advertising in General

Section

17500. False or misleading statements generally ... 284
17500.1. Prohibition against enactment of rule, regulation, or code of ethics restricting or prohibiting advertising not violative of law ... 284
17502. Exemption of broadcasting stations and publishers from provisions of article ... 285
17506.5. "Board within the Department of Consumer Affairs"; "Local consumer affairs agency" ... 285

CIVIL CODE

DIVISION 1. Persons
PART 2. Personal Rights

Section

43.8. Immunity as to communication in aid of evaluation of practitioner of healing or veterinary arts ... 287
47. Privileged publication or broadcast ... 288

CORPORATIONS CODE

TITLE 1. CORPORATIONS
DIVISION 3. Corporations for Specific Purposes
PART 4. Professional Corporations

Section

13401. Definitions ... 291
13401.5. Licensees as shareholders, officers, directors, or employees ... 292

Page

EDUCATION CODE

TITLE 3. Postsecondary Education
DIVISION 5. General Provisions
PART 40. Donahoe Higher Education Act

CHAPTER 9.2. Student Transfer

Article 1.5. Common Course Numbering System

Section

66725. Legislative intent, findings and declarations 300
66725.3. Common course numbering system; Report; Date for incorporation into catalogue 300
66725.5. Common course numbering system in California Community Colleges 301

Article 2. Transfer Functions

Section

66739.5. Legislative findings and declarations; Legislative intent; Construction; Program with purpose of enabling community college students to earn baccalaureate degree at a campus of California State University 302

GOVERNMENT CODE

TITLE 1. GENERAL
DIVISION 7. Miscellaneous
CHAPTER 3.5. Inspection of Public Records

Article 1. General Provisions

Section

6250. Legislative finding and declaration [Repealed effective January 1, 2023] 308
6251. Citation of chapter [Repealed effective January 1, 2023] .. 308
6252. Definitions [Repealed effective January 1, 2023] 308
6252.5. Elected member or officer's access to public records [Repealed effective January 1, 2023] 308
6252.6. Disclosure of name, date of birth and date of death of minor foster child [Repealed effective January 1, 2023] 308
6252.7. Discrimination in allowing access of members of legislative body of local agency to writing or portion thereof prohibited [Repealed effective January 1, 2023] 308
6253. Time for inspection of public records; Unusual circumstances; Posting of public record on internet website [Repealed effective January 1, 2023] 309
6253.1. Agency to assist in inspection of public record [Repealed effective January 1, 2023] 309
6253.3. Control of disclosure by another party [Repealed effective

Page
January 1, 2023] 309
6253.31. Contract of state or local agency requiring private entity to review, audit or report on agency [Repealed effective January 1, 2023] 309
6253.4. Records to be made available [Repealed effective January 1, 2023] 309
6254.5. Confidentiality of state employee home addresses, telephone numbers, birth dates, and personal email addresses [Repealed effective January 1, 2023] 310

TITLE 2. Government of the State of California
DIVISION 3. Executive Department
PART 1. State Departments and Agencies

CHAPTER 1. State Agencies

Article 9. Meetings

Section
11120. Legislative finding and declaration; Open proceedings; Citation of article 313
11121. "State body" 313
11121.9. Providing copy of article to members of state bodies 314
11122. "Action taken" 314
11123. Open meeting requirement for state bodies; Meetings by teleconference; Public reporting requirement for actions at meeting 314
11123.5. Teleconference meeting 315
11124. Prohibited conditions to attendance 316
11124.1. Recording of proceedings; Inspection of recording 317
11125. Notice of meeting 317
11125.1. Agendas of public meetings and other "writings" as public record; Exemptions; Public inspection; Alternative format requirements; Fee 318
11125.2. Public report of action taken regarding public employee 319
11125.5. Emergency meetings; Notification of media 319
11125.7. Opportunity for public to address state body 320
11126. Closed session on issues relating to public employee; Employee's right to public hearing; Closed sessions not prohibited by article; Abrogation of lawyer-client privilege 321
11126.1. Minute book of closed session 328
11126.2. Closed session for response to final draft audit report 328
11126.3. Disclosure of items to be discussed in closed session; Discussion of additional pending litigation matters arising after disclosure 328
11126.5. Clearing room when meeting wilfully interrupted 329
11126.7. Fees 330
11127. State bodies subject to article 330
11128. When closed sessions held 330
11128.5. Adjournment of meeting; Posting of copy of order or notice

Page

of adjournment ... 330
11129. Continuance or recontinuance of hearing ... 331
11130. Action to stop or prevent violations of article; Order for recording of closed sessions; Discovery of recording ... 331
11130.3. Cause of action to void action taken by state agency in violation of open meeting requirements ... 332
11130.5. Costs and attorney fees ... 332
11130.7. Offenses ... 333
11131. Prohibition against use of certain facilities ... 333
11132. Prohibition against closed sessions except as expressly authorized ... 333
11133. Public meetings through teleconference or other electronic means [Repealed effective January 31, 2022] ... 333

PART 2.8. Department of Fair Employment and Housing

CHAPTER 6. Discrimination Prohibited

Article 1. Unlawful Practices, Generally

Section
12944. Discrimination by "licensing board" ... 335

PART 5.5. Department of General Services

CHAPTER 7. Printing

Article 6. Distribution of State Publications

Section
14911. Correction of mailing lists ... 337

TITLE 3. Government of Counties
DIVISION 2. Officers
PART 3. Other Officers

CHAPTER 1. District Attorney

Article 1. Duties as Public Prosecutor

Section
26509. Consumer fraud investigations; Access by district attorney to records of other agencies ... 338

HEALTH AND SAFETY CODE

DIVISION 2. Licensing Provisions
CHAPTER 1. Clinics

Page

Article 1. Definitions and General Provisions

Section
1204. Clinics eligible for licensure 341
1204.2. Written transfer agreement not condition of licensure; Medical records related to transfer; Primary care clinic providing services as alternative birth center 343
1204.3. Alternative birth centers 344

CHAPTER 2. Health Facilities

Article 1. General

Section
1250. Definitions 345
1253.7. Observation services 349
1257.7. Security and safety assessment; Security plan; Guidelines and standards on violence; Reporting 350

Article 2. Administration

Section
1267.61. Written notice of proposed changes to licensee or management companies of skilled nursing facilities 352

Article 3. Regulations

Section
1276.4. Nurse to patient ratios 353

Article 9. Training Programs in Skilled Nursing and Intermediate Care Facilities

Section
1337.1. Approved training programs 354
1337.15. Two year licensed vocational or registered nurse; Qualified instructor 356
1337.16. Online or distance learning nurse assistant training program; Requirements 356
1338.2. Work group for investigation and recommendations 357
1338.4. Access to online learning tool "Building Respect for LGBT Older Adults" [Repealed] 358

CHAPTER 2.2. Health Care Service Plans

Article 2. Administration

Section
1348.8. Requirements for telephone medical advice services;

Page

Forwarding of data to Department of Consumer Affairs ... 358

Article 5. Standards

Section

1373. Required or prohibited contract provisions ... 360

1373.8. Contractees' right to select licensed professionals in California to perform contract services ... 366

1374.55. Coverage for treatment of infertility; "Subsidiary" ... 366

1374.57. Exclusion of dependent child ... 367

DIVISION 10. Uniform Controlled Substances Act

CHAPTER 1. General Provisions and Definitions

Section

11027. "Prescription"; Definitions relating to electronic transmission ... 368

DIVISION 106. Personal Health Care (Including Maternal, Child, and Adolescent)

PART 2. Maternal, Child, and Adolescent Health

CHAPTER 2. Maternal Health

Article 2. Abortion

Section

123420. Misdemeanors; Employers requiring participation in abortion; Discrimination against employee for refusal ... 369

DIVISION 107. Healthy Care Access and Information

PART 3. Health Professions Development

CHAPTER 1. Health Professions Planning

Article 1. Health Personnel Planning [Repealed]

Section

127760. Legislative findings and declarations [Repealed] ... 372

127765. Collection of data from licentiates [Repealed] ... 372

127770. Contents of data [Repealed] ... 372

127775. Confidentiality of data in transmission [Repealed] ... 372

127780. Confidentiality of information received [Repealed] ... 372

127785. Collection of data on health care trainees [Repealed] ... 372

127790. Contents of data on health care trainees [Repealed] ... 372

127795. Implementation of data collection process [Repealed] ... 372

127800. Provision of information as condition of relicensure [Repealed] ... 373

CHAPTER 4. Health Care Workforce Training Programs

Page

Article 4. Midwifery Workforce Training Act

Section
128297. Definitions 373
128298. Program to contract with certified nurse-midwives and licensed midwives training programs 374

CHAPTER 5. Health Professions Education Programs

Article 1. Health Professions Education Programs

Section
128330. Definitions 376
128335. Health Professions Education Foundation [Repealed] 376
128337. Dissolution of Health Professions Education Foundation .. 377
128338. Post-dissolution reference to Health Professions Education Foundation as reference to department 377
128340. Board members [Repealed] 377
128345. Duties and powers of department 377
128350. Duties of Department of Health Care Access and Information 378
128355. Health Professions Education Fund 378
128360. Exemption from certain regulations and rulemaking requirements; Notice to public of Health Professions Education Programs information; Repeal of prior regulations 379
128365. Financial assistance applications and other private documentation exempt from disclosure provisions 379
128370. Exemption of donation-related documents from public disclosure 379
128371. Legislative findings and declarations; Denial of admission to certain programs on the basis on immigration or citizenship status 380

Article 2. California Registered Nurse Education Program

Section
128375. Legislative findings and declarations 381
128380. Legislative intent 381
128385. Registered Nurse Education Program 382
128390. Use of funds 383
128395. Solicitation of advice [Repealed] 383
128400. Registered Nurse Education Fund 383

Article 3. Geriatric Nurse Practitioner and Clinical Nurse Specialist Scholarship Program [Repealed]

Section
128425. Legislative findings and declarations [Repealed] 383
128430. Definitions [Repealed] 384

Page
128435. Creation of program [Repealed] 384
128440. Coordination of awards with other financial assistance [Repealed] 384
128445. Solicitation of advice from other professional and educational groups [Repealed] 384
128450. Funding of program [Repealed] 384

INSURANCE CODE

DIVISION 2. Classes of Insurance
PART 2. Life And Disability Insurance

CHAPTER 1. The Contract

Article 4. Payment and Proceeds

Section
10176. Freedom to choose specified health care professionals 385
10176.7. Mental health or respiratory care licensure requirements for out of state disability policies 387
10177. Professional mental health expenses under self-insured plan 388
10177.8. Mental health care licensure requirements for out of state self-insured plans 389

CHAPTER 4. Standard Provisions in Disability Policies

Article 1. Scope of Chapter and Definitions

Section
10279. Requirements for telephone medical advice services 390

PENAL CODE

PART 1. Of Crimes and Punishments
TITLE 13. Of Crimes Against Property
CHAPTER 4. Forgery and Counterfeiting

Section
471.5. Falsification of medical records 391

PART 4. Prevention of Crimes and Apprehension of Criminals
TITLE 1. Investigation and Control of Crimes and Criminals
CHAPTER 2. Control of Crimes and Criminals

Page

Article 2. Reports of Injuries

Section
11160. Injuries required to be reported; Method of reporting; Team reports; Internal procedures 392
11161. Report by physician or surgeon; Medical records; Referrals 395
11161.5. Legislative intent regarding development of protocols for interagency investigations of a physician's prescription of medication to patients 395
11161.9. Immunity from liability 396
11162. Violation of article; Punishment 396
11162.5. Definitions 396
11162.7. Application of article when reports required under other provisions 397
11163. Claim for attorney's fees incurred in action based on reporting 397
11163.2. Application of privileges; Confidentiality of reports 398

Article 2.5. Child Abuse and Neglect Reporting Act

Section
11165.2. "Neglect"; "Severe neglect"; "General neglect" 398
11165.7. "Mandated reporter"; Training 399
11166.5. Statement acknowledging awareness of reporting duties and promising compliance; Exemptions; Distribution in connection with licensure or certification 404
11167.5. Confidentiality and disclosure of reports 405

UNEMPLOYMENT INSURANCE CODE

DIVISION 1. Unemployment and Disability Compensation
PART 2. Disability Compensation

CHAPTER 2. Disability Benefits

Article 4. Filing, Determination and Payment of Disability Benefit Claims

Section
2708. Medical practitioner's certificate; "Physician"; "Practitioner" 409

WELFARE AND INSTITUTIONS CODE

DIVISION 9. Public Social Services
PART 3. Aid and Medical Assistance

CHAPTER 7. Basic Health Care

Page

Article 3. Administration

Section
14111. Delegation of duties to nurse practitioner in long-term health care facility 414
14111.5. Tasks of nurse practitioner in long-term health care facility 414

Article 4. The Medi-Cal Benefits Program

Section
14132.06. Medi-Cal benefits provided by local educational agency 415

CHAPTER 11. Elder Abuse and Dependent Adult Civil Protection Act

Article 2. Definitions

Section
15610. Construction of chapter 419
15610.02. Legislative findings, declarations, and intent 419
15610.05. "Abandonment" 419
15610.07. "Abuse of an elder or a dependent adult" 420
15610.10. "Adult protective services" 420
15610.13. "Adult protective services agency" 420
15610.15. Division 420
15610.17. "Care custodian" 420
15610.20. "Clients' rights advocate" 421
15610.23. "Dependent adult" 422
15610.25. "Developmentally disabled person" 422
15610.27. "Elder" 422
15610.30. "Financial abuse" of elder or dependent adult 422
15610.35. "Goods and services necessary to avoid physical harm or mental suffering" 423
15610.37. "Health practitioner" 423
15610.40. "Investigation" 424
15610.43. "Isolation" 424
15610.47. "Long-term care facility" 424
15610.50. "Long-term care ombudsman" 425
15610.53. "Mental suffering" 425
15610.57. "Neglect" 425
15610.60. "Patients' rights advocate" 426
15610.63. "Physical abuse" 426
15610.65. "Reasonable suspicion" 427
15610.67. "Serious bodily injury" 427
15610.70. Undue influence 427

Page

Article 3. Mandatory and Nonmandatory Reports of Abuse

Section
15630. Duties of mandated reporter; Punishment for failure to report ... 428
15630.1. Civil penalty for failure to report financial abuse ... 434
15630.2. Report suspected financial abuse by mandated reporter; Elder or dependent adult; Liability; Definitions ... 436
15631. Other persons who may report abuse ... 439
15632. Application of physician-patient or psychotherapist-patient privilege ... 440

Article 4. Confidentiality

Section
15633. Disclosure; Penalties ... 440
15633.5. Other persons to whom disclosure may be made ... 441
15634. Immunity from liability of persons authorized to report abuse; Attorney fees ... 442

Article 8. Prosecution of Elder and Dependent Adult Abuse Cases

Section
15656. Penalties for abuse of elder or dependent adult ... 443

Article 10. Employee Statement

Section
15659. Statement as to knowledge of compliance with reporting requirements ... 444

CODE OF CIVIL PROCEDURE

Part 4. Miscellaneous Provisions
TITLE 3. Of the Production of Evidence
CHAPTER 2. Means of Production

1985. "Subpoena"; Issuance; Affidavit ... 447
1985.1. Agreement to appear at time not specified in subpoena ... 448
1985.2. Subpoena requiring attendance of witness; Notice ... 448
1985.3. Subpoena duces tecum for production of personal records; Definitions; Application of section ... 449
1985.4. Production of consumer records maintained by state or local agency ... 451
1985.6. Subpoena duces tecum for production of employment records; Definitions, Procedures and requirements; Application of section and exceptions ... 452
1987. Service of subpoena, or of written notice ... 454

GOVERNMENT CODE

Page

TITLE 2. Government of the State of California
DIVISION 3. Executive Department
PART 1. State Departments and Agencies
CHAPTER 3.5. Administrative Regulations and Rulemaking

Article 1. General

Section		
11340.	Legislative Findings and Declarations	458
11340.1.	Declarations and intent regarding establishment of Office of Administrative Law	459
11340.2.	Office of Administrative Law; Director and deputy director	459
11340.3.	Employment and compensation of assistants and other employees	459
11340.4.	Recommendations on administrative rulemaking	460
11340.5.	Adoption of guidelines, bulletins and manuals as regulations	460
11340.6.	Petition requesting adoption, amendment, or repeal of regulation; Contents	461
11340.7.	Procedure upon petition requesting adoption, amendment or repeal of regulation	461
11340.85.	Electronic communications	462
11340.9.	Inapplicable provisions	463
11341.	Identification numbers	464
11342.1.	Authority not conferred on state agencies	464
11342.2.	Consistency with statute; Effectuation of purpose of statute	464
11342.4.	Regulations	464

Article 2. Definitions

Section		
11342.510.	Governing definitions	465
11342.520.	"Agency"	465
11342.530.	"Building standard"	465
11342.535.	"Cost impact"	465
11342.540.	"Director"	466
11342.545.	"Emergency"	466
11342.548.	"Major regulation"	466
11342.550.	"Office"	466
11342.560.	"Order of repeal"	466
11342.570.	"Performance standard"	466
11342.580.	"Plain English"	466
11342.590.	"Prescriptive standard"	466
11342.595.	"Proposed action"	467
11342.600.	"Regulation"	467
11342.610.	"Small Business"	467

Page

Article 3. Filing and Publication

Section

11343. Procedure 468
11343.1. Style of regulations; Endorsement 469
11343.2. Endorsement of time and date of filing and maintenance of file for public inspection 469
11343.3. Vehicle weight impacts and ability of vehicle manufacturers or operators to comply with laws limiting weight of vehicles to be taken into account when promulgating administrative regulations 469
11343.4. Effective date of regulation or order of repeal; Applicability 470
11343.5. Filing copies of Code of Regulations or Regulatory Code Supplement 470
11343.6. Rebuttable presumptions raised by filing of certified copy 471
11343.8. Filing and publication of regulation or order of repeal not required to be filed 471

Article 4. The California Code of Regulations, the California Code of Regulations Supplement, and the California Regulatory Notice Register

Section

11344. Publication of Code of Regulations and Code of Regulations Supplement; Availability of regulations on internet 472
11344.1. Publication of Regulatory Notice Register 472
11344.2. Furnishing Code and Supplement to county clerks or delegatees 473
11344.3. Time of publication of documents 473
11344.4. Sale of Code, Supplement and Regulatory Notice Register 474
11344.6. Rebuttable presumption raised by publication of regulations 474
11344.7. Authority of state agencies to purchase copies of Code, Supplement, or Register or to print and distribute special editions 474
11344.9. "California Administrative Code"; "California Administrative Notice Register"; "California Administrative Code Supplement" 474
11345. Identification number not required 475

Article 5. Public Participation: Procedure for Adoption of Regulations

Section

11346. Purpose and applicability of article; Subsequent legislation 475

		Page
11346.1.	Emergency regulations and orders of repeal	476
11346.2.	Availability to public of copy of proposed regulation; Initial statement of reasons for proposed action	477
11346.3.	Assessment of potential for adverse economic impact on businesses and individuals	480
11346.36.	Adoption of regulations for conducting standardized regulatory impact analyses; Submission; Publication	482
11346.4.	Notice of proposed action	483
11346.45.	Increased public participation	484
11346.5.	Contents of notice of proposed adoption, amendment, or repeal of regulation	484
11346.6.	Duty of agency, upon request from person with certain disability, to provide narrative description of proposed regulation	488
11346.7.	Link on website	489
11346.8.	Hearing	489
11346.9.	Final statements of reasons for proposing adoption or amendment of regulation; Informative digest	490
11347.	Decision not to proceed with proposed action	492
11347.1.	Addition to rulemaking file	492
11347.3.	File of rulemaking; Contents and availability of file	493
11348.	Rulemaking records	494

Article 6. Review of Proposed Regulations

Section		
11349.	Definitions	495
11349.1.	Review of regulations; Regulations to govern review process; Return to adopting agency	495
11349.1.5.	Review of standardized regulatory impact analyses; Report; Notice of noncompliance	497
11349.2.	Adding material to file	498
11349.3.	Time for review of regulations; Procedure on disapproval; Return of regulations	498
11349.4.	Rewriting and resubmission of regulation; Review	498
11349.5.	Governor's review of decisions	499
11349.6.	Review by office of emergency regulation	500

Article 7. Review of Existing Regulations

Section		
11349.7.	Priority review of regulations	501
11349.8.	Repeal of regulation for which statutory authority is repealed, ineffective or inoperative	502
11349.9.	Review of notice of repeal	503

Article 8. Judicial Review

Section		
11350.	Judicial declaration regarding validity of regulation;	

		Page
	Grounds for invalidity	504
11350.3.	Judicial declaration as to validity of disapproved or repealed regulation	505

Article 9. Special Procedures

Section		
11351.	Applicability of specified provisions to Public Utilities Commission and Workers' Compensation Appeals Board	506
11352.	Applicability of chapter	506
11353.	Application of chapter to water quality control policy, plans, or guidelines	507
11354.	Effect of certain sections on court determination of applicability of chapter	508
11354.1.	Application of chapter to certain policies, plans and guidelines of San Francisco Bay Conservation and Development Commission	508
11356.	Applicability of articles to building standards	510
11357.	Instructions for determining impact of proposed action on local or state agencies or on school districts	510
11359.	Regulations relating to fire and panic safety	511
11361.	Applicability of chapter; Adoption or revision of regulations, guidelines, or criteria	511

CHAPTER 4. Office of Administration Hearings

Article 1. General Provisions

Section		
11370.	Chapters constituting Administrative Procedure Act	512
11370.1.	"Director"	512
11370.2.	Office of Administrative Hearings in Department of General Services; Director	513
11370.3.	Appointment and assignment of administrative law judges and other personnel	513
11370.4.	Determination and collection of costs	513
11370.5.	Recommendations on administrative adjudication	513

Article 2. Medical Quality Hearing Panel

Section		
11371.	Members of panel; Published decisions; Experts	514
11372.	Conduct of hearing by administrative law judge	515
11373.	Conduct of proceedings under Administrative Procedure Act	515
11373.3.	Facilities and support personnel for review committee panel	515

Page

Article 3. State Agency Reports and Forms Appeals

Section
11380. Appeal filed by business 516

CHAPTER 4.5. Administrative Adjudication: General Provisions

Article 1. Preliminary Provisions

Section
11400. Administrative Procedure Act; References to superseded provisions 517
11400.10. Operative date of chapter; Applicability 517
11400.20. Adoption of interim or permanent regulations 517

Article 2. Definitions

Section
11405.10. Definitions governing construction of chapter 518
11405.20. "Adjudicative proceeding" 518
11405.30. "Agency" 518
11405.40. "Agency head" 519
11405.50. "Decision" 519
11405.60. "Party" 519
11405.70. "Person" 519
11405.80. "Presiding officer" 519

Article 3. Application of Chapter

Section
11410.10. Decision requiring evidentiary hearing 520
11410.20. Applicability to agencies 520
11410.30. Applicability to local agencies 520
11410.40. Adoption of chapter by exempt agency 520
11410.50. Applicability to specified proceedings 521
11410.60. Quasi-public entity 521

Article 4. Governing Procedure

Section
11415.10. Determination of procedure 522
11415.20. Statute to prevail over provision of chapter 522
11415.30. Actions by Governor to avoid loss or delay of federal funds 522
11415.40. Waiver of right conferred by provisions 522
11415.50. Procedure for decision for which adjudicative proceeding not required 523
11415.60. Decision by settlement 523

Page

Article 5. Alternative Dispute Resolution

Section
11420.10. Mediation or arbitration 523
11420.20. Model regulations for alternative dispute resolution 524
11420.30. Protection of communications 524

Article 6. Administrative Adjudication Bill of Rights

Section
11425.10. Required procedures and rights of persons affected 525
11425.20. Hearings open to the public; Order for closure 526
11425.30. Specified persons not to serve as presiding officer 527
11425.40. Disqualification of presiding officer 527
11425.50. Decision to be in writing; Statement of factual and legal basis 527
11425.60. Decisions relied on as precedents; Index of precedent decisions 528

Article 7. Ex Parte Communications

Section
11430.10. Ex parte communications 529
11430.20. Permissible ex parte communications 529
11430.30. Permissible ex parte communication from agency that is party 529
11430.40. Disclosure of communication received while proceeding is pending 530
11430.50. Communication in violation of provisions 530
11430.60. Prohibited communication as grounds to disqualify presiding officer 531
11430.70. Agency head delegated to hear or decide proceeding 531
11430.80. Communication between presiding officer and agency head delegated to hear proceeding 531

Article 8. Language Assistance

Section
11435.05. "Language assistance" 532
11435.10. Interpretation for deaf or hard-of-hearing persons 532
11435.15. Provision of language assistance by state agencies 532
11435.20. Hearing or medical examination to be conducted in English 533
11435.25. Cost of providing interpreter 533
11435.30. Publication of list of certified interpreters 534
11435.35. Publication of list of certified medical examination interpreters 534
11435.40. Designation of languages for certification 535
11435.45. Application fees to take interpreter examinations 535
11435.50. Removal of person from list of certified interpreters 536

Page
11435.55. Qualification and use of noncertified interpreters 536
11435.60. Party to be advised of right to interpreter 536
11435.65. Rules of confidentiality applicable to interpreters 537

Article 9. General Procedural Provisions

Section
11440.10. Review of decision 537
11440.20. Service of writing or electronic document; Notice 537
11440.30. Conduct of hearing by telephone, television, or other electronic means 538
11440.40. Proceedings involving sexual offenses; Limitations on evidence 538
11440.45. Benevolent gestures as admission of liability; Limitations on evidence 539
11440.50. Intervention; Grant of motion; Conditions 539
11440.60. Indication of person paying for written communication 540

Article 10. Informal Hearing

Section
11445.10. Legislative findings and declarations 541
11445.20. Circumstances permitting use of informal hearing procedure 541
11445.30. Notice of informal procedure 542
11445.40. Application of procedures otherwise required 542
11445.50. Denial of use of informal procedure; Conversion to formal hearing; Cross-examination 543
11445.60. Identity of witnesses or other sources 543

Article 11. Subpoenas

Section
11450.05. Application of article 544
11450.10. Issuance for attendance or production of documents 544
11450.20. Persons who may issue subpoenas; Service 544
11450.30. Objection to subpoena; Motion for protective order; Motion to quash 545
11450.40. Witness's mileage and fees 545
11450.50. Written notice to witness to attend; Service 545

Article 12. Enforcement of Orders and Sanctions

Section
11455.10. Grounds for contempt sanction 546
11455.20. Certification of facts to justify contempt sanction; Other procedure 546
11455.30. Bad faith actions; Order to pay expenses including attorney's fees 546

Page

Article 13. Emergency Decision

Section

11460.10. Conduct of proceeding under emergency procedure 547
11460.20. Emergency decision 547
11460.30. Conditions for issuance of emergency decision 547
11460.40. Notice and hearing prior to decision 548
11460.50. Statement of factual and legal basis and reasons for emergency decision 548
11460.60. Formal or informal proceeding after issuance of emergency decision 548
11460.70. Agency record 549
11460.80. Judicial review of decision 549

Article 14. Declaratory Decision

Section

11465.10. Conduct of proceeding under declaratory decision procedure 549
11465.20. Application; Issuance of decision 550
11465.30. Notice of application for decision 550
11465.40. Applicable hearing procedure 550
11465.50. Actions of agency after receipt of application 550
11465.60. Contents of decision; Status and binding effect of decision 551
11465.70. Model regulations 551

Article 15. Conversion of Proceeding

Section

11470.10. Conversion into another type of proceeding 552
11470.20. Appointment of successor to preside over new proceeding 552
11470.30. Record of original proceeding 552
11470.40. Duties of presiding officer of new proceeding 552
11470.50. Adoption of regulations to govern conversion 553

Article 16. Administrative Adjudication Code of Ethics

Section

11475. Name of rules 553
11475.10. Application 553
11475.20. Law governing conduct 553
11475.30. Definitions 554
11475.40. Inapplicable provisions of Code of Judicial Ethics 554
11475.50. Violations 554
11475.60. Compliance requirements 554
11475.70. Construction and intent 555

CHAPTER 5. Administrative Adjudication: Formal Hearing

		Page
11500.	Definitions	556
11501.	Application of chapter to agency	556
11502.	Administrative law judges	556
11503.	Accusation or District Statement of Reduction in Force	557
11504.	Statement of issues	557
11504.5.	Applicability of references to accusations to statements of issues	558
11505.	Service of accusation or District Statement of Reduction in Force and accompanying papers; Notice of defense or notice of participation; Request for hearing	558
11506.	Filing of notice of defense or notice of participation; Contents; Right to hearing on the merits	559
11507.	Amended or supplemental accusation or District Statement of Reduction in Force; Objections	560
11507.3.	Consolidated proceedings; Separate hearings	560
11507.5.	Exclusivity of discovery provisions	561
11507.7.	Motion to compel discovery; Order	561
11508.	Time and place of hearing	562
11509.	Notice of hearing	562
11511.	Depositions	563
11511.5.	Prehearing conference; Conduct by telephone or other electronic means; Conversion to ADR or informal hearing; Prehearing order	563
11511.7.	Settlement conference	564
11512.	Administrative law judge to preside over hearing; Disqualification; Reporting of proceedings	564
11513.	Evidence	565
11514.	Affidavits	566
11515.	Official notice	567
11516.	Amendment of accusation or District Statement of Reduction in Force after submission	567
11517.	Contested cases	567
11518.	Copies of decision to parties	569
11518.5.	Application to correct mistake or error in decision; Modification; Service after correction	569
11519.	Effective date of decision; Stay of execution; Notice of suspension or revocation; Restitution; Actual knowledge as condition of enforcement	569
11519.1.	Order of restitution for financial loss or damages	570
11520.	Defaults and uncontested cases	570
11521.	Reconsideration	571
11522.	Reinstatement of license or reduction of penalty	571
11523.	Judicial review	572
11524.	Continuances; Requirement of good cause; Judicial review of denial	572
11526.	Voting by mail	573
11527.	Charge against funds of agency	573
11528.	Oaths	573
11529.	Interim orders	573

Page

CALIFORNIA CODE OF REGULATIONS

TITLE 1. General Provisions
DIVISION 2. Office of Administrative Hearings
CHAPTER 1. General APA Hearing Procedures

Section

1000. Purpose ... 577
1002. Definitions ... 578
1004. Construction of Regulations ... 578
1006. Format and Filing of Papers ... 579
1008. Service; Proof of Service ... 580
1012. Ex Parte Petitions and Applications for Temporary or Interim Orders ... 581
1014. Pleadings; Notice of Defense; Withdrawal of Notice of Defense ... 581
1015. Notice of Representation and Withdrawal of Counsel or Other Representative ... 582
1016. Consolidated Proceedings; Separate Hearings ... 582
1018. Agency Request for Hearing; Required Documents ... 583
1019. Request for Security ... 584
1020. Motion for Continuance of Hearing ... 584
1022. Motions ... 585
1024. Subpoenas; Motion for a Protective Order ... 586
1026. Prehearing Conferences ... 587
1027. Informal Hearings ... 588
1028. Settlement Conferences; Settlements ... 588
1030. Conduct of Hearing; Protective Orders ... 589
1032. Interpreters and Accommodation ... 590
1034. Peremptory Challenge ... 591
1038. Ordering the Record ... 592
1040. Monetary Sanctions ... 593
1042. Cost Recovery ... 593
1044. Request for Expenses After Default ... 594
1046. Amicus Briefs ... 594
1048. Technical and Minor Changes to Proposed and Final Decisions ... 595
1050. Remand or Reconsideration ... 596

TABLE OF CODE SECTIONS ADDED, AMENDED, REPEALED, OR OTHERWISE AFFECTED

Business and Professions Code

Section Affected	Type of Change	Chapter Number
114.3	Amended	386
205	Amended	511
1246	Amended	685
2701	Amended	413
2706	Amended	413
2708	Amended	413
2717	Amended	413
2725.4	Amended	631
2746.51	Amended	413
2746.53	Amended	413
2746.55	Amended	511
2746.6	Added	565
2761.1	Added	565
2785.6	Added	413
2786	Amended	413
2786.2	Amended	413
2786.3	Amended	413
2786.4	Amended	413
2786.5	Amended	413
2815	Amended	413
2815.5	Amended	413
2836.3	Amended	413
2837.103.5	Added	413
2837.104	Amended	413
4999.2	Amended	684

Corporations Code

Section Affected	Type of Change	Chapter Number
13401	Amended	290
13401.5	Amended	290

Government Code

Section Affected	Type of Change	Chapter Number
6253.4	Amended	169
6254.5	Amended	251
6254.5	Amended	452
11133	Added	48
12944	Amended	48
12944	Amended	630
11343	Amended	48
11346.3	Amended	478

11512	Amended	48

Health and Safety Code

Section Affected	Type of Change	Chapter Number
1422	Amended	277
1423	Amended	28
128365	Amended	28

Penal Code

Section Affected	Type of Change	Chapter Number
11165.2	Amended	770

Welfare and Institutions Code

Section Affected	Type of Change	Chapter Number
15610.63	Amended	197
15630.2	Amended	452
15633	Amended	506

NURSING PRACTICE ACT
EXTRACTED FROM
BUSINESS & PROFESSIONS CODE

Division
2. Healing Arts.

DIVISION 2
HEALING ARTS

Chapter
6. Nursing.

CHAPTER 6
NURSING

Article
1. Administration.
1.5. Nursing Shortage [Repealed.]
2. Scope of Regulation.
2.5. Nurse-Midwives.
3. Disciplinary Proceedings.
3.1. Intervention Program.
3.5. Nursing Corporations.
4. Nursing Schools.
5. Penal Provisions.
6. Revenue.
6.5. Public Health Nurse Certification.
7. Nurse Anesthetists.
8. Nurse Practitioners.
8.5. Advanced Practice Registered Nurses.
9. Clinical Nurse Specialists.

HISTORY: Added Stats 1939 ch 807 § 2. Former Chapter 6, also entitled "Nursing", consisting of §§ 2700–2784, was added Stats 1937 ch 416 and repealed Stats 1939 ch 807 § 1.

ARTICLE 1
ADMINISTRATION

Section
2700. Citation.
2701. Board of Registered Nursing; Authority [Repealed effective January 1, 2027].
2701.5. Board subject to review.
2702. Membership qualifications.
2703. Appointments, terms, vacancies.
2706. Removal from office.
2707. Elections of officers.
2708. Executive officer; Appointment; Duties; Interim executive officer [Repealed effective January 1, 2027].

Section
2708.1. Priority of board; Protection of the public.
2709. Regular meetings.
2709.5. Mediums of exchange.
2710. Special meetings.
2710.5. Advisory committees.
2712. Quorum.
2713. Records.
2714. Offices; Venue.
2715. Prosecutions; Employment matters; Seal; Rule-making authority.
2716. Compensation and expenses.
2717. Plan to address nursing shortage.
2718. Performance audit of enforcement program [Repealed].

§ 2700. Citation

This chapter of the Business and Professions Code constitutes the chapter on professional nursing and shall be construed as revisory and amendatory of the laws heretofore enacted. It may be cited as the Nursing Practice Act.

HISTORY:
Added Stats 1939 ch 807 § 2.

§ 2701. Board of Registered Nursing; Authority [Repealed effective January 1, 2027]

(a) There is in the Department of Consumer Affairs the Board of Registered Nursing consisting of nine members.

(b) For purposes of this chapter, "board" means the Board of Registered Nursing. Any reference in state law to the Board of Nurse Examiners of the State of California or the California Board of Nursing Education and Nurse Registration shall be construed to refer to the Board of Registered Nursing.

(c) The board shall have all authority vested in the previous board under this chapter. The board may enforce all disciplinary actions undertaken by the previous board.

(d) This section shall remain in effect only until January 1, 2027, and as of that date is repealed, unless a later enacted statute that is enacted before January 1, 2027, deletes or extends that date.

HISTORY:
Added Stats 2012 ch 4 § 2 (SB 98), effective February 14, 2012, repealed January 1, 2016. Amended Stats 2015 ch 489 § 1 (SB 466), effective January 1, 2016, repealed January 1, 2018; Stats 2017 ch 520 § 2 (SB 799), effective January 1, 2018, repealed January 1, 2022. Repealed Stats 2021 ch 628 § 1 (AB 1532), effective January 1, 2023. Amended Stats 2021 ch 628 § 1 (AB 1532), effective January 1, 2022; Stats 2022 ch 413 § 4 (AB 2684), effective January 1, 2023, repealed January 1, 2027.

§ 2701.5. Board subject to review

Notwithstanding any other law, the repeal of Section 2701 renders the board subject to review by the appropriate policy committees of the Legislature.

HISTORY:
Added Stats 2021 ch 628 § 2 (AB 1532), effective January 1, 2022.

§ 2702. Membership qualifications

(a) Each member of the board shall be a resident of the state.

(b) Four members shall represent the public at large, and shall not be licensed under any board under this division or any board referred to in Section 1000 or 3600 and shall have no pecuniary interests in the provision of health care services.

(c) Two members shall be licensed registered nurses under the provisions of this chapter, each of whom shall be active in the practice of their profession engaged primarily in direct patient care with at least five continuous years of experience, and who shall not be engaged as an educator or administrator of a nursing education program under the provisions of this chapter.

(d) One member shall be a licensed registered nurse who shall be active as an advanced practice registered nurse as defined in Section 2725.5.

(e) One member shall be a licensed registered nurse under the provisions of this chapter who shall be active as an educator or administrator in an approved program to train registered nurses.

(f) One member shall be a licensed registered nurse who is an administrator of a nursing service with at least five continuous years of experience.

HISTORY:

Added Stats 1939 ch 807 § 2. Amended Stats 1961 ch 1821 § 18; Stats 1972 ch 847 § 3; Stats 1974 ch 632 § 3; Stats 1976 ch 1188 § 12; Stats 2003 ch 640 § 2 (SB 358); Stats 2012 ch 4 § 3 (SB 98), effective February 14, 2012; Stats 2021 ch 628 § 3 (AB 1532), effective January 1, 2022.

§ 2703. Appointments, terms, vacancies

(a) Except as provided in subdivision (c), all appointments shall be for a term of four years and vacancies shall be filled for the unexpired term. No person shall serve more than two consecutive terms.

(b) The Governor shall appoint two of the public members and the licensed members of the board qualified as provided in Section 2702. The Senate Committee on Rules and the Speaker of the Assembly shall each appoint a public member.

(c) The initial appointments shall be for the following terms:

(1) One public member appointed by the Governor shall serve a term of one year. The other public member appointed by the Governor shall serve a term of five years.

(2) One licensed member described in subdivision (c) of Section 2702 shall serve a term of two years. The other licensed member described in subdivision (c) of Section 2702 shall serve a term of three years. The licensed member described in subdivision (e) of Section 2702 shall serve a term of four years. Of the two remaining licensed members, one shall serve a term of two years, and the other shall serve a term of three years.

(3) Each public member appointed by the Senate Committee on Rules or the Speaker of the Assembly shall serve a term of four years.

HISTORY:

Added Stats 1939 ch 807 § 2. Amended Stats 1961 ch 1821 § 19; Stats 1972 ch 847 § 4; Stats 1974 ch 632 § 4; Stats 1976 ch 1188 § 13; Stats 1982 ch 676 § 10; Stats 2003 ch 640 § 3 (SB 358); Stats 2012 ch 4 § 4 (SB 98), effective February 14, 2012.

§ 2706. Removal from office

Pursuant to Section 106, each appointing authority has the power to remove from office, at any time, any member of the board appointed by that authority under Section 2703 for continued neglect of duties required by law, or for incompetence, or unprofessional or dishonorable conduct.

HISTORY:

Added Stats 1939 ch 807 § 2. Amended Stats 2022 ch 413 § 5 (AB 2684), effective January 1, 2023.

§ 2707. Elections of officers

The board shall annually elect from its members a president, vice president, and any other officers as it may deem necessary. The officers of the board shall hold their respective positions during its pleasure.

HISTORY:

Added Stats 1939 ch 807 § 2. Amended Stats 1994 ch 1275 § 11 (SB 2101).

§ 2708. Executive officer; Appointment; Duties; Interim executive officer [Repealed effective January 1, 2027]

(a) The board shall appoint an executive officer who shall perform the duties delegated by the board and be responsible to the board for the accomplishment of those duties.

(b) The executive officer shall be a nurse currently licensed under this chapter and shall possess other qualifications as determined by the board.

(c) The executive officer shall not be a member of the board.

(d) The executive officer is authorized to adopt a decision entered by default and a stipulation for surrender of a license.

(e) This section shall remain in effect only until January 1, 2027, and as of that date is repealed, unless a later enacted statute that is enacted before January 1, 2027, deletes or extends that date.

HISTORY:

Added Stats 2012 ch 4 § 5 (SB 98), effective February 14, 2012, repealed January 1, 2016. Amended Stats 2015 ch 489 § 2 (SB 466), effective January 1, 2016, repealed January 1, 2018; Stats 2017 ch 520 § 3 (SB 799), effective January 1, 2018, repealed January 1, 2022; Stats 2018 ch 571 § 12 (SB 1480), effective January 1, 2019, repealed January 1, 2022; Stats 2021 ch 628 § 4 (AB 1532), effective January 1, 2022, repealed January 1, 2023; Stats 2022 ch 413 § 6 (AB 2684), effective January 1, 2023, repealed January 1, 2027.

§ 2708.1. Priority of board; Protection of the public

Protection of the public shall be the highest priority for the Board of Registered Nursing in exercising its licensing, regulatory, and disciplinary functions. Whenever the protection of the public is inconsistent with other interests sought to be promoted, the protection of the public shall be paramount.

HISTORY:

Added Stats 2002 ch 107 § 10 (AB 269).

§ 2709. Regular meetings

The board for the purpose of transacting its business shall meet at least once every three months, at times and places it designates by resolution. Meetings shall be held in northern and southern California.

HISTORY:

Added Stats 1939 ch 807 § 2. Amended Stats 2012 ch 789 § 2 (SB 122), effective January 1, 2013.

§ 2709.5. Mediums of exchange

The board shall accept in payment of any fee required by this chapter cash or any customary or generally accepted medium of exchange, including check, cashier's check, certified check or money order. For the purposes of this section, customary or generally accepted medium of exchange does not include postage stamps.

HISTORY:
Added Stats 1957 ch 1468 § 1. Amended Stats 2002 ch 810 § 23 (SB 2022).

§ 2710. Special meetings

Special meetings may be held at such times as the board may elect, or on the call of the president of the board, or of not less than three members thereof.

A written notice of the time, place and object of any special meeting shall be mailed by the executive officer to all members of the board who are not parties to the call, at least fifteen days before the day of the meeting.

HISTORY:
Added Stats 1939 ch 807 § 2. Amended Stats 1983 ch 742 § 2.

§ 2710.5. Advisory committees

The board, with permission of the Director of the Department of Consumer Affairs, may form advisory committees to advise the board on the implementation of this chapter. Members of such advisory committees shall be entitled to a per diem and expenses as provided in Section 103.

HISTORY:
Added Stats 1974 ch 632 § 5.

§ 2712. Quorum

Five members of the board constitute a quorum for the transaction of business at any meeting.

HISTORY:
Added Stats 1939 ch 807 § 2. Amended Stats 1961 ch 1821 § 20; Stats 1985 ch 220 § 1, ch 1055 § 1.

§ 2713. Records

The board shall keep a record of all its proceedings, including a register of all applicants for licenses under this chapter and the action of the board upon each application.

HISTORY:
Added Stats 1939 ch 807 § 2. Amended Stats 1951 ch 1659 § 2; Stats 1983 ch 742 § 4.

§ 2714. Offices; Venue

The office of the board shall be in the city of Sacramento. Suboffices may be established in Los Angeles and San Francisco and such records as may be necessary may be transferred temporarily to them. Legal proceedings against the board may be instituted in any county in which any of the three cities above mentioned is located.

HISTORY:
Added Stats 1939 ch 807 § 2.

§ 2715. Prosecutions; Employment matters; Seal; Rule-making authority

(a) The board shall prosecute all persons guilty of violating this chapter.

(b) Except as provided by Section 159.5, the board, in accordance with the Civil Service Law, may employ personnel, including legal counsel, as it deems necessary to carry into effect this chapter.

(c) The board shall have and use a seal bearing the name "Board of Registered Nursing." The board may adopt, amend, or repeal, in accordance with the Administrative Procedure Act (Chapter 3.5 (commencing with Section 11340) of Part 1 of Division 3 of Title 2 of the Government Code), the rules and regulations that may be reasonably necessary to enable it to carry into effect this chapter.

HISTORY:
Added Stats 1939 ch 807 § 2. Amended Stats 1951 ch 1659 § 1; Stats 1957 ch 2084 § 5; Stats 1961 ch 1823 § 3; Stats 1971 ch 716 § 39; Stats 1974 ch 632 § 6; Stats 2016 ch 86 § 5 (SB 1171), effective January 1, 2017; Stats 2017 ch 429 § 7 (SB 547), effective January 1, 2018.

§ 2716. Compensation and expenses

Each member of the board shall receive a per diem and expenses as provided in Section 103.

HISTORY:
Added Stats 1959 ch 1645 § 10.

§ 2717. Plan to address nursing shortage

(a) The board shall incorporate regional forecasts into its biennial analyses of the nursing workforce conducted pursuant to Section 502.

(b) The board shall develop a plan to address regional areas of shortage identified by its nursing workforce forecast.

HISTORY:
Added Stats 2021 ch 591 § 1 (AB 1015), effective January 1, 2022. Amended Stats 2022 ch 413 § 7 (AB 2684), effective January 1, 2023.

§ 2718. Performance audit of enforcement program [Repealed]

HISTORY:
Added Stats 2015 ch 489 § 3 (SB 466), effective January 1, 2016. Repealed Stats 2017 ch 520 § 4 (SB 799), effective January 1, 2018.

ARTICLE 1.5

NURSING SHORTAGE [REPEALED.]

HISTORY: Article 1.5, consisting of §§ 2720–2722, was added Stats 1988 ch 1421 § 2. Repealed July 1, 1990, by the terms of § 2722.

ARTICLE 2

SCOPE OF REGULATION

Section
2725. Legislative intent; Practice of nursing defined.

Section
2725.1. Dispensation of drugs or devices by registered nurse; Construction.
2725.2. Dispensation of self-administered hormonal contraceptives; Injections; Standardized procedure.
2725.3. Functions performed by unlicensed personnel.
2725.4. Abortion by aspiration techniques; Requirements.
2725.5. "Advanced practice registered nurse" defined.
2726. Unauthorized practices.
2727. Practices not prohibited.
2727.5. Liability for emergency care.
2728. Services by attendants and psychiatric technicians; Supervised services of unlicensed graduates of accredited psychiatric technician training programs.
2728.5. Utilization of licensed psychiatric technicians and psychiatric technician interim permittees.
2729. Services by student nurses.
2730. Nurses qualified outside state and engaged to care for patient temporarily in California.
2731. Nonprofit religious care.
2732. Licensure requirement; Use of "R.N.".
2732.05. Verification of current R.N. status.
2732.1. Applications; Interim permits; Waiver of examination; Fees.
2733. Issuance of temporary license where examination waived.
2734. Inactive licenses.
2736. Qualifications generally.
2736.1. Training in detection and treatment of client abuse, and alcohol and chemical substance dependency.
2736.5. Continuing education courses regarding implicit bias.
2736.6. Eligibility of vocational nurse to take examination for licensure as registered nurse.
2737. Application fee.
2738. Holding of examinations.
2740. Conduct of examinations; Finality of decisions.
2741. Fees with application for reexamination.
2742. Issuance of license.

HISTORY: Added Stats 1939 ch 807 § 2.

§ 2725. Legislative intent; Practice of nursing defined

(a) In amending this section at the 1973–74 session, the Legislature recognizes that nursing is a dynamic field, the practice of which is continually evolving to include more sophisticated patient care activities. It is the intent of the Legislature in amending this section at the 1973–74 session to provide clear legal authority for functions and procedures that have common acceptance and usage. It is the legislative intent also to recognize the existence of overlapping functions between physicians and registered nurses and to permit additional sharing of functions within organized health care systems that provide for collaboration between physicians and registered nurses. These organized health care systems include, but are not limited to, health facilities licensed pursuant to Chapter 2 (commencing with Section 1250) of Division 2 of the Health and Safety Code, clinics, home health agencies, physicians' offices, and public or community health services.

(b) The practice of nursing within the meaning of this chapter means those functions, including basic health care, that help people cope with difficulties in daily living that are associated with their actual or potential health or illness problems or the treatment thereof, and that require a substantial amount of scientific knowledge or technical skill, including all of the following:

(1) Direct and indirect patient care services that ensure the safety, comfort, personal hygiene, and protection of patients; and the performance of disease prevention and restorative measures.

(2) Direct and indirect patient care services, including, but not limited to, the administration of medications and therapeutic agents, necessary to implement a treatment, disease prevention, or rehabilitative regimen ordered by and within the scope of licensure of a physician, dentist, podiatrist, or clinical psychologist, as defined by Section 1316.5 of the Health and Safety Code.

(3) The performance of skin tests, immunization techniques, and the withdrawal of human blood from veins and arteries.

(4) Observation of signs and symptoms of illness, reactions to treatment, general behavior, or general physical condition, and (A) determination of whether the signs, symptoms, reactions, behavior, or general appearance exhibit abnormal characteristics, and (B) implementation, based on observed abnormalities, of appropriate reporting, or referral, or standardized procedures, or changes in treatment regimen in accordance with standardized procedures, or the initiation of emergency procedures.

(c) "Standardized procedures," as used in this section, means either of the following:

(1) Policies and protocols developed by a health facility licensed pursuant to Chapter 2 (commencing with Section 1250) of Division 2 of the Health and Safety Code through collaboration among administrators and health professionals including physicians and nurses.

(2) Policies and protocols developed through collaboration among administrators and health professionals, including physicians and nurses, by an organized health care system which is not a health facility licensed pursuant to Chapter 2 (commencing with Section 1250) of Division 2 of the Health and Safety Code.

The policies and protocols shall be subject to any guidelines for standardized procedures that the Division of Licensing of the Medical Board of California and the Board of Registered Nursing may jointly promulgate. If promulgated, the guidelines shall be administered by the Board of Registered Nursing.

(d) Nothing in this section shall be construed to require approval of standardized procedures by the Division of Licensing of the Medical Board of California, or by the Board of Registered Nursing.

(e) No state agency other than the board may define or interpret the practice of nursing for those licensed pursuant to the provisions of this chapter, or develop standardized procedures or protocols pursuant to this chapter, unless so authorized by this chapter, or specifically required under state or federal statute. "State agency" includes every state office, officer, department, division, bureau, board, authority, and commission.

HISTORY:

Added Stats 1939 ch 807 § 2. Amended Stats 1968 ch 348 § 1; Stats 1974 ch 355 § 1, ch 913 § 1; Stats 1978 ch 1161 § 172; Stats 1980 ch 406 § 1; Stats 1989 ch 886 § 52; Stats 1995 ch 279 § 15 (AB 1471); Stats 1996 ch 124 § 2 (AB 3470); Stats 2003 ch 640 § 5 (SB 358).

§ 2725.1. Dispensation of drugs or devices by registered nurse; Construction

(a) Notwithstanding any other provision of law, a registered nurse may dispense drugs or devices upon an order by a licensed physician and surgeon or an order by a certified nurse-midwife, nurse practitioner, or physician assistant issued pursuant to Section 2746.51, 2836.1, or 3502.1, respectively, if the registered nurse is functioning within a licensed primary care clinic as defined in subdivision (a) of Section 1204 of, or within a clinic as defined in subdivision (b), (c), (h), or (j) of Section 1206 of, the Health and Safety Code.

(b) No clinic shall employ a registered nurse to perform dispensing duties exclusively. No registered nurse shall dispense drugs in a pharmacy, keep a pharmacy, open shop, or drugstore for the retailing of drugs or poisons. No registered nurse shall compound drugs. Dispensing of drugs by a registered nurse, except a certified nurse-midwife who functions pursuant to a standardized procedure or protocol described in Section 2746.51 or a nurse practitioner who functions pursuant to a standardized procedure described in Section 2836.1, or protocol, shall not include substances included in the California Uniform Controlled Substances Act (Division 10 (commencing with Section 11000) of the Health and Safety Code). Nothing in this section shall exempt a clinic from the provisions of Article 13 (commencing with Section 4180) of Chapter 9.

(c) Nothing in this section shall be construed to limit any other authority granted to a certified nurse-midwife pursuant to Article 2.5 (commencing with Section 2746), to a nurse practitioner pursuant to Article 8 (commencing with Section 2834), or to a physician assistant pursuant to Chapter 7.7 (commencing with Section 3500).

(d) Nothing in this section shall be construed to affect the sites or types of health care facilities at which drugs or devices are authorized to be dispensed pursuant to Chapter 9 (commencing with Section 4000).

HISTORY:

Added Stats 1986 ch 493 § 1. Amended Stats 1999 ch 83 § 3 (SB 966) (ch 914 prevails), ch 914 § 1 (AB 1545); Stats 2001 ch 289 § 2 (SB 298); Stats 2012 ch 460 § 1 (AB 2348), effective January 1, 2013.

§ 2725.2. Dispensation of self-administered hormonal contraceptives; Injections; Standardized procedure

(a) Notwithstanding any other provision of law, a registered nurse may dispense self-administered hormonal contraceptives approved by the federal Food and Drug Administration (FDA) and may administer injections of hormonal contraceptives approved by the FDA in strict adherence to standardized procedures developed in compliance with subdivision (c) of Section 2725.

(b) The standardized procedure described in subdivision (a) shall include all of the following:

(1) Which nurse, based on successful completion of training and competency assessment, may dispense or administer the hormonal contraceptives.

(2) Minimum training requirements regarding educating patients on medical standards for ongoing women's preventive health, contraception options education and counseling, properly eliciting, documenting, and assessing patient and family health history, and utilization of the United States Medical Eligibility Criteria for Contraceptive Use.

(3) Demonstration of competency in providing the appropriate prior examination comprised of checking blood pressure, weight, and patient and family health history, including medications taken by the patient.

(4) Which hormonal contraceptives may be dispensed or administered under specified circumstances, utilizing the most recent version of the United States Medical Eligibility Criteria for Contraceptive Use.

(5) Criteria and procedure for identification, documentation, and referral of patients with contraindications for hormonal contraceptives and patients in need of a followup visit to a physician and surgeon, nurse practitioner, certified nurse-midwife, or physician assistant.

(6) The extent of physician and surgeon supervision required.

(7) The method of periodic review of the nurse's competence.

(8) The method of periodic review of the standardized procedure, including, but not limited to, the required frequency of review and the person conducting that review.

(9) Adherence to subdivision (a) of Section 2242 in a manner developed through collaboration with health care providers, including physicians and surgeons, certified nurse-midwives, nurse practitioners, physician assistants, and registered nurses. The appropriate prior examination shall be consistent with the evidence-based practice guidelines adopted by the federal Centers for Disease Control and Prevention in conjunction with the United States Medical Eligibility Criteria for Contraceptive Use.

(10) If a patient has been seen exclusively by a registered nurse for three consecutive years, the patient shall be evaluated by a physician and surgeon, nurse practitioner, certified nurse-midwife, or physician assistant prior to continuing the dispensation or administration of hormonal contraceptives.

(c) Nothing in this section shall be construed to affect the sites or types of health care facilities at which drugs or devices are authorized to be dispensed pursuant to Chapter 9 (commencing with Section 4000).

HISTORY:

Added Stats 2012 ch 460 § 2 (AB 2348), effective January 1, 2013.

§ 2725.3. Functions performed by unlicensed personnel

(a) A health facility licensed pursuant to subdivision (a), (b), or (f), of Section 1250 of the Health and Safety Code shall not assign unlicensed personnel to perform nursing functions in lieu of a registered nurse and may not allow unlicensed personnel to perform functions under the direct clinical supervision of a registered nurse that require a substantial amount of scientific knowledge and technical skills, including, but not limited to, any of the following:

(1) Administration of medication.

(2) Venipuncture or intravenous therapy.

(3) Parenteral or tube feedings.

(4) Invasive procedures including inserting nasogastric tubes, inserting catheters, or tracheal suctioning.

(5) Assessment of patient condition.

(6) Educating patients and their families concerning the patient's health care problems, including postdischarge care.

(7) Moderate complexity laboratory tests.

(b) This section shall not preclude any person from performing any act or function that he or she is authorized to perform pursuant to Division 2 (commencing with Section 500) or pursuant to existing statute or regulation as of July 1, 1999.

HISTORY:
Added Stats 1999 ch 945 § 2 (AB 394).

§ 2725.4. Abortion by aspiration techniques; Requirements

Notwithstanding any other provision of this chapter, the following shall apply:

(a) In order to perform an abortion by aspiration techniques pursuant to Section 2253, a person with a license or certificate to practice as a nurse practitioner practicing pursuant to a standardized procedure, or a qualified nurse practitioner functioning pursuant to Section 2837.103 or 2837.104, shall achieve clinical competency by successfully completing requisite training, which shall include both a clinical and didactic component, in performing these procedures provided by any of the following:

(1) A board-approved nurse practitioner program or in a course offered by an accredited nurse practitioner program.

(2) A course offered by a board-approved continuing education provider that reflects evidence-based curriculum and training guidelines or a course approved for Category I continuing medical education.

(3) A course offered by a state or national health care professional or accreditation organization.

(4) Training based on the competency-based training protocols established by the Health Workforce Pilot Project (HWPP) No. 171 through the Office of Statewide Health Planning and Development, now known as the Department of Health Care Access and Information.

(5) Training and evaluation of clinical competency, performed at a clinic or hospital, on performing abortion by aspiration techniques that is provided by any of the following who have performed the procedure themselves:

(A) A physician and surgeon.

(B) A nurse practitioner or certified nurse midwife authorized to perform abortion by aspiration techniques pursuant to this section.

(C) A physician assistant authorized to perform abortion by aspiration techniques pursuant to Section 3502.4.

(b) In order to perform an abortion by aspiration techniques pursuant to Section 2253, a person with a license or certificate to practice as a certified nurse-midwife shall achieve clinical competency by successfully completing requisite training, which shall include both a clinical and didactic component, in performing these procedures provided by any of the following:

(1) A board-approved nurse-midwifery program or in a course offered by an accredited nurse-midwifery program.

(2) A course offered by a Board-approved continuing education provider that reflects evidence-based curriculum and training guidelines or a course approved for Category I continuing medical education.

(3) A course offered by a state or national health care professional or accreditation organization.

(4) Training based on the competency-based training protocols established by the Health Workforce Pilot Project (HWPP) No. 171 through the Office of Statewide Health Planning and Development, now known as the Department of Health Care Access and Information.

(5) Training and evaluation of clinical competency, performed at a clinic or hospital, on performing abortion by aspiration techniques that is provided by any of the following who have performed the procedure themselves:

(A) A physician and surgeon.

(B) A nurse practitioner or certified nurse midwife authorized to perform abortion by aspiration techniques pursuant to this section.

(C) A physician assistant authorized to perform abortion by aspiration techniques pursuant to Section 3502.4.

(c) A violation of this section by a nurse practitioner or certified nurse midwife constitutes unprofessional conduct.

(d) A nurse practitioner who has completed training required in this section and is functioning pursuant to Section 2837.103 or 2837.104 may perform an abortion by aspiration techniques pursuant to Section 2253 without supervision by a physician or surgeon.

(e) A nurse practitioner shall practice abortion by aspiration techniques pursuant to Section 2253 consistent with applicable standards of care and within the scope of their clinical and professional education and training.

(f) A person authorized to perform abortion by aspiration techniques described in paragraph (5) of subdivision (a) and paragraph (5) of subdivision (b) shall not be punished, held liable for damages in a civil action, or denied any right or privilege for any action relating to the evaluation of clinical competency of a nurse practitioner pursuant to paragraph (5) of subdivision (a) or a certified nurse-midwife pursuant to paragraph (5) of subdivision (b).

(g) This section shall not be interpreted to authorize a person with a license or certificate to practice as a nurse practitioner or certified nurse-midwife to perform abortion by aspiration techniques after the first trimester of pregnancy.

(h) For purposes of this section, exclusively online or simulation-based training programs that do not include mandatory clinical hours involving direct patient care shall not meet the clinical training requirements in subdivisions (a) and (b).

HISTORY:

Added Stats 2013 ch 662 § 2 (AB 154), effective January 1, 2014. Amended Stats 2022 ch 631 § 1 (SB 1375), effective January 1, 2023.

§ 2725.5. "Advanced practice registered nurse" defined

"Advanced practice registered nurse" means those licensed registered nurses who have met the requirements of Article 2.5 (commencing with Section 2746), Article 7 (commencing with Section 2825), Article 8 (commencing with Section 2834), or Article 9 (commencing with Section 2838).

HISTORY:

Added Stats 2003 ch 640 § 6 (SB 358).

§ 2726. Unauthorized practices

Except as otherwise provided herein, this chapter confers no authority to practice medicine or surgery.

HISTORY:
Added Stats 1939 ch 807 § 2. Amended Stats 1974 ch 355 § 2.

§ 2727. Practices not prohibited

This chapter does not prohibit:

(a) Gratuitous nursing of the sick by friends or members of the family.

(b) Incidental care of the sick by domestic workers or by persons primarily employed as housekeepers as long as they do not practice nursing within the meaning of this chapter.

(c) Domestic administration of family remedies by any person.

(d) Nursing services in case of an emergency. "Emergency," as used in this subdivision includes an epidemic, pandemic, or other public disaster.

(e) The performance by a person of the duties required in the physical care of a patient or carrying out medical orders prescribed by a licensed physician, provided the person shall not in any way assume to practice as a professional, registered, graduate, or trained nurse.

HISTORY:
Added Stats 1939 ch 807 § 2. Amended Stats 1943 ch 573 § 1; Stats 2021 ch 628 § 5 (AB 1532), effective January 1, 2022.

§ 2727.5. Liability for emergency care

A person licensed under this chapter who in good faith renders emergency care at the scene of an emergency which occurs outside both the place and the course of that person's employment shall not be liable for any civil damages as the result of acts or omissions by that person in rendering the emergency care.

This section shall not grant immunity from civil damages when the person is grossly negligent.

HISTORY:
Added Stats 1963 ch 698 § 1. Amended Stats 1984 ch 1391 § 2.

§ 2728. Services by attendants and psychiatric technicians; Supervised services of unlicensed graduates of accredited psychiatric technician training programs

If adequate medical and nursing supervision by a professional nurse or nurses is provided, nursing service may be given by attendants, psychiatric technicians, or psychiatric technician interim permittees in institutions under the jurisdiction of the State Department of State Hospitals or the State Department of Developmental Services or subject to visitation by the State Department of Public Health or the Department of Corrections and Rehabilitation. Services so given by a psychiatric technician shall be limited to services which he or she is authorized to perform by his or her license as a psychiatric technician. Services so given by a psychiatric technician interim permittee shall be limited to skills included in his or her basic course of study and performed under the supervision of a licensed psychiatric technician or registered nurse.

The Director of State Hospitals, the Director of Developmental Services, and the State Public Health Officer shall determine what shall constitute adequate medical and nursing supervision in any institution under the jurisdiction of the State Department of State Hospitals or the State Department of Developmental Services or subject to visitation by the State Department of Public Health.

Notwithstanding any other provision of law, institutions under the jurisdiction of the State Department of State Hospitals or the State Department of Developmental Services may utilize graduates of accredited psychiatric technician training programs who are not licensed psychiatric technicians or psychiatric technician interim permittees to perform skills included in their basic course of study when supervised by a licensed psychiatric technician or registered nurse, for a period not to exceed nine months.

HISTORY:

Added Stats 1939 ch 807 § 2. Amended Stats 1957 ch 558 § 1; Stats 1971 ch 1593 § 30 (ch 1007 prevails), ch 1007 § 1, operative July 1, 1973; Stats 1973 ch 142 § 7, effective June 30, 1973, operative July 1, 1973; Stats 1977 ch 1252 § 32, operative July 1, 1978; Stats 1987 ch 464 § 1, effective September 9, 1987; Stats 2012 ch 24 § 1 (AB 1470), effective June 27, 2012.

§ 2728.5. Utilization of licensed psychiatric technicians and psychiatric technician interim permittees

Except for those provisions of law relating to directors of nursing services, nothing in this chapter or any other provision of law shall prevent the utilization of a licensed psychiatric technician or psychiatric technician interim permittee in performing services used in the care, treatment, and rehabilitation of mentally ill, emotionally disturbed, or developmentally disabled persons within the scope of practice for which he or she is licensed or authorized in facilities under the jurisdiction of the State Department of State Hospitals or the State Department of Developmental Services or licensed by the State Department of Public Health, that he or she is licensed to perform as a psychiatric technician, or authorized to perform as a psychiatric technician interim permittee including any nursing services under Section 2728, in facilities under the jurisdiction of the State Department of State Hospitals or the State Department of Developmental Services or subject to visitation by the State Department of Public Health.

HISTORY:

Added Stats 1971 ch 1007 § 2. Amended Stats 1973 ch 142 § 8, effective June 30, 1973, operative July 1, 1973; Stats 1977 ch 1252 § 33, operative July 1, 1978; Stats 1978 ch 429 § 15, effective July 17, 1978, operative July 1, 1978; Stats 1987 ch 464 § 2, effective September 9, 1987; Stats 2012 ch 24 § 2 (AB 1470), effective June 27, 2012.

§ 2729. Services by student nurses

Nursing services may be rendered by a student when these services are incidental to the course of study of one of the following:

(a) A student enrolled in a board-approved prelicensure program or school of nursing.

(b) A nurse licensed in another state or country taking a board-approved continuing education course or a postlicensure course.

HISTORY:

Added Stats 1939 ch 807 § 2. Amended Stats 1953 ch 1174 § 4; Stats 1978 ch 212 § 1, effective June 6, 1978.

§ 2730. Nurses qualified outside state and engaged to care for patient temporarily in California

If he does not represent or hold himself out as a professional nurse licensed to practice in this State and if he has an engagement, made in another State or country, requiring him to accompany and care for a patient temporarily residing in this State during the period of such engagement, a nurse legally qualified by another State or country may give nursing care to such patient in this State.

HISTORY:

Added Stats 1939 ch 807 § 2.

§ 2731. Nonprofit religious care

This chapter does not prohibit nursing or the care of the sick, with or without compensation or personal profit, when done by the adherents of and in connection with the practice of the religious tenets of any well recognized church or denomination, so long as they do not otherwise engage in the practice of nursing.

HISTORY:

Added Stats 1939 ch 807 § 2.

§ 2732. Licensure requirement; Use of "R.N."

No person shall engage in the practice of nursing, as defined in Section 2725, without holding a license which is in an active status issued under this chapter except as otherwise provided in this act.

Every licensee may be known as a registered nurse and may place the letter "R.N." after his name.

HISTORY:

Added Stats 1939 ch 807 § 2. Amended Stats 1976 ch 1053 § 1, effective September 28, 1976.

§ 2732.05. Verification of current R.N. status

(a) Every employer of a registered nurse, every employer of a registered nurse required to hold any board-issued certification, and every person acting as an agent for such a nurse in obtaining employment, shall ascertain that the nurse is currently authorized to practice as a registered nurse or as a registered nurse pursuant to a board-issued certification within the provisions of this chapter. As used in this section, "board-issued certification" includes, but is not limited to, certification as a nurse practitioner, nurse practitioner with a furnishing number, nurse anesthetist, nurse midwife, nurse midwife with a furnishing number, public health nurse, clinical nurse specialist, or board listed psychiatric mental health nurse.

(b) Every employer of a temporary licensee or interim permittee and every person acting as an agent for a temporary licensee or interim permittee in obtaining employment shall ascertain that the person is currently authorized to practice as a temporary licensee or interim permittee.

(c) As used in this section, the term "agent" includes, but is not limited to, a nurses registry and a traveling nurse agency.

Examination by an employer or agent of evidence satisfactory to the board showing the nurse's, licensee's, or permittee's current authority to practice under this chapter, prior to employment, shall constitute a determination of authority to so practice.

Nothing in this section shall apply to a patient, or other person acting for a specific patient, who engages the services of a registered nurse or temporary licensee to provide nursing care to a single patient.

HISTORY:

Added Stats 1961 ch 1110 § 1. Amended Stats 1965 ch 680 § 1, ch 727 § 1; Stats 1970 ch 524 § 1; Stats 2007 ch 588 § 37 (SB 1048), effective January 1, 2008.

§ 2732.1. Applications; Interim permits; Waiver of examination; Fees

(a) An applicant for license by examination shall submit a written application in the form prescribed by the board.

Upon approval of the application, the board may issue an interim permit authorizing the applicant to practice nursing pending the results of the first licensing examination following completion of his or her nursing course or for a maximum period of six months, whichever occurs first.

If the applicant passes the examination, the interim permit shall remain in effect until a regular renewable license is issued by the board. If the applicant fails the examination, the interim permit shall terminate upon notice thereof by first-class mail.

(b) The board upon written application may issue a license without examination to any applicant who is licensed or registered as a nurse in a state, district or territory of the United States or Canada having, in the opinion of the board, requirements for licensing or registration equal to or higher than those in California at the time the application is filed with the Board of Registered Nursing, if he or she has passed an examination for the license or registration that is, in the board's opinion, comparable to the board's examination, and if he or she meets all the other requirements set forth in Section 2736.

(c) Each application shall be accompanied by the fee prescribed by this chapter for the filing of an application for a regular renewable license.

The interim permit shall terminate upon notice thereof by first-class mail, if it is issued by mistake or if the application for permanent licensure is denied.

HISTORY:

Added Stats 1953 ch 1174 § 5. Amended Stats 1959 ch 190 § 1; Stats 1965 ch 727 § 2; Stats 1972 ch 668 § 1; Stats 1987 ch 850 § 10; Stats 1992 ch 1289 § 20 (AB 2743); Stats 1994 ch 26 § 57.5 (AB 1807), effective March 30, 1994.

§ 2733. Issuance of temporary license where examination waived

(a)(1)(A) Upon approval of an application filed pursuant to subdivision (b) of Section 2732.1, and upon the payment of the fee prescribed by subdivision (k) of Section 2815, the board may issue a temporary license to practice professional nursing, and a temporary certificate to practice as a certified public health nurse for a period of six months from the date of issuance.

(B) Upon approval of an application filed pursuant to subdivision (b) of Section 2732.1, and upon the payment of the fee prescribed by subdivision (d) of Section 2838.2, the board may issue a temporary certificate to practice as a certified clinical nurse specialist for a period of six months from the date of issuance.

(C) Upon approval of an application filed pursuant to subdivision (b) of Section 2732.1, and upon the payment of the fee prescribed by subdivision (e) of Section 2815.5, the board may issue a temporary certificate to practice as a certified nurse-midwife for a period of six months from the date of issuance.

(D) Upon approval of an application filed pursuant to subdivision (b) of Section 2732.1, and upon the payment of the fee prescribed by subdivision (d) of Section 2830.7, the board may issue a temporary certificate to practice as a certified nurse anesthetist for a period of six months from the date of issuance.

(E) Upon approval of an application filed pursuant to subdivision (b) of Section 2732.1, and upon the payment of the fee prescribed by subdivision (p) of Section 2815, the board may issue a temporary certificate to practice as a certified nurse practitioner for a period of six months from the date of issuance.

(2) A temporary license or temporary certificate shall terminate upon notice thereof by certified mail, return receipt requested, if it is issued by mistake or if the application for permanent licensure is denied.

(b) Upon written application, the board may reissue a temporary license or temporary certificate to any person who has applied for a regular renewable license pursuant to subdivision (b) of Section 2732.1 and who, in the judgment of the board has been excusably delayed in completing their application for or the minimum requirements for a regular renewable license, but the board may not reissue a temporary license or temporary certificate more than twice to any one person.

(c) The board shall prominently display on the front page of its website the availability of temporary licenses and certificates pursuant to this section.

HISTORY:

Added Stats 1953 ch 1174 § 7, as B & P C § 2733.1. Amended Stats 1963 ch 1400 § 1; Amended and renumbered by Stats 1965 ch 727 § 4; Amended Stats 1978 ch 1161 § 172.5; Stats 1987 ch 850 § 11; Stats 1992 ch 1135 § 2.3 (SB 2044); Stats 1994 ch 26 § 58 (AB 1807); Stats 2000 ch 568 § 7 (AB 2888); Stats 2016 ch 799 § 12 (SB 1039), effective January 1, 2017; Stats 2021 ch 628 § 6 (AB 1532), effective January 1, 2022.

§ 2734. Inactive licenses

Upon application in writing to the board and payment of the biennial renewal fee, a licensee may have his license placed in an inactive status for an indefinite period of time. A licensee whose license is in an inactive status may not practice nursing. However, such a licensee does not have to comply with the continuing education standards of Section 2811.5.

HISTORY:

Added Stats 1976 ch 1053 § 2, effective September 28, 1976.

§ 2736. Qualifications generally

(a) An applicant for licensure as a registered nurse shall comply with each of the following:

(1) Have completed such general preliminary education requirements as shall be determined by the board.

(2) Have successfully completed the courses of instruction prescribed by the board for licensure, in a program in this state accredited by the board for training registered nurses, or have successfully completed courses of instruction in a school of nursing outside of this state which, in the opinion of the board at the time the application is filed with the Board of Registered Nursing, are equivalent to the minimum requirements of the board for licensure established for an accredited program in this state.

(3) Not be subject to denial of licensure under Section 480.

(b) An applicant who has received his or her training from a school of nursing in a country outside the United States and who has complied with the provisions of subdivision (a), or has completed training equivalent to that required by subdivision (a), shall qualify for licensure by successfully passing the examination prescribed by the board.

HISTORY:

Added Stats 1939 ch 807 § 2. Amended Stats 1945 ch 1249 § 1; Stats 1953 ch 1174 § 8; Stats 1957 ch 2084 § 6; Stats 1963 ch 1537 § 1.5; Stats 1965 ch 727 § 5; Stats 1969 ch 1541 § 1; Stats 1972 ch 463 § 1; Stats 1974 ch 516 § 1; Stats 1977 ch 1130 § 2; Stats 1978 ch 1161 § 173; Stats 1992 ch 1289 § 21 (AB 2743).

§ 2736.1. Training in detection and treatment of client abuse, and alcohol and chemical substance dependency

(a) The course of instruction for an applicant who matriculates on or after September 1, 1985, shall include training in the detection and treatment of alcohol and chemical substance dependency.

(b) The course of instruction for an applicant who matriculates on or after January 1, 1995, shall include training in the detection and treatment of client abuse, including, but not limited to, spousal or partner abuse. The requirement for coursework in spousal or partner abuse detection and treatment shall be satisfied by, and the board shall accept in satisfaction of the requirement, a certification from the chief academic officer of the educational institution from which the applicant graduated that the required coursework is included within the institution's required curriculum for graduation.

HISTORY:

Added Stats 1984 ch 1149 § 4. Amended Stats 1993 ch 1234 § 5 (AB 890).

§ 2736.5. Continuing education courses regarding implicit bias

(a)(1) The board shall adopt regulations to require that, on and after January 1, 2022, all continuing education courses for licensees under this chapter contain curriculum that includes the understanding of implicit bias.

(2) Beginning January 1, 2023, continuing education providers shall ensure compliance with paragraph (1). Beginning January 1, 2023, the board shall audit continuing education providers, pursuant to Section 2811.5.

(b) Notwithstanding the provisions of subdivision (a), a continuing education course dedicated solely to research or other issues that does not include a direct patient care component is not required to contain curriculum that includes implicit bias in the practice of nursing.

(c) In order to satisfy the requirements of subdivision (a), continuing education courses shall address at least one or a combination of the following:

(1) Examples of how implicit bias affects perceptions and treatment decisions of licensees, leading to disparities in health outcomes.

(2) Strategies to address how unintended biases in decisionmaking may contribute to health care disparities by shaping behavior and producing differences in medical treatment along lines of race, ethnicity, gender identity, sexual orientation, age, socioeconomic status, or other characteristics.

HISTORY:
Added Stats 2019 ch 417 § 3 (AB 241), effective January 1, 2020.

§ 2736.6. Eligibility of vocational nurse to take examination for licensure as registered nurse

The board shall determine by regulation the additional preparation in nursing, in a school approved by the board, which is required for a vocational nurse, licensed under Chapter 6.5 (commencing with Section 2840) of this division, to be eligible to take the examination for licensure under this chapter as a registered nurse. The board shall not require more than 30 units in nursing and related science subjects to satisfy such preparation.

HISTORY:
Added Stats 1969 ch 1541 § 2.

§ 2737. Application fee

An applicant for a license authorizing him to practice nursing in this State under this chapter, upon the filing of his application shall pay the fee required by this chapter.

HISTORY:
Added Stats 1939 ch 807 § 2.

§ 2738. Holding of examinations

The board shall hold not less than two examinations each year at such times and places as the board may determine.

HISTORY:
Added Stats 1939 ch 807 § 2. Amended Stats 1953 ch 1174 § 10.

§ 2740. Conduct of examinations; Finality of decisions

Examinations shall be written, but in the discretion of the board may be supplemented by an oral or practical examination in such subjects as the board determines. All examinations shall be conducted by such persons and in such manner and under such rules and regulations as the board may prescribe.

The board shall finally pass or reject all applicants. Its actions shall be final and conclusive and not subject to review by any court or other authority.

HISTORY:
Added Stats 1939 ch 807 § 2.

§ 2741. Fees with application for reexamination

An application for reexamination shall be accompanied by the fees prescribed by this chapter.

HISTORY:

Added Stats 1939 ch 807 § 2. Amended Stats 1953 ch 1174 § 11; Stats 1965 ch 727 § 7; Stats 1972 ch 901 § 1; Stats 1979 ch 933 § 1; Stats 1981 ch 437 § 1; Stats 1987 ch 850 § 12; Stats 1994 ch 26 § 60 (AB 1807), effective March 30, 1994; Stats 2005 ch 621 § 38 (SB 1111), effective January 1, 2006.

§ 2742. Issuance of license

The board shall issue a license to each applicant who passes the examination and meets all other licensing requirements. The form of the license shall be determined in accordance with Section 164.

HISTORY:

Added Stats 1939 ch 807 § 2. Amended Stats 1971 ch 716 § 40; Stats 1987 ch 850 § 13.

ARTICLE 2.5

NURSE-MIDWIVES

Section

2746. Issuance of certificates.
2746.1. Compliance with article required.
2746.2. Educational prerequisites; Nurse-midwifery committee.
2746.3. Renewal of midwife's certificates.
2746.4. Practice of midwifery by midwife's certificates.
2746.5. Authority conferred by certificate; Required supervision.
2746.51. When nurse-midwife may furnish drugs or devices.
2746.52. Authority to perform episiotomies and repair lacerations of perineum.
2746.53. Furnishing number fees.
2746.54. Obtaining informed consent.
2746.55. Data collected after transfer to hospital or maternal, fetal, or neonatal death that occurred in the out-of-hospital setting.
2746.6. Discipline for performance of abortion.
2746.7. Applications and fees.
2746.8. Renewal of nurse-midwifery certificates.

HISTORY: Added Stats 1974 ch 1407 § 1.

§ 2746. Issuance of certificates

The board shall issue a certificate to practice nurse-midwifery to any person who qualifies under this article and is licensed pursuant to the provisions of this chapter.

HISTORY:

Added Stats 1974 ch 1407 § 1.

§ 2746.1. Compliance with article required

Every applicant for a certificate to practice nurse-midwifery shall comply with all the provisions of this article in addition to the provisions of this chapter.

HISTORY:
Added Stats 1974 ch 1407 § 1.

§ 2746.2. Educational prerequisites; Nurse-midwifery committee

(a) An applicant shall show by evidence satisfactory to the board that they have met the educational standards established by the board or have at least the equivalent thereof.

(b)(1) The board shall appoint a committee of qualified physicians and surgeons and nurses called the Nurse-Midwifery Advisory Committee.

(2) The committee shall make recommendations to the board on all matters related to midwifery practice, education, appropriate standard of care, and other matters as specified by the board. The committee shall provide recommendations or guidance on care when the board is considering disciplinary action against a certified nurse-midwife.

(3) The committee shall consist of four qualified nurse-midwives, two qualified physicians and surgeons, including, but not limited to, obstetricians or family physicians, and one public member.

(4) If the board is unable, despite good faith efforts, to solicit and appoint committee members pursuant to the specifications in paragraph (3), the committee may continue to make recommendations pursuant to paragraph (2).

HISTORY:
Added Stats 1974 ch 1407 § 1. Amended Stats 2019 ch 632 § 4 (AB 1622), effective January 1, 2020; Stats 2020 ch 88 § 3 (SB 1237), effective January 1, 2021.

§ 2746.3. Renewal of midwife's certificates

Midwife's certificates issued by the Medical Board of California prior to the effective date of this article shall be renewable only by such board.

HISTORY:
Added Stats 1974 ch 1407 § 1. Amended Stats 1978 ch 1161 § 174; Stats 1989 ch 886 § 53.

§ 2746.4. Practice of midwifery by midwife's certificates

Nothing in this article shall be construed to prevent the practice of midwifery by a person possessing a midwife's certificate issued by the Medical Board of California on the effective date of this article.

HISTORY:
Added Stats 1974 ch 1407 § 1. Amended Stats 1978 ch 1161 § 175; Stats 1989 ch 886 § 54.

§ 2746.5. Authority conferred by certificate; Required supervision

(a) The certificate to practice nurse-midwifery authorizes the holder to attend cases of low-risk pregnancy and childbirth and to provide prenatal, intrapartum, and postpartum care, including interconception care, family-planning care, and immediate care for the newborn, consistent with the Core Competencies for Basic Midwifery Practice adopted by the American College of Nurse-Midwives, or its successor national professional organization, as approved by the board. For purposes of this subdivision, "low-risk pregnancy" means a pregnancy in which all of the following conditions are met:

(1) There is a single fetus.

(2) There is a cephalic presentation at onset of labor.

(3) The gestational age of the fetus is greater than or equal to 37 weeks and zero days and less than or equal to 42 weeks and zero days at the time of delivery.

(4) Labor is spontaneous or induced.

(5) The patient has no preexisting disease or condition, whether arising out of the pregnancy or otherwise, that adversely affects the pregnancy and that the certified nurse-midwife is not qualified to independently address consistent with this section.

(b)(1) The certificate to practice nurse-midwifery authorizes the holder to practice with a physician and surgeon under mutually agreed-upon policies and protocols that delineate the parameters for consultation, collaboration, referral, and transfer of a patient's care, signed by both the certified nurse-midwife and a physician and surgeon to do either of the following:

(A) Provide a patient with care that falls outside the scope of services specified in subdivision (a).

(B) Provide intrapartum care to a patient who has had a prior cesarean section or surgery that interrupts the myometrium.

(2) If a physician and surgeon assumes care of the patient, the certified nurse-midwife may continue to attend the birth of the newborn and participate in physical care, counseling, guidance, teaching, and support, as indicated by the mutually agreed-upon policies and protocols signed by both the certified nurse-midwife and a physician and surgeon.

(3) After a certified nurse-midwife refers a patient to a physician and surgeon, the certified nurse-midwife may continue care of the patient during a reasonable interval between the referral and the initial appointment with the physician and surgeon.

(c)(1) If a nurse-midwife does not have in place mutually agreed-upon policies and protocols that delineate the parameters for consultation, collaboration, referral, and transfer of a patient's care, signed by both the certified nurse-midwife and a physician and surgeon pursuant to paragraph (1) of subdivision (b), the patient shall be transferred to the care of a physician and surgeon to do either or both of the following:

(A) Provide a patient with care that falls outside the scope of services specified in subdivision (a).

(B) Provide intrapartum care to a patient who has had a prior cesarean section or surgery that interrupts the myometrium.

(2) After the certified nurse-midwife initiates the process of transfer pursuant to paragraph (1), for a patient who otherwise meets the definition of a low-risk pregnancy but no longer meets the criteria specified in paragraph (3) of subdivision (a) because the gestational age of the fetus is greater than 42 weeks and zero days, if there is inadequate time to effect safe transfer to a hospital prior to delivery or transfer may pose a threat to the health and safety of the patient or the unborn child, the certified nurse-midwife may continue care of the patient consistent with the transfer plan described in subdivision (a) of Section 2746.54.

(3) A patient who has been transferred from the care of a certified nurse-midwife to that of a physician and surgeon may return to the care of the certified nurse-midwife after the physician and surgeon has determined

that the condition or circumstance that required, or would require, the transfer from the care of the nurse-midwife pursuant to paragraph (1) is resolved.

(d) The certificate to practice nurse-midwifery authorizes the holder to attend pregnancy and childbirth in an out-of-hospital setting if consistent with subdivisions (a), (b), and (c).

(e) This section shall not be interpreted to deny a patient's right to self-determination or informed decisionmaking with regard to choice of provider or birth setting.

(f) The certificate to practice nurse-midwifery does not authorize the holder of the certificate to assist childbirth by vacuum or forceps extraction, or to perform any external cephalic version.

(g) A certified nurse-midwife shall document all consultations, referrals, and transfers in the patient record.

(h)(1) A certified nurse-midwife shall refer all emergencies to a physician and surgeon immediately.

(2) A certified nurse-midwife may provide emergency care until the assistance of a physician and surgeon is obtained.

(i) This chapter does not authorize a nurse-midwife to practice medicine or surgery.

(j) This section shall not be construed to require a physician and surgeon to sign protocols and procedures for a nurse-midwife or to permit any action that violates Section 2052 or 2400.

(k) This section shall not be construed to require a nurse-midwife to have mutually agreed-upon, signed policies and protocols for the provision of services described in subdivision (a).

HISTORY:

Added Stats 1974 ch 1407 § 1. Amended Stats 2002 ch 764 § 1 (SB 993); Stats 2020 ch 88 § 4 (SB 1237), effective January 1, 2021.

§ 2746.51. When nurse-midwife may furnish drugs or devices

(a) Neither this chapter nor any other law shall be construed to prohibit a certified nurse-midwife from furnishing or ordering drugs or devices, including controlled substances classified in Schedule II, III, IV, or V under the California Uniform Controlled Substances Act (Division 10 (commencing with Section 11000) of the Health and Safety Code), when all of the following apply:

(1) The drugs or devices are furnished or ordered incidentally to the provision of any of the following:

(A) The care and services described in Section 2746.5.

(B) Care rendered, consistent with the certified nurse-midwife's educational preparation or for which clinical competency has been established and maintained, to persons within a facility specified in subdivision (a), (b), (c), (d), (i), or (j) of Section 1206 of the Health and Safety Code, a clinic as specified in Section 1204 of the Health and Safety Code, a general acute care hospital as defined in subdivision (a) of Section 1250 of the Health and Safety Code, a licensed birth center as defined in Section 1204.3 of the Health and Safety Code, or a special hospital specified as a maternity hospital in subdivision (f) of Section 1250 of the Health and Safety Code.

(C) Care rendered in an out-of-hospital setting pursuant to subdivision (d) of Section 2746.5.

(2) The furnishing or ordering of drugs or devices by a certified nurse-midwife for services that do not fall within the scope of services specified in subdivision (a) of Section 2746.5, and Schedule IV or V controlled substances by a nurse-midwife for any condition, including, but not limited to, Schedule IV or V controlled substances for services that fall within the scope of services specified in subdivision (a) of Section 2746.5, are in accordance with the standardized procedures or protocols. For purposes of this section, standardized procedure means a document, including protocols, developed in collaboration with, and approved by, a physician and surgeon and the certified nurse-midwife. The standardized procedure covering the furnishing or ordering of drugs or devices shall specify all of the following:

(A) Which certified nurse-midwife may furnish or order drugs or devices.

(B) Which drugs or devices may be furnished or ordered and under what circumstances.

(C) The method of periodic review of the certified nurse-midwife's competence, including peer review, and review of the provisions of the standardized procedure.

(3) If Schedule II or III controlled substances, as defined in Sections 11055 and 11056 of the Health and Safety Code, are furnished or ordered by a certified nurse-midwife for any condition, including, but not limited to, Schedule II or III controlled substances for services that fall within the scope of services specified in subdivision (a) of Section 2746.5, the controlled substances shall be furnished or ordered in accordance with a patient-specific protocol approved by a physician and surgeon. For Schedule II controlled substance protocols, the provision for furnishing the Schedule II controlled substance shall address the diagnosis of the illness, injury, or condition for which the Schedule II controlled substance is to be furnished.

(b)(1) The furnishing or ordering of drugs or devices by a certified nurse-midwife is conditional on the issuance by the board of a number to the applicant who has successfully completed the requirements of paragraph (2). The board may issue a furnishing number upon initial application and, if approved by the board, the applicant shall not be required to make a separate application. The number shall be included on all transmittals of orders for drugs or devices by the certified nurse-midwife. The board shall maintain a list of the certified nurse-midwives that it has certified pursuant to this paragraph and the number it has issued to each one. The board shall make the list available to the California State Board of Pharmacy upon its request. Every certified nurse-midwife who is authorized pursuant to this section to furnish or issue a drug order for a controlled substance shall register with the United States Drug Enforcement Administration and the Controlled Substance Utilization Review and Enforcement System (CURES) pursuant to Section 11165.1 of the Health and Safety Code.

(2) The board has certified in accordance with paragraph (1) that the certified nurse-midwife has satisfactorily completed a course in pharmacology covering the drugs or devices to be furnished or ordered under this section, including the risks of addiction and neonatal abstinence syndrome

associated with the use of opioids. The board shall establish the requirements for satisfactory completion of this paragraph.

(3) A copy of the standardized procedure or protocol relating to the furnishing or ordering of controlled substances by a certified nurse-midwife shall be provided upon request to any licensed pharmacist who is uncertain of the authority of the certified nurse-midwife to perform these functions.

(4) Certified nurse-midwives who are certified by the board and hold an active furnishing number, who are currently authorized through standardized procedures or protocols to furnish Schedule II controlled substances, and who are registered with the United States Drug Enforcement Administration shall provide documentation of continuing education specific to the use of Schedule II controlled substances in settings other than a hospital based on standards developed by the board.

(c) Drugs or devices furnished or ordered by a certified nurse-midwife may include Schedule II controlled substances under the California Uniform Controlled Substances Act (Division 10 (commencing with Section 11000) of the Health and Safety Code) under the following conditions:

(1) The drugs and devices are furnished or ordered in accordance with requirements referenced in subdivisions (a) and (b).

(2) When Schedule II controlled substances, as defined in Section 11055 of the Health and Safety Code, are furnished or ordered by a certified nurse-midwife, the controlled substances shall be furnished or ordered in accordance with a patient-specific protocol approved by a physician and surgeon.

(d) Furnishing of drugs or devices by a certified nurse-midwife means the act of making a pharmaceutical agent or agents available to the patient. Use of the term "furnishing" in this section shall include the following:

(1) The ordering of a nonscheduled drug or device for services that fall within the scope of services specified in subdivision (a) of Section 2746.5.

(2) The ordering of a nonscheduled drug or device for services that fall outside the scope of services specified in subdivision (a) of Section 2746.5 in accordance with standardized procedures or protocols pursuant to paragraph (2) of subdivision (a).

(3) The ordering of a Schedule IV or V drug for any condition, including, but not limited to, for care that falls within the scope of services specified in subdivision (a) of Section 2746.5, in accordance with standardized procedures or protocols pursuant to paragraph (2) of subdivision (a).

(4) The ordering of a Schedule II or III drug in accordance with a patient-specific protocol approved by a physician and surgeon pursuant to paragraph (3) of subdivision (a).

(5) Transmitting an order of a physician and surgeon.

(e) "Drug order" or "order" for purposes of this section means an order for medication or for a drug or device that is dispensed to or for an ultimate user, issued by a certified nurse-midwife as an individual practitioner, within the meaning of Section 1306.03 of Title 21 of the Code of Federal Regulations. Notwithstanding any other provision of law, (1) a drug order issued pursuant to this section shall be treated in the same manner as a prescription of the supervising physician; (2) all references to "prescription" in this code and the Health and Safety Code shall include drug orders issued by certified nurse-midwives; and (3) the signature of a certified nurse-midwife on a drug order issued in accordance with this section shall be deemed to be the signature of a prescriber for purposes of this code and the Health and Safety Code.

(f) Notwithstanding any other law, a certified nurse-midwife may directly procure supplies and devices, obtain and administer diagnostic tests, directly obtain and administer nonscheduled drugs consistent with the provision of services that fall within the scope of services specified in subdivision (a) of Section 2746.5, order laboratory and diagnostic testing, and receive reports that are necessary to their practice as a certified nurse-midwife within their scope of practice, consistent with Section 2746.5.

HISTORY:

Added Stats 1991 ch 870 § 2 (AB 1350). Amended Stats 2001 ch 289 § 3 (SB 298); Stats 2002 ch 764 § 2 (SB 993); Stats 2005 ch 266 § 1 (SB 614), effective January 1, 2006; Stats 2012 ch 796 § 1 (SB 1524), effective January 1, 2013; Stats 2018 ch 693 § 7 (SB 1109), effective January 1, 2019; Stats 2020 ch 88 § 5 (SB 1237), effective January 1, 2021; Stats 2022 ch 413 § 8 (AB 2684), effective January 1, 2023.

§ 2746.52. Authority to perform episiotomies and repair lacerations of perineum

(a) Notwithstanding Section 2746.5, the certificate to practice nurse-midwifery authorizes the holder to perform and repair episiotomies, and to repair first-degree and second-degree lacerations of the perineum.

(b) A certified nurse-midwife performing and repairing first-degree and second-degree lacerations of the perineumshall do both of the following:

(1) Ensure that all complications are referred to a physician and surgeon immediately.

(2) Ensure immediate care of patients who are in need of care beyond the scope of practice of the certified nurse-midwife, or emergency care for times when a physician and surgeon is not on the premises.

HISTORY:

Added Stats 1996 ch 158 § 1 (SB 1738), effective July 12, 1996. Amended Stats 2020 ch 88 § 6 (SB 1237), effective January 1, 2021.

§ 2746.53. Furnishing number fees

The board may charge the applicant a fee to cover all necessary costs to implement Section 2746.51, that shall be not more than one thousand five hundred dollars ($1,500) for an initial application, nor more than one thousand dollars ($1,000) for an application for renewal. The board may charge a penalty fee for failure to renew a furnishing number within the prescribed time that shall be not more than five hundred dollars ($500).

HISTORY:

Added Stats 2016 ch 799 § 13 (SB 1039), effective January 1, 2017. Amended Stats 2022 ch 413 § 9 (AB 2684), effective January 1, 2023.

§ 2746.54. Obtaining informed consent

(a) A certified nurse-midwife shall disclose in oral and written form to a prospective patient as part of a patient care plan, and obtain informed consent for, all of the following:

(1) The patient is retaining a certified nurse-midwife and the certified nurse-midwife is not supervised by a physician and surgeon.

(2) The certified nurse-midwife's current licensure status and license number.

(3) The practice settings in which the certified nurse-midwife practices.

(4) If the certified nurse-midwife does not have liability coverage for the practice of midwifery, the certified nurse-midwife shall disclose that fact.

(5) There are conditions that are outside of the scope of practice of a certified nurse-midwife that will result in a referral for a consultation from, or transfer of care to, a physician and surgeon.

(6) The specific arrangements for the referral of complications to a physician and surgeon for consultation. The certified nurse-midwife shall not be required to identify a specific physician and surgeon.

(7) The specific arrangements for the transfer of care during the prenatal period, hospital transfer during the intrapartum and postpartum periods, and access to appropriate emergency medical services for mother and baby if necessary, and recommendations for preregistration at a hospital that has obstetric emergency services and is most likely to receive the transfer.

(8) If, during the course of care, the patient is informed that the patient has or may have a condition indicating the need for a mandatory transfer, the certified nurse-midwife shall initiate the transfer.

(9) The availability of the text of laws regulating certified nurse-midwifery practices and the procedure for reporting complaints to the Board of Registered Nursing, which may be found on the Board of Registered Nursing's internet website.

(10) Consultation with a physician and surgeon does not alone create a physician-patient relationship or any other relationship with the physician and surgeon. The certified nurse-midwife shall inform the patient that certified nurse-midwife is independently licensed and practicing midwifery and in that regard is solely responsible for the services the certified nurse-midwife provides.

(b) The disclosure and consent shall be signed by both the certified nurse-midwife and the patient and a copy of the disclosure and consent shall be placed in the patient's medical record.

(c) The Nurse-Midwifery Advisory Committee, in consultation with the board, may recommend to the board the form for the written disclosure and informed consent statement required to be used by a certified nurse-midwife under this section.

(d) This section shall not apply when the intended site of birth is the hospital setting.

HISTORY:

Added Stats 2020 ch 88 § 7 (SB 1237), effective January 1, 2021.

§ 2746.55. Data collected after transfer to hospital or maternal, fetal, or neonatal death that occurred in the out-of-hospital setting

(a) For all maternal or neonatal transfers to the hospital setting during labor or the immediate postpartum period, for which the intended place of birth was an out-of-hospital setting at the onset of labor, or for any maternal, fetal, or neonatal death that occurred in the out-of-hospital setting during labor or the immediate postpartum period, and for which the intended birth care provider is a certified nurse-midwife in the out-of-hospital setting, the department shall collect, and the certified nurse-midwife shall be required to submit, within 90 days of the transfer or death, the following data in the form determined by the department. The data shall include all of the following:

(1) Attendant's name, for the certified nurse-midwife who attended the patient at the time of transfer, or who attended the patient at the time of maternal, fetal, or neonatal death.

(2) Attendant's license number, for the certified nurse-midwife who attended the patient at the time of transfer, or who attended the patient at the time of maternal, fetal, or neonatal death.

(3) The child's date of delivery for births attended by the nurse-midwife.

(4) The sex of the child, for births attended by the nurse-midwife.

(5) The date of birth of the parent giving birth.

(6) The date of birth of the parent not giving birth.

(7) The residence ZIP Code of the parent giving birth.

(8) The residence county of the parent giving birth.

(9) The weight of the parent giving birth (prepregnancy weight and delivery weight of parent giving birth).

(10) The height of the parent giving birth.

(11) The race and ethnicity of the genetic parents, unless the parent declines to disclose.

(12) The obstetric estimate of gestation (completed weeks), at time of transfer.

(13) The total number of prior live births.

(14) The principal source of payment code for delivery.

(15) Any complications and procedures of pregnancy and concurrent illnesses up until time of transfer or death.

(16) Any complications and procedures of labor and delivery up until time of transfer or death.

(17) Any abnormal conditions and clinical procedures related to the newborn up until time of transfer or death.

(18) Fetal presentation at birth, or up until time of transfer.

(19) Whether this pregnancy is a multiple pregnancy (more than one fetus this pregnancy).

(20) Whether the patient has had a previous cesarean section.

(21) If the patient had a previous cesarean, indicate how many.

(22) The intended place of birth at the onset of labor, including, but not limited to, home, freestanding birth center, hospital, clinic, doctor's office, or other location.

(23) Whether there was a maternal death.

(24) Whether there was a fetal death.

(25) Whether there was a neonatal death.

(26) Hospital transfer during the intrapartum or postpartum period, including, who was transferred (mother, infant, or both) and the complications, abnormal conditions, or other indications that resulted in the transfer.

(27) The name of the transfer hospital, or other hospital identification method as required, such as the hospital identification number.

(28) The county of the transfer hospital.

(29) The ZIP Code of the transfer hospital.

(30) The date of the transfer.

(31) Other information as prescribed by the State Department of Public Health.

(b) In the event of a maternal, fetal, or neonatal death that occurred in an out-of-hospital setting during labor or the immediate postpartum period, a certified nurse-midwife shall submit to the department, within 90 days of the death, all of the following data in addition to the data required in subdivision (a):

(1) The date of the maternal, neonatal, or fetal death.

(2) The place of delivery, for births attended by the nurse-midwife.

(3) The county of the place of delivery, for births attended by the nurse-midwife.

(4) The ZIP Code of the place of delivery, for births attended by the nurse-midwife.

(5) The APGAR scores, for births attended by the nurse-midwife.

(6) The birthweight, for births attended by the nurse-midwife.

(7) The method of delivery, for births attended by the nurse-midwife.

(c) The data submitted pursuant to subdivisions (a) and (b) shall be in addition to the certificate of live birth information required pursuant to Sections 102425 and 102426 of the Health and Safety Code.

(d) For those cases that involve a hospital transfer, the department shall link the data submitted by the certified nurse-midwife, pursuant to subdivision (a), to the live birth data reported by hospitals to the department, pursuant to Sections 102425 and 102426 of the Health and Safety Code, and to the patient discharge data that reflects the birth hospitalization and reported by hospitals to the Department of Health Care Access and Information, so that additional data reflecting the outcome can be incorporated into the aggregated reports submitted pursuant to subdivision (i).

(e) The department may adjust, improve, or expand the data elements required to be reported pursuant to subdivisions (a) and (b) to better coordinate with other data collection and reporting systems, or in order to collect more accurate data, as long as the minimum data elements in subdivisions (a) and (b) are preserved.

(f) The department shall treat the information and data gathered pursuant to this section, for the creation of the reports described in subdivision (i), as confidential records, and shall not permit the disclosure of any patient or certified nurse-midwife information to any law enforcement or regulatory agency for any purpose, including, but not limited to, investigations for licensing, certification, or regulatory purposes. This subdivision shall not prevent the department from responding to inquiries from the Board of Registered Nursing as to whether a licensee has reported pursuant to this section.

(g) The information collected by the department pursuant to this section, and not otherwise subject to current confidentiality requirements, shall be treated as confidential records and shall only be made available for use consistent with paragraph (1) of, paragraph (4) of, and subparagraph (A) of paragraph (8) of, subdivision (a) of Section 102430 of the Health and Safety Code and pursuant to the application, review, and approval process established by the department pursuant to Section 102465 of the Health Safety Code.

(h) At the time of each certified nurse-midwife's license renewal, the Board of Registered Nursing shall send a written notification to the certified nurse-midwife notifying them of the mandated vital records reporting requirements for out-of-hospital births pursuant to subdivisions (a) and (b) and Section 102415 of the Health and Safety Code and that a violation of this section shall subject the certified nurse-midwife to disciplinary or administrative action by the board.

(i)(1) The department shall report to the Legislature on the data collected pursuant to this section. The report shall include the aggregate information, including, but not limited to, birth outcomes of patients under the care of a certified nurse-midwife in an out-of-hospital setting at the onset of labor, collected pursuant to this section and Sections 102425 and 102426 of the Health and Safety Code.

(2) The first report, to reflect a 12-month period of time, shall be submitted no later than four and one-half years after the State Department of Public Health receives an appropriation as specified in subdivision (m) and each subsequent report reflecting a 12-month reporting period shall be submitted annually to the Legislature every year thereafter.

(3) A report required under this subdivision shall be submitted in compliance with Section 9795 of the Government Code.

(j) All reports, including those submitted to the Legislature or made publicly available, shall utilize standard public health reporting practices for accurate dissemination of these data elements, specifically in regards to the reporting of small numbers in a way that does not risk a confidentiality or other disclosure breach. No identifying information in regards to the patient or the nurse-midwife shall be disclosed in the reports submitted pursuant to subdivision (i).

(k) A violation of this section shall subject the certified nurse-midwife to disciplinary or administrative action by the Board of Registered Nursing.

(*l*) For purposes of this section, "department" means the State Department of Public Health.

(m) This section shall become operative only upon the Legislature making an appropriation to implement the provisions of this section.

HISTORY:

Added Stats 2020 ch 88 § 8 (SB 1237), effective January 1, 2021. Amended Stats 2022 ch 511 § 14 (SB 1495), effective January 1, 2023.

§ 2746.6. Discipline for performance of abortion

(a) The board shall not suspend or revoke a certificate to practice nurse-midwifery solely for performing an abortion if the holder performed the abortion in accordance with the provisions of this chapter and the Reproductive Privacy Act (Article 2.5 (commencing with Section 123460) of Chapter 2 of Part 2 of Division 106 of the Health and Safety Code).

(b) Notwithstanding any other law, including, but not limited to, Sections 141, 480, 490, and 2761, the board shall not deny an application for certification as a certified nurse-midwife, or suspend, revoke, or otherwise impose discipline upon a person certified in this state to practice nurse-midwifery under either of the following circumstances:

(1) The person is licensed or certified to practice nurse-midwifery in another state and was disciplined in that state solely for performing an abortion in that state.

(2) The person is licensed or certified to practice nurse-midwifery in another state and was convicted in that state for an offense related solely to the performance of an abortion in that state.

HISTORY:
Added Stats 2022 ch 565 § 2 (AB 2626), effective September 27, 2022.

§ 2746.7. Applications and fees

An applicant for certification pursuant to this article shall submit a written application in the form prescribed by the board, accompanied by the fee prescribed by Section 2815.5.

HISTORY:
Added Stats 1974 ch 1407 § 1.

§ 2746.8. Renewal of nurse-midwifery certificates

Each certificate issued pursuant to this article shall be renewable biennially, and each person holding a certificate under this article shall apply for a renewal of his certificate and pay the biennial renewal fee required by Section 2815.5 every two years on or before the last day of the month following the month in which his birthday occurs, beginning with the second birthday following the date on which the certificate was issued, whereupon the board shall renew the certificate.

Each such certificate not renewed in accordance with this section shall expire but may within a period of eight years thereafter be reinstated upon payment of the biennial renewal fee and penalty fee required by Section 2815.5 and upon submission of such proof of the applicant's qualifications as may be required by the board, except that during such eight-year period no examination shall be required as a condition for the reinstatement of any such expired certificate which has lapsed solely by reason of nonpayment of the renewal fee. After the expiration of such eight-year period the board may require as a condition of reinstatement that the applicant pass such examination as it deems necessary to determine his present fitness to resume the practice of nurse-midwifery.

HISTORY:
Added Stats 1974 ch 1407 § 1.

ARTICLE 3

DISCIPLINARY PROCEEDINGS

Section

2750. Persons subject to discipline; Conduct of proceedings.
2751. Acceptance of surrender of license through stipulated agreement.
2759. Scope of discipline.
2760. Effect of suspension; Conditions of reinstatement.
2760.1. Petition for reinstatement or modification of penalty; Notice to Attorney General; Hearing.
2761. Grounds for action.
2761.1. Performance of abortion.
2761.5. Reporting mechanisms.
2762. Drug-related transgressions.

Section
2764. Jurisdiction in event license suspended or surrendered.
2765. What deemed conviction.

HISTORY: Added Stats 1939 ch 807 § 2.

§ 2750. Persons subject to discipline; Conduct of proceedings

Every certificate holder or licensee, including licensees holding temporary licenses, or licensees holding licenses placed in an inactive status, may be disciplined as provided in this article. As used in this article, "license" includes certificate, registration, or any other authorization to engage in practice regulated by this chapter. The proceedings under this article shall be conducted in accordance with Chapter 5 (commencing with Section 11500) of Part 1 of Division 3 of Title 2 of the Government Code, and the board shall have all the powers granted therein.

HISTORY:

Added Stats 1939 ch 807 § 2. Amended Stats 1945 ch 895 § 1; Stats 1965 ch 727 § 8; Stats 1976 ch 1053 § 3, effective September 28, 1976; Stats 1983 ch 696 § 1; Stats 1984 ch 144 § 10; Stats 1994 ch 1275 § 13 (SB 2101).

§ 2751. Acceptance of surrender of license through stipulated agreement

(a) Notwithstanding any other law, the board may, in its discretion, accept the surrender of a license through a stipulated agreement in the absence of a pleading when the ability of a registered nurse to practice nursing safely is impaired due to mental or physical illness.

(b) This alternative proceeding shall apply only to cases that would otherwise have been processed pursuant to Section 820.

(c) Until the time that the licensee signs the stipulated agreement for license surrender, he or she may elect to have the disciplinary process conducted pursuant to Chapter 5 (commencing with Section 11500) of Part 1 of Division 3 of Title 2 of the Government Code.

(d) The stipulated agreement in this alternative proceeding shall specify that:

(1) The license surrender shall be public information and shall be considered a disciplinary action.

(2) The licensee may petition the board for reinstatement after a period of not less than one year after the effective date of the decision.

(3) Any reinstatement proceeding shall be conducted pursuant to Section 2760.1.

(4) Upon seeking reinstatement, it is the responsibility of the former licensee to submit competent evidence of the ability to safely and competently practice as a registered nurse.

HISTORY:

Added Stats 2002 ch 1011 § 6 (SB 2021).

§ 2759. Scope of discipline

The board shall discipline the holder of any license, whose default has been entered or who has been heard by the board and found guilty, by any of the following methods:

(a) Suspending judgment.

(b) Placing him or her upon probation.

(c) Suspending his or her right to practice nursing for a period not exceeding one year.

(d) Revoking his or her license.

(e) Taking other action in relation to disciplining him or her as the board in its discretion may deem proper.

HISTORY:

Added Stats 1939 ch 807 § 2. Amended Stats 2016 ch 86 § 6 (SB 1171), effective January 1, 2017.

§ 2760. Effect of suspension; Conditions of reinstatement

If the holder of a license is suspended, he or she shall not be entitled to practice nursing during the term of suspension.

Upon the expiration of the term of suspension, he or she shall be reinstated by the board and shall be entitled to resume his or her practice of nursing unless it is established to the satisfaction of the board that he or she has practiced nursing in this state during the term of suspension. In this event, the board shall revoke his or her license.

HISTORY:

Added Stats 1939 ch 807 § 2. Amended Stats 1972 ch 300 § 1; Stats 1994 ch 1275 § 14 (SB 2101).

§ 2760.1. Petition for reinstatement or modification of penalty; Notice to Attorney General; Hearing

(a) A registered nurse whose license has been revoked or suspended or who has been placed on probation may petition the board for reinstatement or modification of penalty, including reduction or termination of probation, after a period not less than the following minimum periods has elapsed from the effective date of the decision ordering that disciplinary action, or if the order of the board or any portion of it is stayed by the board itself or by the superior court, from the date the disciplinary action is actually implemented in its entirety, or for a registered nurse whose initial license application is subject to a disciplinary decision, from the date the initial license was issued:

(1) Except as otherwise provided in this section, at least three years for reinstatement of a license that was revoked, except that the board may, in its sole discretion, specify in its order a lesser period of time provided that the period shall be not less than one year.

(2) At least two years for early termination of a probation period of three years or more.

(3) At least one year for modification of a condition, or reinstatement of a license revoked for mental or physical illness, or termination of probation of less than three years.

(b) The board shall give notice to the Attorney General of the filing of the petition. The petitioner and the Attorney General shall be given timely notice by letter of the time and place of the hearing on the petition, and an opportunity to present both oral and documentary evidence and argument to the board. The petitioner shall at all times have the burden of proof to establish by clear and convincing evidence that he or she is entitled to the relief sought in the petition.

(c) The hearing may be continued from time to time as the board deems appropriate.

(d)(1) The petition may be heard by the board or the board may assign the petition to an administrative law judge of the Office of Administrative Hearings.

(2) If the board assigns the petition to an administrative law judge, the administrative law judge shall submit a proposed decision, as specified in Section 11517 of the Government Code, to the board for its consideration, which shall include reasons supporting the proposed decision.

(e) The board may grant or deny the petition, or may impose any terms and conditions that it reasonably deems appropriate as a condition of reinstatement or reduction of penalty.

(f) In considering a petition for reinstatement or modification of a penalty, the board or the administrative law judge shall evaluate and consider evidence of rehabilitation submitted by the petitioner using criteria specified in regulations promulgated by the board.

(g) The board may impose, or the administrative law judge may recommend, terms and conditions on the petitioner in reinstating a license, certificate, or permit or in modifying a penalty.

(h) The petitioner shall provide a current set of fingerprints accompanied by the necessary fingerprinting fee.

(i) No petition shall be considered while the petitioner is under sentence for any criminal offense, including any period during which the petitioner is on court-imposed probation or parole, or subject to an order of registration pursuant to Section 290 of the Penal Code. No petition shall be considered while there is an accusation or petition to revoke probation pending against the petitioner.

(j) Except in those cases where the petitioner has been disciplined pursuant to Section 822, the board may in its discretion deny without hearing or argument any petition that is filed pursuant to this section within a period of two years from the effective date of a prior decision following a hearing under this section.

HISTORY:

Added Stats 1994 ch 1275 § 15 (SB 2101). Amended Stats 1997 ch 758 § 33 (SB 1346); Stats 1998 ch 970 § 11 (AB 2802); Stats 2009 ch 308 § 33 (SB 819), effective January 1, 2010; Stats 2017 ch 429 § 8 (SB 547), effective January 1, 2018.

§ 2761. Grounds for action

The board may take disciplinary action against a certified or licensed nurse or deny an application for a certificate or license for any of the following:

(a) Unprofessional conduct, which includes, but is not limited to, the following:

(1) Incompetence, or gross negligence in carrying out usual certified or licensed nursing functions.

(2) A conviction of practicing medicine without a license in violation of Chapter 5 (commencing with Section 2000), in which event the record of conviction shall be conclusive evidence thereof.

(3) The use of advertising relating to nursing which violates Section 17500.

(4) Denial of licensure, revocation, suspension, restriction, or any other disciplinary action against a health care professional license or certificate by another state or territory of the United States, by any other government agency, or by another California health care professional licensing board. A certified copy of the decision or judgment shall be conclusive evidence of that action.

(b) Procuring his or her certificate or license by fraud, misrepresentation, or mistake.

(c) Procuring, or aiding, or abetting, or attempting, or agreeing, or offering to procure or assist at a criminal abortion.

(d) Violating or attempting to violate, directly or indirectly, or assisting in or abetting the violating of, or conspiring to violate any provision or term of this chapter or regulations adopted pursuant to it.

(e) Making or giving any false statement or information in connection with the application for issuance of a certificate or license.

(f) Conviction of a felony or of any offense substantially related to the qualifications, functions, and duties of a registered nurse, in which event the record of the conviction shall be conclusive evidence thereof.

(g) Impersonating any applicant or acting as proxy for an applicant in any examination required under this chapter for the issuance of a certificate or license.

(h) Impersonating another certified or licensed practitioner, or permitting or allowing another person to use his or her certificate or license for the purpose of nursing the sick or afflicted.

(i) Aiding or assisting, or agreeing to aid or assist any person or persons, whether a licensed physician or not, in the performance of, or arranging for, a violation of any of the provisions of Article 12 (commencing with Section 2220) of Chapter 5.

(j) Holding oneself out to the public or to any practitioner of the healing arts as a "nurse practitioner" or as meeting the standards established by the board for a nurse practitioner unless meeting the standards established by the board pursuant to Article 8 (commencing with Section 2834) or holding oneself out to the public as being certified by the board as a nurse anesthetist, nurse midwife, clinical nurse specialist, or public health nurse unless the person is at the time so certified by the board.

(k) Except for good cause, the knowing failure to protect patients by failing to follow infection control guidelines of the board, thereby risking transmission of blood-borne infectious diseases from licensed or certified nurse to patient, from patient to patient, and from patient to licensed or certified nurse. In administering this subdivision, the board shall consider referencing the standards, regulations, and guidelines of the State Department of Health Services developed pursuant to Section 1250.11 of the Health and Safety Code and the standards, guidelines, and regulations pursuant to the California Occupational Safety and Health Act of 1973 (Part 1 (commencing with Section 6300), Division 5, Labor Code) for preventing the transmission of HIV, hepatitis B, and other blood-borne pathogens in health care settings. As necessary, the board shall consult with the Medical Board of California, the Board of Podiatric Medicine, the Dental Board of California, and the Board of Vocational Nursing and Psychiatric Technicians, to encourage appropriate consistency in the implementation of this subdivision.

The board shall seek to ensure that licentiates and others regulated by the board are informed of the responsibility of licentiates to minimize the risk of transmission of blood-borne infectious diseases from health care provider to patient, from patient to patient, and from patient to health care provider, and of the most recent scientifically recognized safeguards for minimizing the risks of transmission.

HISTORY:

Added Stats 1939 ch 807 § 2. Amended Stats 1953 ch 1053 § 1; Stats 1977 ch 439 § 1; Stats 1978 ch 212 § 2, effective June 6, 1978; Stats 1979 ch 933 § 2; Stats 1983 ch 696 § 2; Stats 1984 ch 144 § 11; Stats 1987 ch 850 § 15; Stats 1991 ch 1180 § 4 (SB 1070); Stats 1992 ch 1350 § 4 (SB 1813); Stats 1994 ch 26 § 61 (AB 1807), effective March 30, 1994, ch 1275 § 16 (SB 2101); Stats 1997 ch 759 § 17 (SB 827); Stats 2000 ch 568 § 8 (AB 2888).

§ 2761.1. Performance of abortion

(a) The board shall not suspend or revoke the certification or license of a nurse practitioner solely for performing an abortion if the holder performed the abortion in accordance with the provisions of this chapter and the Reproductive Privacy Act (Article 2.5 (commencing with Section 123460) of Chapter 2 of Part 2 of Division 106 of the Health and Safety Code).

(b) Notwithstanding any other law, including, but not limited to, Sections 141, 480, 490, and 2761, the board shall not deny an application for certification or licensure as a nurse practitioner, or suspend, revoke, or otherwise impose discipline upon a person certified or licensed in this state as a nurse practitioner under either of the following circumstances:

(1) The person is licensed or certified as a nurse practitioner in another state and was disciplined in that state solely for performing an abortion in that state.

(2) The person is licensed or certified as a nurse practitioner in another state and was convicted in that state for an offense related solely to the performance of an abortion in that state.

HISTORY:

Added Stats 2022 ch 565 § 3 (AB 2626), effective September 27, 2022.

§ 2761.5. Reporting mechanisms

It is the intent of the Legislature to provide for a study of reporting mechanisms to the board so that it can identify methods of receiving timely information on nurses who may have violated this chapter. The California Research Bureau shall prepare and deliver a report to the Legislature by January 1, 2019, that evaluates to what extent employers voluntarily report disciplined nurses to the board and offers options for consistent and reasonable reporting mechanisms. The report shall include, but not be limited to, the following:

(a) A review of existing mandatory reporting requirements that alert the board to nurses who may have violated this chapter.

(b) A review of existing laws permitting, prohibiting, encouraging, or discouraging voluntary reporting to the board.

(c) An analysis of the number of employer reports to the board, the number of those reports investigated by the board, and the final action taken by the board for each report.

(d) Employer reporting requirements of other boards within the department.

(e) Nursing reporting requirements of other states.

HISTORY:

Added Stats 2017 ch 520 § 5 (SB 799), effective January 1, 2018.

§ 2762. Drug-related transgressions

In addition to other acts constituting unprofessional conduct within the meaning of this chapter it is unprofessional conduct for a person licensed under this chapter to do any of the following:

(a) Obtain or possess in violation of law, or prescribe, or except as directed by a licensed physician and surgeon, dentist, or podiatrist administer to himself or herself, or furnish or administer to another, any controlled substance as defined in Division 10 (commencing with Section 11000) of the Health and Safety Code or any dangerous drug or dangerous device as defined in Section 4022.

(b) Use any controlled substance as defined in Division 10 (commencing with Section 11000) of the Health and Safety Code, or any dangerous drug or dangerous device as defined in Section 4022, or alcoholic beverages, to an extent or in a manner dangerous or injurious to himself or herself, any other person, or the public or to the extent that such use impairs his or her ability to conduct with safety to the public the practice authorized by his or her license.

(c) Be convicted of a criminal offense involving the prescription, consumption, or self-administration of any of the substances described in subdivisions (a) and (b) of this section, or the possession of, or falsification of a record pertaining to, the substances described in subdivision (a) of this section, in which event the record of the conviction is conclusive evidence thereof.

(d) Be committed or confined by a court of competent jurisdiction for intemperate use of or addiction to the use of any of the substances described in subdivisions (a) and (b) of this section, in which event the court order of commitment or confinement is prima facie evidence of such commitment or confinement.

(e) Falsify, or make grossly incorrect, grossly inconsistent, or unintelligible entries in any hospital, patient, or other record pertaining to the substances described in subdivision (a) of this section.

HISTORY:

Added Stats 1953 ch 1053 § 2. Amended Stats 1957 ch 923 § 1; Stats 1961 ch 378 § 1; Stats 1978 ch 1161 § 178; Stats 1984 ch 1635 § 4; Stats 1998 ch 970 § 12 (AB 2802).

§ 2764. Jurisdiction in event license suspended or surrendered

The lapsing or suspension of a license by operation of law or by order or decision of the board or a court of law, or the voluntary surrender of a license by a licentiate shall not deprive the board of jurisdiction to proceed with any investigation of or action or disciplinary proceeding against such license, or to render a decision suspending or revoking such license.

HISTORY:
Added Stats 1953 ch 1053 § 4.

§ 2765. What deemed conviction

A plea or verdict of guilty or a conviction following a plea of nolo contendere made to a charge substantially related to the qualifications, functions and duties of a registered nurse is deemed to be a conviction within the meaning of this article. The board may order the license or certificate suspended or revoked, or may decline to issue a license or certificate, when the time for appeal has elapsed, or the judgment of conviction has been affirmed on appeal or when an order granting probation is made suspending the imposition of sentence, irrespective of a subsequent order under the provisions of Section 1203.4 of the Penal Code allowing such person to withdraw his or her plea of guilty and to enter a plea of not guilty, or setting aside the verdict of guilty, or dismissing the accusation, information or indictment.

HISTORY:
Added Stats 1955 ch 336 § 1. Amended Stats 1978 ch 1161 § 179; Stats 1983 ch 696 § 3.

ARTICLE 3.1
INTERVENTION PROGRAM

Section
2770. Legislative intent.
2770.1. Definitions.
2770.2. Intervention evaluation committees; Composition; Appointments.
2770.3. Per diem and expenses of committee members.
2770.4. Quorum; Majority vote requirement.
2770.5. Election of chairperson and vice chairperson.
2770.6. Administration of article.
2770.7. Establishment of criteria for acceptance, denial, or termination of registered nurses in program; Investigations; Disciplinary actions.
2770.8. Intervention program manager responsibilities; Duties and responsibilities of committees.
2770.9. Informing participants of procedures, rights, and responsibilities.
2770.10. Authority of committee to convene in closed session.
2770.11. Termination of participation for noncompliance with provisions of program.
2770.12. Purging of records following intervention program.
2770.13. Provision of representation in defamation action resulting from reports or information given to committee.
2770.14. Board reports.

HISTORY: Added Stats 1984 ch 865 § 1. The heading of Article 3.1, which formerly read "Diversion Program," amended to read as above by Stats 2015 ch 426 § 21 (SB 800), effective January 1, 2016.

§ 2770. Legislative intent

It is the intent of the Legislature that the Board of Registered Nursing seek ways and means to identify and rehabilitate registered nurses whose competency may be impaired due to abuse of alcohol and other drugs, or due to mental illness so that registered nurses so afflicted may be rehabilitated and returned to the practice of nursing in a manner that will not endanger the public health and safety. It is also the intent of the Legislature that the Board of Registered Nursing shall implement this legislation by establishing an intervention program as a voluntary alternative to traditional disciplinary actions.

HISTORY:

Added Stats 1984 ch 865 § 1. Amended Stats 2015 ch 426 § 22 (SB 800), effective January 1, 2016.

§ 2770.1. Definitions

As used in this article:

(a) "Board" means the Board of Registered Nursing.

(b) "Committee" means an intervention evaluation committee created by this article.

(c) "Program manager" means the staff manager of the intervention program, as designated by the executive officer of the board. The program manager shall have background experience in dealing with substance abuse issues.

HISTORY:

Added Stats 1984 ch 865 § 1. Amended Stats 2008 ch 548 § 17 (SB 1441), effective January 1, 2009; Stats 2015 ch 426 § 23 (SB 800), effective January 1, 2016.

§ 2770.2. Intervention evaluation committees; Composition; Appointments

(a) One or more intervention evaluation committees is hereby created in the state to be established by the board. Each committee shall be composed of five persons appointed by the board. No board member shall serve on any committee.

(b) Each committee shall have the following composition:

(1) Three registered nurses, holding active California licenses, who have demonstrated expertise in the field of chemical dependency or psychiatric nursing.

(2) One physician, holding an active California license, who specializes in the diagnosis and treatment of addictive diseases or mental illness.

(3) One public member who is knowledgeable in the field of chemical dependency or mental illness.

(c) It shall require a majority vote of the board to appoint a person to a committee. Each appointment shall be at the pleasure of the board for a term not to exceed four years. In its discretion the board may stagger the terms of the initial members appointed.

HISTORY:

Added Stats 1984 ch 865 § 1. Amended Stats 1999 ch 655 § 36 (SB 1308); Stats 2015 ch 426 § 24 (SB 800), effective January 1, 2016.

§ 2770.3. Per diem and expenses of committee members

Each member of a committee shall receive per diem and expenses as provided in Section 103.

HISTORY:
Added Stats 1984 ch 865 § 1.

§ 2770.4. Quorum; Majority vote requirement

Three members of a committee shall constitute a quorum for the transaction of business at any meeting. Any action requires a majority vote of the committee.

HISTORY:
Added Stats 1984 ch 865 § 1.

§ 2770.5. Election of chairperson and vice chairperson

Each committee shall elect from its membership a chairperson and a vice chairperson.

HISTORY:
Added Stats 1984 ch 865 § 1.

§ 2770.6. Administration of article

The board shall administer the provisions of this article.

HISTORY:
Added Stats 1984 ch 865 § 1.

§ 2770.7. Establishment of criteria for acceptance, denial, or termination of registered nurses in program; Investigations; Disciplinary actions

(a) The board shall establish criteria for the acceptance, denial, or termination of registered nurses in the intervention program. Only those registered nurses who have voluntarily requested to participate in the intervention program shall participate in the program.

(b) A registered nurse under current investigation by the board may request entry into the intervention program by contacting the board. Prior to authorizing a registered nurse to enter into the intervention program, the board may require the registered nurse under current investigation for any violations of this chapter or any other provision of this code to execute a statement of understanding that states that the registered nurse understands that his or her violations that would otherwise be the basis for discipline may still be investigated and may be the subject of disciplinary action in accordance with this section.

(c)(1) Neither acceptance nor participation in the intervention program shall preclude the board from investigating or continuing to investigate, or, except as provided in this subdivision, taking disciplinary action or continuing to take disciplinary action against, any registered nurse for any unprofessional conduct committed before, during, or after participation in the intervention program.

(2) The board may investigate at its discretion complaints against registered nurses participating in the intervention program.

(3) Disciplinary action with regard to acts committed before or during participation in the intervention program shall not take place unless the registered nurse withdraws or is terminated from the program.

(d) All registered nurses shall sign an agreement of understanding that the withdrawal or termination from the intervention program at a time when the program manager or intervention evaluation committee determines the licentiate presents a threat to the public's health and safety shall result in the utilization by the board of intervention program treatment records in disciplinary or criminal proceedings.

(e) Any registered nurse terminated from the intervention program for failure to comply with program requirements is subject to disciplinary action by the board for acts committed before, during, and after participation in the intervention program. A registered nurse who has been under investigation by the board and has been terminated from the intervention program by an intervention evaluation committee shall be reported by the intervention evaluation committee to the board.

HISTORY:

Added Stats 1984 ch 865 § 1. Amended Stats 2008 ch 548 § 18 (SB 1441), effective January 1, 2009; Stats 2015 ch 426 § 25 (SB 800), effective January 1, 2016; Stats 2017 ch 520 § 6 (SB 799), effective January 1, 2018.

§ 2770.8. Intervention program manager responsibilities; Duties and responsibilities of committees

A committee created under this article operates under the direction of the intervention program manager. The program manager has the primary responsibility to review and evaluate recommendations of the committee. Each committee shall have the following duties and responsibilities:

(a) To evaluate those registered nurses who request participation in the program according to the guidelines prescribed by the board, and to make recommendations.

(b) To review and designate those treatment services to which registered nurses in an intervention program may be referred.

(c) To receive and review information concerning a registered nurse participating in the program.

(d) To consider in the case of each registered nurse participating in a program whether he or she may with safety continue or resume the practice of nursing.

(e) To call meetings as necessary to consider the requests of registered nurses to participate in an intervention program, and to consider reports regarding registered nurses participating in a program.

(f) To make recommendations to the program manager regarding the terms and conditions of the intervention agreement for each registered nurse participating in the program, including treatment, supervision, and monitoring requirements.

HISTORY:

Added Stats 1984 ch 865 § 1. Amended Stats 1999 ch 655 § 37 (SB 1308); Stats 2008 ch 548 § 19 (SB 1441), effective January 1, 2009; Stats 2015 ch 426 § 26 (SB 800), effective January 1, 2016.

§ 2770.9. Informing participants of procedures, rights, and responsibilities

The committee shall inform each registered nurse who requests participation in a program of the procedures followed in the program, of the rights and responsibilities of the registered nurse in the program, and of the possible results of noncompliance with the program.

HISTORY:

Added Stats 1984 ch 865 § 1.

§ 2770.10. Authority of committee to convene in closed session

Notwithstanding Article 9 (commencing with Section 11120) of Chapter 1 of Part 1 of Division 3 of Title 2 of the Government Code, relating to public meetings, a committee may convene in closed session to consider reports pertaining to any registered nurse requesting or participating in an intervention program. A committee shall only convene in closed session to the extent that it is necessary to protect the privacy of such a licentiate.

HISTORY:

Added Stats 1984 ch 865 § 1. Amended Stats 1993 ch 589 § 6 (AB 2211); Stats 2015 ch 426 § 27 (SB 800), effective January 1, 2016.

§ 2770.11. Termination of participation for noncompliance with provisions of program

(a) Each registered nurse who requests participation in an intervention program shall agree to cooperate with the rehabilitation program designed by the committee and approved by the program manager. Any failure to comply with a rehabilitation program may result in termination of the registered nurse's participation in a program. The name and license number of a registered nurse who is terminated for any reason, other than successful completion, shall be reported to the board's enforcement program.

(b) If the program manager determines that a registered nurse, who is denied admission into the program or terminated from the program, presents a threat to the public or his or her own health and safety, the program manager shall report the name and license number, along with a copy of all intervention program records for that registered nurse, to the board's enforcement program. The board may use any of the records it receives under this subdivision in any disciplinary proceeding.

HISTORY:

Added Stats 1984 ch 865 § 1. Amended Stats 1999 ch 655 § 38 (SB 1308); Stats 2002 ch 1011 § 7 (SB 2021); Stats 2008 ch 548 § 20 (SB 1441), effective January 1, 2009; Stats 2015 ch 426 § 28 (SB 800), effective January 1, 2016.

§ 2770.12. Purging of records following intervention program

(a) After the committee and the program manager in their discretion have determined that a registered nurse has successfully completed the intervention program, all records pertaining to the registered nurse's participation in the intervention program shall be purged.

(b) All board and committee records and records of a proceeding pertaining to the participation of a registered nurse in the intervention program shall be kept confidential and are not subject to discovery or subpoena, except as specified in subdivision (b) of Section 2770.11 and subdivision (c).

(c) A registered nurse shall be deemed to have waived any rights granted by any laws and regulations relating to confidentiality of the intervention program, if he or she does any of the following:

(1) Presents information relating to any aspect of the intervention program during any stage of the disciplinary process subsequent to the filing of an accusation, statement of issues, or petition to compel an examination pursuant to Article 12.5 (commencing with Section 820) of Chapter 1. The waiver shall be limited to information necessary to verify or refute any information disclosed by the registered nurse.

(2) Files a lawsuit against the board relating to any aspect of the intervention program.

(3) Claims in defense to a disciplinary action, based on a complaint that led to the registered nurse's participation in the intervention program, that he or she was prejudiced by the length of time that passed between the alleged violation and the filing of the accusation. The waiver shall be limited to information necessary to document the length of time the registered nurse participated in the intervention program.

HISTORY:

Added Stats 1999 ch 655 § 39.1 (SB 1308). Amended Stats 2008 ch 548 § 21 (SB 1441), effective January 1, 2009; Stats 2015 ch 426 § 29 (SB 800), effective January 1, 2016.

§ 2770.13. Provision of representation in defamation action resulting from reports or information given to committee

The board shall provide for the legal representation of any person making reports under this article to a committee or the board in any action for defamation directly resulting from those reports regarding a registered nurse's participation in an intervention program.

HISTORY:

Added Stats 1984 ch 865 § 1. Amended Stats 1999 ch 655 § 40 (SB 1308); Stats 2015 ch 426 § 30 (SB 800), effective January 1, 2016.

§ 2770.14. Board reports

(a) The board shall produce reports which include, but are not limited to, information concerning the number of cases accepted, denied, or terminated with compliance or noncompliance.

(b) The board shall conduct a periodic cost analysis of the program.

HISTORY:

Added Stats 1984 ch 865 § 1. Amended Stats 1999 ch 655 § 41 (SB 1308).

ARTICLE 3.5

NURSING CORPORATIONS

Section

2775. Definition.
2776. Individual unprofessional conduct.
2777. Corporate unprofessional conduct.
2778. Name.
2779. Shareholders, directors and officers.
2780. Income while shareholder is disqualified.
2781. Regulations.

HISTORY: Added Stats 1981 ch 621 § 1.

§ 2775. Definition

A nursing corporation is a corporation which is authorized to render professional services, as defined in Section 13401 of the Corporations Code, so long as that corporation and its shareholders, officers, directors, and employees rendering professional services who are registered nurses are in compliance with the Moscone-Knox Professional Corporation Act, the provisions of this article and all other statutes and regulations now or hereafter enacted or adopted pertaining to such corporation and the conduct of its affairs.

With respect to a nursing corporation, the governmental agency referred to in the Moscone-Knox Professional Corporation Act is the Board of Registered Nursing.

HISTORY:
Added Stats 1981 ch 621 § 1.

§ 2776. Individual unprofessional conduct

It shall constitute unprofessional conduct and a violation of this chapter for any person licensed under this chapter to violate, attempt to violate, directly or indirectly, or assist in or abet the violation of, or conspire to violate any provision or term of this article, the Moscone-Knox Professional Corporation Act, or any regulations duly adopted under those laws.

HISTORY:
Added Stats 1981 ch 621 § 1.

§ 2777. Corporate unprofessional conduct

A nursing corporation shall not do or fail to do any act the doing of which or the failure to do which would constitute unprofessional conduct under any statute or regulation, now or hereafter in effect. In the conduct of its practice, it shall observe and be bound by such statutes and regulations to the same extent as a person holding a license under this chapter.

HISTORY:
Added Stats 1981 ch 621 § 2.

§ 2778. Name

The name of a nursing corporation and any name or names under which it may render professional services shall contain the words "nursing" or "registered nursing," and wording or abbreviations denoting corporate existence.

HISTORY:
Added Stats 1981 ch 621 § 1.

§ 2779. Shareholders, directors and officers

Except as provided in Sections 13401.5 and 13403 of the Corporations Code, each shareholder, director and officer of a nursing corporation, except an assistant secretary and an assistant treasurer, shall be a licensed person as defined in Section 13401 of the Corporations Code.

HISTORY:
Added Stats 1981 ch 621 § 1.

§ 2780. Income while shareholder is disqualified

The income of a nursing corporation attributable to professional services rendered while a shareholder is a disqualified person, as defined in Section 13401 of the Corporations Code, shall not in any manner accrue to the benefit of such shareholder or his or her shares in the nursing corporation.

HISTORY:
Added Stats 1981 ch 621 § 1.

§ 2781. Regulations

The board may adopt and enforce regulations to carry out the purposes and objectives of this article, including regulations requiring (a) that the bylaws of a nursing corporation shall include a provision whereby the capital stock of such corporation owned by a disqualified person (as defined in Section 13401 of the Corporations Code), or a deceased person, shall be sold to the corporation or to the remaining shareholders of such corporation within such time as such regulations may provide, and (b) that a nursing corporation shall provide adequate security by insurance or otherwise for claims against it by its patients arising out of the rendering of professional services.

HISTORY:
Added Stats 1981 ch 621 § 1.

ARTICLE 4
NURSING SCHOOLS

Section
2785. List of approved schools.
2785.5. Board to facilitate efficient transfer agreements between associate degree nursing programs and baccalaureate degree nursing programs.
2785.6. Nursing Education and Workforce Advisory Committee.
2786. Approved school requirements; Analysis of practice of registered nurse; Implicit bias training requirement.
2786.1. Denial or revocation for school not giving credit for military education and experience; Regulations; Review of school's policies and practices regarding credit for military education and experience and posting of information on Web site.
2786.2. Private postsecondary school of nursing; Memorandum of understanding; Actively accredited approved schools.
2786.3. Nursing programs affected by interruptions due to state of emergency; Requests submitted to board of nursing education; Approval.
2786.4. Payments for student clinical experience placements prohibited.
2786.5. Fees.
2786.6. Grounds for denial of approval.
2788. Inspections; Approval of schools meeting requirements; Notice of defects.
2789. Exempt schools.

HISTORY: Added Stats 1939 ch 807 § 2.

§ 2785. List of approved schools

The board shall prepare and maintain a list of approved schools of nursing in this state whose graduates, if they have the other necessary qualifications provided in this chapter, shall be eligible to apply for a license to practice nursing in this state.

HISTORY:
Added Stats 1939 ch 807 § 2. Amended Stats 1983 ch 742 § 5.

§ 2785.5. Board to facilitate efficient transfer agreements between associate degree nursing programs and baccalaureate degree nursing programs

The board shall establish a workgroup, or use an existing committee, to encourage and facilitate efficient transfer agreements or other enrollment models between associate degree nursing programs and baccalaureate degree nursing programs so students are able to complete the baccalaureate program without unnecessary repetition of coursework.

HISTORY:
Added Stats 2004 ch 271 § 1 (AB 2839).

§ 2785.6. Nursing Education and Workforce Advisory Committee

There is created within the jurisdiction of the board a Nursing Education and Workforce Advisory Committee, which shall solicit input from approved nursing programs and members of the nursing and health care professions to study and recommend nursing education standards and solutions to workforce issues to the board.

(a) The committee shall be comprised of the following:

(1) One nursing program director representative of a statewide association for associate's degrees in nursing programs.

(2) One nursing program director representative of a statewide association representing bachelor's degrees in nursing programs.

(3) One California Community Colleges Chancellor's Office representative.

(4) One California State University Office of the Chancellor representative.

(5) One currently practicing registered nurse representative.

(6) Two currently practicing advanced practice registered nurse representatives.

(7) Two registered nurse employer representatives in nursing service administration.

(8) One professional nursing organization representative.

(9) Three nursing union organization representatives.

(10) One public representative.

(11) One Health Workforce Development Division representative.

(12) One board research vendor.

(13) Any other members representing an organization in the nursing education or workforce field that the board determines is necessary for the work of the committee and is not listed under this subdivision.

(b)(1) Except as provided in paragraph (2), all appointments shall be for a term of four years and vacancies shall be filled for the unexpired term. No person shall serve more than two consecutive terms except for the representatives from organizations.

(2)(A) The initial appointments for the education representatives shall be for the following terms:

(i) One Nursing Program Director who is a member of a statewide association for associate's degrees in nursing programs shall serve three years.

(ii) One nursing program director who is a member of a statewide association representing bachelor's degrees in nursing programs shall serve a term of two years.

(iii) One California Community Colleges Chancellor's Office representative shall serve a term of four years.

(B) The initial appointments for the workforce representatives shall be for the following terms:

(i) One practicing registered nurse representative shall serve a term of four years.

(ii) One of the two practicing advanced practice registered nurse representatives shall serve a term of three years and the other shall serve a term of two years.

(C) The initial appointments for the employer representatives shall be for the following terms:

(i) One of the two registered nurse employer representatives shall serve a term of three years and the other shall serve a term of four years.

(ii) One professional nursing organization representative shall serve a term of two years.

(D) The public member shall serve a term of four years.

(c) The committee shall meet a minimum of two times per year and shall appoint officers annually.

(d)(1) The committee shall dedicate a minimum of one meeting each towards nursing education issues and nursing workforce issues.

(2) The committee may establish subcommittees to study issues specific to education, workforce, or any other topic relevant to the purpose of the committee.

(e) The committee may refer information and recommendations to the board or other committees of the board.

(f)(1) The board may implement, interpret, or make specific this section by means of a charter, or other similar document, approved by the board.

(2) The board may revise the charter, or other similar document, developed pursuant to this section, as necessary. The development or revision of the charter, or other similar document, shall be exempt from the requirements of the Administrative Procedure Act (Chapter 3.5 (commencing with Section 11340) of Part 1 of Title 2 of the Government Code).

(g) The committee shall study and recommend standards for simulated clinical experiences based on the best practices published by the International Nursing Association for Clinical Simulation and Learning, the National Council of State Boards of Nursing, the Society for Simulation in Healthcare, or equivalent standards.

HISTORY:

Added Stats 2022 ch 413 § 10 (AB 2684), effective January 1, 2023.

§ 2786. Approved school requirements; Analysis of practice of registered nurse; Implicit bias training requirement

(a)(1) An approved school of nursing, or an approved nursing program, is one that has been approved by the board, gives the course of instruction approved by the board, covering not fewer than two academic years, is affiliated or conducted in connection with one or more hospitals, and is an institution of higher education. For purposes of this section, "institution of higher education" includes, but is not limited to, community colleges offering an associate of arts or associate of science degree and private postsecondary institutions offering an associate of arts, associate of science, or baccalaureate degree or an entry-level master's degree, and is an institution that is not subject to the California Private Postsecondary Education Act of 2009 (Chapter 8 (commencing with Section 94800) of Part 59 of Division 10 of Title 3 of the Education Code).

(2) An approved school of nursing or nursing program shall meet a minimum of 500 direct patient care clinical hours in a board-approved clinical setting with a minimum of 30 hours of supervised direct patient care clinical hours dedicated to each nursing area specified by the board.

(A) Additional clinical hours required by the program for nursing education preparation in each nursing area as specified by the board shall be identified and documented in the curriculum plan for each area.

(B) An approved school of nursing or nursing program shall not be required to track the minimum clinical hours by individual students.

(3) An approved school of nursing or nursing program may cover fewer than two academic years if approved to providing a course of instruction that prepares a licensed vocational nurse licensed under the Vocational Nursing Practice Act (commencing with Section 2840) for a license under this chapter.

(b) A school of nursing that is affiliated with an institution that is subject to the California Private Postsecondary Education Act of 2009 (Chapter 8 (commencing with Section 94800) of Part 59 of Division 10 of Title 3 of the Education Code), may be approved by the board to grant an associate of arts or associate of science degree to individuals who graduate from the school of nursing or to grant a baccalaureate degree in nursing with successful completion of an additional course of study as approved by the board and the institution involved.

(c)(1) The board shall determine by regulation the required subjects of instruction to be completed in an approved school of nursing for licensure as a registered nurse and shall include the minimum units of theory and clinical experience necessary to achieve essential clinical competency at the entry level of the registered nurse. The board's regulations shall be designed to require all schools to provide clinical instruction in all phases of the educational process, except as necessary to accommodate military education and experience as specified in Section 2786.1.

(2) Notwithstanding paragraph (1), whenever an agency or facility used by an approved nursing program for direct patient care clinical practice is no longer available or sufficient, the director of the approved nursing program may submit to a board nursing education consultant a request that the approved nursing program allow theory to precede clinical practice if all of the following conditions are met:

(A) No alternative agency or facility located within 25 miles of the impacted approved nursing program, campus, or location, as applicable, has a sufficient number of open placements that are available and accessible to the approved nursing program for direct patient care clinical practice hours in the same subject matter area. An approved program shall not be required to submit more than required under subparagraph (A) of paragraph (3) of subdivision (a) of Section 2786.3.

(B) Clinical practice takes place in the academic term immediately following theory.

(C) Theory is taught concurrently with clinical practice not in direct patient care if no direct patient care experiences are available.

(3)(A) The board shall annually collect, analyze, and report information related to the number of clinical placement slots that are available and the location of those clinical placement slots within the state, including, but not limited to, information concerning the total number of placement slots a clinical facility can accommodate and how many slots the programs that use the facility will need.

(B) The board shall utilize data from available regional or individual institution databases.

(C) The board shall place the annual report on its internet website.

(d) The board shall perform or cause to be performed an analysis of the practice of the registered nurse no less than every five years. Results of the analysis shall be utilized to assist in the determination of the required subjects of instruction, validation of the licensing examination, and assessment of the current practice of nursing.

(e)(1) The executive officer shall develop a uniform method for evaluating requests and granting approvals pursuant to this section.

(2) The executive officer may revise the uniform method developed pursuant to this subdivision, as necessary. The development or revision of the uniform method shall be exempt from the requirements of the Administrative Procedure Act (Chapter 3.5 (commencing with Section 11340) of Part 1 of Title 2 of the Government Code).

(3) The board's nursing education consultants shall use the uniform method to evaluate requests and grant approvals pursuant to this section.

(4) The board shall post the approved method and any revisions on the board's website.

(f)(1) Graduation requirements for an approved school of nursing, or an approved nursing program, shall include one hour of direct participation in an implicit bias training which shall include all of the following:

(A) Identification of previous or current unconscious biases and misinformation.

(B) Identification of personal, interpersonal, institutional, structural, and cultural barriers to inclusion.

(C) Corrective measures to decrease implicit bias at the interpersonal and institutional levels, including ongoing policies and practices for that purpose.

(D) Information on the effects, including, but not limited to, ongoing personal effects, of historical and contemporary exclusion and oppression of minority communities.

(E) Information about cultural identity across racial or ethnic groups.

(F) Information about communicating more effectively across identities, including racial, ethnic, religious, and gender identities.

(G) Discussion on power dynamics and organizational decisionmaking.

(H) Discussion on health inequities within the perinatal care field, including information on how implicit bias impacts maternal and infant health outcomes.

(I) Perspectives of diverse, local constituency groups and experts on particular racial, identity, cultural, and provider-community relations issues in the community.

(J) Information on reproductive justice.

(2) This subdivision shall not be construed to do any of the following:

(A) Affect the requirements for licensure under this chapter.

(B) Require a curriculum revision.

(C) Affect licensure by endorsement under this chapter.

HISTORY:

Added Stats 1939 ch 807 § 2. Amended Stats 1951 ch 1748 § 1; Stats 1953 ch 1032 § 1; Stats 1974 ch 516 § 2; Stats 1975 ch 87 § 1, effective May 17, 1975; Stats 1983 ch 742 § 6; Stats 1985 ch 1055 § 2; Stats 2001 ch 435 § 6 (SB 349); Stats 2010 ch 208 § 1 (AB 2344), effective January 1, 2011; Stats 2012 ch 789 § 3 (SB 122), effective January 1, 2013; Stats 2015 ch 489 § 5 (SB 466), effective January 1, 2016; Stats 2021 ch 445 § 1 (AB 1407), effective January 1, 2022; Stats 2022 ch 413 § 11 (AB 2684), effective January 1, 2023.

§ 2786.1. Denial or revocation for school not giving credit for military education and experience; Regulations; Review of school's policies and practices regarding credit for military education and experience and posting of information on Web site

(a) The board shall deny the application for approval made by, and shall revoke the approval given to, any school of nursing that does not give student applicants credit in the field of nursing for military education and experience by the use of challenge examinations or other methods of evaluation.

(b) The board shall adopt regulations by January 1, 2017, requiring schools to have a process to evaluate and grant credit for military education and experience. The regulations shall be adopted pursuant to the Administrative Procedure Act (Chapter 3.5 (commencing with Section 11340) of Part 1 of Division 3 of Title 2 of the Government Code). The word "credit," as used in this subdivision, is limited to credit for licensure only. The board is not authorized to prescribe the credit that an approved school of nursing shall give toward an academic certificate or degree.

(c) The board shall review a school's policies and practices regarding granting credit for military education and experience at least once every five years to ensure consistency in evaluation and application across schools. The board shall post on its Internet Web site information related to the acceptance of military coursework and experience at each approved school.

HISTORY:

Added Stats 2015 ch 489 § 6 (SB 466), effective January 1, 2016.

§ 2786.2. Private postsecondary school of nursing; Memorandum of understanding; Actively accredited approved schools

(a) A private postsecondary school of nursing approved by the board pursuant to subdivision (b) of Section 2786 shall comply with Chapter 8 of Part 59 of Division 10 of Title 3 of the Education Code. The board shall have a memorandum of understanding with the Bureau for Private Postsecondary Education to delineate the powers of the board to review and approve schools of nursing and the powers of the bureau to protect the interest of students attending institutions governed by the California Private Postsecondary Education Act of 2009, Chapter 8 (commencing with Section 94800) of Division 10 of Title 3 of the Education Code.

(b)(1) For approved schools of nursing that are actively accredited by an institutional or programmatic accreditor recognized by the United States Department of Education, the board shall, without requiring additional documentation or action, do the following, unless unrelated to the scope of accreditation:

(A) Perform site inspections jointly with accreditors.

(B) Accept continuing accreditation decisions from accreditors.

(C) Accept faculty hiring decisions made by the approved program director.

(D) Accept the self-study required by programmatic accreditors as a substitute for board self-study or data collection if the following are met:

(i) The program provides a crosswalk connecting the items in the report to the board's regulatory requirements.

(ii) If the report does not address any of the board's regulatory requirements, the program provides an addendum to the report to address those requirements.

(E) Accept substantive change requests, as defined under the uniform method developed under subdivision (e) of Section 2786, if approved by the accreditor unless the request is a request to increase enrollment or perform a major curriculum revision.

(F) When considering a request to increase enrollment, the board may consider only the following factors related to the ability to adequately train additional students:

(i) Adequacy of resources, including, but not limited to, faculty, facilities, equipment, and supplies.

(ii) Availability of clinical placements.

(iii) Complaints that have been verified by the board from students, faculty, or other interested parties.

(iv) Licensing examination pass rates, graduation rates, and retention rates.

(v) Any other similar factors specified by the board in regulations. The board shall not consider nursing workforce issues, including those identified under Section 2717, as factors for purposes of this subparagraph.

(2) Upon complaint or other evidence that an approved school of nursing does not meet the board's standards, the board may withhold approval under this subdivision or perform additional site inspections pursuant to Section 2788.

(3) The board may make or withhold approvals under this subdivision prior to the adoption of implementing regulations.

HISTORY:

Added Stats 2012 ch 789 § 4 (SB 122), effective January 1, 2013. Amended Stats 2022 ch 413 § 12 (AB 2684), effective January 1, 2023.

§ 2786.3. Nursing programs affected by interruptions due to state of emergency; Requests submitted to board of nursing education; Approval

(a) Until the end of the 2023-24 academic year, or whenever the Governor declares a state of emergency for a county in which an agency or facility used by an approved nursing program for direct patient care clinical practice is no longer available, the director of the approved nursing program may submit to a board nursing education consultant requests to do any of the following:

(1) Utilize a clinical setting until the end of the academic term without the following:

(A) Approval by the board.

(B) Written agreements with the clinical facility.

(C) Submitting evidence of compliance with board regulations relating to the utilization of clinical settings, except as necessary for a board nursing education consultant to ensure course objectives and faculty responsibilities will be met.

(2) Utilize preceptorships until the end of the academic term without having to maintain written policies relating to the following:

(A) Identification of criteria used for preceptor selection.

(B) Provision for a preceptor orientation program that covers the policies of the preceptorship and preceptor, student, and faculty responsibilities.

(C) Identification of preceptor qualifications for both the primary and the relief preceptor.

(D) Description of responsibilities of the faculty, preceptor, and student for the learning experiences and evaluation during preceptorship.

(E) Maintenance of preceptor records that includes names of all current preceptors, registered nurse licenses, and dates of preceptorships.

(F) Plan for an ongoing evaluation regarding the continued use of preceptors.

(3) Subject to subparagraph (F), request that the approved nursing program be allowed to reduce the required number of direct patient care hours to 50 percent in geriatrics and medical-surgical and 25 percent in mental health-psychiatric nursing, obstetrics, and pediatrics if all of the following conditions are met:

(A) No alternative agency or facility has a sufficient number of open placements that are available and accessible within 25 miles of the approved nursing program for direct patient care clinical practice hours in the same subject matter area. An approved nursing program shall submit, and not be required to provide more than, the following:

(i) The list of alternative agencies or facilities listed within 25 miles of the impacted approved nursing program, campus, or location, as applicable, using the facility finder on the Department of Health Care Access and Information website.

(ii) The list of courses impacted by the loss of clinical placements and the academic term the courses are offered.

(iii) Whether each of the listed alternative agencies or facilities would meet the course objectives for the courses requiring placements.

(iv) Whether the approved nursing program has contacted each of the listed alternative agencies or facilities about the availability of clinical placements. The approved nursing program shall not be required to contact a clinical facility that would not meet course objectives.

(v) The date of contact or attempted contact.

(vi) The number of open placements at each of the listed alternative agencies or facilities that are available for the academic term for each course. If an alternative agency or facility does not respond within 48 hours, the approved nursing program may list the alternative agency or facility as unavailable. If the alternative agency or facility subsequently responds prior to the submission of the request to a board nursing education consultant, the approved nursing program shall update the list to reflect the response.

(vii) Whether the open and available placements are accessible to the students and faculty. An open and available placement is accessible if there are no barriers that otherwise prohibit a student from entering the facility, including, but not limited to, the lack of personal protective equipment or cost-prohibitive infectious disease testing. An individual's personal unwillingness to enter an alternative agency or facility does not make a placement inaccessible.

(viii) The total number of open and available placements that are accessible to the students and faculty compared to the total number of placements needed.

(B) The substitute clinical practice hours not in direct patient care provide a learning experience, as defined by the board consistent with Section 2708.1, that is at least equivalent to the learning experience provided by the direct patient care clinical practice hours.

(C) The temporary reduction provided in paragraph (3) shall cease as soon as practicable or by the end of the academic term, whichever is sooner.

(D) The substitute clinical practice hours not in direct patient care that are simulation experiences are based on the best practices published by the International Nursing Association for Clinical Simulation and Learning, the National Council of State Boards of Nursing, the Society for Simulation in Healthcare, or equivalent standards approved by the board.

(E) A maximum of 25 percent of the direct patient care hours specified in paragraph (3) in geriatrics and medical-surgical may be completed via telehealth.

(F) Notwithstanding subdivision (a), no new requests under this paragraph shall be approved after the 2023–2024 academic year and any requests approved under this paragraph shall expire at the end of the 2023–24 academic year.

(b) If the conditions in paragraph (1), (2), or (3) of subdivision (a), as applicable to the request, are met, a board nursing education consultant shall approve the request. If an approved nursing program fails to submit information satisfactory to the board nursing education consultant, or fails to meet the conditions specified, the board nursing education consultant shall deny the request. If the request is not approved or denied on or before 5:00 p.m. on the date seven business days after receipt of the request, the request shall be deemed approved.

(c)(1) Within 30 days of the effective date of this section, the board's executive officer shall develop a uniform method for evaluating requests and granting approvals pursuant to this section.

(2) The executive officer may revise the uniform method developed pursuant to this subdivision from time to time, as necessary. The development or revision of the uniform method shall be exempt from the requirements of the Administrative Procedure Act (Chapter 3.5 (commencing with Section 11340) of Part 1 of Title 2 of the Government Code).

(3) The board's nursing education consultants shall use the uniform method to evaluate requests and grant approvals pursuant to this section.

(4) The board shall post the uniform method and any revisions on the board's website.

HISTORY:

Added Stats 2020 ch 282 § 2 (AB 2288), effective September 29, 2020. Amended Stats 2021 ch 628 § 7 (AB 1532), effective January 1, 2022; Stats 2022 ch 413 § 13 (AB 2684), effective January 1, 2023.

§ 2786.4. Payments for student clinical experience placements prohibited

(a) An institution of higher education or a private postsecondary school of nursing subject to Section 2786, or an entity affiliated with the institution or school of nursing, shall not make a payment to any clinical agency or facility in exchange for clinical experience placements for students enrolled in a nursing program offered by or affiliated with the institution or private postsecondary school of nursing.

(b) A payment shall be deemed a violation of subdivision (a) if made within two years of a clinical experience placement at a facility.

(c) The payment of reasonable administrative fees for purposes of credentialing, databank registration, purchasing supplies, or similar costs or reimbursements does not constitute a violation of subdivision (a).

HISTORY:

Added Stats 2022 ch 413 § 14 (AB 2684), effective January 1, 2023.

§ 2786.5. Fees

(a) Subject to the provisions of Section 128.5, an institution of higher education or a private postsecondary school of nursing approved by the board pursuant to subdivision (b) of Section 2786 shall remit to the board for deposit in the Board of Registered Nursing Fund the following fees, in accordance with the following schedule:

(1) The fee for approval of a school of nursing shall be fixed by the board at not more than eighty thousand dollars ($80,000).

(2) The processing fee for authorization of a substantive change to an approval of a school of nursing shall be fixed by the board at not more than five thousand dollars ($5,000). The board shall not require a fee for substantive changes approved under subparagraph (E) of paragraph (1) of

subdivision (b) of Section 2786.2 or curriculum revisions, as defined under the uniform method developed under subdivision (e) of Section 2786.

(b) If the board determines that the cost of providing oversight and review of a school of nursing, as required by this article, is less than the amount of any fees required to be paid by that institution pursuant to this article, the board may decrease the fees applicable to that institution to an amount that is proportional to the board's costs associated with that institution.

HISTORY:

Added Stats 2012 ch 789 § 5 (SB 122). Amended Stats 2016 ch 799 § 14 (SB 1039), effective January 1, 2017; Stats 2022 ch 413 § 15 (AB 2684), effective January 1, 2023.

§ 2786.6. Grounds for denial of approval

The board shall deny the application for approval made by, and shall revoke the approval given to, any school of nursing which:

(a) Does not give to student applicants credit, in the field of nursing, for previous education and the opportunity to obtain credit for other acquired knowledge by the use of challenge examinations or other methods of evaluation; or,

(b) Is operated by a community college and discriminates against an applicant for admission to a school solely on the grounds that the applicant is seeking to fulfill the units of nursing required by Section 2736.6.

The board shall prescribe, by regulation, the education for which credit is to be given and the amount of credit which is to be given for each type of education. The word "credit," as used in the preceding sentence, is limited to credit for licensure only. The board is not authorized to prescribe the credit which an approved school of nursing shall give toward an academic certificate or degree.

HISTORY:

Added Stats 1969 ch 1541 § 3. Amended Stats 1976 ch 1405 § 1; Stats 1983 ch 742 § 8.

§ 2788. Inspections; Approval of schools meeting requirements; Notice of defects

It shall be the duty of the board, through its executive officer, to inspect all schools of nursing in this state at such times as the board shall deem necessary. Written reports of the executive officer's visits shall be made to the board, which shall thereupon approve those schools of nursing that meet the requirements provided by the board.

Upon receiving the report of the executive officer, if the board determines that any approved school of nursing is not maintaining the standard required by the board, notice thereof in writing specifying the defect or defects shall be immediately given to the school. If the defects are not corrected within a reasonable time, the school of nursing may be removed from the approved list and notice thereof in writing given to it.

HISTORY:

Added Stats 1939 ch 807 § 2. Amended Stats 1983 ch 742 § 10.

§ 2789. Exempt schools

None of the provisions of this chapter shall be applicable to any school or schools conducted by any well recognized church or denomination for the purpose of training the adherents of such church or denomination in the care of the sick in accordance with its religious tenets.

HISTORY:
Added Stats 1939 ch 807 § 2.

ARTICLE 5
PENAL PROVISIONS

Section
2795. Unlawful practice; Misrepresentation of licensee status.
2796. Use of "R. N.", etc.
2797. Impersonation of applicants or examinees.
2798. Conduct of unapproved school; Unprofessional conduct for registered nurse.
2799. Penalty for violations.
2800. Applicability of article.

HISTORY: Added Stats 1939 ch 807 § 2.

§ 2795. Unlawful practice; Misrepresentation of licensee status

Except as provided in this chapter, it is unlawful for any person to do any of the following:

(a) To practice or to offer to practice nursing in this state unless the person holds a license in an active status.

(b) To use any title, sign, card, or device to indicate that he or she is qualified to practice or is practicing nursing, unless the person has been duly licensed or certified under this chapter.

HISTORY:
Added Stats 1939 ch 807 § 2. Amended Stats 1976 ch 1053 § 5, effective September 28, 1976; Stats 1983 ch 696 § 4; Stats 1990 ch 350 § 2 (SB 2084).

§ 2796. Use of "R. N.", etc.

It is unlawful for any person or persons not licensed or certified as provided in this chapter to use the title "registered nurse," the letters "R.N. ," or the words "graduate nurse," "trained nurse," or "nurse anesthetist."

It is unlawful for any person or persons not licensed or certified as provided in this chapter to impersonate a professional nurse or pretend to be licensed to practice professional nursing as provided in this chapter.

HISTORY:
Added Stats 1939 ch 807 § 2. Amended Stats 1965 ch 727 § 9; Stats 1983 ch 696 § 5.

§ 2797. Impersonation of applicants or examinees

It is unlawful for a person to wilfully make any false representation or to impersonate any other person or permit or aid any person in any manner to impersonate him in connection with any examination or application for a license, or request to be examined or licensed.

HISTORY:
Added Stats 1939 ch 807 § 2.

§ 2798. Conduct of unapproved school; Unprofessional conduct for registered nurse

(a) It is unlawful for anyone to conduct a school of nursing unless the school has been approved by the board.

(b) If the board has a reasonable belief, either by complaint or otherwise, that a school is allowing students to apply for its nursing program and that nursing program does not have the approval of the board, the board shall immediately order the school to cease and desist from offering students the ability to enroll in its nursing program. The board shall also notify the Bureau for Private Postsecondary Education and the Attorney General's office that the school is offering students the ability to enroll in a nursing program that does not have the approval of the board.

(c) It shall be unprofessional conduct for any registered nurse to violate or attempt to violate, either directly or indirectly, or to assist or abet the violation of, this section.

(d) This section is not applicable to schools conducted under Section 2789 of this chapter.

HISTORY:

Added Stats 1939 ch 807 § 2. Amended Stats 1947 ch 504 § 1; Stats 1961 ch 1823 § 6; Stats 2012 ch 789 § 6 (SB 122), effective January 1, 2013.

§ 2799. Penalty for violations

Any person who violates any of the provisions of this chapter is guilty of a misdemeanor and upon a conviction thereof shall be punished by imprisonment in the county jail for not less than 10 days nor more than one year, or by a fine of not less than twenty dollars ($20) nor more than one thousand dollars ($1,000), or by both such fine and imprisonment.

HISTORY:

Added Stats 1939 ch 807 § 2. Amended Stats 1983 ch 1092 § 10, effective September 27, 1983, operative January 1, 1984.

§ 2800. Applicability of article

None of the sections in this article, except Sections 2796 and 2797, shall be applicable to any person or persons specifically exempted from the general provisions of this act by Section 2731 hereof, or to schools conducted by any well recognized church or denomination for the purpose of training the adherents of such church or denomination in the care of the sick in accordance with its religious tenets; and any adherent of any well recognized church or denomination who engages in nursing or the care of the sick in connection with the practice of the religious tenets of such well recognized church or denomination may use the word "nurse" in connection with or following his or her name, provided he or she shall not use the title "registered nurse," the letters "R.N.," the words "graduate nurse," "trained nurse," "nurse anesthetist," or any other name, word or symbol in connection with or following his or her name so as to lead another or others to believe that he or she is a professional nurse licensed under the provisions of this chapter.

HISTORY:

Added Stats 1939 ch 807 § 2. Amended Stats 1983 ch 696 § 6.

ARTICLE 6
REVENUE

Section
2810. Board of Registered Nursing Fund.
2811. Renewal of licenses; Expiration and reinstatement; Restoration of license in inactive status to active status.
2811.5. Continuing education as prerequisite for renewal.
2811.6. Availability of continuing education course records for board inspection.
2812. Reports; Deposit of funds.
2814. Use of funds.
2815. Fee schedule for registered nurses.
2815.1. Increase in license renewal fee.
2815.5. Fee schedule for nurse-midwives.
2815.7. Report to the legislature upon proposal or adoption of fee increase.

HISTORY: Added Stats 1939 ch 807 § 2.

§ 2810. Board of Registered Nursing Fund

There is established in the State Treasury a Board of Registered Nursing Fund. The California Board of Nursing Education and Nurse Registration Fund of the State of California is abolished. The Controller, on, January 1, 1975, shall transfer any balance in that fund to the Board of Registered Nursing Fund. Any reference in state law to the Board of Nurse Examiners Fund or the Board of Nurse Examiners Fund of the State of California shall be construed to refer to the Board of Registered Nursing Fund.

HISTORY:
Added Stats 1939 ch 807 § 2. Amended Stats 1961 ch 1823 § 7; Stats 1974 ch 632 § 8.

§ 2811. Renewal of licenses; Expiration and reinstatement; Restoration of license in inactive status to active status

(a) Each person holding a regular renewable license under this chapter, whether in an active or inactive status, shall apply for a renewal of his or her license and pay the biennial renewal fee required by this chapter each two years on or before the last day of the month following the month in which his or her birthday occurs, beginning with the second birthday following the date on which the license was issued, whereupon the board shall renew the license.

(b) Each such license not renewed in accordance with this section shall expire but may within a period of eight years thereafter be reinstated upon payment of the fee required by this chapter and upon submission of such proof of the applicant's qualifications as may be required by the board, except that during such eight-year period no examination shall be required as a condition for the reinstatement of any such expired license which has lapsed solely by reason of nonpayment of the renewal fee. After the expiration of such eight-year period the board may require as a condition of reinstatement that the applicant pass such examination as it deems necessary to determine his present fitness to resume the practice of professional nursing.

(c) A license in an inactive status may be restored to an active status if the licensee meets the continuing education standards of Section 2811.5.

HISTORY:

Added Stats 1939 ch 807 § 2. Amended Stats 1945 ch 1249 § 2; Stats 1953 ch 1174 § 12; Stats 1957 ch 1626 § 1; Stats 1963 ch 599 § 1; Stats 1965 ch 727 § 10; Stats 1971 ch 1516 § 2; Stats 1972 ch 919 § 3; Stats 1974 ch 923 § 2; Stats 1976 ch 1053 § 6, effective September 28, 1976; Stats 2016 ch 799 § 15, effective January 1, 2017 (SB 1039).

§ 2811.5. Continuing education as prerequisite for renewal

(a) Each person renewing their license under Section 2811 shall submit proof satisfactory to the board that, during the preceding two-year period, they have been informed of the developments in the registered nurse field or in any special area of practice engaged in by the licensee, occurring since the last renewal thereof, either by pursuing a course or courses of continuing education in the registered nurse field or relevant to the practice of the licensee, and approved by the board, or by other means deemed equivalent by the board.

(b) Notwithstanding Section 10231.5 of the Government Code, the board, in compliance with Section 9795 of the Government Code, shall do the following:

(1) By January 1, 2019, deliver a report to the appropriate legislative policy committees detailing a comprehensive plan for approving and disapproving continuing education opportunities.

(2) By January 1, 2020, report to the appropriate legislative committees on its progress implementing this plan.

(c) For purposes of this section, the board shall, by regulation, establish standards for continuing education. The standards shall be established in a manner to ensure that a variety of alternative forms of continuing education are available to licensees, including, but not limited to, online, academic studies, in-service education, institutes, seminars, lectures, conferences, workshops, extension studies, and home study programs. The standards shall take cognizance of specialized areas of practice, and content shall be relevant to the practice of nursing and shall be related to the scientific knowledge or technical skills required for the practice of nursing or be related to direct or indirect patient or client care. The continuing education standards established by the board shall not exceed 30 hours of direct participation in a course or courses approved by the board, or its equivalent in the units of measure adopted by the board.

(d) The board shall audit continuing education providers at least once every five years to ensure adherence to regulatory requirements, and shall withhold or rescind approval from any provider that is in violation of the regulatory requirements.

(e) The board shall encourage continuing education in spousal or partner abuse detection and treatment. In the event the board establishes a requirement for continuing education coursework in spousal or partner abuse detection or treatment, that requirement shall be met by each licensee within no more than four years from the date the requirement is imposed.

(f) In establishing standards for continuing education, the board shall consider including a course in the special care needs of individuals and their families, including, but not limited to, all of the following:

(1) Pain and symptom management, including palliative care.

(2) The psychosocial dynamics of death.

(3) Dying and bereavement.

(4) Hospice care.

(g) This section shall not apply to licensees during the first two years immediately following their initial licensure in California or any other governmental jurisdiction, except that, beginning January 1, 2023, those licensees shall complete one hour of direct participation in an implicit bias course offered by a continuing education provider approved by the board that meets all the same requirements outlined in paragraph (1) of subdivision (e) of Section 2786, including, but not limited to, the identification of the licensees previous or current unconscious biases and misinformation and corrective measures to decrease implicit bias at the interpersonal and institutional levels, including ongoing policies and practices for that purpose.

(h) The board may, in accordance with the intent of this section, make exceptions from continuing education requirements for licensees residing in another state or country, or for reasons of health, military service, or other good cause.

HISTORY:

Added Stats 1974 ch 923 § 4. Amended Stats 1976 ch 1053 § 7, effective September 28, 1976, operative July 1, 1978; Stats 1978 ch 212 § 3, effective June 6, 1978; Stats 1990 ch 1207 § 2 (AB 3242); Stats 1993 ch 1234 § 6 (AB 890); Stats 1998 ch 791 § 3 (SB 1140); Stats 2016 ch 799 § 16 (SB 1039), effective January 1, 2017; Stats 2017 ch 520 § 7 (SB 799), effective January 1, 2018; Stats 2021 ch 445 § 2 (AB 1407), effective January 1, 2022.

§ 2811.6. Availability of continuing education course records for board inspection

Providers of continuing education programs approved by the board pursuant to Section 2811.5 shall make available for board inspection records of continuing education courses given to registered nurses.

HISTORY:

Added Stats 1978 ch 167 § 1.

§ 2812. Reports; Deposit of funds

Within 10 days after the beginning of each month, the board shall report to the State Controller the amount and source of all collections made under this chapter. At the same time, all amounts shall be paid into the State Treasury, where they shall be placed to the credit of the Board of Registered Nursing Fund and to the Registered Nurse Education Fund, as specified in Section 128400 of the Health and Safety Code.

HISTORY:

Added Stats 1939 ch 807 § 2. Amended Stats 1961 ch 1823 § 8; Stats 1974 ch 632 § 9; Stats 1988 ch 252 § 1; Stats 1996 ch 1023 § 11 (SB 1497), effective September 29, 1996.

§ 2814. Use of funds

All money in the Board of Registered Nursing Fund shall be available, upon appropriation by the Legislature, to carry out this chapter and the promotion of nursing education in this state.

HISTORY:

Added Stats 1939 ch 807 § 2. Amended Stats 1941 ch 1081 § 1; Stats 1961 ch 1823 § 9; Stats 1974 ch 632 § 10; Stats 2017 ch 520 § 8 (SB 799), effective January 1, 2018.

§ 2815. Fee schedule for registered nurses

Subject to the provisions of Section 128.5, the amount of the fees prescribed by this chapter in connection with the issuance of licenses for registered nurses under its provisions is that fixed by the following schedule:

(a)(1) The fee to be paid upon the filing by a graduate of an approved school of nursing in this state of an application for a licensure by examination shall be fixed by the board at not more than one thousand dollars ($1,000).

(2) The fee to be paid upon the filing by a graduate of a school of nursing in another state, district, or territory of the United States of an application for a licensure by examination shall be fixed by the board at not more than one thousand dollars ($1,000).

(3) The fee to be paid upon the filing by a graduate of a school of nursing in another country of an application for a licensure by examination shall be fixed by the board at not more than one thousand five hundred dollars ($1,500).

(4) The fee to be paid upon the filing of an application for licensure by a repeat examination shall be fixed by the board at not more than one thousand dollars ($1,000).

(b) The fee to be paid for taking each examination shall be the actual cost to purchase an examination from a vendor approved by the board.

(c)(1) The fee to be paid for application by a person who is licensed or registered as a nurse in another state, district, or territory of the United States for licensure by endorsement shall be fixed by the board at not more than one thousand dollars ($1,000).

(2) The fee to be paid for application by a person who is licensed or registered as a nurse in another country for licensure by endorsement shall be fixed by the board at not more than one thousand five hundred dollars ($1,500).

(d)(1) The biennial fee to be paid upon the filing of an application for renewal of the license shall be not more than seven hundred fifty dollars ($750). In addition, an assessment of ten dollars ($10) shall be collected and credited to the Registered Nurse Education Fund, pursuant to Section 2815.1.

(2) The fee to be paid upon the filing of an application for reinstatement pursuant to subdivision (b) of Section 2811 shall be not more than one thousand dollars ($1,000).

(e) The penalty fee for failure to renew a license within the prescribed time shall be fixed by the board at not more than 50 percent of the regular renewal fee, but not more than three hundred seventy-five dollars ($375).

(f) The fee to be paid for approval of a continuing education provider shall be fixed by the board at not more than one thousand dollars ($1,000).

(g) The biennial fee to be paid upon the filing of an application for renewal of provider approval shall be fixed by the board at not more than one thousand dollars ($1,000).

(h) The penalty fee for failure to renew provider approval within the prescribed time shall be fixed at not more than 50 percent of the regular renewal fee, but not more than five hundred dollars ($500).

(i) The penalty for submitting insufficient funds or fictitious check, draft or order on any bank or depository for payment of any fee to the board shall be fixed at not more than thirty dollars ($30).

(j) The fee to be paid for an interim permit shall be fixed by the board at not more than two hundred fifty dollars ($250).

(k) The fee to be paid for a temporary license shall be fixed by the board at not more than two hundred fifty dollars ($250).

(*l*) The fee to be paid for processing endorsement papers to other states shall be fixed by the board at not more than two hundred dollars ($200).

(m) The fee to be paid for a certified copy of a school transcript shall be fixed by the board at not more than one hundred dollars ($100).

(n)(1) The fee to be paid for a duplicate pocket license shall be fixed by the board at not more than seventy-five dollars ($75).

(2) The fee to be paid for a duplicate wall certificate shall be fixed by the board at not more than one hundred dollars ($100).

(o)(1) The fee to be paid by a registered nurse for an evaluation of their qualifications to use the title "nurse practitioner" shall be fixed by the board at not more than one thousand five hundred dollars ($1,500).

(2) The fee to be paid by a registered nurse for a temporary certificate to practice as a nurse practitioner shall be fixed by the board at not more than five hundred dollars ($500).

(3) The fee to be paid upon the filing of an application for renewal of a certificate to practice as a nurse practitioner shall be not more than one thousand dollars ($1,000).

(4) The penalty fee for failure to renew a certificate to practice as a nurse practitioner within the prescribed time shall be not more than five hundred dollars ($500).

(p) The fee to be paid by a registered nurse for listing as a "psychiatric mental health nurse" shall be fixed by the board at not than seven hundred fifty dollars ($750).

(q) The fee to be paid for duplicate National Council Licensure Examination for registered nurses (NCLEX-RN) examination results shall be not more than one hundred dollars ($100).

(r) The fee to be paid for a letter certifying a license shall be not more than thirty dollars ($30).

(s) The fee to be paid for a certificate issued pursuant to Section 2837.103 shall be an amount sufficient to cover the reasonable regulatory cost of issuing the certificate.

(t) The fee to be paid for a certificate issued pursuant to Section 2837.104 shall be an amount sufficient to cover the reasonable regulatory cost of issuing the certificate.

No further fee shall be required for a license or a renewal thereof other than as prescribed by this chapter.

HISTORY:

Added Stats 1939 ch 807 § 2. Amended Stats 1953 ch 1174 § 13; Stats 1955 ch 1769 § 1; Stats 1959 ch 1578 § 1; Stats 1963 ch 1400 § 2; Stats 1965 ch 1191 § 13; Stats 1974 ch 1407 § 2; Stats 1975 ch 999 § 1; Stats 1978 ch 1161 § 180; Stats 1979 ch 933 § 3; Stats 1981 ch 437 § 2; Stats 1984 ch 525 § 1; Stats 1988 ch 252 § 2; Stats 1991 ch 352 § 1 (AB 485); Stats 2003 ch 640 § 7 (SB 358); Stats 2016 ch 799 § 17 (SB 1039), effective January 1, 2017; Stats 2022 ch 413 § 16 (AB 2684), effective January 1, 2023.

§ 2815.1. Increase in license renewal fee

As provided in subdivision (d) of Section 2815, the Board of Registered Nursing shall collect an additional ten dollar ($10) assessment at the time of the biennial licensure renewal. This amount shall be credited to the Registered Nurse Education Fund. This assessment is separate from those fees prescribed in Section 2815.

HISTORY:

Added Stats 1988 ch 252 § 3. Amended Stats 1991 ch 352 § 2 (AB 485); Stats 1999 ch 146 § 1 (AB 1107), effective July 22, 1999, ch 149 § 1 (SB 308), effective July 22, 1999; Stats 2003 ch 640 § 8 (SB 358).

§ 2815.5. Fee schedule for nurse-midwives

The amount of the fees prescribed by this chapter in connection with the issuance of certificates as nurse-midwives is that fixed by the following schedule:

(a) The fee to be paid upon the filing of an application for a certificate shall be fixed by the board at not more than one thousand five hundred dollars ($1,500).

(b) The biennial fee to be paid upon the application for a renewal of a certificate shall be fixed by the board at not more than one thousand dollars ($1,000).

(c) The penalty fee for failure to renew a certificate within the prescribed time shall be 50 percent of the renewal fee in effect on the date of the renewal of the license, but not more than five hundred dollars ($500).

(d) The fee to be paid upon the filing of an application for the nurse-midwife equivalency examination shall be fixed by the board at not more than two hundred dollars ($200).

(e) The fee to be paid for a temporary certificate shall be fixed by the board at not more than five hundred dollars ($500).

HISTORY:

Added Stats 1974 ch 1407 § 3. Amended Stats 1978 ch 1161 § 181; Stats 1981 ch 437 § 3; Stats 1991 ch 352 § 3 (AB 485); Stats 2016 ch 799 § 18 (SB 1039), effective January 1, 2017; Stats 2022 ch 413 § 17 (AB 2684), effective January 1, 2023.

§ 2815.7. Report to the legislature upon proposal or adoption of fee increase

The board shall report to the appropriate policy and fiscal committees of each house of the Legislature whenever the board proposes or adopts an increase in any fee imposed pursuant to this chapter. The board shall specify the reasons for each fee increase and shall identify the percentage of the funds derived from an increase in any fee that will be used for investigational or enforcement related activities by the board.

HISTORY:

Added Stats 1991 ch 352 § 4 (AB 485).

ARTICLE 6.5
PUBLIC HEALTH NURSE CERTIFICATION

Section
2816. Fee.

Section
2817. Child abuse and neglect detection training requirement.
2818. Legislative findings; Use of title "public health nurse".
2819. Repeal and adoption of regulations.
2820. Scope of practice.

HISTORY: Added Stats 1992 ch 1135 § 2.8. Former Article 6.5, entitled "Nursing Education Programs", consisting of §§ 2816–2822, was added Stats 1970 ch 995 § 1 and repealed Stats 1992 ch 1135 § 2.6.

§ 2816. Fee

The nonrefundable fee to be paid by a registered nurse for an evaluation of his or her qualifications to use the title "public health nurse" shall not be less than three hundred dollars ($300) or more than one thousand dollars ($1,000). The fee to be paid upon the application for renewal of the certificate to practice as a public health nurse shall not be less than one hundred twenty-five dollars ($125) and not more than five hundred dollars ($500). The penalty fee for failure to renew a certificate to practice as a public health nurse within the prescribed time shall be 50 percent of the renewal fee in effect on the date of renewal of the certificate, but not less than sixty-two dollars and fifty cents ($62.50), and not more than two hundred fifty dollars ($250). All fees payable under this section shall be collected by and paid to the Board of Registered Nursing Fund. It is the intention of the Legislature that the costs of carrying out the purposes of this article shall be covered by the revenue collected pursuant to this section. The board shall refund any registered nurse who paid more than three hundred dollars ($300) for an evaluation of his or her qualifications to use the title "public health nurse" between April 5, 2018, and December 31, 2018.

HISTORY:

Added Stats 1992 ch 1135 § 2.8 (SB 2044). Amended Stats 2016 ch 799 § 19 (SB 1039), effective January 1, 2017; Stats 2018 ch 571 § 13 (SB 1480), effective January 1, 2019.

§ 2817. Child abuse and neglect detection training requirement

The qualifications prescribed by the board under this article shall include a requirement that an applicant for employment as a public health nurse and all public health nurses employed on or after January 1, 1981, acquire training in child abuse and neglect detection.

HISTORY:

Added Stats 1992 ch 1135 § 2.8 (SB 2044).

§ 2818. Legislative findings; Use of title "public health nurse"

(a) The Legislature recognizes that public health nursing is a service of crucial importance for the health, safety, and sanitation of the population in all of California's communities. These services currently include, but are not limited to:

(1) Control and prevention of communicable disease.

(2) Promotion of maternal, child, and adolescent health.

(3) Prevention of abuse and neglect of children, elders, and spouses.

(4) Outreach screening, case management, resource coordination and assessment, and delivery and evaluation of care for individuals, families, and communities.

(b) The Legislature also finds that conflicting definitions of "public health nurse" have been created by various state and local agencies within California. The Legislature also finds that the public is harmed by the conflicting usage of the title "public health nurse" and lack of consistency between the use of the term and the qualifications required in state law and in administrative regulations. Therefore, the Legislature finds that the public interest would be served by determining the conditions for the legitimate use by registered nurses of a title which includes the term "public health nurse."

(c) No individual shall hold himself or herself out as a public health nurse or use a title which includes the term "public health nurse" unless that individual is in possession of a valid California public health nurse certificate issued pursuant to this article.

(d) No employer subject to regulation by Section 602 of the Health and Safety Code shall hold out any employee to be a public health nurse or grant a title to any employee including the term "public health nurse" unless that employee holds a valid California public health nurse certificate pursuant to this article.

HISTORY:
Added Stats 1992 ch 1135 § 2.8 (SB 2044).

§ 2819. Repeal and adoption of regulations

In order to effect a speedy and efficient transfer of public health nurse certification from the State Department of Health Services to the board, existing Sections 4500 to 4504, inclusive, of Title 17 of the California Code of Regulations shall be repealed by the State Department of Health Services and adopted by the board to place them in Chapter 14 of Title 16 of the California Code of Regulations, and any reference to the State Department of Health Services in those regulations shall be changed to refer to the board. The repeal of the regulations and adoption of the revised regulations pursuant to this section shall be exempt from the Administrative Procedure Act, Chapter 3.5 (commencing with Section 11340) of Part 1 of Division 3 of Title 2 of the Government Code, except that the repealed and adopted regulations shall be filed with the Office of Administrative Law for publication in the California Code of Regulations.

HISTORY:
Added Stats 1992 ch 1135 § 2.8 (SB 2044).

§ 2820. Scope of practice

Nothing in this article shall be construed as expanding the scope of practice of a registered nurse beyond that which is authorized under Section 2725.

HISTORY:
Added Stats 1992 ch 1135 § 2.8 (SB 2044).

ARTICLE 7
NURSE ANESTHETISTS

Section
2825. Citation of article.
2826. Definitions.
2827. Anesthesia services; Approval; Permit.
2828. Nonemployee nurse anesthetists working in acute care facilities.
2829. Unlawful use of title "nurse anesthetist".
2830. Certificate to practice.
2830.5. Evidence that applicant has met requirements.
2830.6. Certification.
2830.7. Fee schedule for nurse anesthetists.
2831. Written application; Fee.
2832. Applicant to comply with all provisions of article.
2833. Renewal of certificate; Reinstatement of expired certificate.
2833.3. Article not limitation on ability to practice nursing.
2833.5. Practice not authority to practice medicine or surgery.
2833.6. Effect of provisions on existing scope of practice.

HISTORY: Added Stats 1983 ch 696 § 7. Former Article 7, entitled "Temporary Provisions," consisting of §§ 2825–2830, was added Stats 1939 ch 807 § 2 and repealed Stats 1982 ch 454 § 1.

§ 2825. Citation of article

This article may be cited as the Nurse Anesthetists Act.

HISTORY:
Added Stats 1983 ch 696 § 7.

§ 2826. Definitions

As used in this article:

(a) "Nurse anesthetist" means a person who is a registered nurse, licensed by the board and who has met standards for certification from the board. In the certification and recertification process the board shall consider the standards of the Council on Certification of Nurse Anesthetists and the Council on Recertification of Nurse Anesthetists and may develop new standards if there is a public safety need for standards more stringent than the councils' standards. In determining the adequacy for public safety of the councils' standards or in developing board standards, the board shall comply with the provisions of Chapter 3.5 (commencing with Section 11340) of Part 1 of Division 3 of Title 2 of the Government Code.

(b) "Accredited Program" means a program for the education of nurse anesthetists which has received approval from the board. In the approval process the board shall consider the standards of the Council on Accreditation of Nurse Anesthesia Education Programs and Schools and may develop new standards if the councils' standards are determined to be inadequate for public safety. In determining the adequacy for public safety of the councils' standards or in developing board standards, the board shall comply with the provisions of Chapter 3.5 (commencing with Section 11340) of Part 1 of Division 3 of Title 2 of the Government Code.

(c) "Appropriate committee" means the committee responsible for anesthesia practice which is responsible to the executive committee of the medical staff.

(d) "Trainee" means a registered nurse enrolled in an accredited program of nurse anesthesia.

(e) "Graduate" means a nurse anesthetist who is a graduate of an accredited program of nurse anesthesia awaiting initial certification results for not more than one year from the date of graduation.

HISTORY:

Added Stats 1983 ch 696 § 7.

§ 2827. Anesthesia services; Approval; Permit

The utilization of a nurse anesthetist to provide anesthesia services in an acute care facility shall be approved by the acute care facility administration and the appropriate committee, and at the discretion of the physician, dentist or podiatrist. If a general anesthetic agent is administered in a dental office, the dentist shall hold a permit authorized by Article 2.7 (commencing with Section 1646) of Chapter 4 or, commencing January 1, 2022, Article 2.75 (commencing with Section 1646) of Chapter 4.

HISTORY:

Added Stats 1983 ch 696 § 7. Amended Stats 2018 ch 929 § 16 (SB 501), effective January 1, 2019.

§ 2828. Nonemployee nurse anesthetists working in acute care facilities

In an acute care facility, a nurse anesthetist who is not an employee of the facility shall, nonetheless, be subject to the bylaws of the facility and may be required by the facility to provide proof of current professional liability insurance coverage. Notwithstanding any other provision of law, a nurse anesthetist shall be responsible for his or her own professional conduct and may be held liable for those professional acts.

HISTORY:

Added Stats 1983 ch 696 § 7.

§ 2829. Unlawful use of title "nurse anesthetist"

It is unlawful for any person or persons to advertise, use any title, sign, card, or device, or to otherwise hold himself or herself out as a "nurse anesthetist" unless the person meets the requirements of subdivision (a) of Section 2826 and has been so certified under the provisions of this article.

HISTORY:

Added Stats 1983 ch 696 § 7.

§ 2830. Certificate to practice

The board shall issue a certificate to practice nurse anesthesia to any person who qualifies under this article and is licensed pursuant to the provisions of this chapter.

HISTORY:

Added Stats 1983 ch 696 § 7.

§ 2830.5. Evidence that applicant has met requirements

Every applicant shall show by evidence satisfactory to the board that he or she has met the requirements of this article.

HISTORY:

Added Stats 1983 ch 696 § 7.

§ 2830.6. Certification

Notwithstanding Section 2830, the board shall certify all applicants who can show certification by the Council on Certification of Nurse Anesthetists or the Council on Recertification of Nurse Anesthetists as of the effective date of this chapter. This certification shall be documented to the board in a manner to be determined by the board. Proof of certification shall be filed with the board within six months from the effective date of this article and the board shall, within one year from the effective date of this article, issue a certificate to applicants who have filed proof of certification within that six-month period.

HISTORY:

Added Stats 1983 ch 696 § 7.

§ 2830.7. Fee schedule for nurse anesthetists

The amount of the fees prescribed by this chapter in connection with the issuance of certificates as nurse anesthetists is that fixed by the following schedule:

(a) The fee to be paid upon the filing of an application for a certificate shall be fixed by the board at not less than five hundred dollars ($500) nor more than one thousand five hundred dollars ($1,500).

(b) The biennial fee to be paid upon the application for a renewal of a certificate shall be fixed by the board at not less than one hundred fifty dollars ($150) nor more than one thousand dollars ($1,000).

(c) The penalty fee for failure to renew a certificate within the prescribed time shall be 50 percent of the renewal fee in effect on the date of the renewal of the license, but not less than seventy-five dollars ($75) nor more than five hundred dollars ($500).

(d) The fee to be paid for a temporary certificate shall be fixed by the board at not less than one hundred fifty dollars ($150) nor more than five hundred dollars ($500).

HISTORY:

Added Stats 1991 ch 352 § 4.5 (AB 485). Amended Stats 2016 ch 799 § 20 (SB 1039), effective January 1, 2017.

§ 2831. Written application; Fee

An applicant for certification pursuant to this article shall submit a written application in the form prescribed by the board, accompanied by the fee prescribed by Section 2830.7 which shall also apply to the issuance of a certificate under the provisions of this article.

HISTORY:

Added Stats 1983 ch 696 § 7. Amended Stats 1991 ch 352 § 5 (AB 485).

§ 2832. Applicant to comply with all provisions of article

Every applicant for a certificate to practice nurse anesthesia shall comply with all the provisions of this article in addition to the provisions of this chapter.

HISTORY:

Added Stats 1983 ch 696 § 7.

§ 2833. Renewal of certificate; Reinstatement of expired certificate

Each certificate issued pursuant to this article shall be renewable biennially, and each person holding a certificate under this article shall apply for a renewal of his or her certificate and pay the biennial renewal fee required by Section 2830.7 every two years on or before the last day of the month following the month in which his or her birthday occurs, beginning with the second birthday following the date on which the certificate was issued, whereupon the board shall renew the certificate.

Each certificate not renewed in accordance with this section shall expire but may within a period of eight years thereafter be reinstated upon payment of the biennial renewal fee and penalty fee required by Section 2830.7 and upon submission of such proof of the applicant's qualifications as may be required by the board, except that during that eight-year period no examination shall be required as a condition for the reinstatement of any expired certificate which has lapsed solely by reason of nonpayment of the renewable fee. After the expiration of the eight-year period the board may require as a condition of reinstatement that the applicant pass an examination as it deems necessary to determine his or her present fitness to resume the practice of nurse anesthesia.

HISTORY:

Added Stats 1983 ch 696 § 7. Amended Stats 1991 ch 352 § 6 (AB 485).

§ 2833.3. Article not limitation on ability to practice nursing

Nothing in this article shall be construed to limit a certified nurse anesthetist's ability to practice nursing.

HISTORY:

Added Stats 1983 ch 696 § 7.

§ 2833.5. Practice not authority to practice medicine or surgery

Except as provided in Section 2725 and in this section, the practice of nurse anesthetist does not confer authority to practice medicine or surgery.

HISTORY:

Added Stats 1983 ch 696 § 7.

§ 2833.6. Effect of provisions on existing scope of practice

This chapter is not intended to address the scope of practice of, and nothing in this chapter shall be construed to restrict, expand, alter, or modify the existing scope of practice of, a nurse anesthetist.

HISTORY:

Added Stats 1983 ch 696 § 7.

ARTICLE 8
NURSE PRACTITIONERS

Section
2834. Legislative finding of conflicting definitions and usage.
2835. License requirement.
2835.5. Requirements for initial qualification or certification as nurse practitioner.
2835.7. Authorized standardized procedures.
2836. Establishment of categories and standards.
2836.1. Furnishing or ordering of drugs or devices by nurse practitioners.
2836.2. What constitutes furnishing or ordering of drugs or devices.
2836.3. Issuance of number to nurse practitioners dispensing drugs or devices.
2836.4. Furnishing or ordering buprenorphine.
2837. Registered nursing practice not limited.

HISTORY: Added Stats 1977 ch 439 § 2.

§ 2834. Legislative finding of conflicting definitions and usage

The Legislature finds that various and conflicting definitions of the nurse practitioner are being created by state agencies and private organizations within California. The Legislature also finds that the public is harmed by conflicting usage of the title of nurse practitioner and lack of correspondence between use of the title and qualifications of the registered nurse using the title. Therefore, the Legislature finds the public interest served by determination of the legitimate use of the title "nurse practitioner" by registered nurses.

HISTORY:
Added Stats 1977 ch 439 § 2.

§ 2835. License requirement

No person shall advertise or hold himself out as a "nurse practitioner" who is not a nurse licensed under this chapter and does not, in addition, meet the standards for a nurse practitioner established by the board.

HISTORY:
Added Stats 1977 ch 439 § 2.

§ 2835.5. Requirements for initial qualification or certification as nurse practitioner

On and after January 1, 2008, an applicant for initial qualification or certification as a nurse practitioner under this article who has not been qualified or certified as a nurse practitioner in California or any other state shall meet the following requirements:

(a) Hold a valid and active registered nursing license issued under this chapter.

(b) Possess a master's degree in nursing, a master's degree in a clinical field related to nursing, or a graduate degree in nursing.

(c) Satisfactorily complete a nurse practitioner program approved by the board.

HISTORY:
Added Stats 1984 ch 525 § 2. Amended Stats 2004 ch 344 § 1 (AB 2226); Stats 2015 ch 426 § 31 (SB 800), effective January 1, 2016.

§ 2835.7. Authorized standardized procedures

(a) Notwithstanding any other provision of law, in addition to any other practices that meet the general criteria set forth in statute or regulation for inclusion in standardized procedures developed through collaboration among administrators and health professionals, including physicians and surgeons and nurses, pursuant to Section 2725, standardized procedures may be implemented that authorize a nurse practitioner to do any of the following:

(1) Order durable medical equipment, subject to any limitations set forth in the standardized procedures. Notwithstanding that authority, nothing in this paragraph shall operate to limit the ability of a third-party payer to require prior approval.

(2) After performance of a physical examination by the nurse practitioner and collaboration with a physician and surgeon, certify disability pursuant to Section 2708 of the Unemployment Insurance Code.

(3) For individuals receiving home health services or personal care services, after consultation with the treating physician and surgeon, approve, sign, modify, or add to a plan of treatment or plan of care.

(b) Nothing in this section shall be construed to affect the validity of any standardized procedures in effect prior to the enactment of this section or those adopted subsequent to enactment.

HISTORY:
Added Stats 2009 ch 308 § 34 (SB 819), effective January 1, 2010.

§ 2836. Establishment of categories and standards

(a) The board shall establish categories of nurse practitioners and standards for nurses to hold themselves out as nurse practitioners in each category. Such standards shall take into account the types of advanced levels of nursing practice which are or may be performed and the clinical and didactic education, experience, or both needed to practice safely at those levels. In setting such standards, the board shall consult with nurse practitioners, physicians and surgeons with expertise in the nurse practitioner field, and health care organizations utilizing nurse practitioners. Established standards shall apply to persons without regard to the date of meeting such standards. If the board sets standards for use of nurse practitioner titles which include completion of an academically affiliated program, it shall provide equivalent standards for registered nurses who have not completed such a program.

(b) Any regulations promulgated by a state department that affect the scope of practice of a nurse practitioner shall be developed in consultation with the board.

HISTORY:
Added Stats 1977 ch 39 § 2. Amended Stats 2002 ch 764 § 3 (SB 993).

§ 2836.1. Furnishing or ordering of drugs or devices by nurse practitioners

Neither this chapter nor any other provision of law shall be construed to prohibit a nurse practitioner from furnishing or ordering drugs or devices when all of the following apply:

(a) The drugs or devices are furnished or ordered by a nurse practitioner in accordance with standardized procedures or protocols developed by the nurse practitioner and the supervising physician and surgeon when the drugs or devices furnished or ordered are consistent with the practitioner's educational preparation or for which clinical competency has been established and maintained.

(b) The nurse practitioner is functioning pursuant to standardized procedure, as defined by Section 2725, or protocol. The standardized procedure or protocol shall be developed and approved by the supervising physician and surgeon, the nurse practitioner, and the facility administrator or the designee.

(c)(1) The standardized procedure or protocol covering the furnishing of drugs or devices shall specify which nurse practitioners may furnish or order drugs or devices, which drugs or devices may be furnished or ordered, under what circumstances, the extent of physician and surgeon supervision, the method of periodic review of the nurse practitioner's competence, including peer review, and review of the provisions of the standardized procedure.

(2) In addition to the requirements in paragraph (1), for Schedule II controlled substance protocols, the provision for furnishing Schedule II controlled substances shall address the diagnosis of the illness, injury, or condition for which the Schedule II controlled substance is to be furnished.

(d) The furnishing or ordering of drugs or devices by a nurse practitioner occurs under physician and surgeon supervision. Physician and surgeon supervision shall not be construed to require the physical presence of the physician, but does include (1) collaboration on the development of the standardized procedure, (2) approval of the standardized procedure, and (3) availability by telephonic contact at the time of patient examination by the nurse practitioner.

(e) For purposes of this section, no physician and surgeon shall supervise more than four nurse practitioners at one time.

(f)(1) Drugs or devices furnished or ordered by a nurse practitioner may include Schedule II through Schedule V controlled substances under the California Uniform Controlled Substances Act (Division 10 (commencing with Section 11000) of the Health and Safety Code) and shall be further limited to those drugs agreed upon by the nurse practitioner and physician and surgeon and specified in the standardized procedure.

(2) When Schedule II or III controlled substances, as defined in Sections 11055 and 11056, respectively, of the Health and Safety Code, are furnished or ordered by a nurse practitioner, the controlled substances shall be furnished or ordered in accordance with a patient-specific protocol approved by the treating or supervising physician. A copy of the section of the nurse practitioner's standardized procedure relating to controlled substances shall be provided, upon request, to any licensed pharmacist who dispenses drugs or devices, when there is uncertainty about the nurse practitioner furnishing the order.

(g)(1) The board has certified in accordance with Section 2836.3 that the nurse practitioner has satisfactorily completed a course in pharmacology covering the drugs or devices to be furnished or ordered under this section.

(2) A physician and surgeon may determine the extent of supervision necessary pursuant to this section in the furnishing or ordering of drugs and devices.

(3) Nurse practitioners who are certified by the board and hold an active furnishing number, who are authorized through standardized procedures or protocols to furnish Schedule II controlled substances, and who are registered with the United States Drug Enforcement Administration, shall complete, as part of their continuing education requirements, a course including Schedule II controlled substances, and the risks of addiction associated with their use, based on the standards developed by the board. The board shall establish the requirements for satisfactory completion of this subdivision.

(h) Use of the term "furnishing" in this section, in health facilities defined in Section 1250 of the Health and Safety Code, shall include (1) the ordering of a drug or device in accordance with the standardized procedure and (2) transmitting an order of a supervising physician and surgeon.

(i) "Drug order" or "order" for purposes of this section means an order for medication which is dispensed to or for an ultimate user, issued by a nurse practitioner as an individual practitioner, within the meaning of Section 1306.02 of Title 21 of the Code of Federal Regulations. Notwithstanding any other provision of law, (1) a drug order issued pursuant to this section shall be treated in the same manner as a prescription of the supervising physician; (2) all references to "prescription" in this code and the Health and Safety Code shall include drug orders issued by nurse practitioners; and (3) the signature of a nurse practitioner on a drug order issued in accordance with this section shall be deemed to be the signature of a prescriber for purposes of this code and the Health and Safety Code.

HISTORY:

Added Stats 1986 ch 493 § 2. Amended Stats 1991 ch 870 § 3 (AB 1350); Stats 1996 ch 455 § 1 (AB 1077); Stats 1999 ch 749 § 1 (SB 816); Stats 2002 ch 764 § 4 (SB 993); Stats 2003 ch 748 § 1 (AB 1196); Stats 2004 ch 205 § 1 (AB 2560); Stats 2012 ch 796 § 2 (SB 1524), effective January 1, 2013; Stats 2018 ch 693 § 8 (SB 1109), effective January 1, 2019.

§ 2836.2. What constitutes furnishing or ordering of drugs or devices

Furnishing or ordering of drugs or devices by nurse practitioners is defined to mean the act of making a pharmaceutical agent or agents available to the patient in strict accordance with a standardized procedure. All nurse practitioners who are authorized pursuant to Section 2836.1 to furnish or issue drug orders for controlled substances shall register with the United States Drug Enforcement Administration.

HISTORY:

Added Stats 1986 ch 493 § 3. Amended Stats 1999 ch 749 § 2 (SB 816); Stats 2011 ch 350 § 20 (SB 943), effective January 1, 2012.

§ 2836.3. Issuance of number to nurse practitioners dispensing drugs or devices

(a) The furnishing of drugs or devices by nurse practitioners is conditional on issuance by the board of a number to the nurse applicant who has successfully completed the requirements of subdivision (g) of Section 2836.1. The board may issue a furnishing number upon initial application and, if approved by the board, the applicant shall not be required to make a separate application. The number shall be included on all transmittals of orders for drugs or devices by the nurse practitioner. The board shall make the list of numbers issued available to the Board of Pharmacy. The board may charge the applicant a fee to cover all necessary costs to implement this section, that shall be not more than one thousand five hundred dollars ($1,500) for an initial application, nor more than one thousand dollars ($1,000) for an application for renewal. The board may charge a penalty fee for failure to renew a furnishing number within the prescribed time that shall be not more than five hundred dollars ($500).

(b) The number shall be renewable at the time of the applicant's registered nurse license renewal.

(c) The board may revoke, suspend, or deny issuance of the numbers for incompetence or gross negligence in the performance of functions specified in Sections 2836.1 and 2836.2.

HISTORY:

Added Stats 1986 ch 493 § 4. Amended Stats 2016 ch 799 § 21 (SB 1039), effective January 1, 2017; Stats 2022 ch 473 § 18 (AB 2684), effective January 1, 2023.

§ 2836.4. Furnishing or ordering buprenorphine

Neither this chapter nor any other provision of law shall be construed to prohibit a nurse practitioner from furnishing or ordering buprenorphine when done in compliance with the provisions of the Comprehensive Addiction Recovery Act (Public Law 114-198), as enacted on July 22, 2016, including the following:

(a) The requirement that the nurse practitioner complete not fewer than 24 hours of initial training provided by an organization listed in sub-subclause (aa) of subclause (II) of clause (iv) of subparagraph (G) of paragraph (2) of subdivision (g) of Section 823 of Title 21 of the United States Code, or any other organization that the United States Secretary of Health and Human Services determines is appropriate for the purposes of that sub-subclause, that addresses the following:

(1) Opioid maintenance and detoxification.

(2) Appropriate clinical use of all drugs approved by the Food and Drug Administration for the treatment of opioid use disorder.

(3) Initial and periodic patient assessments, including substance use monitoring.

(4) Individualized treatment planning, overdose reversal, and relapse prevention.

(5) Counseling and recovery support services.

(6) Staffing roles and considerations.

(7) Diversion control.

(8) Other best practices, as identified by the United States Secretary of Health and Human Services.

(b) The alternative requirement that the nurse practitioner have other training or experience that the United States Secretary of Health and

Human Services determines will demonstrate the ability of the nurse practitioner to treat and manage opiate-dependent patients.

(c) The requirement that the nurse practitioner be supervised by, or work in collaboration with, a licensed physician and surgeon.

HISTORY:

Added Stats 2017 ch 242 § 1 (SB 554), effective January 1, 2018.

§ 2837. Registered nursing practice not limited

Nothing in this article shall be construed to limit the current scope of practice of a registered nurse authorized pursuant to this chapter.

HISTORY:

Added Stats 1977 ch 439 § 2.

ARTICLE 8.5

ADVANCED PRACTICE REGISTERED NURSES

Section

2837.100. Legislative intent.
2837.101. Definitions.
2837.102. Nurse Practitioner Advisory Committee.
2837.103. Requirements to perform, in certain settings or organizations, specified functions without standardized procedures.
2837.103.5. Conditional authority of nurse practitioner to prescribe, order, dispense, procure, and furnish pharmacological agents.
2837.104. Requirements to perform, outside of certain settings or organizations, specified functions without standardized procedures.
2837.105. Occupational analysis of nurse practitioners performing certain functions.

HISTORY: Added Stats 2020 ch 265 § 4 (AB 890), effective January 1, 2021.

§ 2837.100. Legislative intent

It is the intent of the Legislature that the requirements under this article shall not be an undue or unnecessary burden to licensure or practice. The requirements are intended to ensure the new category of licensed nurse practitioners has the least restrictive amount of education, training, and testing necessary to ensure competent practice.

HISTORY:

Added Stats 2020 ch 265 § 4 (AB 890), effective January 1, 2021.

§ 2837.101. Definitions

For purposes of this article, the following terms have the following meanings:

(a) "Committee" means the Nurse Practitioner Advisory Committee.

(b) "Standardized procedures" has the same meaning as that term is defined in Section 2725.

(c) "Transition to practice" means additional clinical experience and mentorship provided to prepare a nurse practitioner to practice independently. "Transition to practice" includes, but is not limited to, managing a panel of patients, working in a complex health care setting, interpersonal communication, interpersonal collaboration and team-based care, professionalism, and business management of a practice. The board shall, by regulation, define minimum standards for transition to practice. Clinical experience may include experience obtained before January 1, 2021, if the experience meets the requirements established by the board.

HISTORY:
Added Stats 2020 ch 265 § 4 (AB 890), effective January 1, 2021.

§ 2837.102. Nurse Practitioner Advisory Committee

(a) The board shall establish a Nurse Practitioner Advisory Committee to advise and make recommendations to the board on all matters relating to nurse practitioners, including, but not limited to, education, appropriate standard of care, and other matters specified by the board. The committee shall provide recommendations or guidance to the board when the board is considering disciplinary action against a nurse practitioner.

(b) The committee shall consist of four qualified nurse practitioners, two physicians and surgeons with demonstrated experience working with nurse practitioners, and one public member.

HISTORY:
Added Stats 2020 ch 265 § 4 (AB 890), effective January 1, 2021.

§ 2837.103. Requirements to perform, in certain settings or organizations, specified functions without standardized procedures

(a)(1) Notwithstanding any other law, a nurse practitioner may perform the functions specified in subdivision (c) pursuant to that subdivision, in a setting or organization specified in paragraph (2) pursuant to that paragraph, if the nurse practitioner has successfully satisfied the following requirements:

(A) Passed a national nurse practitioner board certification examination and, if applicable, any supplemental examination developed pursuant to paragraph (4) of subdivision (a) of Section 2837.105.

(B) Holds a certification as a nurse practitioner from a national certifying body accredited by the National Commission for Certifying Agencies or the American Board of Nursing Specialties and recognized by the board.

(C) Provides documentation that educational training was consistent with standards established by the board pursuant to Section 2836 and any applicable regulations as they specifically relate to requirements for clinical practice hours. Online educational programs that do not include mandatory clinical hours shall not meet this requirement.

(D) Has completed a transition to practice in California of a minimum of three full-time equivalent years of practice or 4600 hours.

(2) A nurse practitioner who meets all of the requirements of paragraph (1) may practice, including, but not limited to, performing the functions authorized pursuant to subdivision (c), in one of the following settings or organizations in which one or more physicians and surgeons practice with the nurse practitioner without standardized procedures:

(A) A clinic, as defined in Section 1200 of the Health and Safety Code.

(B) A health facility, as defined in Section 1250 of the Health and Safety Code, except for the following:

(i) A correctional treatment center, as defined in paragraph (1) of subdivision (j) of Section 1250 of the Health and Safety Code.

(ii) A state hospital, as defined in Section 4100 of the Welfare and Institutions Code.

(C) A facility described in Chapter 2.5 (commencing with Section 1440) of Division 2 of the Health and Safety Code.

(D) A medical group practice, including a professional medical corporation, as defined in Section 2406, another form of corporation controlled by physicians and surgeons, a medical partnership, a medical foundation exempt from licensure, or another lawfully organized group of physicians and surgeons that provides health care services.

(E) A home health agency, as defined in Section 1727 of the Health and Safety Code.

(F) A hospice facility licensed pursuant to Chapter 8.5 (commencing with Section 1745) of Division 2 of the Health and Safety Code.

(3) In health care agencies that have governing bodies, as defined in Division 5 of Title 22 of the California Code of Regulations, including, but not limited to, Sections 70701and 70703 of Title 22 of the California Code of Regulations, the following apply:

(A) A nurse practitioner shall adhere to all applicable bylaws.

(B) A nurse practitioner shall be eligible to serve on medical staff and hospital committees.

(C) A nurse practitioner shall be eligible to attend meetings of the department to which the nurse practitioner is assigned. A nurse practitioner shall not vote at department, division, or other meetings unless the vote is regarding the determination of nurse practitioner privileges with the organization, peer review of nurse practitioner clinical practice, whether a licensee's employment is in the best interest of the communities served by a hospital pursuant to Section 2401, or the vote is otherwise allowed by the applicable bylaws.

(b) An entity described in subparagraphs (A) to (F), inclusive, of paragraph (2) of subdivision (a) shall not interfere with, control, or otherwise direct the professional judgment of a nurse practitioner functioning pursuant to this section in a manner prohibited by Section 2400 or any other law.

(c) In addition to any other practices authorized by law, a nurse practitioner who meets the requirements of paragraph (1) of subdivision (a) may perform the following functions without standardized procedures in accordance with their education and training:

(1) Conduct an advanced assessment.

(2)(A) Order, perform, and interpret diagnostic procedures.

(B) For radiologic procedures, a nurse practitioner can order diagnostic procedures and utilize the findings or results in treating the patient. A nurse practitioner may perform or interpret clinical laboratory procedures that they are permitted to perform under Section 1206 and under the federal Clinical Laboratory Improvement Act (CLIA).

(3) Establish primary and differential diagnoses.

(4) Prescribe, order, administer, dispense, procure, and furnish therapeutic measures, including, but not limited to, the following:

(A) Diagnose, prescribe, and institute therapy or referrals of patients to health care agencies, health care providers, and community resources.

(B) Prescribe, administer, dispense, and furnish pharmacological agents, including over-the-counter, legend, and controlled substances.

(C) Plan and initiate a therapeutic regimen that includes ordering and prescribing nonpharmacological interventions, including, but not limited to, durable medical equipment, medical devices, nutrition, blood and blood products, and diagnostic and supportive services, including, but not limited to, home health care, hospice, and physical and occupational therapy.

(5) After performing a physical examination, certify disability pursuant to Section 2708 of the Unemployment Insurance Code.

(6) Delegate tasks to a medical assistant pursuant to Sections 1206.5, 2069, 2070, and 2071, and Article 2 (commencing with Section 1366) of Chapter 3 of Division 13 of Title 16 of the California Code of Regulations.

(d) A nurse practitioner shall verbally inform all new patients in a language understandable to the patient that a nurse practitioner is not a physician and surgeon. For purposes of Spanish language speakers, the nurse practitioner shall use the standardized phrase "enfermera especializada."

(e) A nurse practitioner shall post a notice in a conspicuous location accessible to public view that the nurse practitioner is regulated by the Board of Registered Nursing. The notice shall include the board's telephone number and the internet website where the nurse practitioner's license may be checked and complaints against the nurse practitioner may be made.

(f) A nurse practitioner shall refer a patient to a physician and surgeon or other licensed health care provider if a situation or condition of a patient is beyond the scope of the education and training of the nurse practitioner.

(g) A nurse practitioner practicing under this section shall have professional liability insurance appropriate for the practice setting.

(h) Any health care setting operated by the Department of Corrections and Rehabilitation is exempt from this section.

HISTORY:

Added Stats 2020 ch 265 § 4 (AB 890), effective January 1, 2021. Amended Stats 2021 ch 124 § 1 (AB 938), effective January 1, 2022.

§ 2837.103.5. Conditional authority of nurse practitioner to prescribe, order, dispense, procure, and furnish pharmacological agents

(a) Notwithstanding paragraph (1) of subdivision (a) of Section 2837.103, the authority for a nurse practitioner to prescribe, order, dispense, procure, and furnish pharmacological agents pursuant to subparagraph (B) of paragraph (4) of subdivision (c) of Section 2837.103 is conditional on all of the following:

(1) The issuance of a furnishing number by the board pursuant to Section 2836.3.

(2) If prescribing, ordering, dispensing, procuring, or furnishing controlled substances, registration with the United States Drug Enforcement Administration.

(3) If prescribing, ordering, dispensing, procuring, or furnishing Schedule II controlled substances, as part of their continuing education requirements,

completion of a course including Schedule II controlled substances, and the risks of addiction associated with their use, based on the standards developed by the board. The board shall establish the requirements for satisfactory completion of this paragraph.

(b) This section shall not be construed to require a nurse practitioner practicing pursuant to Sections 2837.103 or 2837.104 to practice under standardized procedures or physician supervision.

HISTORY:

Added Stats 2022 ch 413 § 19 (AB 2684), effective January 1, 2023.

§ 2837.104. Requirements to perform, outside of certain settings or organizations, specified functions without standardized procedures

(a) Beginning January 1, 2023, notwithstanding any other law, the following apply to a nurse practitioner who holds an active certification issued by the board pursuant to subdivision (b):

(1) The nurse practitioner may perform the functions specified in subdivision (c) of Section 2837.103 pursuant to that subdivision outside of the settings or organizations specified under subparagraphs (A) to (F), inclusive, of paragraph (2) of subdivision (a) of Section 2837.103.

(2) Subject to subdivision (f) and any applicable conflict of interest policies of the bylaws, the nurse practitioner shall be eligible for membership of an organized medical staff.

(3) Subject to subdivision (f) and any applicable conflict of interest policies of the bylaws, a nurse practitioner member may vote at meetings of the department to which nurse practitioners are assigned.

(b) The board shall issue a certificate to perform the functions specified in subdivision (c) of Section 2837.103 pursuant to that subdivision outside of the settings and organizations specified under subparagraphs (A) to (F), inclusive, of paragraph (2) of subdivision (a) of Section 2837.103, if the nurse practitioner satisfies all of the following requirements:

(1) Meets all of the requirements specified in paragraph (1) of subdivision (a) of Section 2837.103.

(2) Holds a valid and active license as a registered nurse in California and a master's degree in nursing or in a clinical field related to nursing or a doctoral degree in nursing.

(3) Has practiced as a nurse practitioner in good standing for at least three years, not inclusive of the transition to practice required pursuant to subparagraph (D) of paragraph (1) of subdivision (a) of Section 2837.103. The board may, at its discretion, lower this requirement for a nurse practitioner holding a Doctorate of Nursing Practice degree (DNP) based on practice experience gained in the course of doctoral education experience.

(c) A nurse practitioner authorized to practice pursuant to this section shall comply with all of the following:

(1) The nurse practitioner, consistent with applicable standards of care, shall not practice beyond the scope of their clinical and professional education and training, including specific areas of concentration and shall only practice within the limits of their knowledge and experience and national certification.

(2) The nurse practitioner shall consult and collaborate with other healing arts providers based on the clinical condition of the patient to whom health care is provided. Physician consultation shall be obtained as specified in the individual protocols and under the following circumstances:

(A) Emergent conditions requiring prompt medical intervention after initial stabilizing care has been started.

(B) Problem which is not resolving as anticipated after an ongoing evaluation and management of the situation.

(C) History, physical, or lab findings inconsistent with the clinical perspective.

(D) Upon request of patient.

(3) Nurse practitioner consultation with a physician and surgeon alone shall not create a physician-patient relationship. The nurse practitioner shall be solely responsible for the services they provide.

(4) The nurse practitioner shall establish a plan for referral of complex medical cases and emergencies to a physician and surgeon or other appropriate healing arts providers. The nurse practitioner shall have an identified referral plan specific to the practice area, that includes specific referral criteria. The referral plan shall address the following:

(A) Whenever situations arise which go beyond the competence, scope of practice, or experience of the nurse practitioner.

(B) Whenever patient conditions fail to respond or the patient is acutely decompensating in a manner that is not consistent with the progression of the disease and corresponding treatment plan.

(C) Any patient with a rare condition.

(D) Any patient conditions that do not fit the commonly accepted diagnostic pattern for a disease or disorder.

(E) All emergency situations after initial stabilizing care has been started.

(d) A nurse practitioner shall verbally inform all new patients in a language understandable to the patient that a nurse practitioner is not a physician and surgeon. For purposes of Spanish language speakers, the nurse practitioner shall use the standardized phrase "enfermera especializada."

(e) A nurse practitioner shall post a notice in a conspicuous location accessible to public view that the nurse practitioner is regulated by the Board of Registered Nursing. The notice shall include the board's telephone number and internet website where the nurse practitioner's license may be checked and complaints against the nurse practitioner may be made.

(f) A nurse practitioner practicing pursuant to this section shall maintain professional liability insurance appropriate for the practice setting.

(g) For purposes of this section, corporations and other artificial legal entities shall have no professional rights, privileges, or powers.

(h) Subdivision (g) shall not apply to a nurse practitioner if either of the following apply:

(1) The certificate issued pursuant to this section is inactive, surrendered, revoked, or otherwise restricted by the board.

(2) The nurse practitioner is employed pursuant to the exemptions under Section 2401.

HISTORY:
Added Stats 2020 ch 265 § 4 (AB 890), effective January 1, 2021. Amended Stats 2022 ch 413 § 20 (AB 2684), effective January 1, 2023.

§ 2837.105. Occupational analysis of nurse practitioners performing certain functions

(a)(1) The board shall request the department's Office of Professional Examination Services, or an equivalent organization, to perform an occupational analysis of nurse practitioners performing the functions specified in subdivision (c) of Section 2837.103 pursuant to that subdivision.

(2) The board, together with the Office of Professional Examination Services, shall assess the alignment of the competencies tested in the national nurse practitioner certification examination required by subparagraph (A) of paragraph (1) of subdivision (a) of Section 2837.103 with the occupational analysis performed according to paragraph (1).

(3) The occupational analysis shall be completed by January 1, 2023.

(4) If the assessment performed according to paragraph (2) identifies additional competencies necessary to perform the functions specified in subdivision (c) of Section 2837.103 pursuant to that subdivision that are not sufficiently validated by the national nurse practitioner board certification examination required by subparagraph (A) of paragraph (1) of subdivision (a) of Section 2837.103, the board shall identify and develop a supplemental exam that properly validates identified competencies.

(b) The examination process shall be regularly reviewed pursuant to Section 139.

HISTORY:
Added Stats 2020 ch 265 § 4 (AB 890), effective January 1, 2021.

ARTICLE 9

CLINICAL NURSE SPECIALISTS

Section
2838. License required.
2838.1. Qualifications and credentials.
2838.2. Standards and fees.
2838.3. Operative date of article.
2838.4. Effect of article.

HISTORY: Added Stats 1997 ch 159 § 3, operative July 1, 1998.

§ 2838. License required

No person shall advertise or hold himself or herself out as a "clinical nurse specialist" unless he or she is a nurse licensed under this chapter, and meets the standards for a clinical nurse specialist established by the board.

HISTORY:
Added Stats 1997 ch 159 § 3 (AB 90), operative July 1, 1998.

§ 2838.1. Qualifications and credentials

(a) On and after July 1, 1998, any registered nurse who holds himself or herself out as a clinical nurse specialist or who desires to hold himself or herself out as a clinical nurse specialist shall, within the time prescribed by the board and prior to his or her next license renewal or the issuance of an initial license, submit his or her education, experience, and other credentials, and any other information as required by the board to determine that the person qualifies to use the title "clinical nurse specialist."

(b) Upon finding that a person is qualified to hold himself or herself out as a clinical nurse specialist, the board shall appropriately indicate on the license issued or renewed that the person is qualified to use the title "clinical nurse specialist." The board shall also issue to each qualified person a certificate indicating that the person is qualified to use the title "clinical nurse specialist."

HISTORY:

Added Stats 1997 ch 159 § 3 (AB 90), operative July 1, 1998.

§ 2838.2. Standards and fees

(a) A clinical nurse specialist is a registered nurse with advanced education, who participates in expert clinical practice, education, research, consultation, and clinical leadership as the major components of his or her role.

(b) The board may establish categories of clinical nurse specialists and the standards required to be met for nurses to hold themselves out as clinical nurse specialists in each category. The standards shall take into account the types of advanced levels of nursing practice that are or may be performed and the clinical and didactic education, experience, or both needed to practice safety at those levels. In setting the standards, the board shall consult with clinical nurse specialists, physicians and surgeons appointed by the Medical Board of California with expertise with clinical nurse specialists, and health care organizations that utilize clinical nurse specialists.

(c) A registered nurse who meets one of the following requirements may apply to become a clinical nurse specialist:

(1) Possession of a master's degree in a clinical field of nursing.

(2) Possession of a master's degree in a clinical field related to nursing with coursework in the components referred to in subdivision (a).

(3) On or before July 1, 1998, meets the following requirements:

(A) Current licensure as a registered nurse.

(B) Performs the role of a clinical nurse specialist as described in subdivision (a).

(C) Meets any other criteria established by the board.

(d)(1) A nonrefundable fee of not less than five hundred dollars ($500), but not to exceed one thousand five hundred dollars ($1,500) shall be paid by a registered nurse applying to be a clinical nurse specialist for the evaluation of his or her qualifications to use the title "clinical nurse specialist."

(2) The fee to be paid for a temporary certificate to practice as a clinical nurse specialist shall be not less than thirty dollars ($30) nor more than fifty dollars ($50).

(3) A biennial renewal fee shall be paid upon submission of an application to renew the clinical nurse specialist certificate and shall be established by the board at no less than one hundred fifty dollars ($150) and no more than one thousand dollars ($1,000).

(4) The penalty fee for failure to renew a certificate within the prescribed time shall be 50 percent of the renewal fee in effect on the date of the renewal of the license, but not less than seventy-five dollars ($75) nor more than five hundred dollars ($500).

(5) The fees authorized by this subdivision shall not exceed the amount necessary to cover the costs to the board to administer this section.

HISTORY:

Added Stats 1997 ch 159 § 3 (AB 90), operative July 1, 1998. Amended Stats 2016 ch 799 § 22 (SB 1039), effective January 1, 2017.

§ 2838.3. Operative date of article

This article shall become operative on July 1, 1998.

HISTORY:

Added Stats 1997 ch 159 § 3 (AB 90), operative July 1, 1998.

§ 2838.4. Effect of article

Nothing in this article shall be construed to limit, revise, or expand the current scope of practice of a registered nurse.

HISTORY:

Added Stats 1997 ch 159 § 3 (AB 90), operative July 1, 1998.

Resolution of Chapter 156

Assembly Concurrent Resolution No. 103 - Relative to nursing.

[Filed with Secretary of State November 27, 1972.]

WHEREAS, The licensing laws for physicians, registered nurses, and licensed vocational nurses are ambiguous concerning the performance of certain roles by registered nurses and vocational nurses, and of the congruent roles of nurses and physicians; and

WHEREAS, commencing in 1957, the California Nurses' Association, the California Medical Association, and the California Hospital Association have developed and distributed a series of joint statements on the role of the registered nurse in meeting new and changing needs of patient care and on the congruent roles of the nurse and the physician; and

WHEREAS, the joint statements have primarily functioned to validate developments in practice after the changes have become common practice, and have not been used to anticipate new needs or to encourage responsible innovative demonstrations of methods and practice for registered nurses and licensed vocational nurses; now, therefore, be it

Resolved by the Assembly of the State of California, the Senate thereof concurring,

That it will best serve the public interest if such joint statements are utilized in cases of conflicting or absent statutory definition to validate generally accepted practices or patterns of care, and in addition, to assist the Legislature, licensing boards, other appropriate agencies, and responsible professional associations in anticipating new needs, making responsible innovations in practice patterns, and developing demonstration projects, all in the interest of patient care; and be it further

Resolved, That it is in the public interest that such joint statements are made a matter of public record for information and guidance to educators, practitioners, the public and the Legislature, and it is therefore directed that permanent files of such joint statements be maintained by the State Department of Public Health, the Board of Medical Examiners of the State of California, the California Board of Nursing Education and Nurse Registration and the Board of Vocational Nurse and Psychiatric Technician Examiners of the State of California, for public inspection; and it is further directed that the State Department of Public Health report annually to the Legislature as to new joint statements or modifications of existing joint statements; and be it further

Resolved, That the appropriate professional organizations representing physicians, registered nurses, vocational nurses, and hospitals are encouraged to form a joint practice commission which shall have as one of its purposes the encouragement, development, modification and publication of joint statements and interdisciplinary accords relating to needs and methodology of better and more effective nursing care.

EXTRACTED FROM
CALIFORNIA CODE OF REGULATIONS

TITLE 16
PROFESSIONAL AND VOCATIONAL REGULATIONS

Division
14. Board of Registered Nursing

DIVISION 14
BOARD OF REGISTERED NURSING

Article
1. General Provisions Section
2. Registration and Examination
3. Prelicensure Nursing Programs
3.5. Citations and Fines
4. Grounds for Discipline, Disciplinary Proceedings and Rehabilitation
4.1. Intervention Program Guidelines
5. Continuing Education
6. Nurse-Midwives
7. Standardized Procedure Guidelines
8. Standards for Nurse Practitioners
9. Public Health Nurse
10. Sponsored Free Health Care Events— Requirements for Exemption

ARTICLE 1
GENERAL PROVISIONS SECTION

Section
1402. Definitions.
1403. Delegation of Certain Functions.
1405. Authority of Executive Officer.

§ 1402. Definitions.

For the purpose of this chapter, the term "board" means the California Board of Registered Nursing; and the term "code" means the Business and Professions Code.

Authority cited: Section 2715, Business and Professions Code. Reference: Section 2715, Business and Professions Code.

History

1. Amendment filed 8-28-61 as procedural and organizational; designated effective 9-15-61 (Register 61, No. 17).
2. Amendment filed 3-28-75 as procedural and organizational; effective upon filing (Register 75, No. 13).
3. Amendment filed 9-27-85; effective thirtieth day thereafter (Register 85, No. 39).

§ 1403. Delegation of Certain Functions.

(a) The power and discretion conferred by law upon the board to receive and file accusations; issue notices of hearing, statements to respondent and statements of issues; receive and file notices of defense; determine the time and place of hearings under Section 11508 of the Government Code; issue subpoenas and subpoenas duces tecum; set and calendar cases for hearing and perform other functions necessary to the efficient dispatch of the business of the board in connection with proceedings under the provisions of Sections 11500 through 11528 of the Government Code, prior to the hearing of such proceedings; to approve settlement agreements for the revocation, surrender or interim suspension of a license; and the certification and delivery or mailing of copies of decisions under Section 11518 of said code are hereby delegated to and conferred upon the executive officer, or, in his/her absence from the office of the board, his/her designee.

(b) All settlement agreements for the revocation, surrender, or interim suspension of a license approved pursuant to section 1403(a) shall be reported at regularly scheduled board meetings.

Authority cited: Section 2715, Business and Professions Code. Reference: Section 2708, Business and Professions Code.

History

1. Amendment filed 5-22-84; effective thirtieth day thereafter (Register 84, No. 21).

2. Amendment filed 7-23-2014; operative 7-23-2014 pursuant to Government Code section 11343.4(b)(3) (Register 2014, No. 30).

§ 1405. Authority of Executive Officer.

The executive officer is authorized to:

(a) Plan, direct supervise and organize the work of the staff of the board.

(b) Research nursing practice issues and proposed positions to the board based on the board's interpretation of the Nursing Practice Act and other related statutes or regulations.

(c) Implement regulations adopted by the board.

(d) Administer examinations, collect fees, issue licenses and permits and investigate complaints.

(e) Implement and enforce all standards including those set for schools of nursing, which include inspecting and evaluating schools of nursing and making recommendations on accreditation.

(f) Manage funds and administer the fund and budget according to board directions.

(g) Report to the board on implementation of board policies and responses to board activity.

(h) Represent the board, as appropriate, to the public and the media.

Authority cited: Section 2715, Business and Professions Code. Reference: Section 2708, Business and Professions Code.

History

1. New section filed 10-14-53 as procedural and organizational; effective upon filing (Register 53, No. 18).

2. Renumbering from 1410.5 to 1405 and amendment filed 2-5-64; effective thirtieth day thereafter (Register 64, No. 3).

3. Amendment filed 9-27-85; effective thirtieth day thereafter (Register 85, No. 39).

ARTICLE 2
REGISTRATION AND EXAMINATION

Section

1409. Issuance of License.
1409.1. Filing of Names and Addresses.
1410. Application.
1410.1. Application Processing Times.
1410.4. Abandonment of Application.
1411.5. Examination Procedure.
1411.6. Examination Disclosure.
1412. High School Education or the Equivalent.
1413. English Comprehension.
1414. Interim Permits.
1414.1. Foreign Licensees.
1414.5. Temporary License.
1417. Fees.
1418. Eligibility for Licensure of Applicants Who Have Military Education and Experience.
1419. Renewal of License.
1419.1. Inactive License.
1419.2. Renewal Processing Times.
1419.3. Reinstatement of Expired License.
1419.4. Issuance of Duplicate License.

§ 1409. Issuance of License.

A license as a registered nurse shall be issued only by examination except as provided in Section 2732.1(b) of the code.

History

1. Amendment filed 2-23-66; effective thirtieth day thereafter (Register 66, No. 6).
2. Amendment refiled 3-8-66; effective thirtieth day thereafter (Register 66, No. 7).

§ 1409.1. Filing of Names and Addresses.

Each person holding a certificate, license or any other authority to practice nursing or engage in any activity under any laws administered by the board shall file his/her current name and mailing address with the board at its office in Sacramento within thirty (30) days after any change of name or mailing address, giving both old and new name, and address, as appropriate.

Authority cited: Section 2715, Business and Professions Code. Reference: Section 2715, Business and Professions Code.

History

1. Renumbering of former Section 1419.2 to Section 1409.1 filed 4-7-87; operative 5-7-87 (Register 87, No. 16).

§ 1410. Application.

(a) An application for a license as a registered nurse by examination shall be submitted on an application form provided by the board, and filed with the board at its office in Sacramento. An application shall be accompanied by the fee and such evidence, statements or documents as therein required including evidence of eligibility to take the examination. The applicant shall submit an additional application and fee for the examination to the board or to its examination contractor, as directed by the board.The Board shall provide the contractor's application to the applicant.No license shall be issued without a complete transcript on file indicating successful completion of the courses prescribed by the board for licensure or documentation deemed equivalent by the Board.

(b) An application for a license as a registered nurse without examination under the provisions of Section 2732.1(b) of the code shall be submitted on an application form prescribed and provided by the board, accompanied by the appropriate fee and by such evidence, statements, or documents as therein required, and filed with the board at its office in Sacramento.

(c) The applicant shall be notified in writing of the results of the evaluation of his/her application for license if the application is rejected.

Authority cited: Section 2715, Business and Professions Code. Reference: Sections 480, 2729, 2732.1, 2733, 2736, 2736.5, 2736.6, 2737 and 2815, Business and Professions Code.

History

1. Amendment filed 1-27-70; effective thirtieth day thereafter (Register 70, No. 5). For prior history, see Register 66, No. 7.
2. Amendment of subsection (a) filed 10-10-75; effective thirtieth day thereafter (Register 75, No. 41).
3. Amendment of subsection (a) filed 5-14-76; effective thirtieth day thereafter (Register 76, No. 20).
4. Amendment of subsection (a) filed 9-27-85; effective thirtieth day thereafter (Register 85, No. 39).
5. Amendment of subsections (a) and (c) and amendment of Note filed 10-2-96; operative 11-1-96 (Register 96, No. 40).
6. Amendment of subsection (a) and repealer of subsection (d) filed 5-20-98; operative 6-19-98 (Register 98, No. 21).

§ 1410.1. Application Processing Times.

(a) Within 90 calendar days of receipt of an application for original licensure as a registered nurse, provided under the provisions of section 2732.1 of the Code, the board shall inform the applicant in writing that it is either complete and accepted for filing or that it is deficient and what specific information or documentation is required to complete the application.

(b) Within 390 calendar days from the date of filing of a completed examination application for original licensure as a registered nurse, the board shall inform the applicant in writing of its decision regarding the application. This time period applies to applicants whose application is complete on the examination deadline date and who take the first available examination.

(c) Within 365 calendar days from the date of filing a completed application for original licensure as a registered nurse without examination, the board shall inform applicant in writing of its decision regarding the application.

(d) The board's actual time periods for processing an application for original licensure as a registered nurse, from the receipt of the initial application to the final decision, based on the two years preceding the proposal of this section were as follows:

Application By Examination			Application Without Examination		
Minimum	-	127 days	Minimum	-	11 days
Median	-	183 days	Median	-	62 days
Maximum	-	387 days	Maximum	-	332 days

Time periods take into account section 1410.4 (e) which provides for abandonment of incomplete applications after one year.

Authority cited: Section 2715, Business and Professions Code; and Section 15376, Government Code. Reference: Section 2732.1, Business and Professions Code; and Section 15376, Government Code.

History

1. New section filed 2-13-91; operative 3-15-91 (Register 91, No. 12).

§ 1410.4. Abandonment of Application.

(a) An applicant whose application for examination has been accepted shall be deemed to have abandoned the application if he/she does not take such examination within a two-year period from the date of the written notice of eligibility to take the examination.

(b) An applicant whose application for examination has been rejected shall be deemed to have abandoned the application if he/she does not submit evidence that he/she has removed the deficiencies specified in the written evaluation notice and take an examination within a three-year period from the date of the written evaluation notice.

(c) An applicant whose application for license without examination has been rejected shall be deemed to have abandoned the application if he/she does not submit evidence that he/she has removed the deficiencies specified in the written evaluation notice within a three-year period from the date of the written evaluation notice.

(d) Submission of additional data, requests for reconsideration or re-evaluation, or other inquiries or statements involving an application shall not extend the respective time periods specified in subdivisions (a), (b), (c), and (e) of this section.

(e) An applicant whose application for license is incomplete shall be deemed to have abandoned the application if he/she does not submit all required documents, data and information within a period of one year from the date of mailing to him/her by the board of a written notice addressed to the last address on file with the board.

(f) An application submitted subsequent to the abandonment of a former application shall be treated as a new application.The applicant must meet all current requirements in effect at the time of reapplication.

Authority cited: Section 2715, Business and Professions Code. Reference: Section 2732.1, Business and Professions Code.

History

1. Amendment filed 10-17-66; effective thirtieth day thereafter (Register 66, No. 36). For prior history, see Register 66, No. 7.
2. Repealer of subsection (f) and renumbering of subsection (g) to (f) filed 10-10-75; effective thirtieth day thereafter (Register 75, No. 41).
3. Amendment filed 9-27-85; effective thirtieth day thereafter (Register 85, No. 39).
4. Amendment of subsections (a) and (f) filed 10-2-96; operative 11-1-96 (Register 96, No. 40).

§ 1411.5. Examination Procedure.

The examination for licensure as a registered nurse shall be a written examination as determined by the board. The board may enter into a contractual agreement for said examination with a public or private organization.

Authority cited: Section 2715, Business and Professions Code. Reference: Sections 2738 and 2740, Business and Professions Code.

History

1. New section filed 1-27-70; effective thirtieth day thereafter (Register 70, No. 5).
2. Amendment filed 2-9-73; effective thirtieth day thereafter (Register 73, No. 6).
3. Amendment filed 3-23-84; effective upon filing pursuant to Government Code Section 11346.2(d) (Register 84, No. 12).

Regulations

§ 1411.6. Examination Disclosure.

An applicant who takes the examination shall not disclose the contents of the written examination questions to anyone other than a person authorized by the Board. No one except as authorized by the Board shall solicit, accept, or compile information regarding the contents of written examination questions, either before, during or after the administration of any examination.

Authority cited: Section 2715, Business and Professions Code. Reference: Section 2740, Business and Professions Code.

History

1. New section filed 3-22-82; effective thirtieth day thereafter (Register 82, No. 13).

§ 1412. High School Education or the Equivalent.

An applicant must meet the general preliminary education requirement of a high school education in the United States or the equivalent. Upon request of the Board, an applicant shall provide evidence of education equivalent to completion of a high school course of study in the United States by submitting one of the following:

(a) A high school diploma received from a U.S. high school.

(b) A General Education Development Certificate.

(c) A degree from any junior college, college or university accredited by a state agency authorized to accredit such institutions.

(d) An evaluation by a high school, unified school district, junior college, college, university or board of education which the board determines, after review, establishes that an education equivalent to a high school education in the United States was obtained in this or another state or in any foreign country.

Authority cited: Section 2715, Business and Professions Code. Reference: Section 2736, Business and Professions Code.

History

1. Amendment filed 1-27-70; effective thirtieth day thereafter (Register 70, No. 5). For prior history, see Register 66, No. 7.
2. Amendment filed 3-16-77; effective thirtieth day thereafter (Register 77, No. 12).
3. Amendment filed 9-27-85; effective thirtieth day thereafter (Register 85, No. 39).
4. Amendment of subsection (b) filed 4-7-87; operative 5-7-87 (Register 87, No. 16).
5. Amendment filed 9-21-99; operative 10-21-99 (Register 99, No. 39).

§ 1413. English Comprehension.

When the Board has reasonable doubt of an applicant's ability to comprehend the English language to a degree sufficient to permit him to discharge his duties as a Professional Nurse in this State with safety to the public, the Board shall require him to pass an examination to demonstrate such ability.

History

1. New section filed 2-5-64; effective thirtieth day thereafter (Register 64, No. 3). For history of former Section 1413 see Register 27, No. 5.

§ 1414. Interim Permits.

(a) An applicant whose application for licensure in California by examination has been approved will be eligible for an interim permit if the applicant has completed the educational requirements for licensure in nursing. (If the applicant is taking the examination as a graduate, the interim permit may be issued upon graduation. If the applicant is taking the examination as a non-graduate, the interim permit may be issued upon completion of the educational requirements for licensure.)

(b) An interim permit is not renewable and is in effect to the expiration date or until the results of the examination are mailed, at which time it becomes null and void.

(c) A permittee shall practice under the direct supervision of a registered nurse who shall be present and available on the patient care unit during all the time the permittee is rendering professional services. The supervising registered nurse may delegate to the permittee any function taught in the permittee's basic nursing program which, in the judgment of the supervising registered nurse, the permittee is capable of performing.

(d) An interim permittee is not authorized to use any other title or designation than "I.P." or "permittee" or "nurse permittee" or "nurse interim permittee."

(e) As an applicant for a license, the permittee is subject to the disciplinary provisions of Sections 2761and 2762 of the Business and Professions Code as is the Registered Nurse.

Authority cited: Section 2715, Business and Professions Code. Reference: Section 2732.1, Business and Professions Code.

History

1. New section filed 4-6-79; effective thirtieth day thereafter (Register 79, No. 14).
2. Amendment of subsection (c) filed 6-17-85; effective thirtieth day thereafter (Register 85, No. 25).
3. Amendment of subsection (c) filed 9-27-85; effective thirtieth day thereafter (Register 85, No. 39).
4. Amendment of subsection (a) filed 4-7-87; operative 5-7-87 (Register 87, No. 16).
5. Amendment of subsections (a) and (b) filed 10-2-96; operative 11-1-96 (Register 96, No. 40).

§ 1414.1. Foreign Licensees.

An applicant who is currently licensed in a foreign country and who meets the educational requirements in Section 2736 may be issued an interim permit, subject to the conditions set forth in subsections (b), (c), (d), and (e) of Section 1414.

Authority cited: Section 2715, Business and Professions Code. Reference: Sections 2732.1, 2732.15 and 2736, Business and Professions Code.

History

1. New section filed 5-22-80; effective thirtieth day thereafter (Register 80, No. 21).
2. Amendment filed 9-27-85; effective thirtieth day thereafter (Register 85, No. 39).

§ 1414.5. Temporary License.

(a) A person who meets the requirements of Section 2733 of the code may apply for a temporary license.

(b) An applicant whose application for a temporary license has been rejected shall be deemed to have abandoned the application if he/she does not submit evidence that he/she has removed the deficiencies specified in the written evaluation notice within a one-year period from the date of the written evaluation notice.

Authority cited: Sections 2715 and 2733, Business and Professions Code. Reference: Section 2732.1, Business and Professions Code.

History

1. New section filed 9-27-85; effective thirtieth day thereafter (Register 85, No. 39).

§ 1417. Fees.

Pursuant to sections 2746.53, 2786.5, 2815, 2815.1, 2815.5, 2815.7, 2816, 2830.7, 2831, 2833, 2836.3 and 2838.2 of the code, the following fees are established:

(a)	Interim Permit Fee	$100

Regulations

(b)	Application Fee for Licensure by Examination for a California Graduate from an Approved California School	$300
(c)	Application Fee for Licensure by Examination from a Graduate in Another State, District or Territory of the United States	$350
(d)	Application Fee for Licensure by Examination by an International Graduate	$750
(e)	Application Fee for Repeat Examination	$250
(f)	Temporary License Fee	$100
(g)	Application Fee for Endorsement by a Registered Nurse in Another State, District or Territory of the United States	$350
(h)	Application Fee for Endorsement by an International RN	$750
(i)	Biennial Registered Nurse Renewal Fee	$190
	(1) Renewal fee - BRN	$180
	(2) RN Education Fund Administered by Office of Statewide Health Planning and Development	$10
(j)	Penalty Fee for Failure to Timely Renew a Registered Nurse License	$90
(k)	Application Fee for Reinstatement of Lapsed License	$350
(*l*)	Temporary Nurse Practitioner Certification Fee	$150
(m)	Nurse Practitioner Certification Application Fee	$500
(n)	Biennial Nurse Practitioner Renewal Fee	$150
(o)	Penalty Fee for Failure to Timely Renew Nurse Practitioner certification	$75
(p)	Application Fee for Certified Nurse Practitioner Furnishing	$400
(q)	Biennial Certified Nurse Practitioner Furnishing Fee	$162
	(1) Renewal Fee - BRN	$150
	(2) Controlled Substance Utilization Review and Evaluation System Fee	$12
(r)	Penalty Fee for Failure to Timely Renew Certified Nurse Practitioner Furnishing	$75
(s)	Temporary Nurse-Midwife Certification Fee	$150
(t)	Nurse-Midwife Certification Application Fee	$500
(u)	Fee for Application for Nurse-Midwife Equivalency Examination	$200
(v)	Biennial Nurse-Midwife Certification Renewal Fee	$150
(w)	Penalty Fee for Failure to Timely Renew Nurse-Midwife Certification	$75
(x)	Application Fee for Certified Nurse-Midwife $150 Furnishing	$400
(y)	Biennial Certified Nurse-Midwife Furnishing Fee	$162
	(1) Renewal Fee - BRN	$150
	(2) Controlled Substance Utilization Review and Evaluation System Fee	$12
(z)	Penalty Fee for Failure to Timely Renew Certified Nurse-Midwife Furnishing	$75
(aa)	Temporary Nurse Anesthetists Certification Fee	$150
(ab)	Nurse Anesthetists Certification Application Fee	$500
(ac)	Biennial Nurse Anesthetists Certification Renewal Fee	$150
(ad)	Penalty Fee for Failure to Timely Renew Nurse Anesthetists Certification	$75
(ae)	Temporary Clinical Nurse Specialist Fee	$30
(af)	Clinical Nurse Specialist Application Fee	$500

(ag)	Biennial Clinical Nurse Specialist Renewal Fee	$150
(ah)	Penalty Fee for Failure to Timely Renew Clinical Nurse Specialist	$75
(ai)	Temporary Public Health Nurse Fee	$150
(aj)	Public Health Nurse Application Fee	$500
(ak)	Biennial Public Health Nurse Renewal Fee	$125
(al)	Psychiatric/Mental Health Nurse Application Fee	$350
(am)	Application Fee for Continuing Education Provider Approval	$750
(an)	Biennial Continuing Education Provider Renewal Fee	$750
(ao)	Penalty Fee for Failure to Timely Renew a Continuing Education Provider Approval	$375
(ap)	Application Fee for an Institution of Higher Education or a Private Postsecondary School of Nursing Approval	$40,000
(aq)	Fee for Continuing Approval of a Nursing Program Established After January 1, 2013	$15,000
(ar)	Fee for Authorizing of a Substantive Change to an Approval of a School of Nursing	$2,500
(as)	Duplicate License Fee	$50
(at)	Duplicate Wall Certification Fee	$60
(au)	Copy of NCLEX-RN Results	$60
(av)	Certified Copy of a School Transcript	$50
(aw)	Fee for Processing Endorsement Papers to Other States	$100
(ax)	Confirmation of License Certification	$20
(ay)	Penalty Fee for Dishonored Check	$30

Regulations

Authority cited: Section 2715, Business and Professions Code. Reference: Sections 163.5, 208(a), 2733, 2746.53, 2786.5, 2811, 2811.5, 2815, 2815.1, 2815.5, 2815.7, 2816, 2830.7, 2831, 2833, 2836.1, 2836.2, 2836.3 and 2838.2, Business and Professions Code.

History

1. Amendment of subsections (b), (c) and (g) filed 9-3-85; effective upon filing pursuant to Government Code section 11346.2(d) (Register 85, No. 36). For prior history, see Register 84, No. 42.

2. Amendment filed 4-27-87; operative 5-27-87 (Register 87, No. 19).

3. Amendment of subsections (b) and (c) filed 9-27-89; operative 9-27-89 pursuant to Government Code section 11346.2(d) (Register 89, No. 40).

4. Amendment of subsections (a), (b), (c) and (g) filed 2-4-91; operative 7-1-91 (Register 91, No. 10).

5. Change without regulatory effect amending section filed 1-8-92 pursuant to section 100, title 1, California Code of Regulations; operative 1-1-92 (Register 92, No. 11).

6. Amendment of subsection (a), new subsection (a)(25) and amendment of Note filed 9-2-98; operative 10-2-98 (Register 98, No. 36).

7. Amendment of section and Note filed 11-24-2010; operative 12-24-2010 (Register 2010, No. 48).

8. Amendment filed 8-20-2015 as an emergency; operative 8-20-2015 (Register 2015, No. 34). A Certificate of Compliance must be transmitted to OAL by 2-16-2016 or emergency language will be repealed by operation of law on the following day.

9. Amendment refiled 2-8-2016 as an emergency; operative 2-16-2016 (Register 2016, No. 7). A Certificate of Compliance must be transmitted to OAL by 5-16-2016 or emergency language will be repealed by operation of law on the following day.

10. Certificate of Compliance as to 2-16-2016 order, including further amendment of subsection (23), new subsections (23)(a)-(b) and amendment of Note, transmitted to OAL 3-18-2016 and filed 4-28-2016; amendments operative 4-28-2016 pursuant to Government Code section 11343.4(b)(3) (Register 2016, No. 18).

11. Amendment of section and Note filed 10-15-2018; operative 10-15-2018 pursuant to Government Code section 11343.4(b)(3) (Register 2018, No. 42).

Regulations

§ 1418. Eligibility for Licensure of Applicants Who Have Military Education and Experience.

An applicant who presents with relevant military education and experience, and who presents documentation from a board-approved registered prelicensure nursing program of equivalency credit evaluation that provides evidence of meeting, in whole or in part, the minimum standards for competency set forth in Section 1443.5 and minimum education requirements of licensure listed pursuant to Sections 1426(c)(1) to (3), utilizing challenge examination or other evaluative methods, will be considered to meet, in whole or in part, the education requirements for licensure.

Authority cited: Sections 2715 and 2786.1, Business and Professions Code. Reference: Sections 2786 and 2786.1, Business and Professions Code.

History

1. New section filed 10-28-76; effective thirtieth day thereafter (Register 76, No. 44).
2. Amendment filed 9-27-85; effective thirtieth day thereafter (Register 85, No. 39).
3. Repealer and new section filed 3-9-2000; operative 4-8-2000 (Register 2000, No. 10).
4. Amendment of section heading, repealer and new section and amendment of Note filed 10-8-2018; operative 10-8-2018 pursuant to Government Code section 11343.4(b)(3) (Register 2018, No. 41).

§ 1419. Renewal of License.

(a)A renewal application shall be on the form provided by the board, accompanied by the fee specified in Section 1417(a)(3) and required information and filed with the board at its office in Sacramento.

(b) For a license that expires on or after March 1, 2009, as a condition of renewal, an applicant for renewal not previously fingerprinted by the board, or for whom a record of the submission of fingerprints no longer exists, is required to furnish to the Department of Justice, as directed by the board, a full set of fingerprints for the purpose of conducting a criminal history record check and to undergo a state and federal level criminal offender record information search conducted through the Department of Justice. Failure to submit a full set of fingerprints to the Department of Justice on or before the date required for renewal of a license is grounds for discipline by the board. It shall be certified on the renewal form whether the fingerprints have been submitted. This requirement is waived if the license is renewed in an inactive status, or the licensee is actively serving in the military outside the country.

(c) As a condition of renewal, an applicant for renewal shall disclose on the renewal form whether, since he or she last renewed his or her license, he or she has been convicted of any violation of the law in this or any other state, the United States or its territories, military court, or other country, omitting traffic infractions under $1,000 not involving alcohol, dangerous drugs, or a controlled substance.

(d) As a condition of renewal, an applicant for renewal shall disclose on the renewal form whether, since he or she last renewed his or her license, he or she has had a license disciplined by a government agency or other disciplinary body. Discipline includes, but is not limited to, suspension, revocation, voluntary surrender, probation, reprimand, or any other restriction on a license held.

(e) Failure to provide all of the information required by this section renders any application for renewal incomplete and not eligible for renewal.

Authority cited: Sections 2708.1, 2715, 2761(a)(4) and 2761(f), Business and Professions Code. Reference: Sections 2715, 2761(f), 2765 and 2811, Business and Professions Code; and Section 11105(b)(10), Penal Code.

History

1. New section filed 9-27-85; effective thirtieth day thereafter (Register 85, No. 39). For history of former Section 1419, see Registers 64, No. 3, and 27, No. 5.
2. Amendment filed 2-1-96; operative 3-2-96 (Register 96, No. 5).
3. Amendment of section and Note filed 11-24-2008 as an emergency; operative 11-24-2008 (Register 2008, No. 48). A Certificate of Compliance must be transmitted to OAL by 5-26-2009 or emergency language will be repealed by operation of law on the following day.
4. Certificate of Compliance as to 11-24-2008 order, including further amendment of section and Note, transmitted to OAL 4-29-2009 and filed 6-2-2009 (Register 2009, No. 23).
5. Editorial correction of subsection (b) (Register 2009, No. 25).
6. Amendment of subsection (c) filed 4-22-2014; operative 4-22-2014 pursuant to Government Code section 11343.4(b)(3) (Register 2014, No. 17).

§ 1419.1. Inactive License.

A license may be maintained in an inactive status by paying the renewal fee as it becomes due. The licensee shall not practice nursing during the time the license is inactive.

To activate an inactive license, the licensee must submit a written request and evidence of 30 hours of approved continuing education taken during the two year period immediately preceding the request for activation. A licensee activating a license pursuant to this section shall furnish a full set of fingerprints as required by and set out in section 1419(b) as a condition of activation.

Authority cited: Sections 2708.1, 2715 and 2761(f), Business and Professions Code. Reference: Sections 2734 and 2761(f), Business and Professions Code; and Section 11105(b)(10), Penal Code.

History

1. New section filed 9-27-85; effective thirtieth day thereafter (Register 85, No. 39).
2. Amendment of second paragraph and Note filed 11-24-2008 as an emergency; operative 11-24-2008 (Register 2008, No. 48). A Certificate of Compliance must be transmitted to OAL by 5-26-2009 or emergency language will be repealed by operation of law on the following day.
3. Certificate of Compliance as to 11-24-2008 order transmitted to OAL 4-29-2009 and filed 6-2-2009 (Register 2009, No. 23).

§ 1419.2. Renewal Processing Times.

(a) Within 60 calendar days of receipt of a renewal form from a registered nurse, the board shall inform the nurse in writing that it is either complete and accepted for processing or that it is deficient and what specific information or documentation is required to complete the renewal form.

(b) Within 60 calendar days of receipt of a completed renewal form from a registered nurse, the board shall inform the nurse in writing of the renewal decision.

(c) The board's actual time periods for processing registered nurse renewals, from the receipt of the initial renewal form to the final decision, based on the two years preceding the proposal of this section were as follows:

Minimum	-	9 days
Median	-	19 days
Maximum	-	107 days

Authority cited: Section 2715, Business and Professions Code; and Section 15376, Government Code. Reference: Section 2811, Business and Professions Code; and Section 15376, Government Code.

Regulations

History
1. New section filed 2-13-91 section filed 2; operative 3-15-91 (Register 91, No. 12).

§ 1419.3. Reinstatement of Expired License.

In the event a licensee does not renew his/her license as provided in Section 2811 of the code, the license expires. A licensee renewing pursuant to this section shall furnish a full set of fingerprints as required by and set out in section 1419(b) as a condition of renewal.

(a) A licensee may renew a license that has not been expired for more than eight years by paying the renewal and penalty fees as specified in Section 1417 and providing evidence of 30 hours of continuing education taken within the prior two-year period.

(b) A licensee may renew a license that has been expired for more than eight years by paying the renewal and penalty fees specified in Section 1417 and providing evidence that he or she holds a current valid active and clear registered nurse license in another state, a United States territory, or Canada, or by passing the Board's current examination for licensure.

Authority cited: Sections 2708.1, 2715, 2761(f) and 2811.5, Business and Professions Code. Reference: Sections 2761(f), 2811 and 2811.5, Business and Professions Code; and Section 11105(b)(10), Penal Code.

History
1. New section filed 9-27-85; effective thirtieth day thereafter (Register 85, No. 39).
2. Change without regulatory effect amending section filed 12-29-98 pursuant to section 100, title 1, California Code of Regulations (Register 99, No. 1).
3. Amendment filed 9-19-2001; operative 10-19-2001 (Register 2001, No. 38).
4. Amendment of first paragraph and Note filed 11-24-2008 as an emergency; operative 11-24-2008 (Register 2008, No. 48). A Certificate of Compliance must be transmitted to OAL by 5-26-2009 or emergency language will be repealed by operation of law on the following day.
5. Certificate of Compliance as to 11-24-2008 order transmitted to OAL 4-29-2009 and filed 6-2-2009 (Register 2009, No. 23).

§ 1419.4. Issuance of Duplicate License.

A licensee shall report a lost or stolen license within ten (10) days of the loss and shall request, in writing, replacement of the lost license and pay the fee specified in Section 1417 (a)(13). A licensee may be required to submit a notarized statement explaining the circumstances of the loss, and/or file a license renewal form provided by the board.

Authority cited: Section 2715, Business and Professions Code. Reference: Section 2815, Business and Professions Code.

History
1. New section filed 9-27-85; effective thirtieth day thereafter (Register 85, No. 39).
2. Amendment filed 4-7-87; operative 5-7-87 (Register 87, No. 16).
3. Amendment filed 2-1-96; operative 3-2-96 (Register 96, No. 5).

ARTICLE 3
PRELICENSURE NURSING PROGRAMS

Section
1420. Definitions.
1421. Application for Approval.
1422. Certificate of Approval.
1423. Approval Requirements.
1423.1. Grounds for Denial or Removal of Board Approval.
1423.2. Denial or Revocation of Approval of a Nursing Program.

1424. Administration and Organization of the Nursing Program.
1425. Faculty—Qualifications and Changes.
1425.1. Faculty Responsibilities.
1426. Required Curriculum.
1426.1. Preceptorship.
1427. Clinical Facilities.
1428. Student Participation.
1428.6. Policies Relating to Establishing Eligibility for Examination.
1429. Licensed Vocational Nurses, Thirty (30) Semester or Forty-Five (45) Quarter Unit Option.
1430. Previous Education Credit.
1431. Licensing Examination Pass Rate Standard.
1432. Changes to an Approved Program.

§ 1420. Definitions.

For purposes of this article, the term:

(a) "Affiliated institution" means a non-institution of higher education, such as a hospital, that is approved or has applied for board approval for a nursing program and is affiliated with an institution of higher education pursuant to section 2786 of the code;

(b) "Approved nursing program" means a school, program, department or division of nursing in this state approved under the provisions of sections 2785 through 2789 of the code and this article;

(c) "Assistant Director" means a registered nurse administrator or faculty member who meets the qualifications of section 1425(b) and is designated by the director to assist in the administration of the program and perform the functions of the director when needed;

(d) "Clinically competent" means that the nursing program faculty member possesses and exercises the degree of learning, skill, care and experience ordinarily possessed and exercised by staff level registered nurses of the nursing area to which the faculty member is assigned;

(e) "Clinical practice" means the planned learning experiences designed for students to apply nursing knowledge and skills to meet course objectives in a variety of board-approved clinical settings. Clinical practice includes learning experiences provided in various health care agencies as well as nursing skills labs, simulation labs, and computer labs;

(f) "Content expert" means an instructor who has the responsibility to review and monitor the program's entire curricular content for a designated nursing area of geriatrics, medical-surgical, mental health/psychiatric nursing, obstetrics, or pediatrics;

(g) "Course of instruction" means the minimum education program that meets the requirements of section 1426 for eligibility to take the licensing examination and that is not less than two (2) academic years or equivalent;

(h) "Director" means the registered nurse administrator or faculty member who meets the qualifications of section 1425(a) and has the authority and responsibility to administer the program. The director coordinates and directs all activities in developing, implementing, and managing a nursing program, including its fiscal planning;

(i) "Faculty" means all registered nurses who teach in an approved nursing program;

(j) "Institution of higher education" means an educational setting that provides post-secondary or higher education, such as a university, a community college offering an associate degree, or other collegial institution that grants associate of arts degrees or baccalaureate or higher degrees to graduates of the nursing program;

(k) "Learning experience" means those activities planned for students by the faculty that are designed to meet the objectives of the required course of instruction, including the basic standards of competent performance in section 1443.5;

(*l*) "Nursing process" means the application of scientific, evidence-based knowledge in the identification and treatment of actual or potential patient health problems. The nursing process includes assessment, nursing diagnosis, planning and outcome identification, implementation, and evaluation;

(m) "Non-faculty" means all persons other than faculty members who meet the minimum qualifications of clinical teaching assistant and are selected by the nursing program to teach or supervise nursing students in designated nursing areas;

(n) "Preceptor" means a registered nurse who meets the qualifications set out in section 1426.1(b)(3)(A) through (D), employed by a health care agency, who is assigned to assist and supervise nursing students in an educational experience that is designed and directed by a faculty member;

(o) "Prelicensure registered nursing program" means an institution of higher education or affiliated institution that offers a course of instruction to prepare students for entry level registered nurse practice and to take the licensing examination;

(p) "Technology" means equipment, tools, and devices that are used to facilitate and support the teaching and learning of the nursing program's board-approved curriculum;

(q) "Year" means an academic year, unless otherwise specified.

Authority cited: Section 2715, Business and Professions Code. Reference: Sections 2785-2788, Business and Professions Code.

History

1. Repealer of Article 3 (Sections 1420-1435.5, not consecutive) and new Article 3 (Sections 1420-1430, not consecutive) filed 9-27-85; effective thirtieth day thereafter (Register 85, No. 39). For prior history, including former Sections 1419, 1422.2, 1422.3, 1424, 1425.5, 1426, 1427.5, 1427.6, 1429, 1430, 1433.05, 1433.1-1433.3, 1436 and 1437, see Registers 85, No. 25; 78, No. 9; 77, Nos. 47 and 34; 76, No. 47; 75, Nos. 41 and 33; 74, No. 13; 73, No. 40; 72, No. 53; 70, No. 5; 68, No. 24; 66, Nos. 37, 7 and 6; 64, No. 3; 61, Nos. 13 and 7; 60, No. 21; 57, No. 15; 55, No. 4; 54, No. 8; 53, No. 18; 27, No. 5; 26, No. 4 and 20, No. 1.

2. Amendment of article heading and section filed 9-21-2010; operative 10-21-2010 (Register 2010, No. 39).

§ 1421. Application for Approval.

(a) An institution of higher education or affiliated institution applying for approval of a new prelicensure registered nursing program (program applicant) shall be in the state and shall comply with the requirements specified in the board's document entitled, "Instructions for Institutions Seeking Approval of a New Prelicensure Registered Nursing Program", (EDP-I-01Rev 03/10), ("Instructions"), which is hereby incorporated by reference, including:

(1) Notify the board in writing of its intent to offer a new program that complies with board requirements;

(2) Submit a feasibility study in accordance with the requirements specified in the "Instructions";

(3) Appoint a director who meets the requirements of section 1425(a). Such appointment shall be made upon board acceptance of the feasibility study for the proposed program.

(4) After acceptance of the feasibility study by the board, and no later than six (6) months prior to the proposed date for enrollment of students, submit a self-study to the board in accordance with the requirements specified in the "Instructions" demonstrating how the program will meet the requirements of sections 1424 through 1432 of this article and sections 2786.6(a) and (b) of the code.

(5) Have a representative at public meetings of the board and board committee pursuant to the "Instructions" when the feasibility study and self-study are considered.

(b) The board shall consider the feasibility study and accept, reject, or defer action on the study to permit the program applicant time to provide additional information to be considered, based upon the following criteria:

(1) Evidence of initial and sustainable budgetary provisions for the proposed program;

(2) Institution of higher education's authority to grant an associate of arts, baccalaureate, or higher degree;

(3) For an affiliated institution, an agreement with an institution of higher education in the same general location authorized to grant an associate of arts, baccalaureate, or higher degree to students successfully completing the nursing program;

(4) Evidence of availability of clinical placements for students of the proposed program;

(5) Plans for administrative and faculty recruitment to staff the proposed program.

(c) The board's designee shall review the self-study, conduct a site visit of the proposed program, and submit a written report to the board that contains findings as to whether the application and supporting documentation for the proposed program comply with the requirements set forth in (a)(4).

(d) The board shall consider the application along with the written report and may thereafter grant or deny approval, or defer action on the application. The board's decision is based on the applicant's demonstration that it meets the requirements of sections 1424 through 1432 and sections 2786.6(a) and (b) of the code.

Authority cited: Sections 2715, 2786 and 2786.6, Business and Professions Code. Reference: Sections 2786 and 2786.6, Business and Professions Code.

History

1. Amendment of section heading and section filed 9-21-2010; operative 10-21-2010 (Register 2010, No. 39).

§ 1422. Certificate of Approval.

(a) A certificate of approval shall be issued to each nursing program when it is initially approved by the board.

(b) The board shall revoke a nursing program's approval, and the program shall return the certificate of approval to the board under the following conditions:

(1) The institution of higher education cannot grant degrees; or

(2) The board determines that the nursing program is in non-compliance with the requirements set forth in this article or sections 2786 through 2788 of the code.

Authority cited: Section 2715, Business and Professions Code. Reference: Sections 2786-2788, Business and Professions Code.

History

1. Amendment of section heading and section filed 9-21-2010; operative 10-21-2010 (Register 2010, No. 39)

§ 1423. Approval Requirements.

(a) In order for a program to be approved by the board or to retain its approval, it shall comply with all requirements set forth in this article and in sections 2786 through 2788 of the code.

(b) A material misrepresentation of fact by a program applicant or an approved nursing program in any information required to be submitted to the board is grounds for denial of approval or revocation of the program's approval.

Authority cited: Section 2715, Business and Professions Code. Reference: Sections 2786-2788, Business and Professions Code.

History

1. Amendment of section heading and section filed 9-21-2010; operative 10-21-2010 (Register 2010, No. 39)

§ 1423.1. Grounds for Denial or Removal of Board Approval.

The board shall deny approval and shall remove approval of a prelicensure nursing program that:

(a) Fails to provide evidence of granting credit, in the field of nursing, for previous education, including military education and experience, through an established policy and procedure, to evaluate and grant credit.

(1) Each prelicensure program shall have a policy and procedures that describe the process to award credits for specific course(s), including the prior military education and experience, through challenge examinations or other methods of evaluation for meeting academic credits and licensure requirements.

(2) Each program shall make information regarding evaluation of and granting credit in the field of nursing for previous education, including military education and experience, for purpose of establishing equivalency or granting credit, available to applicants in published documents, such as college catalog or student handbook and online, so that it is available to the public and to the board.

(3) Each program shall maintain a record that shows applicants and results of transferred/challenged credits, including applicants who applied for transfer of military education and experience.

(b) Fails to provide opportunity for applicants with military education and experience for equivalent academic credit through challenge examination or other method of evaluation.

Authority cited: Sections 2786, 2786.1 and 2788, Business and Professions Code. Reference: Sections 2786.1 and 2786.6, Business and Professions Code.

History

1. New section filed 10-8-2018; operative 10-8-2018 pursuant to Government Code section 11343.4(b)(3) (Register 2018, No. 41).

§ 1423.2. Denial or Revocation of Approval of a Nursing Program.

(a) Upon presenting evidence of noncompliance with Article 3 and lack of demonstrated corrective actions to remove noncompliance, the board may take actions to:

(1) Deny approval of a nursing program; or

(2) Revoke approval from a nursing program; or

(3) Place a nursing program on a warning status with intent to revoke approval; or

(4) Revoke approval when a program has been on a warning status for one year and the program fails to show substantive corrective changes.

(b) The board shall provide specific requirements for correction of noncompliance findings and a return date for review of the program's approval status.

Authority cited: Sections 2786, 2786.1 and 2788, Business and Professions Code. Reference: Section 2786.1, Business and Professions Code.

History

1. New section filed 10-8-2018; operative 10-8-2018 pursuant to Government Code section 11343.4(b)(3) (Register 2018, No. 41).

§ 1424. Administration and Organization of the Nursing Program.

(a) There shall be a written statement of philosophy and objectives that serves as a basis for curriculum structure. Such statement shall take into consideration the individual difference of students, including their cultural and ethnic background, learning styles, goals, and support systems. It shall also take into consideration the concepts of nursing and man in terms of nursing activities, the environment, the health-illness continuum, and relevant knowledge from related disciplines.

(b) The policies and procedures by which the program is administered shall be in writing, shall reflect the philosophy and objectives of the program, and shall be available to all students.

(1) The nursing program shall have a written plan for evaluation of the total program, including admission and selection procedures, attrition and retention of students, and performance of graduates in meeting community needs.

(2) The program shall have a procedure for resolving student grievances.

(3) The program shall have policies and procedures regarding the granting of credit for military education and acquired knowledge by providing opportunity to obtain credit by the following methods, including but not limited to the listed methods:

(A) the use of challenge examinations; or

(B) the use of evaluative methods to validate achievement of course objectives and competencies.

(4) The program shall make available the policies and procedures, including the acceptance of military coursework and experience, on the school's website.

(c) There shall be an organizational chart which identifies the relationships, lines of authority and channels of communication within the program, between the program and other administrative segments of the institution with which it is affiliated, and between the program, the institution and clinical agencies.

(d) The program shall have sufficient resources, including faculty, library, staff and support services, physical space and equipment, including technology, to achieve the program's objectives.

(e) The director and the assistant director shall dedicate sufficient time for the administration of the program.

(f) The program shall have a board-approved assistant director who is knowledgeable and current regarding the program and the policies and procedures by which it is administered, and who is delegated the authority to perform the director's duties in the director's absence.

(g) Faculty members shall have the primary responsibility for developing policies and procedures, planning, organizing, implementing and evaluating all aspects of the program.

(h) The faculty shall be adequate in type and number to develop and implement the program approved by the board, and shall include at least one qualified instructor in each of the areas of nursing required by section 1426(d) who will be the content expert in that area. Nursing faculty members whose teaching responsibilities include subject matter directly related to the practice of nursing shall be clinically competent in the areas to which they are assigned.

(i) When a non-faculty individual participates in the instruction and supervision of students obtaining clinical experience, his or her responsibilities shall be described in writing and kept on file by the nursing program.

(j) The assistant director shall function under the supervision of the director. Instructors shall function under the supervision of the director or the assistant director. Assistant instructors and clinical teaching assistants shall function under the supervision of an instructor.

(k) The student/teacher ratio in the clinical setting shall be based on the following criteria:

(1) Acuity of patient needs;

(2) Objectives of the learning experience;

(3) Class level of the students;

(4) Geographic placement of students;

(5) Teaching methods; and

(6) Requirements established by the clinical agency.

Authority cited: Sections Sections 2715, 2786, 2786.1 and 2786.6, Business and Professions Code. Reference: Sections 2786-2788, Business and Professions Code.

History

1. Amendment of subsections (b) and (g) filed 4-27-87; operative 5-27-87 (Register 87, No. 18).
2. Amendment filed 9-21-2010; operative 10-21-2010 (Register 2010, No. 39).
3. New subsections (b)(3)-(4) and amendment of Note filed 10-8-2018; operative 10-8-2018 pursuant to Government Code section 11343.4(b)(3) (Register 2018, No. 41).
4. Editorial correction reinstating inadvertently omitted subsection (i) (Register 2019, No. 3).

§ 1425. Faculty—Qualifications and Changes.

All faculty, the director, and the assistant director shall be approved by the board pursuant to the document, "Faculty Qualifications and Changes Explanation of CCR 1425 (EDP-R-02 Rev 09/2012), which is incorporated herein by reference. A program shall report to the board all changes in faculty, including changes in teaching areas, prior to employment of, or within 30 days after, termination of employment of a faculty member. Such changes shall be reported on forms provided by the board: Faculty Approval/Resignation Notification form (EDP-P-02, Rev 09/2012) and Director or Assistant Director Approval form (EDP-P-03, Rev 09/2012), which are herein incorporated by reference. Each faculty member, director, and assistant director shall hold a clear and active license issued by the board and shall possess the following qualifications:

(a) The director of the program shall meet the following minimum qualifications:

(1) A master's or higher degree from an accredited college or university which includes course work in nursing, education or administration;

(2) One (1) year's experience as an administrator with validated performance of administrative responsibilities consistent with section 1420(h);

(3) Two (2) years' experience teaching in pre-or post-licensure registered nursing programs; and

(4) One (1) year's continuous, full-time or its equivalent experience direct patient care as a registered nurse; or

(5) Equivalent experience and/or education, as determined by the board.

(b) The assistant director shall meet the education requirements set forth in subsection (a)(1) above and the experience requirements set forth in subsections (a)(3) and (a)(4) above, or such experience as the board determines to be equivalent.

(c) An instructor shall meet the following minimum qualifications:

(1) The education requirements set forth in subsection (a)(1); and

(2) Direct patient care experience within the previous five (5) years in the nursing area to which he or she is assigned, which can be met by:

(A) One (1) year's continuous, full-time or its equivalent experience providing direct patient care as a registered nurse in the designated nursing area; or

(B) One (1) academic year of registered nurse level clinical teaching experience in the designated nursing area or its equivalent that demonstrates clinical competency; and

(3) Completion of at least one (1) year's experience teaching courses related to registered nursing or completion of a post-baccalaureate course which includes practice in teaching registered nursing.

(d) An assistant instructor shall meet the following minimum qualifications:

(1) A baccalaureate degree from an accredited college which shall include courses in nursing, or in natural, behavioral or social sciences relevant to nursing practice;

(2) Direct patient care experience within the previous five (5) years in the nursing area to which he or she will be assigned, which can be met by:

(A) One (1) year's continuous, full-time or its equivalent experience providing direct patient care as a registered nurse in the designated nursing area; or

(B) One (1) academic year of registered nurse level clinical teaching experience in the designated nursing area or its equivalent that demonstrates clinical competency.

(e) A clinical teaching assistant shall have at least one (1) year continuous, full-time or its equivalent experience in the designated nursing area within the previous five (5) years as a registered nurse providing direct patient care.

(f) A content expert shall be an instructor and shall possess the following minimum qualifications:

(1) A master's degree in the designated nursing area; or

(2) A master's degree that is not in the designated nursing area and shall:

(A) Have completed thirty (30) hours of continuing education or two (2) semester units or three (3) quarter units of nursing education related to the designated nursing area; or have national certification in the designated nursing area from an accrediting organization, such as the American Nurses Credentialing Center (ANCC); and

(B) Have a minimum of two hundred forty (240) hours of clinical experience within the previous three (3) years in the designated nursing area; or have a minimum of one (1) academic year of registered nurse level clinical teaching experience in the designated nursing area within the previous five (5) years.

Authority cited: Sections 2715 and 2786, Business and Professions Code. Reference: Sections 2786-2788, Business and Professions Code.

History

1. Amendment filed 3-24-86; effective thirtieth day thereafter (Register 86, No. 13).
2. Amendment of first paragraph and subsection (b)(5) filed 4-27-87; operative 5-27-87 (Register 87, No. 18).
3. Amendment filed 9-21-2010; operative 10-21-2010 (Register 2010, No. 39).
4. Change without regulatory effect amending incorporated by reference forms and amending first paragraph filed 10-31-2012 pursuant to section 100, title 1, California Code of Regulations (Register 2012, No. 44).

§ 1425.1. Faculty Responsibilities.

(a) Each faculty member shall assume responsibility and accountability for instruction, evaluation of students, and planning and implementing curriculum content.

(b) Each faculty member shall participate in an orientation program, including, but not limited to, the program's curriculum, policies and procedures, strategies for teaching, and student supervision and evaluation.

(c) A registered nurse faculty member shall be responsible for clinical supervision only of those students enrolled in the registered nursing program.

(d) Each faculty member shall be clinically competent in the nursing area in which he or she teaches. The board document, "Faculty Remediation Guidelines" (EDP-R-08 Rev. 02/09), which provides guidelines for attaining and documenting clinical competency, is herein incorporated by reference.

Authority cited: Sections 2715, 2786 and 2786.6, Business and Professions Code. Reference: Sections 2786-2788, Business and Professions Code.

History

1. Amendment of subsection (a) filed 4-27-87; operative 5-27-87 (Register 87, No. 18).
2. Amendment filed 9-21-2010; operative 10-21-2010 (Register 2010, No. 39).

§ 1426. Required Curriculum.

(a) The curriculum of a nursing program shall be that set forth in this section, and shall be approved by the board. Any revised curriculum shall be approved by the board prior to its implementation.

(b) The curriculum shall reflect a unifying theme, which includes the nursing process as defined by the faculty, and shall be designed so that a student who completes the program will have the knowledge, skills, and abilities necessary to function in accordance with the registered nurse scope of practice as defined in code section 2725, and to meet minimum competency standards of a registered nurse.

(c) The curriculum shall consist of not less than fifty-eight (58) semester units, or eighty-seven (87) quarter units, which shall include at least the following number of units in the specified course areas:

(1) Art and science of nursing, thirty-six (36) semester units or fifty-four (54) quarter units, of which eighteen (18) semester or twenty-seven (27) quarter

units will be in theory and eighteen (18) semester or twenty-seven (27) quarter units will be in clinical practice.

(2) Communication skills, six (6) semester or nine (9) quarter units. Communication skills shall include principles of oral, written, and group communication.

(3) Related natural sciences (anatomy, physiology, and microbiology courses with labs), behavioral and social sciences, sixteen (16) semester or twenty-four (24) quarter units.

(d) Theory and clinical practice shall be concurrent in the following nursing areas: geriatrics, medical-surgical, mental health/psychiatric nursing, obstetrics, and pediatrics. Instructional outcomes will focus on delivering safe, therapeutic, effective, patient-centered care; practicing evidence-based practice; working as part of interdisciplinary teams; focusing on quality improvement; and using information technology. Instructional content shall include, but is not limited to, the following: critical thinking, personal hygiene, patient protection and safety, pain management, human sexuality, client abuse, cultural diversity, nutrition (including therapeutic aspects), pharmacology, patient advocacy, legal, social and ethical aspects of nursing, and nursing leadership and management.

(1) Theory and clinical practice requirements of the curriculum will be adjusted in recognition of military education and experiences of the student, when applicable, through an individualized process for evaluating and granting equivalency credit for military education and experience that results in meeting the same course objectives and competency standards.

(e) The following shall be integrated throughout the entire nursing curriculum:

(1) The nursing process;

(2) Basic intervention skills in preventive, remedial, supportive, and rehabilitative nursing;

(3) Physical, behavioral, and social aspects of human development from birth through all age levels;

(4) Knowledge and skills required to develop collegial relationships with health care providers from other disciplines;

(5) Communication skills including principles of oral, written, and group communications;

(6) Natural science, including human anatomy, physiology, and microbiology; and

(7) Related behavioral and social sciences with emphasis on societal and cultural patterns, human development, and behavior relevant to health-illness.

(f) The program shall have tools to evaluate a student's academic progress, performance, and clinical learning experiences that are directly related to course objectives.

(g) The course of instruction shall be presented in semester or quarter units or the equivalent under the following formula:

(1) One (1) hour of instruction in theory each week throughout a semester or quarter equals one (1) unit.

(2) Three (3) hours of clinical practice each week throughout a semester or quarter equals one (1) unit. With the exception of an initial nursing course that teaches basic nursing skills in a skills lab, 75% of clinical hours in a course

must be in direct patient care in an area specified in section 1426(d) in a board-approved clinical setting.

Authority cited: Sections 2715, 2786.1 and 2786.6, Business and Professions Cod. Reference: Sections 2785-2788, Business and Professions Code.

History

1. Amendment of subsection (d) filed 4-27-87; operative 5-27-87 (Register 87, No. 18).
2. Amendment of section heading and section filed 9-21-2010; operative 10-21-2010 (Register 2010, No. 39).
3. New subsection (d)(1) and amendment of Note filed 10-8-2018; operative 10-8-2018 pursuant to Government Code section 11343.4(b)(3) (Register 2018, No. 41).
4. Editorial correction removing erroneously inserted subsections (Register 2019, No. 5).

§ 1426.1. Preceptorship.

A preceptorship is a course, or component of a course, presented at the end of a board-approved curriculum, that provides students with a faculty-planned and supervised experience comparable to that of an entry-level registered nurse position. A program may choose to include a preceptorship in its curriculum. The following shall apply:

(a) The course shall be approved by the board prior to its implementation.

(b) The program shall have written policies and shall keep policies on file for conducting the preceptorship that include all of the following:

(1) Identification of criteria used for preceptor selection;

(2) Provision for a preceptor orientation program that covers the policies of the preceptorship and preceptor, student, and faculty responsibilities;

(3) Identification of preceptor qualifications for both the primary and the relief preceptor that include the following requirements:

(A) An active, clear license issued by the board;

(B) Clinically competent, and meet the minimum qualifications specified in section 1425(e);

(C) Employed by the health care agency for a minimum of one (1) year; and

(D) Completed a preceptor orientation program prior to serving as a preceptor.

(E) A relief preceptor, who is similarly qualified to be the preceptor is present and available on the primary preceptor's days off.

(4) Communication plan for faculty, preceptor, and student to follow during the preceptorship that addresses:

(A) The frequency and method of faculty/preceptor/student contact;

(B) Availability of faculty and preceptor to the student during his or her preceptorship experience;

1. Preceptor is present and available on the patient care unit the entire time the student is rendering nursing services during the preceptorship.

2. Faculty is available to the preceptor and student during the entire time the student is involved in the preceptorship learning activity.

(5) Description of responsibilities of the faculty, preceptor, and student for the learning experiences and evaluation during preceptorship, that include the following activities:

(A) Faculty member conducts periodic on-site meetings/conferences with the preceptor and the student;

(B) Faculty member completes and conducts the final evaluation of the student with input from the preceptor;

(6) Maintenance of preceptor records that includes names of all current preceptors, registered nurse licenses, and dates of preceptorships; and

(7) Plan for an ongoing evaluation regarding the continued use of preceptors.

(c) Faculty/student ratio for preceptorship shall be based on the following criteria:

(1) Student/preceptor needs;

(2) Faculty's ability to effectively supervise;

(3) Students' assigned nursing area; and

(4) Agency/facility requirements.

Authority cited: Sections 2715 and 2786.6, Business and Professions Code. Reference: Sections 2785-2788, Business and Professions Code.

History

1. New section filed 9-21-2010; operative 10-21-2010 (Register 2010, No. 39).

§ 1427. Clinical Facilities.

(a) A nursing program shall not utilize any agency or facility for clinical experience without prior approval by the board. Each program must submit evidence that it has complied with the requirements of subdivisions (b), (c), and (d) of this section and the policies outlined by the board.

(b) A program that utilizes an agency or facility for clinical experience shall maintain written objectives for student learning in such facilities, and shall assign students only to facilities that can provide the experience necessary to meet those objectives.

(c) Each such program shall maintain written agreements with such facilities and such agreements shall include the following:

(1) Assurance of the availability and appropriateness of the learning environment in relation to the program's written objectives;

(2) Provision for orientation of faculty and students;

(3) A specification of the responsibilities and authority of the facility's staff as related to the program and to the educational experience of the students;

(4) Assurance that staff is adequate in number and quality to ensure safe and continuous health care services to patients;

(5) Provisions for continuing communication between the facility and the program; and

(6) A description of the responsibilities of faculty assigned to the facility utilized by the program.

(d) In selecting a new clinical agency or facility for student placement, the program shall take into consideration the impact that an additional group of students would have on students of other nursing programs already assigned to the agency or facility.

Authority cited: Sections 2715 and 2786, Business and Professions Code. Reference: Sections 2786-2788, Business and Professions Code.

History

1. Amendment filed 9-21-2010; operative 10-21-2010 (Register 2010, No. 39).

§ 1428. Student Participation.

Students shall be provided opportunity to participate with the faculty in the identification of policies and procedures related to students including but not limited to:

(a) Philosophy and objectives;

(b) Learning experience; and

(c) Curriculum, instruction, and evaluation of the various aspects of the program, including clinical facilities.

Authority cited: Sections 2715 and 2786, Business and Professions Code. Reference: Sections 2786-2788, Business and Professions Code.

History

1. Amendment filed 9-21-2010; operative 10-21-2010 (Register 2010, No. 39).

§ 1428.6. Policies Relating to Establishing Eligibility for Examination.

(a) At least four (4) weeks prior to its established graduation date, the nursing program shall submit to the board a roster of names of those students and their expected date to successfully complete required course work. Except as provided below such a student shall be deemed eligible to take the examination after the date on which the student successfully completed the required course work.

(b) The nursing program shall notify the board immediately by telephone, facsimile, or e-mail of any student who fails to maintain eligibility and such individuals shall be deemed ineligible to take the examination.

Authority cited: Sections 2715 and 2786, Business and Professions Code. Reference: Sections 2786-2788, Business and Professions Code.

History

1. Amendment filed 10-2-96; operative 11-1-96 (Register 96, No. 40).
2. Amendment filed 9-21-2010; operative 10-21-2010 (Register 2010, No. 39).

§ 1429. Licensed Vocational Nurses, Thirty (30) Semester or Forty-Five (45) Quarter Unit Option.

(a) An applicant who is licensed in California as a vocational nurse is eligible to apply for licensure as a registered nurse if such applicant has successfully completed the courses prescribed below and meets all the other requirements set forth in section 2736 of the code. Such applicant shall submit evidence to the board, including a transcript, of successful completion of the requirements set forth in subsection (c) and of successful completion or challenge of courses in physiology and microbiology comparable to such courses required for licensure as a registered nurse.

(b) The school shall offer objective counseling of this option and evaluate each licensed vocational nurse applicant for admission to its registered nursing program on an individual basis. A school's determination of the prerequisite courses required of a licensed vocational nurse applicant shall be based on an analysis of each applicant's academic deficiencies, irrespective of the time such courses were taken.

(c) The additional education required of licensed vocational nurse applicants shall not exceed a maximum of thirty (30) semester or forty-five (45) quarter units. Courses required for vocational nurse licensure do not fulfill the additional education requirement. However, other courses comparable to those required for licensure as a registered nurse, as specified in section 1426, may fulfill the additional education requirement.

Nursing courses shall be taken in an approved nursing program and shall be beyond courses equivalent to the first year of professional nursing courses. The nursing content shall include nursing intervention in acute, preventive, remedial, supportive, rehabilitative and teaching aspects of nursing. Theory and courses with concurrent clinical practice shall include advanced medical-surgical, mental health, psychiatric nursing and geriatric nursing. The nursing content shall include the basic standards for competent performance prescribed in section 1443.5 of these regulations.

Authority cited: Section 2715, Business and Professions Code. Reference: Sections 2736, 2736.6 and 2786, Business and Professions Code.

History

1. Amendment of section heading and section filed 9-21-2010; operative 10-21-2010 (Register 2010, No. 39).

§ 1430. Previous Education Credit.

An approved nursing program shall have a process for a student to obtain credit for previous education or for other acquired knowledge in the field of nursing, including military education and experience, through equivalence, challenge examinations, or other methods of evaluation. The program shall make the information available in published documents, such as college catalog or student handbook, and online.

Authority cited: Sections 2715, 2786.1 and 2786.6, Business and Professions Code. Reference: Sections 2736, 2786.1, 2786.6 and 2788, Business and Professions Code.

History

1. Renumbering of former section 1430 to new section 1432 and new section 1430 filed 9-21-2010; operative 10-21-2010 (Register 2010, No. 39).

2. Amendment of section and Note filed 10-8-2018; operative 10-8-2018 pursuant to Government Code section 11343.4(b)(3) (Register 2018, No. 41).

§ 1431. Licensing Examination Pass Rate Standard.

The nursing program shall maintain a minimum pass rate of seventy-five percent (75%) for first time licensing examination candidates.

(a) A program exhibiting a pass rate below seventy-five percent (75%) for first time candidates in an academic year shall conduct a comprehensive program assessment to identify variables contributing to the substandard pass rate and shall submit a written report to the board. The report shall include the findings of the assessment and a plan for increasing the pass rate including specific corrective measures to be taken, resources, and timeframe.

(b) A board-approval visit will be conducted if a program exhibits a pass rate below seventy-five percent (75%) for first time candidates for two (2) consecutive academic years.

(c) The board may place a program on warning status with intent to revoke the program's approval and may revoke approval if a program fails to maintain the minimum pass rate pursuant to section 2788 of the code.

Authority cited: Sections 2715 and 2788, Business and Professions Code. Reference: Section 2788, Business and Professions Code.

History

1. New section filed 9-21-2010; operative 10-21-2010 (Register 2010, No. 39).

§ 1432. Changes to an Approved Program.

(a) Each nursing program holding a certificate of approval shall:

(1) File its legal name and current mailing address with the board at its principal office and shall notify the board at said office of any change of name or mailing address within thirty (30) days prior to such change. It shall give both the old and the new name or address.

(2) Notify the board within ten (10) days of any:

(A) Change in fiscal condition that will or may potentially adversely affect applicants or students enrolled in the nursing program.

(B) Substantive change in the organizational structure, administrative responsibility, or accountability in the nursing program, the institution of higher education in which the nursing program is located or with which it is affiliated that will affect the nursing program.

(b) An approved nursing program shall not make a substantive change without prior board authorization. These changes include:

(1) Change in location.

(2) Change in ownership.

(3) Addition of a new campus or location.

(4) Significant change in the agreement between an approved nursing program that is not an institution of higher education and the institution of higher education with which it is affiliated.

Authority cited: Sections 2715, 2786 and 2788, Business and Professions Code. Reference: Sections 2715, 2786 and 2788, Business and Professions Code.

History

1. Renumbering of former section 1430 to new section 1432, including amendment of section heading, section and Note, filed 9-21-2010; operative 10-21-2010 (Register 2010, No. 39).

ARTICLE 3.5
CITATIONS AND FINES

Section

1435. Citations—Content and Service.
1435.1. Exceptions.
1435.15. Citation Disclosure and Record Purge.
1435.2. Violations and Fines.
1435.3. Citations for Unlicensed Individual.
1435.4. Criteria to be Considered in Assessing a Fine or Order of Abatement.
1435.5. Contested Citations.
1435.6. Compliance with Citation/Order of Abatement.
1435.7. Notification to Other Boards and Agencies.

§ 1435. Citations—Content and Service.

(a) The Executive Officer of the board or his/her designee, in lieu of filing an accusation against any licensee, may issue a citation which may contain an administrative fine and/or order of abatement against that licensee for any violation of law which would be grounds for discipline or of any regulation adopted by the board pursuant thereto.

(b) Each citation shall be in writing and shall describe with particularity the nature and facts of each violation specified in the citation, including a reference to the statute or regulation alleged to have been violated.

(c) The citation may contain an assessment of an administrative fine, an order of abatement fixing a reasonable time for abatement of the violation, or both.

(d) The citation shall inform the cited individual of the right to an informal citation conference concerning the matter and of the right to an administrative hearing.

(e) The citation shall be served upon the individual personally or by certified mail.

Authority cited: Sections 125.9, 148 and 2715, Business and Professions Code.Reference: Sections 125.9 and 148, Business and Professions Code.

History

1. New Article 3.5 (sections 1435-1435.7) and section 1435 filed 7-12-96; operative 8-11-96 (Register 96, No. 28).
2. Amendment of subsection (a) filed 12-16-2002; operative 1-15-2003 (Register 2002, No. 51).

§ 1435.1. Exceptions.

A citation shall not be issued in any of the following circumstances:

(a) The violation is of such a nature and/or severity that revocation of the license or restrictions on the license are necessary in order to ensure consumer protection.

(b) The licensee's conduct displayed a disregard for the patient and/or the patient's rights.This includes but is not limited to physical abuse; neglect; abandonment; fiduciary abuse (as defined in Article 2, Chapter 11 commencing with Section 15610 of the Welfare and Institutions Code with additional modification of the definitions to include all types of patients); or the deprivation of care or services which are necessary to avoid physical harm or mental suffering.

(c) The licensee failed to comply with any requirement of any previous citation, including any order of abatement or fine.

(d) The licensee has been previously disciplined by the board or has previously been denied a license by the board for the same or similar actions.

(e) The violation involves unprofessional conduct related to controlled substances or dangerous drugs.

(f) The violation involves unprofessional conduct related to sexual abuse, misconduct or relations with a patient.

(g) The licensee was convicted of an offense substantially related to the qualifications, functions, and duties of a registered nurse and there is insufficient evidence of rehabilitation.

Authority cited: Sections 125.9, 148 and 2715, Business and Professions Code.Reference: Sections 125.9 and 148, Business and Professions Code; Article 2, Chapter 11 commencing with Section 15610, Welfare and Institutions Code.

History

1. New section filed 7-12-96; operative 8-11-96 (Register 96, No. 28).

§ 1435.15. Citation Disclosure and Record Purge.

(a) Every citation that is issued pursuant to this article shall be disclosed to an inquiring member of the public.

(b) Every citation, once it has been resolved by payment of the administrative fine and/or compliance with the order of abatement, shall be purged three (3) years from the date of resolution, except for citations referenced in subsection (c).

(c) No citation shall be purged if issued pursuant to CCR Section 1435.3, and no citation shall be purged for any citation issued against an unlicensed individual using the title "registered nurse" or the letters "RN" after his or her name.

(d) A citation that has been withdrawn or dismissed shall be purged from the board's file as soon as administratively feasible, but no more than one year.

Authority cited: Sections 125.9, 148 and 2715, Business and Professions Code. Reference: Sections 125.9 and 148, Business and Professions Code.

History

1. New section filed 12-16-2002; operative 1-15-2003 (Register 2002, No. 51).

Regulations

§ 1435.2. Violations and Fines.

(a) In any citation, the Executive Officer of the board or his/her designee may assess a fine for violations of the Nursing Practice Act, any regulation adopted pursuant thereto, or any applicable section of the Business and Profession Code governing the practice of registered nursing.

(b) The range of fines shall be from $0.00 - $2500. Fines shall be assessed based on criteria stated in section 1435.4. In no case shall the total fines exceed $2,500 for each investigation.

(c) Notwithstanding the administrative fine amounts specified in subsection (b), a citation may include a fine between $2,501 and $5,000 if one or more of the following circumstances apply:

1. The citation involves a violation that has an immediate relationship to the health and safety of another person.

2. The cited person has a history of two or more prior citations of the same or similar violations;

3. The citation involves multiple violations that demonstrate a willful disregard of the law.

4. The citation involves a violation or violations perpetrated against a senior citizen or person with disability.

Authority cited: Sections 125.9, 148, 2715 and 2761(d), Business and Professions Code.Reference: Sections 119, 125, 125.6, 125.9, 136, 148, 496, 498, 499, 810 (a), 2725.1, 2732, 2732.05, 2761, 2795, 2796 and 2797, Business and Professions Code and Sections 1411.6, 1414(c), 1414(d), 1443.5, 1451(d), 1451(e), 1453 and 1474, Title 16, California Code ofRegulations.

History

1. New section filed 7-12-96; operative 8-11-96 (Register 96, No. 28).
2. Amendment filed 12-16-2002; operative 1-15-2003 (Register 2002, No. 51).
3. Designation of first and second sentences as subsections (a) and (b), respectively, and new subsections (c)-(c)4. filed 3-12-2008; operative 4-11-2008 (Register 2008, No. 11).

§ 1435.3. Citations for Unlicensed Individual.

The Executive Officer of the board or his/her designee may issue citations, in accordance with Section 148 of the Code, against any individual (as defined in section 302(e) of the Code) who is performing or who has performed services for which licensure is required under the Nursing Practice Act or regulations adopted pursuant thereto.Citations issued under this section shall meet the requirements set forth in subdivisions (b), (c), (d), and (e) of Section 1435 and shall be subject to the provisions of Sections 1435.2, 1435.4, 1435.5 and subdivisions (a), (b), and (c) of Section 1435.6.Each citation issued under this section shall contain an order of abatement.The sanction authorized under this section shall be separate from and in addition to any other civil or criminal remedies.

Authority cited: Sections 125.9, 148 and 2715, Business and Professions Code.Reference: Sections 125.9, 148 and 302(e), Business and Professions Code.

History

1. New section filed 7-12-96; operative 8-11-96 (Register 96, No. 28).
2. Amendment filed 12-16-2002; operative 1-15-2003 (Register 2002, No. 51).

§ 1435.4. Criteria to be Considered in Assessing a Fine or Order of Abatement.

In any citation which includes a fine or order of abatement, the following factors shall be considered in determining the amount of the fine to be assessed or the terms of the order of abatement:

(a) Gravity of the violation.

(b) History of previous violations of the same or similar nature.

(c) Length of time that has passed since the date of the violation.

(d) Consequences of the violation, including potential or actual patient harm.

(e) The good or bad faith exhibited by the cited individual.

(f) Evidence that the violation was willful.

(g) The extent to which the individual cooperated with the board's investigation.

(h) The extent to which the individual has remediated any knowledge and/or skills deficiencies which could have injured a patient.

(i) Any other mitigating or aggravating factors.

Authority cited: Sections 125.9, 148 and 2715, Business and Professions Code.Reference: Sections 125.9 and 148, Business and Professions Code.

History

1. New section filed 7-12-96; operative 8-11-96 (Register 96, No. 28).

§ 1435.5. Contested Citations.

(a) The individual cited may, within 14 calendar days after service of the citation, submit a written request for an informal citation conference with the Executive Officer or his/her designee. The citation decision shall be stayed upon receipt of the written request until a final decision has been issued.

(b) The Executive Officer or his/her designee shall, within 30 calendar days from receipt of the written request, hold an informal citation conference with the individual cited and his/her legal counsel or authorized representative, if desired.

(c) The Executive Officer or his/her designee may affirm, modify or dismiss the citation, including any fine or order of abatement, at the conclusion of the informal citation conference.A written decision, including the reasons for the decision, shall be mailed to the individual and his/her legal counsel, if any, within 14 calendar days from the date of the informal citation conference. If the citation is affirmed or modified, the individual may, within 30 calendar days from the mailing date of the informal citation conference decision, request an administrative hearing. The request for an administrative hearing shall be in writing.

(d) In addition to the appeal rights in (a) through (c) above, the individual may request an administrative hearing provided for in subdivision (b)(4) of Section 125.9 of the Code within 30 days of the date of issuance of the citation or assessment.

Authority cited: Sections 125.9, 148 and 2715, Business and Professions Code.References: Sections 125.9 and 148, Business and Professions Code.

History

1. New section filed 7-12-96; operative 8-11-96 (Register 96, No. 28).
2. Amendment filed 12-16-2002; operative 1-15-2003 (Register 2002, No. 51).

§ 1435.6. Compliance with Citation/Order of Abatement.

(a) Orders of abatement may be extended for good cause.If a cited individual who has been issued an order of abatement is unable to complete the correction within the time set forth in the citation because of conditions beyond his/her control after the exercise of reasonable diligence, then he/she may request from the Executive Officer or his/her designee an extension of time within which to complete the correction.Such a request shall be in writing and shall be made within the time set forth for abatement.

(b) If a citation is not contested, or if the order is appealed and the individual cited does not prevail, failure to abate the violation or to pay the assessed fine within the time allowed shall constitute a violation and a failure to comply with the citation or order of abatement.

(c) Failure to timely comply with an order of abatement or pay an assessed fine may result in disciplinary action being taken by the board or other appropriate judicial relief being taken against the individual cited.

(d) If a fine is not paid after a citation has become final, the fine shall be added to the cited individual's license renewal fee.A license shall not be renewed without payment of renewal fee and fine.

Authority cited: Sections 125.9, 148 and 2715, Business and Professions Code.Reference: Sections 125.9 and 148, Business and Professions Code.

History

1. New section filed 7-12-96; operative 8-11-96 (Register 96, No. 28).
2. Amendment of subsection (a) filed 12-16-2002; operative 1-15-2003 (Register 2002, No. 51).

§ 1435.7. Notification to Other Boards and Agencies.

After a citation has become final, it shall be reported to other boards of registered nursing and other regulatory agencies.

Authority cited: Sections 125.9, 148 and 2715, Business and Professions Code.Reference: Sections 125.9 and 148, Business and Professions Code.

History

1. New section filed 7-12-96; operative 8-11-96 (Register 96, No. 28).

ARTICLE 4
GROUNDS FOR DISCIPLINE, DISCIPLINARY PROCEEDINGS AND REHABILITATION

Section

1441. Unprofessional Conduct.
1442. Gross Negligence.
1443. Incompetence.
1443.5. Standards of Competent Performance.
1444. Substantial Relationship Criteria.
1444.5. Disciplinary Guidelines.
1445. Criteria for Rehabilitation.
1445.1. Petition for Reinstatement.

§ 1441. Unprofessional Conduct.

In addition to the conduct described in Section 2761 (a) of the Code, "unprofessional conduct" also includes, but is not limited to, the following:

(a) As a licensee, failure to provide to the board, as directed, lawfully requested copies of documents within 15 days of receipt of the request or within the time specified in the request, whichever is later, unless the licensee is unable to provide the documents within this time period for good cause, including but not limited to, physical inability to access the records in the time allowed due to illness or travel. This subsection shall not apply to a licensee who does not have access to, and control over, the documents.

(b) Failure to cooperate and participate in any board investigation pending against the licensee. This subsection shall not be construed to deprive a licensee of any privilege guaranteed by the Fifth Amendment to the Constitution of the United States, or any other constitutional or statutory privileges. This subsection shall not be construed to require a licensee to cooperate with a request that would require the licensee to waive any constitutional or statutory privilege or to comply with a request for information or other matters within an unreasonable period of time in light of the time constraints of the licensee's practice. Any exercise by a licensee of any constitutional or statutory privilege shall not be used against the licensee in a regulatory or disciplinary proceeding against the licensee.

(c) Failure to report to the board, within 30 days, any of the following:

(1) The conviction of the licensee, including any verdict of guilty, or pleas of guilty or no contest, of any felony or misdemeanor.

(2) Any disciplinary action taken by another licensing entity or authority of this state or of another state or an agency of the federal government or the United States military.

(d) Failure or refusal to comply with a court order, issued in the enforcement of a subpoena, mandating the release of records to the board.

Authority cited: Section 2715, Business and Professions Code. Reference: Sections 2761 and 2765, Business and Professions Code.

History

1. New section filed 7-23-2014; operative 7-23-2014 pursuant to Government Code section 11343.4(b)(3) (Register 2014, No. 30).

2. Amendment of subsection (a) filed 5-20-2021; operative 5-20-2021 pursuant to Government Code section 11343.4(b)(3) (Register 2021, No. 21).

§ 1442. Gross Negligence.

As used in Section 2761 of the code, "gross negligence" includes an extreme departure from the standard of care which, under similar circumstances, would have ordinarily been exercised by a competent registered nurse. Such an extreme departure means the repeated failure to provide nursing care as required or failure to provide care or to exercise ordinary precaution in a single situation which the nurse knew, or should have known, could have jeopardized the client's health or life.

Authority cited: Section 2715, Business and Professions Code. Reference: Section 2761, Business and Professions Code.

History

1. New Article 4 (Sections 1442 and 1443) filed 3-26-74; effective thirtieth day thereafter. (Register 74, No. 13). For history of former Article 4 (Sections 1442 and 1443), see Registers 57, No. 15, and 64, No. 3.

2. Amendment filed 5-29-81; effective thirtieth day thereafter (Register 81, No. 22).

3. Amendment filed 6-17-85; effective thirtieth day thereafter (Register 85, No. 25).

§ 1443. Incompetence.

As used in Section 2761 of the code, "incompetence" means the lack of possession of or the failure to exercise that degree of learning, skill, care and experience ordinarily possessed and exercised by a competent registered nurse as described in Section 1443.5.

Authority cited: Section 2715, Business and Professions Code. Reference: Section 2761, Business and Professions Code.

History

1. Amendment filed 5-29-81; effective thirtieth day thereafter (Register 81, No. 22).

2. Amendment filed 6-17-85; effective thirtieth day thereafter (Register 85, No. 25).

Regulations

§ 1443.5. Standards of Competent Performance.

A registered nurse shall be considered to be competent when he/she consistently demonstrates the ability to transfer scientific knowledge from social, biological and physical sciences in applying the nursing process, as follows:

(1) Formulates a nursing diagnosis through observation of the client's physical condition and behavior, and through interpretation of information obtained from the client and others, including the health team.

(2) Formulates a care plan, in collaboration with the client, which ensures that direct and indirect nursing care services provide for the client's safety, comfort, hygiene, and protection, and for disease prevention and restorative measures.

(3) Performs skills essential to the kind of nursing action to be taken, explains the health treatment to the client and family and teaches the client and family how to care for the client's health needs.

(4) Delegates tasks to subordinates based on the legal scopes of practice of the subordinates and on the preparation and capability needed in the tasks to be delegated, and effectively supervises nursing care being given by subordinates.

(5) Evaluates the effectiveness of the care plan through observation of the client's physical condition and behavior, signs and symptoms of illness, and reactions to treatment and through communication with the client and health team members, and modifies the plan as needed.

(6) Acts as the client's advocate, as circumstances require, by initiating action to improve health care or to change decisions or activities which are against the interests or wishes of the client, and by giving the client the opportunity to make informed decisions about health care before it is provided.

Authority cited: Section 2715, Business and Professions Code. Reference: Sections 2725 and 2761, Business and Professions Code.

History

1. New section filed 6-17-85; effective thirtieth day thereafter (Register 85, No. 25).

§ 1444. Substantial Relationship Criteria.

(a) For the purposes of denial, suspension, or revocation of a license or certificate pursuant to section 141, Division 1.5 (commencing with section 475), or Sections 2761 or 2765 of the code, a crime, professional misconduct, or act shall be considered to be substantially related to the qualifications, functions or duties of a person holding a license or certificate under the Nursing Practice Act (Chapter 6 of Division 2 of the code), if to a substantial degree it evidences the present or potential unfitness of a person holding a license or certificate to perform the functions authorized and/or mandated by the license or certificate, or in a manner consistent with the public health, safety, or welfare.

(b) In making the substantial relationship determination required under subdivision (a) for a crime, the board shall consider the following criteria:

(1) The nature and gravity of the offense;

(2) The number of years elapsed since the date of the offense; and

(3) The nature and duties of a registered nurse, or the license or certificate type sought or held by the person.

(c) For purposes of subdivision (a), substantially related crimes, professional misconduct, or acts shall include, but are not limited to, the following:

(1) Violating or attempting to violate, directly or indirectly, or assisting in or abetting the violation of or conspiring to violate any provision or term of the Nursing Practice Act and its implementing regulations.

(2) Theft, dishonesty, fraud, deceit, or unprofessional conduct listed in section 2762 of the code.

(3) Child, elder, or dependent adult abuse.

(4) Sex offenses requiring a person to register as a sex offender pursuant to section 290 of the Penal Code.

(5) Lewd conduct or sexual misconduct.

(6) Assault, battery, or other violence including, but not limited to, those violations listed in subdivision (d) of Penal Code section 11160.

(7) Use of drugs or alcohol to an extent or in a manner dangerous to the individual or the public.

(8) Harassment, trespass, or stalking.

(9) Failure to comply with any mandatory reporting requirements.

Authority cited: Sections 481 and 2715, Business and Professions Code. Reference: Sections 141, 480, 481, 490, 493, 2736, 2761, 2762 and 2765, Business and Professions Code; and Sections 290 and 11160, Penal Code.

History

1. New section filed 5-14-75; effective thirtieth day thereafter (Register 75, No. 20).
2. Amendment filed 9-27-85; effective thirtieth day thereafter (Register 85, No. 39).
3. Amendment of first paragraph, repealer of subsections (a)-(e), new subsections (a)-(d), and amendment of Note filed 6-6-2001; operative 7-6-2001 (Register 2001, No. 23).
4. Amendment of section and Note filed 5-20-2021; operative 5-20-2021 pursuant to Government Code section 11343.4(b)(3) (Register 2021, No. 21).

§ 1444.5. Disciplinary Guidelines.

In reaching a decision on a disciplinary action under the administrative adjudication provisions of the Administrative Procedure Act (Government Code Section 11400 et seq.), the board shall consider the disciplinary guidelines entitled: "Recommended Guidelines for Disciplinary Orders and Conditions of Probation" (10/02), which are hereby incorporated by reference. Deviation from these guidelines and orders, including the standard terms of probation, is appropriate where the board, in its sole discretion, determines that the facts of the particular case warrant such a deviation—for example: the presence of mitigating factors; the age of the case; evidentiary problems.

Notwithstanding the disciplinary guidelines, any proposed decision issued in accordance with the procedures set forth in Chapter 5 (commencing with section 11500) of Part 1 of Division 3 of Title 2 of the Government Code that contains any finding of fact that the licensee engaged in any acts of sexual contact, as defined in subdivision (c) of Section 729 of the Business and Professions Code, with a patient, or has committed an act or been convicted of a sex offense as defined in Section 44010 of the Education Code, shall contain an order revoking the license. The proposed decision shall not contain an order staying the revocation of the license.

Authority cited: Section 2715, Business and Professions Code; and Section 11400.20, Government Code. Reference: Sections 726, 729, 2750, 2759, 2761 and 2762, Business and Professions Code; Section 44010, Education Code; and Section 11425.50, Government Code.

History

1. New section filed 6-17-97; operative 6-17-97 pursuant to Government Code section 11343.4(d) (Register 97, No. 25).

2. Amendment of "Recommended Guidelines for Disciplinary Orders and Conditions of Probation" (incorporated by reference) and amendment of section filed 6-14-2000; operative 7-14-2000 (Register 2000, No. 24).

3. Amendment of section and Note filed 4-24-2003; operative 5-24-2003 (Register 2003, No. 17).

4. Amendment of section and Note filed 7-23-2014; operative 7-23-2014 pursuant to Government Code section 11343.4(b)(3) (Register 2014, No. 30).

5. Amendment of first paragraph filed 5-20-2021; operative 5-20-2021 pursuant to Government Code section 11343.4(b)(3) (Register 2021, No. 21)

§ 1445. Criteria for Rehabilitation.

(a) Denial of a license or certificate.

(1) When considering the denial of a license or certificate under Section 480 of the code on the ground that the applicant has been convicted of a crime, the board shall consider whether the applicant has made a showing of rehabilitation if the applicant completed the criminal sentence at issue without a violation of parole or probation. In making this determination, the board shall consider the following criteria:

(A) The nature and gravity of the crime(s).

(B) The reason for granting probation and the length of the applicable parole or probation period(s).

(C) The extent to which the applicable parole or probation period was shortened or lengthened, and the reason(s) the period was modified.

(D) The terms or conditions of parole or probation and the extent to which they bear on the applicant's rehabilitation.

(E) The extent to which the terms or conditions of parole or probation were modified, and the reason(s) for modification.

(2) If the applicant has not completed the criminal sentence at issue without a violation of parole or probation, the board determines that the applicant did not make the showing of rehabilitation based on the criteria in subdivision (a), the denial is based on professional misconduct, or the denial is based on one or more of the grounds specified in Sections 2761 or 2762 of the code, the board shall apply the following criteria in evaluating an applicant's rehabilitation:

(A) The nature and gravity of the act(s), professional misconduct, or crime(s) under consideration as grounds for denial.

(B) Evidence of any act(s), professional misconduct, or crime(s) committed subsequent to the act(s), professional misconduct, or crime(s) under consideration as grounds for denial.

(C) The time that has elapsed since commission of the act(s), professional misconduct, or crime(s) referred to in subdivisions (A) and (B).

(D) Whether the applicant has complied with any terms of parole, probation, restitution or any other sanctions lawfully imposed against the applicant.

(E) The criteria in subdivisions (a)(1)(A) through (E), as applicable.

(F) Evidence, if any, of rehabilitation submitted by the applicant.

(b) Suspension or revocation of a license or certificate.

(1) When considering the suspension or revocation of a license or certificate on the ground that the licensee or certificate holder under the Nursing Practice Act (Chapter 6 of Division 2 of the code) has been convicted of a crime, the board shall consider whether the licensee made a showing of rehabilitation if the licensee completed the criminal sentence at issue without a violation of parole or probation. In making this determination, the board shall consider the following criteria:

(A) The nature and gravity of the crime(s).

(B) The reason for granting probation and the length(s) of the applicable parole or probation period(s).

(C) The extent to which the applicable parole or probation period was shortened or lengthened, and the reason(s) the period was modified.

(D) The terms or conditions of parole or probation and the extent to which they bear on the licensee or certificate holder's rehabilitation.

(E) The extent to which the terms or conditions of parole or probation were modified, and the reason(s) for the modification.

(2) If the licensee or certificate holder has not completed the criminal sentence at issue without a violation of parole or probation, the board determines that the licensee or certificate holder did not make the showing of rehabilitation based on the criteria in subdivision (b)(1), the suspension or revocation is based on a disciplinary action as described in Section 141 of the code, or the suspension or revocation is based on one or more of the grounds specified in Sections 2761 or 2762 of the code, the board shall apply the following criteria in evaluating a licensee or certificate holder's rehabilitation:

(A) The nature and gravity of the acts(s), disciplinary action(s), or crime(s).

(B) The total criminal record.

(C) The time that has elapsed since commission of the act(s), disciplinary action(s), or crime(s).

(D) Whether the licensee or certificate holder has complied with any terms of parole, probation, restitution, or any other sanctions lawfully imposed against such person.

(E) The criteria in subdivisions (b)(1)(A) through (E), as applicable.

(F) If applicable, evidence of dismissal proceedings pursuant to Section 1203.4 of the Penal Code.

(G) Evidence, if any, of rehabilitation submitted by the licensee or certificate holder.

Authority cited: Sections 481, 482 and 2715, Business and Professions Code. Reference: Sections 141, 480, 481, 482, 2736, 2761 and 2762, Business and Professions Code.

History

1. New section filed 5-25-73; effective thirtieth day thereafter (Register 73, No. 21). For history of former section, see Register 70, No. 5.

2. Renumbering from Section 1411 filed 3-26-74; effective thirtieth day thereafter (Register 74, No. 13).

3. Amendment of subsections (a) and (b) and new subsection (c) filed 5-14-75; effective thirtieth day thereafter (Register 75, No. 20).

4. Amendment filed 9-27-85; effective thirtieth day thereafter (Register 85, No. 39).

5. Amendment of section and Note filed 5-20-2021; operative 5-20-2021 pursuant to Government Code section 11343.4(b)(3) (Register 2021, No. 21)

§ 1445.1. Petition for Reinstatement.

(a) A person may petition for reinstatement of a license under the provisions of Section 11522 of the Government Code by:

(1) Obtaining the appropriate forms from the board office in Sacramento and

(2) Submitting the required form of petition and supplementary documentation to the board at least forty-five (45) days in advance of the date on which the person desires to be heard, as directed in the written instructions which accompany the forms.

(b) The burden of proving rehabilitation is upon the petitioner. When considering a petition for reinstatement of a license, the board shall evaluate and consider evidence of rehabilitation submitted by the petitioner, using those criteria specified in Section 1445 of this article.

Authority cited: Section 2715, Business and Professions Code. Reference: Section 11522, Government Code.

History

1. New section filed 9-27-85; effective thirtieth day thereafter (Register 85, No. 39).

ARTICLE 4.1
INTERVENTION PROGRAM GUIDELINES

Section

1446. Definitions.
1447. Criteria for Admission.
1447.1. Procedure for Review of Applicants.
1447.2. Causes for Denial of Admission.
1448. Causes for Termination from the Program.
1448.1. Notification of Termination.
1449. Confidentiality of Records.

§ 1446. Definitions.

As used in this article:

(a) "Program" means the alcohol and drug abuse and mental illness intervention program for registered nurses authorized pursuant to Article 3.1 (commencing with Section 2770) of Chapter 6 of Division 2 of the Business and Professions Code.

(b) "Committee" means intervention evaluation committee consisting of the following members: Three registered nurses, one physician and one public member all of whom have expertise in the area of chemical dependency.

(c) "Board" means Board of Registered Nursing.

Authority cited: Section 2715, Business and Professions Code. Reference: Sections 2770.1 and 2770.2, Business and Professions Code.

History

1. New Article 4.1 (Sections 1446, 1447, 1447.1-1447.2, 1448, 1448.1 and 1449) filed 5-7-85; effective thirtieth day thereafter (Register 85, No. 19).

2. Change without regulatory effect amending article heading and subsections (a) and (b) filed 2-24-2016 pursuant to section 100, title 1, California Code of Regulations (Register 2016, No. 9).

§ 1447. Criteria for Admission.

An applicant shall meet the following criteria for admission to the program:

(a) Is a registered nurse licensed in this state.

(b) Resides in California.

(c) Is mentally ill or abuses alcohol and/or drugs in a manner which may affect the applicant's ability to safely perform the duties of a registered nurse.

(d) Voluntarily requests admission to the program.

(e) Agrees to undergo reasonable medical and/or psychiatric examinations necessary for evaluation for participation in the program.

(f) Cooperates by providing such medical information, disclosure authorizations and releases of liability as may be requested by the committee.

(g) Agrees in writing to comply with all elements of the intervention program.

(h) Has not had her/his license previously disciplined by the Board for substance abuse or mental illness.

(i) Has not been terminated from this or any other intervention program for non-compliance.

Authority cited: Sections 2715 and 2770.7, Business and Professions Code. Reference: Section 2770.7, Business and Professions Code.

History

1. Change without regulatory effect amending subsections (g) and (i) filed 2-24-2016 pursuant to section 100, title 1, California Code of Regulations (Register 2016, No. 9).

§ 1447.1. Procedure for Review of Applicants.

The following procedures shall be used to review applicants for admission to the program:

(a) The program director and a nurse or physician consultant shall interview each applicant. They shall recommend such medical and/or psychiatric examinations as may be necessary to determine the applicant's eligibility for the program and shall request such other information, authorizations and releases as may be necessary for participation in the program. The IEC shall advise the applicant that the applicant is responsible for costs incurred for the examinations and rehabilitation aspects of the program.

(b) The program director and the nurse or physician consultant shall each make a recommendation to the committee as to whether the applicant should be admitted to the program.

(c) The committee shall review each application and make its decision on admission of the applicant based upon its evaluation and the recommendations from the program director and the nurse or physician consultant.

(d) The committee's decision on admission of an applicant shall be final.

Authority cited: Sections 2715 and 2770.7, Business and Professions Code. Reference: Section 2770.7, Business and Professions Code.

History

1. Change without regulatory effect amending subsection (a) filed 2-24-2016 pursuant to section 100, title 1, California Code of Regulations (Register 2016, No. 9).

§ 1447.2. Causes for Denial of Admission.

The committee may deny an applicant admission to the program for any of the following reasons:

(a) The applicant does not meet the requirements set forth in Section 1447.

(b) Information is received by the board which, after investigation, indicates that the applicant may have violated a provision of the laws governing the practice of nursing, Chapter 6 (commencing with Section 2700) of Division 2 of the Code, excluding Section 2762.

(c) The applicant is diverting controlled substances for sale.

(d) The committee determines that the applicant will not substantially benefit from participation in the program or that the applicant's participation in the program creates too great a risk to the public health, safety or welfare.

Authority cited: Sections 2715 and 2770.7, Business and Professions Code. Reference: Section 2770.7, Business and Professions Code.

§ 1448. Causes for Termination from the Program.

The committee may terminate a nurse's participation in the program for any of the following reasons:

(a) Successful completion of the program designated by the committee.

(b) Failure to comply with the rehabilitation program designated by the committee.

(c) Failure to comply with any of the requirements set forth in Section 1447.

(d) Failure to substantially benefit from participation in the program.

(e) Receipt of information by the board which, after investigation, indicates the participant may have violated a provision of the laws governing the practice of nursing, Chapter 6 (commencing with Section 2700) of Division 2 of the Code, excluding Section 2762.

Authority cited: Sections 2715 and 2770.7, Business and Professions Code. Reference: Section 2770.7, Business and Professions Code.

§ 1448.1. Notification of Termination.

Whenever a nurse's participation is terminated for any reasons other than successful completion of the program, the committee shall, within thirty days, report such fact to the board in writing. The committee's written notification to the board shall consist solely of the participant's name and license number.

Authority cited: Section 2715, Business and Professions Code. Reference: Section 2770.11, Business and Professions Code.

§ 1449. Confidentiality of Records.

(a) All board, committee and program records relating to application to and participation in the program shall be kept confidential pursuant to Section 2770.12 of the Code. Such records shall be purged when a nurse's participation in the program is terminated.

(b) Information or records received by the board prior to the acceptance of the applicant into the program or which do not relate to application for the program may be utilized by the board in any disciplinary or criminal proceedings instituted against the participant.

Authority cited: Section 2715, Business and Professions Code. Reference: Section 2770.12, Business and Professions Code.

ARTICLE 5
CONTINUING EDUCATION

Section

1450. Definitions.
1451. License Renewal Requirements.
1451.1. Expiration of Licenses.
1451.2. Continuing Education Courses.
1452. Exemption from Continuing Education Requirements.
1453. Falsifying Renewal Application.
1454. Approved Providers.
1455. Continuing Education Hours.
1456. Continuing Education Courses.
1457. Instructor Qualifications.
1458. Course Verification.
1459. Advertisement.
1459.1. Withdrawal of Approval.

§ 1450. Definitions.

For purposes of this Article:

(a) "Continuing Education" means the variety of forms of learning experiences, including, but not limited to, lectures, conferences, academic studies, in service education, institutes, seminars, workshops, extension studies, and independent/

home study programs undertaken by registered nurses for relicensure. These learning experiences are meant to enhance the knowledge of the registered nurse in the practice of nursing in direct and indirect patient care.

(b) "Course" means a systematic learning experience, at least one hour in length, which deals with and is designed for the acquisition of knowledge, skills, and information in direct and indirect patient care.

(c) "Content Relevant to the Practice of Nursing" means content related to the development and maintenance of current competency in the delivery of nursing care as specified in Section 1456.

(d) "Experimental medical procedure or treatment" means the management and care of a patient involving any of the following:

(1) research approved by an Institutional Review Board as defined in Title 21, Code of Federal Regulations, Section 56.102 (hereby incorporated by reference as of August 8, 2022) involving a clinical trial or human subject as those terms are defined in Title 45, Code of Federal Regulations, Section 46.102 (hereby incorporated by reference as of August 8, 2022);

(2) for drugs, biological products, or devices, the treatment will be considered experimental if the United States Food and Drug Administration approved the drug, biological product, or device for use, but the drug, biological product, or device is used for a purpose other than that for which it was approved; or

(3) any treatment or procedure for which peer-reviewed scientific journals or studies show that the procedure or treatment is the subject of on-going clinical trials.

(e) "Independent/Home Study Courses" means continuing education courses offered for individual study by an approved provider.

(f) "Hour" means at least fifty (50) minutes of participation in an organized learning experience;

(g) "Approved Providers" means those individuals, partnerships, corporations, associations, organizations, organized health care systems, educational institutions, or governmental agencies offering continuing education as approved by the Board.

(h) "Implicit bias" means the attitudes or internalized stereotypes that affect our perceptions, actions, and decisions in an unconscious manner. Implicit bias often contributes to unequal treatment of people based on race, ethnicity, gender identity, sexual orientation, age, disability, and other characteristics.

(i) "Direct patient care" means the provision of health care services directly to individuals being treated for or suspected of having physical or mental illnesses. Direct patient care includes preventative care.

Authority cited: Sections 2715, 2736.5 and 2811.5, Business and Professions Code. Reference: Section 2811.5, Business and Professions Code.

History

1. New Article 5 (Sections 1450-1456) filed 10-10-75; effective thirtieth day thereafter (Register 75, No. 41).
2. Amendment filed 12-18-81; effective thirtieth day thereafter (Register 81, No. 51).
3. Amendment of section and NOTE filed 8-12-2022; operative 10-1-2022 (Register 2022, No. 32).

§ 1451. License Renewal Requirements.

(a) Pursuant to Section 2811 of the Code, each licensee shall pay the renewal fee and submit proof, satisfactory to the Board that during the preceding renewal period or preceding two years, the licensee has started and successfully completed thirty (30) hours of continuing education approved by the Board.

Regulations

(b) Licensees shall submit proof to the Board of successful completion of the required number of approved continuing education hours by signing a statement under penalty of perjury, indicating compliance and agreeing to supply supporting documents on request.

(c) Licensees shall not be allowed to claim partial credit for a continuing education course, however, instructors who participate in a part of an offering may receive full credit if the total offering is attended.

(d) Licensees shall keep the certificates or gradeslips from academic institutions pursuant to Section 1458 (b)(7) for four years from the date they complete approved continuing education courses and must submit such certificates or gradeslips to the Board when requested.

Authority cited: Section 2715, Business and Professions Code. Reference: Section 2811.5, Business and Professions Code.

History

1. Amendment filed 12-18-81; effective thirtieth day thereafter (Register 81, No. 51).

2. Change without regulatory effect repealing subsection (b), relettering subsections, and amending newly designated subsection (d) filed 12-29-98 pursuant to section 100, title 1, California Code of Regulations (Register 99, No. 1).

§ 1451.1. Expiration of Licenses.

(a) Licenses issued by the Board will expire unless renewed. To renew a license, the applicant shall submit proof, satisfactory to the Board of completion of thirty (30) hours of continuing education and shall pay the renewal fee.

(b) A licensee who participates in and successfully completes a continuing education course which overlaps a renewal period may apply the credit earned for the renewal period in which the course ends.

(c) An expired license may, within eight years of the date of expiration, be reinstated by the Board if the applicant meets the requirements of Section 2811 of the Code and is otherwise eligible to obtain a reinstatement, and if the applicant meets the requirements set forth in Section 1419.3.

Authority cited: Section 2715, Business and Professions Code. Reference: Sections 2811 and 2811.5, Business and Professions Code.

History

1. New section filed 12-18-81; effective thirtieth day thereafter (Register 81, No. 51).

2. Amendment of subsection (c) and repealer of subsections (d) and (e) filed 4-7-87; operative 5-7-87 (Register 87, No. 16).

§ 1451.2. Continuing Education Courses.

(a) Continuing Education course credit may be given for the following continuing education courses:

(1) Courses offered by an approved Provider as specified in Section 1454. In addition to classroom courses, courses may be designed by an approved Provider for participation in activities which include nursing practice, publishing and/or research, provided that such courses meet the requirements of Section 1456.

(2) Out of state courses which have been approved for voluntary or mandatory continuing education by Registered Nurse licensing agencies of other states and/or state nurses' associations, as well as offerings by nationally recognized health associations and/or their regional subdivisions provided that such courses meet the requirements of Section 1456.

(3) Out of state academic courses in an accredited* post-secondary institution which are related to the specific knowledge and/or technical skills required for the practice of nursing.

(4) Other courses as may be approved by the Board at its sole discretion.

Authority cited: Section 2715, Business and Professions Code. Reference: Section 2811.5, Business and Professions Code.

History

1. New section filed 12-18-81; effective thirtieth day thereafter (Register 81, No. 51).

§ 1452. Exemption from Continuing Education Requirements.

(a) During the first two years immediately following initial licensure in California or other jurisdictions, licensees shall be exempt from completion of the continuing education requirements specified in Section 1451.

(b) At the time of making application for renewal, an applicant may request exemption from continuing education requirements if:

(1) The licensee is requesting inactive status for the license; or

(2) The licensee can show evidence, satisfactory to the Board that

(A) he or she has been employed overseas for a period of one (1) year or more, or a resident overseas for a period of one (1) year or more and currently employed; or

(B) he or she is employed by a Federal Institution or Agency or one of the Military Services (USA), where that person is practicing nursing outside of the State of California on a California license, or

(C) he or she has had hardship of one or more years' duration, if

1. there is a total physical disability for one (1) year or more and verification of readiness or ability to return to work; or

2. there is a total disability of a member of the immediate family for whom licensee has total responsibility for one (1) year or more.

Authority cited: Section 2715, Business and Professions Code. Reference: Section 2811.5, Business and Professions Code.

History

1. Amendment filed 3-2-78; effective thirtieth day thereafter (Register 78, No. 9).
2. Repealer and new section filed 12-18-81; effective thirtieth day thereafter (Register 81, No. 51).

§ 1453. Falsifying Renewal Application.

A licensee who falsifies or makes a material misrepresentation of fact on a renewal application will be subject to disciplinary action as provided for in Section 2750 of the Business and Professions Code.

Authority cited: Section 2715, Business and Professions Code. Reference: Sections 2761 and 2811.5, Business and Professions Code.

History

1. Amendment filed 3-2-78; effective thirtieth day thereafter (Register 78, No. 9).
2. Repealer and new section filed 12-18-81; effective thirtieth day thereafter (Register 81, No. 51).

§ 1454. Approved Providers.

(a) For the purpose of this Article, the title "approved provider" can only be used when an individual, partnership, corporation, association, organization, organized health care system, educational institution or governmental agency, having committed no act which would lead to disciplinary action pursuant to

*Minimum requirement is regional accreditation.

Section 1459.1, has submitted a provider application on forms supplied by the Board, remitted the appropriate fee and has been issued a provider number.

(b) An individual, partnership, corporation, association, organized health care system, governmental agency, educational institution and other organizations may be issued only one provider number; provided, however, that any autonomous entity within such organization may be issued one provider number.

(c) An approved provider shall have a written and published policy, available on request, which provides information on:

(1) refunds in cases of non-attendance

(2) time period for return of fees

(3) notification if course is cancelled.

(d) The approved provider is required to accept full responsibility for each and every course, including, but not limited to recordkeeping, advertising course content as related to Board standards, issuance of certificates and instructor qualifications. When two or more providers co-sponsor a course, only one provider number shall be used for that course and that provider must assume full responsibility for recordkeeping, advertising course content as related to Board standards, issuance of certificates and instructor(s') qualifications.

(e) Providers may not grant partial credit for continuing education.

(f) Approved providers shall keep the following records for a period of four years in one location within the State of California, or in a place approved by the Board:

(1) course outlines of each course given

(2) record of time and places each course given

(3) course instructor vitaes or resumes

(4) name and license number of registered nurses taking any approved course and a record of any certificate issued to them.

(g) Approved providers must notify the Board, within thirty (30) days, of any changes in organizational structure of a provider and/or the person(s) responsible for the provider's continuing education course(s), including name and address changes.

(h) Provider approval is non-transferable.

(i) The Board shall audit records, courses, instructors and related activities of a provider.

Authority cited: Section 2715, Business and Professions Code. Reference: Section 2811.5, Business and Professions Code.

History

1. Repealer and new section filed 12-18-81; effective thirtieth day thereafter (Register 81, No. 51).
2. Amendment of subsection (a) filed 2-1-96; operative 3-2-96 (Register 96, No. 5).

§ 1455. Continuing Education Hours.

The Board will accept hours of approved continuing education on the following bases:

(a) Each hour of theory shall be accepted as one hour of continuing education.

(b) Each three hours in course-related clinical practice will be accepted as one hour of continuing education.

(c) Courses less than one (1) hour in duration will not be approved.

(d) One (1) CEU (continuing education unit) is equal to ten (10) continuing education contact hours.

(e) One (1) academic quarter unit is equal to ten (10) continuing education hours.

(f) One (1) academic semester unit is equal to fifteen (15) continuing education hours.

Authority cited: Section 2715, Business and Professions Code. Reference: Section 2811.5, Business and Professions Code.

History

1. Renumbering of former Section 1455 to Section 1456 and new section filed 3-2-78; effective thirtieth day thereafter (Register 78, No. 9).

2. Amendment filed 9-15-78; effective thirtieth day thereafter (Register 78, No. 37).

3. Repealer and new section filed 12-18-81; effective thirtieth day thereafter (Register 81, No. 51).

§ 1456. Continuing Education Courses.

(a) The content of all courses of continuing education must be relevant to the practice of nursing and must:

(1) Be related to the scientific knowledge and/or technical skills required for the practice of nursing, or

(2) Be related to direct and/or indirect patient/client care.

(3) Enhance the knowledge of the Registered Nurse at a level above that required for licensure. Courses related to the scientific knowledge for the practice of nursing include basic and advanced courses in the physical, social, and behavioral sciences, as well as advanced nursing in general or specialty areas. Content which includes the application of scientific knowledge to patient care in addition to advanced nursing courses may include courses in related areas, i.e., human sexuality; death, dying, and grief; foreign languages (conversational); therapeutic interpersonal relationship skills; pharmacology; generally accepted experimental medical procedures or treatments; and those related to specialty areas of nursing practice. Courses in nursing administration, management, education, research, or other functional areas of nursing relating to indirect patient/client care would be acceptable.

Courses which deal with self-improvement, changes in attitude, financial gain, and those courses designed for lay people are not acceptable for meeting requirements for license renewal.

(4) Contain curriculum that includes the understanding of implicit bias pursuant to Section 2736.5 of the code, unless the course is dedicated solely to research or other issues that does not include a direct patient care component.

(b) For the purposes of this section, "generally accepted experimental medical procedures or treatments" means:

(1) the efficacy of the procedure(s) or treatment(s) is supported by at least two peer-reviewed, publicly available scientific journals or studies, or is published in medical and/or scientific literature, and

(2) there is no clear and convincing contradictory evidence presented in a major peer reviewed medical journal that the treatment or procedure is not safe and effective.

Authority cited: Sections 2715, 2736.5 and 2811.5, Business and Professions Code. Reference: Sections 2736.5 and 2811.5, Business and Professions Code.

History

1. Renumbering of Section 1455 to Section 1456 filed 3-2-78; effective thirtieth day thereafter (Register 78, No. 9).

2. Repealer and new section filed 12-18-81; effective thirtieth day thereafter (Register 81, No. 51).

3. Amendment of section and NOTE filed 8-12-2022; operative 10-1-2022 (Register 2022, No. 32).

§ 1457. Instructor Qualifications.

(a) It is the responsibility of each approved provider to use qualified instructors.

(b) Instructors teaching approved continuing education courses shall have the following minimum qualifications:

(1) The registered nurse instructor, shall

(A) hold a current valid license to practice as a registered nurse and be free from any disciplinary action by this Board, and

(B) be knowledgeable, current and skillful in the subject matter of the course as evidenced through:

1. holding a baccalaureate or higher degree from an accredited college or university and validated experience in subject matter; or

2. experience in teaching similar subject matter content within the two years preceding the course; or

3. have at least one year's experience within the last two years in the specialized area in which he/she is teaching.

(2) The non-nurse instructor, shall

(A) be currently licensed or certified in his/her area of expertise if appropriate, and

(B) show evidence of specialized training, which may include, but not be limited to a certificate of training or an advanced degree in given subject area, and

(C) have at least one year's experience within the last two years in the practice of teaching of the specialized area in which he/she teaches.

(3) Nothing in this Section exempts an individual from the legal requirements of the California Nursing Practice Act.

Authority cited: Section 2715, Business and Professions Code. Reference: Section 2811.5, Business and Professions Code.

History

1. Renumbering of Section 1456 to Section 1457 filed 3-2-78; effective thirtieth day thereafter (Register 78, No. 9).

2. Repealer and new section filed 12-18-81; effective thirtieth day thereafter (Register 81, No. 51).

§ 1458. Course Verification.

(a) Approved providers shall issue a document of proof, i.e., gradeslip, or transcript to each licensee to show that the individual has met the established criteria for successful completion of a course.

(b) A certificate or diploma documenting successful completion shall contain the following information:

(1) Name of student and registered nurse license number or other identification number.

(2) Course title.

(3) Provider name (as approved by the Board), address, and provider number.

(4) Date of course.

(5) Number of continuing education contact hours.

(6) Signature of instructor and/or provider, or provider designee.

(7) This document must be retained by the licensee for a period of four years after the course concludes.

(c) Course verification must be issued within a reasonable length of time after the completion of the course, not to exceed ninety days.

Authority cited: Section 2715, Business and Professions Code. Reference: Section 2811.5, Business and Professions Code.

History

1. New section filed 5-13-77; effective thirtieth day thereafter (Register 77, No. 20).
2. Renumbering of Section 1457 to Section 1458 filed 3-2-78; effective thirtieth day thereafter (Register 78, No. 9).
3. Repealer and new section filed 12-18-81; effective thirtieth day thereafter (Register 81, No. 51).

§ 1459. Advertisement.

Information disseminated by approved providers publicizing continuing education shall be true and not misleading and shall include the following:

1. The statement "Provider approved by the California Board of Registered Nursing, Provider Number ______ for ______ contact hours."
2. Provider's policy on refunds in cases of non-attendance by the registrant.
3. A clear, concise description of the course content and/or objectives.
4. Provider name as officially on file with the Board.

Authority cited: Section 2715, Business and Professions Code. Reference: Section 2811.5, Business and Professions Code.

History

1. New section filed 12-18-81; effective thirtieth day thereafter (Registered 81, No. 51).

§ 1459.1. Withdrawal of Approval.

(a) The Board may withdraw its approval of a provider or deny a provider application for causes which include, but are not limited to, the following:

(1) Conviction of a felony or any offense substantially related to the activities of a provider.

(2) Failure to comply with any provision of Chapter 6, Division 2, of the Business and Professions Code and/or Chapter 14 of Title 16 of the California Code of Regulations.

(b) Any material misrepresentation of fact by a continuing education provider or applicant in any information required to be submitted to the Board is grounds for withdrawal of approval or denial of an application.

(c) The board may withdraw its approval of a provider after giving the provider written notice setting forth its reason for withdrawal and after affording a reasonable opportunity to be heard by the board or its designee after thirty (30) days written notice of the specific charges to be heard.

(d) Should the BRN deny the provider approval, applicant has the opportunity to formally appeal the action to the Board within a thirty (30) day period.

Authority cited: Section 2715, Business and Professions Code. Reference: Section 2811.5, Business and Professions Code.

History

1. New section filed 12-18-81; effective thirtieth day thereafter (Register 81, No. 51).
2. Amendment of subsection (c) filed 3-23-84; effective upon filing pursuant to Government Code Section 11346.2(d) (Register 84, No. 12).
3. Amendment of subsection (a)(2) filed 2-1-96; operative 3-2-96 (Register 96, No. 5).

ARTICLE 6
NURSE-MIDWIVES

Section

1460. Qualifications for Certification.
1461. Nurse-Midwifery Committee.
1462. Standards for Nurse-Midwifery Programs.

1463. Scope of Practice.
1463.5. Abortion by Aspiration Techniques.
1466. Renewal of Certificates.

§ 1460. Qualifications for Certification.

(a) Initial certification.

(1) An applicant for certification to practice midwifery must meet the following conditions:

(A) Be licensed as a registered nurse under the Nursing Practice Act, Business and Professions Code, Section 2700, et seq. , and

(B) Be a graduate of a Board approved program in nurse-midwifery.

(2) Equivalency. A registered nurse applicant not meeting the above requirements shall be eligible for certification, providing one of the following conditions exists:

(A) A graduate of a nurse-midwifery program not meeting Board of Registered Nursing standards who shows evidence satisfactory to the Board that deficiencies have been corrected in a Board approved nurse-midwifery program, or have been corrected through successful completion of specific courses which have been approved by the Board.

(B) Certification as a nurse-midwife by a national or state organization whose standards are satisfactory to the Board.

Authority cited: Section 2715, Business and Professions Code. Reference: Sections 2746, 2746.2, 2746.5, Business and Professions Code.

History

1. New Article 6 (§§ 1460-1465, not consecutive) filed 10-10-75; effective thirtieth day thereafter (Register 75, No. 41).
2. New subsections (b) and (c) filed 1-9-76; effective thirtieth day thereafter (Register 76, No. 2).
3. Repealer and new section filed 4-7-79; effective thirtieth day thereafter (Register 79, No. 14).
4. Amendment of subsection (a)(2)(A) filed 5-29-81; effective thirtieth day thereafter (Register 81, No. 22).
5. Repealer of subsections (a)(2)(C)-(a)(2)(D)2. filed 1-25-2000; operative 2-24-2000 (Register 2000, No. 4).

§ 1461. Nurse-Midwifery Committee.

The board shall appoint a committee comprised of at least one nurse-midwife and one physician, who have demonstrated familiarity with consumer needs, collegial practice and accompanied liability, and related educational standards in the delivery of maternal-child health care. This committee shall also include at least one public member and may include such other members as the board deems appropriate. The purpose of this committee is to advise the board on all matters pertaining to nurse-midwifery as established by the board, and, if necessary, to assist the board or its designated representatives in the evaluation of applications for nurse-midwifery certification.

Authority cited: Section 2715, Business and Professions Code. Reference: Section 2746.2, Business and Professions Code.

History

1. Renumbering from Section 1461 to Section 1466 filed 4-6-79; effective thirtieth day thereafter (Register 79, No. 14).
2. New section filed 4-6-79; effective thirtieth day thereafter (Register 79, No. 14).
3. Amendment filed 12-4-85; effective thirtieth day thereafter (Register 85, No. 49).

§ 1462. Standards for Nurse-Midwifery Programs.

(a) Program of study. The program of study preparing a nurse-midwife shall:

(1) Have as its primary purpose the preparation of nurse-midwives;

(2) Have its philosophy clearly defined and available in written form;

(3) Have its objectives, reflective of the philosophy, stated in behavioral terms, which describe the theoretical knowledge base and clinical competencies expected of the graduates.

(b) Curriculum.

(1) The curriculum shall be no less than twelve(12) months in length, and shall be specifically designed to provide a knowledge and skills base necessary for nurse-midwifery management of women and neonates. Such content shall include, but not be limited to, the following:

(A) Anatomy; physiology; genetics; obstetrics and gynecology; embryology and fetal development; neonatology; child growth and development; pharmacology; nutrition; laboratory and diagnostic tests and procedures; and physical assessment.

(B) Concepts in psycho-social, emotional, and cultural aspects of maternal/child care; human sexuality; counseling and teaching; maternal/infant/family bonding process; breast feeding; family planning; principles of preventive health; and community health.

(C) All aspects of the management of normal pregnancy, labor and delivery, postpartum period, newborn care, family planning and/or routine gynecological care in alternative birth centers, homes and hospitals.

(2) The program shall provide concurrent theory and clinical practice in a setting in the United States.

(3) The program shall include the nurse-midwifery management process which includes the following steps:

(A) Obtains or updates a defined and relevant data base for assessment of the health status of the client.

(B) Identifies problems/diagnosis based upon correct interpretation of the data base.

(C) Prepares a defined needs/problem list with corroboration from the client.

(D) Consults and collaborates with and refers to, appropriate members of the health care team.

(E) Provides information to enable clients to make appropriate decisions and to assume appropriate responsibility for their own health.

(F) Assumes direct responsibility for the development of comprehensive, supportive care for the client and with the client.

(G) Assumes direct responsibility for implementing the plan of care.

(H) Initiates appropriate measures for obstetrical and neonatal emergencies.

(I) Evaluates, with corroboration from the client, the achievement of health care goals and modifies plan of care appropriately.

(4) The program shall prepare the nurse-midwife to practice as follows:

(A) Management of the normal pregnancy.

(B) Management of normal labor and delivery in all birth settings, including the following when indicated:

1. Administration of intravenous fluids, analgesics, and postpartum oxytocics.

2. Amniotome during labor.

3. Application of external or internal monitoring devices.

4. Administration of local anesthesia: paracervical blocks, pudendal blocks, and local infiltration.

5. Episiotomy.

6. Repair of episiotomies and lacerations.
7. Resuscitation of the newborn.

(C) Management of the normal postpartum period.

(D) Management of the normal newborn care.

(E) Management of family planning and/or routine gynecological care including: fitting vaginal diaphragms, insertion of intrauterine devices, selection of contraceptive agents from approved formulary.

(c) Faculty. Faculty of the nurse-midwifery educational program shall comply with the following requirements:

(1) Faculty shall include one or more nurse-midwives and one or more physicians with current training and practice in obstetrics.

(2) Faculty teaching in the program shall be current in knowledge and practice in the specialty being taught.

(3) Nurse-midwives, clinical instructors, and physicians who participate in teaching, supervising and evaluating students shall show evidence of current practice.

Authority cited: Section 2715, Business and Professions Code. Reference: Sections 2746, 2746.2 and 2746.5, Business and Professions Code.

History

1. New section filed 4-6-79; effective thirtieth day thereafter (Register 79, No. 14).
2. Amendment filed 12-4-85; effective thirtieth day thereafter (Register 85, No. 49).

§ 1463. Scope of Practice.

The scope of nurse-midwifery practice includes:

(a) Providing necessary supervision, care and advice in a variety of settings to women during the antepartal, intrapartal, postpartal, interconceptional periods, and family planning needs.

(b) Conducting deliveries on his or her own responsibility and caring for the newborn and the infant. This care includes preventive measures and the detection of abnormal conditions in mother and child.

(c) Obtaining physician assistance and consultation when indicated.

(d) Providing emergency care until physician assistance can be obtained.

(e) Other practices and procedures may be included when the nurse-midwife and the supervising physician deem appropriate by using the standardized procedures as specified in Section 2725 of the Code.

Authority cited: Section 2715, Business and Professions Code. Reference: Sections 2746, 2746.2 and 2746.5, Business and Professions Code.

History

1. New section filed 4-6-79; effective thirtieth day thereafter (Register 79, No. 14).
2. Editorial correction to subsection designations (Register 79, No. 14).
3. Amendment of subsection (e) and repealer of subsection (f) filed 12-4-85; effective thirtieth day thereafter (Register 85, No. 49).

§ 1463.5. Abortion by Aspiration Techniques.

For the purposes of Section 2725.4 of the Code, after January 1, 2016, certified nurse-midwives may perform an abortion by aspiration techniques in the first trimester of pregnancy if they have completed the requisite training in performing these procedures equivalent to the didactic curriculum and clinical training protocols of the HWPP No. 171 provided by any of the following:

(1) A Board-approved nurse-midwifery program or in a course offered by an accredited nurse-midwifery program;

(2) A course offered by a Board-approved continuing education provider that reflects evidence-based curriculum and training guidelines or a course approved for Category I continuing medical education;

(3) A course offered by a state or national health care professional or accreditation organization.

Authority cited: Section 2715, Business and Professions Code. Reference: Section 2725.4, Business and Professions Code.

History

1. New section filed 3-3-2016; operative 3-3-2016 pursuant to Government Code section 11343.4(b)(3) (Register 2016, No. 10).

§ 1466. Renewal of Certificates.

Certificates to practice nurse-midwifery may be renewed biennially by application for renewal on a form provided by the board and payment of the renewal fee.

Authority cited: Section 2715, Business and Professions Code. Reference: Section 2815.5, Business and Professions Code.

History

1. Renumbering from Section 1461 to Section 1466 filed 4-6-79; effective thirtieth day thereafter (Register 79, No. 14).

2. Amendment filed 12-4-85; effective thirtieth day thereafter (Register 85, No. 49).

ARTICLE 7
STANDARDIZED PROCEDURE GUIDELINES

Section

1470. Purpose.
1471. Definitions.
1472. Standardized Procedure Functions.
1474. Standardized Procedure Guidelines.

§ 1470. Purpose.

The Board of Registered Nursing in conjunction with the Medical Board of California (see the regulations of the Medical Board of California, Article 9.5, Chapter 13, Title 16 of the California Code of Regulations) intends, by adopting the regulations contained in the article, to jointly promulgate guidelines for the development of standardized procedures to be used in organized health care systems which are subject to this rule. The purpose of these guidelines is:

(a) To protect consumers by providing evidence that the nurse meets all requirements to practice safely.

(b) To provide uniformity in development of standardized procedures.

Authority cited: Section 2715, Business and Professions Code. Reference: Sections 2725 and 2811.5, Business and Professions Code.

History

1. New Article 7 (Sections 1470-1474, inclusive) filed 9-8-76; effective thirtieth day thereafter (Register 76, No. 37).

2. Amendment filed 6-17-85; effective thirtieth day thereafter (Register 85, No. 25).

3. Amendment of first paragraph filed 2-1-96; operative 3-2-96 (Register 96, No. 5).

Regulations

§ 1471. Definitions.

For purposes of this article:

(a) "Standardized procedure functions" means those functions specified in Business and Professions Code Section 2725(c) and (d) which are to be performed according to "standardized procedures";

(b) "Organized health care system" means a health facility which is not licensed pursuant to Chapter 2 (commencing with Section 1250), Division 2 of the Health and Safety Code and includes, but is not limited to, clinics, home health agencies, physicians' offices and public or community health services;

(c) "Standardized procedures" means policies and protocols formulated by organized health care systems for the performance of standardized procedure functions.

§ 1472. Standardized Procedure Functions.

An organized health care system must develop standardized procedures before permitting registered nurses to perform standardized procedure functions. A registered nurse may perform standardized procedure functions only under the conditions specified in a health care system's standardized procedures; and must provide the system with satisfactory evidence that the nurse meets its experience, training, and/or education requirements to perform such functions.

§ 1474. Standardized Procedure Guidelines.

Following are the standardized procedure guidelines jointly promulgated by the Medical Board of California and by the Board of Registered Nursing:

(a) Standardized procedures shall include a written description of the method used in developing and approving them and any revision thereof.

(b) Each standardized procedure shall:

(1) Be in writing, dated and signed by the organized health care system personnel authorized to approve it.

(2) Specify which standardized procedure functions registered nurses may perform and under what circumstances.

(3) State any specific requirements which are to be followed by registered nurses in performing particular standardized procedure functions.

(4) Specify any experience, training, and/or education requirements for performance of standardized procedure functions.

(5) Establish a method for initial and continuing evaluation of the competence of those registered nurses authorized to perform standardized procedure functions.

(6) Provide for a method of maintaining a written record of those persons authorized to perform standardized procedure functions.

(7) Specify the scope of supervision required for performance of standardized procedure functions, for example, immediate supervision by a physician.

(8) Set forth any specialized circumstances under which the registered nurse is to immediately communicate with a patient's physician concerning the patient's condition.

(9) State the limitations on settings, if any, in which standardized procedure functions may be performed.

(10) Specify patient record keeping requirements.

(11) Provide for a method of periodic review of the standardized procedures.

Authority cited: Section 2715, Business and Professions Code. Reference: Section 2725, Business and Professions Code.

History

1. Amendment of first paragraph and new Note filed 2-1-96; operative 3-2-96 (Register 96, No. 5).

ARTICLE 8
STANDARDS FOR NURSE PRACTITIONERS

Section

1480. Definitions.
1481. Categories of Nurse Practitioners.
1482. Requirements for Certification As a Nurse Practitioner
1483. Evaluation of Credentials.
1483.1 Requirements for Nurse Practitioner Education Programs in California.
1483.2 Requirements for Reporting Nurse Practitioner Education Program Changes.
1484. Nurse Practitioner Education.
1485. Scope of Practice.
1485.5. Abortion by Aspiration Techniques.
1486 Requirements for Clinical Practice Experience for Nurse Practitioner Students Enrolled in Non-California based Nurse Practitioner Education Programs.

§ 1480. Definitions.

(a) "Acute care" means restorative care provided by the nurse practitionerto patients with rapidly changing, unstable, chronic, complex acute, and critical conditions in a variety of clinical practice settings.

(b) "Advanced health assessment" means the knowledge of advanced processes of collecting and interpreting information regarding a patient's health care status. Advanced health assessment provides the basis for differential diagnoses and treatment plans.

(c) "Advanced pathophysiology" means the advanced knowledge and management of physiological disruptions that accompany a wide range of alterations in health.

(d) "Advanced pharmacology" means the integration of the advanced knowledge of pharmacology, pharmacokinetics, and pharmacodynamics content across the lifespan and prepares the certified nurse practitioner to initiate appropriate pharmacotherapeutics safely and effectively in the management of acute and chronic health conditions.

(e) "California based nurse practitioner education program" means a board approved academic program, physically located in California that offers a graduate degree in nursing or graduate level certificate in nursing to qualified students and is accredited by a nursing organization recognized by the United States Department of Education or the Council of Higher Education Accreditation.

(f) "Category" means the population focused area of practice in which the certified nurse practitioner provides patient care.

(g) "Clinically competent" means the individual possesses and exercises the degree of learning, skill, care, and experience ordinarily possessed and exercised by a certified nurse practitioner providing healthcare in the same nurse practitioner category. The clinical experience must be such that the nurse received intensive experience in performing the diagnostic and treatment procedures essential to the provision of primary care.

(h) “Clinical field related to nursing” means a specialized field of clinical practice in one of the following categories of nurse practitioners as recognized by the National Organization of Nurse Practitioner Faculties (NONPF), which are: Family/Individual across the lifespan; Adult-gerontology, primary care; Adult-gerontology, acute care; Neonatal; Pediatrics, primary care; Pediatrics, acute care; Women’s health/gender-related; and Psychiatric-Mental Health across the lifespan.

(i) “Clinical practice experience” means supervised direct patient care in the clinical setting that provides for the acquisition and application of advanced practice nursing knowledge, skills, and competencies.

(j) “Direct supervision of students” means a clinical preceptor or a faculty member is physically present at the practice site. The clinical preceptor or faculty member retains the responsibility for patient care while overseeing the student.

(k) [reserved]

(l) “Lead nurse practitioner faculty educator” means the nurse practitioner faculty member of the nurse practitioner education program who has administrative responsibility for developing and implementing the curriculum in the nurse practitioner category.

(m) “Major curriculum change” means a substantive change in a nurse practitioner education program curriculum, structure, content, method of delivery, or clinical hours.

(n) “National Certification” means the certified nurse practitioner has passed an examination provided by a national certification organization accredited by the National Commission for Certifying Agencies or the American Board of Nursing Specialties, as approved by the board.

(o) “Nurse practitioner” means an advanced practice registered nurse who meets board education and certification requirements and possesses additional advanced practice educational preparation and skills in physical diagnosis, psycho-social assessment, and management of health-illness needs in primary care, and/or acute care.

(p) “Nurse practitioner curriculum” means a curriculum that consists of the graduate core; advanced practice registered nursing core, and nurse practitioner role and population-focused courses.

(1) “Graduate core” means the foundational curriculum content deemed essential for all students pursuing a graduate degree in nursing.

(2) “Advanced practice registered nursing core” means the essential broad-based curriculum required for all nurse practitioner students in the areas of advanced health assessment, advanced pathophysiology, and advanced pharmacology.

(q) “Nurse practitioner education program director” means the individual responsible for administration, implementation, and evaluation of the nurse practitioner education program and the achievement of the program outcomes in collaboration with program faculty.

(r) “Non-California based nurse practitioner education program” means an academic program accredited by a nursing organization recognized by the United States Department of Education or the Council of Higher Education Accreditation that offers a graduate degree in nursing or graduate level certificate in nursing to qualified students and does not have a physical location in California. Preparation at the graduate level must be comprehensive and focus on the clinical practice of providing direct care to individuals.

(s) "Primary care" means comprehensive and continuous care provided to patients, families, and the community. Primary care focuses on basic preventative care, health promotion, disease prevention, health maintenance, patient education, and the diagnoses and treatment of acute and chronic illnesses in a variety of practice settings.

Authority cited: Sections 2715, 2725 and 2836, Business and Professions Code. Reference: Sections 2725.5, 2834, 2835.5 and 2836.1, Business and Professions Code.

History

1. New Article 8 (Sections 1480-1485) filed 7-13-79; effective thirtieth day thereafter (Register 79, No. 28).

2. Amendment filed 12-7-85; effective thirtieth day thereafter (Register 85, No. 49).

3. Amendment of section and NOTE filed 1-15-2019; operative 1-15-2019 pursuant to Government Code section 11343.4(b)(3) (Register 2019, No. 3).

4. Change without regulatory effect amending section filed 12-23-2021 pursuant to section 100, title 1, California Code of Regulations (Register 2021, No. 52).

§ 1481. Categories of Nurse Practitioners.

(a) Categories of nurse practitioners include:

(1) Family/individual across the lifespan;

(2) Adult-gerontology, primary care or acute care;

(3) Neonatal;

(4) Pediatrics, primary care or acute care;

(5) Women's health/gender-related;

(6) Psychiatric-Mental Health across the lifespan.

(b) A registered nurse who has been certified by the board as a nurse practitioner may use the title, "advanced practice registered nurse" and/or "certified nurse practitioner" and may place the letters APRN-CNP after his or her name or in combination with other letters or words that identify the category.

Authority cited: Sections 2715 and 2836, Business and Professions Code. Reference: Sections 2834, 2835.5, 2836, 2836.1 and 2837, Business and Professions Code.

History

1. Amendment filed 12-4-85; effective thirtieth day thereafter (Register 85, No. 49).

2. Repealer and new section and amendment of Note filed 1-15-2019; operative 1-15-2019 pursuant to Government Code section 11343.4(b)(3) (Register 2019, No. 3).

§ 1482. Requirements for Certification As a Nurse Practitioner

(a) To obtain certification as a Nurse Practitioner, an applicant must hold a valid and active license as a registered nurse in California and possess a master's degree in nursing, a master's degree in a clinical field related to nursing, or a graduate degree in nursing and one of the following:

(1) Successful completion of a nurse practitioner education program approved by the Board;

(2) National certification as a nurse practitioner in one or more categories listed in Section 1481(a) from a national certification organization accredited by the National Commission on Certifying Agencies or the American Board of Nursing Specialties.

(b) A nurse who has not completed an academically affiliated nurse practitioner education program shall provide evidence of having completed equivalent education and supervised clinical practice, as set forth in this article.

(c) Graduates who have completed a nurse practitioner education program in a foreign country shall meet the requirements as set forth in this article. The applicant shall submit the required credential evaluation through a board-approved evaluation service evidencing education equivalent to a master's or doctoral degree in Nursing.

Authority cited: Section 2715, Business and Professions Code. Reference: Sections 2835, 2835.5 and 2836, Business and Professions Code.

History

1. Amendment filed 12-4-85; effective thirtieth day thereafter (Register 85, No. 49).

2. Amendment of section heading, section and Note filed 1-15-2019; operative 1-15-2019 pursuant to Government Code section 11343.4(b)(3) (Register 2019, No. 3).

§ 1483. Evaluation of Credentials.

(a) An application for evaluation of a registered nurse's qualifications to be certified as a nurse practitioner shall be filed with the board by submitting the Application for Nurse Practitioner (NP) Certification (Rev. 03/2019), which is hereby incorporated by reference. A temporary Nurse Practitioner (NP) certificate shall be obtained by submitting the Application for Temporary Nurse Practitioner (NP) Certificate (Rev. 03/2019), which is hereby incorporated by reference. In order to furnish drugs or devices in California as a Nurse Practitioner, the certified nurse practitioner must be issued a Nurse Practitioner Furnishing Number by submitting the Nurse Practitioner Furnishing Number Application (Rev. 03/2019), which is hereby incorporated by reference, for approval. Submission of each application shall be accompanied by the fee prescribed in Section 1417 and such evidence, statements or documents as therein required by the board.

(b) The Application for Nurse Practitioner (NP) Certification, the Application for Temporary Nurse Practitioner (NP) Certificate and the Nurse Practitioner Furnishing Number Application shall include submission of the name of the graduate nurse practitioner education program or post-graduate nurse practitioner education program.

(c) The Application for Nurse Practitioner (NP) Certification shall include submission of an official sealed transcript with the date of graduation or post-graduate program completion, nurse practitioner category, credential conferred, and the specific courses taken to provide sufficient evidence the applicant has completed the required course work including the required number of supervised direct patient care clinical practice hours.

(d) A graduate from a board-approved nurse practitioner education program shall be considered a graduate of a nationally accredited program if the program held national nursing accreditation at the time the graduate completed the program. The program graduate is eligible to apply for nurse practitioner certification with the board regardless of the program's national nursing accreditation status at the time of submission of the application to the Board.

(e) The board shall notify the applicant in writing that the application is complete and accepted for filing or that the application is deficient and what specific information is required within 30 days from the receipt of an application. A decision on the evaluation of credentials shall be reached within 60 days from the filing of a completed application. The median, minimum, and maximum times for processing an application, from the receipt of the initial application to the final decision, shall be 42 days, 14 days, and one year, respectively, taking into account Section 1410.4(e) which provides for abandonment of incomplete applications after one year.

Authority cited: Section 2715, Business and Professions Code. Reference: Sections 2815 and 2835.5, Business and Professions Code.

History

1. Repealer and new section filed 8-21-86; effective thirtieth day (Register 86, No. 34).

2. Amendment of section and Note filed 1-15-2019; operative 1-15-2019 pursuant to Government Code section 11343.4(b)(3) (Register 2019, No. 3).

3. Change without regulatory effect amending subsection (a) filed 4-24-2019 pursuant to section 100, title 1, California Code of Regulations (Register 2019, No. 17).

§ 1483.1 Requirements for Nurse Practitioner Education Programs in California.

(a) The California based nurse practitioner education program shall:

(1) Provide evidence to the board that the nurse practitioner program is in an accredited academic institution located in California.

(2) Be an academic program accredited by a nursing organization recognized by the United States Department of Education or the Council of Higher Education Accreditation that offers a graduate degree in Nursing or graduate level certificate in Nursing to qualified students.

(3) Provide the board with evidence of ongoing continuing nurse practitioner education program accreditation within 30 days of the program receiving this information from the national nursing accreditation body.

(4) Notify the board of changes in the program's institutional and national nursing accreditation status within 30 days.

(b) The board shall grant the nurse practitioner education program initial and continuing approval when the board receives the required accreditation evidence from the program.

(c) The board may change the approval status for a board-approved nurse practitioner education program at any time, if the board determines the program has not provided necessary compliance evidence to meet board regulations notwithstanding institutional and national nursing accreditation status and review schedules.

Authority cited: Section 2715, Business and Professions Code. Reference: Sections 2785, 2786, 2786.5, 2786.6, 2788, 2798, 2815 and 2835.5, Business and Professions Code.

History

1. New section filed 1-15-2019; operative 1-15-2019 pursuant to Government Code section 11343.4(b)(3) (Register 2019, No. 3).

§ 1483.2 Requirements for Reporting Nurse Practitioner Education Program Changes.

(a) A board-approved nurse practitioner education program shall notify the board within thirty (30) days of any of the following changes:

(1) A change of legal name or mailing address prior to making such changes. The program shall file its legal name and current mailing address with the board at its principal office and the notice shall provide both the old and the new name and address as applicable.

(2) A fiscal condition that adversely affects students enrolled in the nursing program.

(3) Substantive changes in the organizational structure affecting the nursing program.

(b) An approved nursing program shall not make a substantive change without prior board notification. Substantive changes include, but are not limited to the following:

(1) Change in location;

(2) Change in ownership;

(3) Addition of a new campus or location;

(4) Major curriculum change.

Authority cited: Section 2715, Business and Professions Code. Reference: Sections 2715, 2785, 2786, 2786.5, 2786.6, 2788, 2798 and 2835.5, Business and Professions Code.

History

1. New section filed 1-15-2019; operative 1-15-2019 pursuant to Government Code section 11343.4(b)(3) (Register 2019, No. 3).

§ 1484. Nurse Practitioner Education.

(a) The program of study preparing a nurse practitioner shall be approved by the board and be consistent with the nurse practitioner curriculum core competencies as specified by the National Organization of Nurse Practitioner Faculties in "Nurse Practitioner Core Competencies Content" (2017), which is hereby incorporated by reference.

(b) The purpose of the nurse practitioner education program shall be to prepare a graduate nurse practitioner to provide competent primary care and/or acute care services in one or more of the categories.

Written program materials shall reflect the mission, philosophy, purposes, and outcomes of the program and be available to students.

Learning outcomes for the nurse practitioner education program shall be measurable and reflect assessment and evaluation of the theoretical knowledge and clinical competencies required of the graduate.

(c) Administration and organization of the nurse practitioner education program shall:

(1) Be taught in a college or university accredited by a nursing organization that is recognized by the United States Department of Education or the Council of Higher Education Accreditation that offers a graduate degree to qualified students.

(2) Prepare graduates for national certification as a certified nurse practitioner in one or more nurse practitioner category by the National Commission on Certifying Agencies or the American Board of Nursing Specialties.

(3) Have admission requirements and policies for withdrawal, dismissal and readmission that are clearly stated and available to the student.

(4) Inform applicants of the academic accreditation and board approval status of the program.

(5) Document the nurse practitioner role and the category of educational preparation on the program's official transcript.

(6) Maintain a method for retrieval of records in the event of program closure.

(7) Have and implement a written total program evaluation plan.

(8) Have sufficient resources to achieve the program outcomes.

(d) Faculty.

(1) There shall be an adequate number of qualified faculty to develop and implement the program and to achieve the stated outcomes.

(2) Each faculty member shall demonstrate current competence in the area in which he or she teaches.

(3) There shall be a lead nurse practitioner faculty educator who meets the faculty qualifications.

(4) Faculty who teach in the nurse practitioner education program shall be educationally qualified and clinically competent in the same category as the theory and clinical areas taught. Faculty shall meet the following requirements:

(A) Hold an active, valid California registered nurse license;

(B) Have a Master's degree or higher degree in nursing;

(C) Have at least two years of clinical experience as a nurse practitioner, certified nurse midwife, clinical nurse specialist, or certified registered nurse anesthetist within the last five (5) years of practice and consistent with the teaching responsibilities.

(5) Faculty teaching in clinical courses shall be current in clinical practice.

(6) Each faculty member shall assume responsibility and accountability for instruction, planning, and implementation of the curriculum, and evaluation of students and the program.

(7) Interdisciplinary faculty who teach non-clinical nurse practitioner nursing courses, such as but not limited to, pharmacology, pathophysiology, and physical assessment, shall have a valid and active California license issued by the appropriate licensing agency and an advanced graduate degree in the appropriate content areas.

(e) Director.

(1) The nurse practitioner education program director shall be responsible and accountable for the nurse practitioner education program within an accredited academic institution including the areas of education program, curriculum design, and resource acquisition, and shall meet the following requirements:

(A) Hold an active, valid California registered nurse license;

(B) Have a Master's or a higher degree in nursing;

(C) Have had one academic year of experience, within the last five (5) years, as an instructor in a school of professional nursing, or in a program preparing nurse practitioners; and

(D) Be certified by the board as a nurse practitioner.

(2) The director, if he or she meets the requirements for the certified nurse practitioner role, may fulfill the lead nurse practitioner faculty educator role and responsibilities.

(f) Clinical Preceptor.

(1) A clinical preceptor in the nurse practitioner education program shall:

(A) Hold an active valid, California license to practice his or her respective profession and demonstrate current clinical competence.

(B) Participate in teaching, supervising, and evaluating students, and shall be competent in the content and skills being taught to the students.

(2) Clinical preceptor functions and responsibilities shall be clearly documented in a written agreement between the agency, the preceptor, and the nurse practitioner education program including the clinical preceptor's role to teach, supervise and evaluate students in the nurse practitioner education program.

(3) A clinical preceptor is oriented to program and curriculum requirements, including responsibilities related to student supervision and evaluation;

(4) A clinical preceptor shall be evaluated by the program faculty at least every two (2) years.

(g) Students shall hold an active, valid California registered nurse license to participate in nurse practitioner education program clinical experiences.

(h) Nurse Practitioner Education Program Curriculum.

The nurse practitioner education program curriculum shall include all theoretical and clinical instruction that meet the standards set forth in this section and be consistent with national standards for graduate and nurse practitioner education, including nationally recognized core role and category competencies and be approved by the board.

(1) The program shall evaluate previous education and experience in health care for the purpose of granting credit for meeting program requirements.

(2) The curriculum shall provide broad educational preparation and include a graduate core, advance practice registered nursing core, the nurse practitioner core role competencies, and the competencies specific to the category.

(3) The program shall prepare the graduate to be eligible to sit for a specific national nurse practitioner category certification examination consistent with educational preparation.

(4) The curriculum plan shall have appropriate course sequencing and progression, which includes, but is not limited to the following:

(A) The advanced practice registered nursing core courses in advanced health assessment, advanced pharmacology, and advanced pathophysiology shall be completed prior to or concurrent with commencing clinical course work.

(B) Instruction and skills practice for diagnostic and treatment procedures shall occur prior to application in the clinical setting.

(C) Concurrent theory and clinical practice courses in the category shall emphasize the management of health-illness needs in primary and/ or acute care.

(D) The supervised direct patient care precepted clinical experiences shall be under the supervision of a certified nurse practitioner.

(5) The program shall meet and may exceed the minimum of 500 clinical hours of supervised direct patient care experiences, as specified in current nurse practitioner standards provided in this section. Additional clinical hours required for preparation in more than one category shall be identified and documented in the curriculum plan for each category.

(6) The nurse practitioner education curriculum shall include content related to California Nursing Practice Act, Business & Professions Code, Division 2, Chapter 6, Article 8, "Nurse Practitioners", and California Code of Regulations Title 16, Division 14, Article 7, "Standardized Procedure Guidelines" and Article 8, "Standards for Nurse Practitioners," including, but not limited to:

(A) Section 2835.7 of Business & Professions Code, "Additional authorized acts; implementation of standardized procedures";

(B) Section 2836.1 of Business & Professions Code, "Furnishing or ordering of drugs or devices."

(7) The program may be full-time or part-time, and shall be consistent with standards as established by The National Organization of Nurse Practitioner Faculties (NONPF) in "Nurse Practitioner Core Competencies

Content" (2017) or the American Association of Colleges of Nursing (AACN) in "Criteria for Evaluation of Nurse Practitioner Programs" (2016), which is hereby incorporated by reference. The program must also include theory and supervised clinical practice.

(8) The course of instruction program units and contact hours shall be calculated using the following formulas:

(A) One (1) hour of instruction in theory each week throughout a semester or quarter equals one (1) unit.

(B) Three (3) hours of clinical practice each week throughout a semester or quarter equals one (1) unit. Academic year means two semesters, where each semester is 15-18 weeks; or three quarters, where each quarter is 10-12 weeks.

(9) Supervised clinical practice shall consist of at least 12 semester units or 18 quarter units.

(10) The duration of clinical experience shall be sufficient for the student to demonstrate clinical competencies in the nurse practitioner category.

(11) The nurse practitioner education program shall arrange for clinical instruction and supervision of the student.

Authority cited: Sections 2715, 2835.7 and 2836, Business and Professions Code. Reference: Sections 2835, 2835.5, 2835.7, 2836, 2836.1, 2836.2, 2836.3 and 2837, Business and Professions Code.

History

1. Amendment of section heading, section and NOTE filed 1-15-2019; operative 1-15-2019 pursuant to Government Code section 11343.4(b)(3) (Register 2019, No. 3).
2. Amendment of subsection (h)(5) filed 2-8-2022; operative 4-1-2022 (Register 2022, No. 6).

§ 1485. Scope of Practice.

Nothing in this article shall be construed to limit the current scope of practice of the registered nurse authorized pursuant to the Business and Professions Code, Division 2, Chapter 6. The nurse practitioner shall function within the scope of practice as specified in the Nursing Practice Act and as it applies to all registered nurses.

Authority cited: Section 2715, Business and Professions Code. Reference: Sections 2834 and 2837, Business and Professions Code.

History

1. Amendment filed 12-4-85; effective thirtieth day thereafter (Register 85, No. 49).

§ 1485.5. Abortion by Aspiration Techniques.

For the purposes of Section 2725.4 of the Code, after January 1, 2016, certified nurse practitioners may perform an abortion by aspiration techniques in the first trimester of pregnancy if they have completed the requisite training in performing these procedures equivalent to the didactic curriculum and clinical training protocols of the HWPP No. 171 provided by any of the following:

(1) A Board-approved nurse practitioner program or in a course offered by an accredited nurse practitioner program;

(2) A course offered by a Board-approved continuing education provider that reflects evidence-based curriculum and training guidelines or a course approved for Category I continuing medical education;

(3) A course offered by a state or national health care professional or accreditation organization.

Authority cited: Section 2715, Business and Professions Code. Reference: Section 2725.4, Business and Professions Code.

History

1. New section filed 3-3-2016; operative 3-3-2016 pursuant to Government Code section 11343.4(b)(3) (Register 2016, No. 10).

§ 1486 Requirements for Clinical Practice Experience for Nurse Practitioner Students Enrolled in Non-California based Nurse Practitioner Education Programs.

(a) The Non-California based Nurse Practitioner education program requesting clinical placements for students in clinical practice settings in California shall:

(1) Obtain prior board approval;

(2) Ensure students have successfully completed prerequisite courses and are enrolled in the nurse practitioner education program;

(3) Secure clinical preceptors who meet board requirements;

(4) Ensure the clinical preceptorship experiences in the program meet all board requirements and national education standards and competencies for the nurse practitioner role and population as outlined by the National Organization of Nurse Practitioner Faculties (NONPF) in "Nurse Practitioner Core Competencies Content" (2017) or the American Association of Colleges of Nursing (AACN) in "Criteria for Evaluation of Nurse Practitioner Programs" (2016);

(5) Demonstrate evidence that the curriculum includes content related to legal aspects of California certified nurse practitioner laws and regulations. The curriculum shall include content related to California Nursing Practice Act, Business & Professions Code, Division 2, Chapter 6, Article 8, "Nurse Practitioners" and California Code of Regulations Title 16, Division 14, Article 7, "Standardized Procedure Guidelines" and Article 8, "Standards for Nurse Practitioners", including, but not limited to:

(A) Section 2835.7 of Business & Professions Code, "Additional authorized acts; implementation of standardized procedures";

(B) Section 2836.1 of Business & Professions Code, "Furnishing or ordering of drugs or devices".

(b) Clinical preceptor functions and responsibilities shall be clearly documented in a written agreement between the agency, the preceptor, and the nurse practitioner education program including the clinical preceptor's role to teach, supervise and evaluate students in the nurse practitioner education program.

(c) A clinical preceptor in the nurse practitioner education program shall:

(1) Hold a valid and active California license to practice their respective profession and demonstrate current clinical competence.

(2) Participate in teaching, supervising, and evaluating students, and shall be competent in the content and skills being taught to the students.

(3) Be a health care provider qualified by education, licensure and clinical competence in the assigned nurse practitioner category to provide direct supervision of the clinical practice experiences for a nurse practitioner student.

(4) Be oriented to program and curriculum requirements, including responsibilities related to student supervision and evaluation;

(5) Be evaluated by the program faculty at least every two (2) years.

(d) Students shall hold an active, valid California registered nurse license to participate in nurse practitioner education program clinical experiences.

(e) The nurse practitioner education program shall notify the board of pertinent changes within 30 days.

(f) The board may withdraw authorization for program clinical placements in California, at any time.

Authority cited: Section 2715, Business and Professions Code. Reference: Sections 2729, 2835, 2835.5 and 2836, Business and Professions Code.

History

1. New section filed 1-15-2019; operative 1-15-2019 pursuant to Government Code section 11343.4(b)(3) (Register 2019, No. 3).

2. Change without regulatory effect amending section filed 8-8-2022 pursuant to section 100, title 1, California Code of Regulations (Register 2022, No. 32).

ARTICLE 9
PUBLIC HEALTH NURSE

Section

1490. Public Health Nurse Certificate.
1491. Qualifications and Requirements.
1492. Application for Public Health Nurse Certificate.
1493. Issuance of Certificate.

§ 1490. Public Health Nurse Certificate.

(a) A Public Health Nurse Certificate shall be issued by the Board to a person who:

(1) Completes and submits an application pursuant to Section 1492; and

(2) Meets the qualifications and requirements specified in Section 1491.

(b) A Public Health Nurse Certificate shall remain valid as long as the person's license to practice as a registered nurse in California is active.

(c) The Board may issue a duplicate certificate to a person who states in writing that his or her certificate has been lost, stolen or destroyed.

Authority cited: Section 2715, Business and Professions Code. Reference: Section 2818, Business and Professions Code.

History

1. Amendment filed 12-8-45 (Register 3).

2. Amendment filed 9-24-51 designated to be effective 1-1-54 (Register 25, No. 6).

3. Amendment filed 12-18-61; effective thirtieth day thereafter (Register 61, No. 26).

4. Repealer of subsection (c) filed 6-9-67; effective thirtieth day thereafter (Register 67, No. 22).

5. Repealer of subsection (d) filed 4-14-72; effective thirtieth day thereafter (Register 72, No. 16).

6. Amendment filed 3-9-87; effective thirtieth day thereafter (Register 87, No. 11).

7. New article 9 and renumbering of former title 17, section 4500 to new title 16, section 1490, and amendment of subsections (a)-(a)(2) and (c) and Note filed 1-26-96; operative 2-28-96. Submitted to OAL for printing only (Register 96, No. 5).

8. Amendment of Note filed 9-2-98; operative 10-2-98 (Register 98, No. 36).

§ 1491. Qualifications and Requirements.

An applicant for a Public Health Nurse Certificate shall have a license, in active status, to practice as a registered nurse in California and shall have met the education and clinical experience requirements as follows:

(1) Possession of a baccalaureate or entry-level master's degree in nursing from a nursing school accredited by a Board-approved accrediting body, such as the National League for Nursing Accrediting Commission, or the Commission on Collegiate Nursing Education. The baccalaureate or entry-level master's

program must have included coursework in public health nursing, including a supervised clinical experience in public health settings; or

(2) Possession of a baccalaureate or entry-level master's degree in nursing from a nursing school which is not accredited by a Board-approved accrediting body, such as the National League for Nursing Accrediting Commission or the Commission on Collegiate Nursing Education, but the Board has determined that the nursing school's public health nursing coursework and the supervised clinical experience are equivalent to that of a nursing school accredited by a Board-approved accrediting body; or

(3) Possession of a baccalaureate degree in a field other than nursing and completion of a specialized public health nursing program that includes a supervised clinical experience at a baccalaureate school of nursing accredited by a Board-approved accrediting body, such as the National League for Nursing Accrediting Commission or the Commission on Collegiate Nursing Education.

(4) Theoretical content for a Public Health Nurse Certificate shall include, but is not limited to, the following areas:

(A) Physical, mental, and developmental assessment: child and adult;

(B) Surveillance and epidemiology: chronic and communicable diseases;

(C) Health promotion and disease prevention;

(D) Multicultural nursing concepts;

(E) Research methodology and statistics;

(F) Health teaching concepts and strategies;

(G) Population based practice: assessment and development of community collaboration at the level of systems, community and family/individual;

(H) Assessment of health needs of individuals and families, to include environment, and interventions across the lifespan;

(I) Legal and health care financing issues;

(J) Family violence, e.g., child, adult, domestic, elder abuse, etc., prevention, detection, intervention, treatment, and California reporting requirements;

(K) Case management/care coordination; and

(L) Emergency preparedness and response.

(5) A faculty member of the nursing program shall be responsible for coordinating students' clinical experience and supervision.

(6) Supervised clinical experience shall be:

(A) In public health settings with individuals, families, and community;

(B) Concurrent with or following acquisition of theoretical knowledge prescribed by the curriculum; and

(C) A minimum of 90 hours.

(7) Training in the prevention, early detection, intervention, California reporting requirements, and treatment of child neglect and abuse that shall be at least seven (7) hours in length and shall be acquired through:

(A) A baccalaureate nursing program or a specialized public health nursing program; or

(B) A course of instruction in the prevention, early detection, intervention, California reporting requirements, and treatment of child neglect and abuse that is offered by a continuing education provider approved by the Board.

Authority cited: Section 2715, Business and Professions Code. Reference: Sections 2817 and 2818, Business and Professions Code.

History

1. New section filed 4-14-72; effective thirtieth day thereafter (Register 72, No. 16).

2. Amendment filed 3-9-87; effective thirtieth day thereafter (Register 87, No. 11).
3. Editorial correction of subsection (a)(2) (Register 90, No. 35).
4. Renumbering and amendment of former title 17, section 4501 to new title 16, section 1491 and amendment of Note filed 1-26-96; operative 2-28-96. Submitted to OAL for printing only (Register 96, No. 5).
5. Amendment of section and Note filed 9-2-98; operative 10-2-98 (Register 98, No. 36).
6. Amendment of section and Note filed 5-12-2005; operative 6-11-2005 (Register 2005, No. 19).

§ 1492. Application for Public Health Nurse Certificate.

(a) A person seeking a Public Health Nurse Certificate shall complete and submit an application on the forms prescribed by the Board and shall submit a nonrefundable fee as prescribed by Section 1417 to the Board of Registered Nursing.

(b) Receipt of an application, information, documents, or fees supporting an application shall be deemed to occur on the date the application, information, documents, or fees are received by the Board.

(c) An application shall be considered complete when all required documents, information, and fees have been received by the Board.

(d) The applicant shall sign a statement contained on the application form prescribed by the Board that certifies under penalty of perjury pursuant to the laws of the State of California that the information contained in the application is true and correct.

Authority cited: Sections 2715 and 2816, Business and Professions Code. Reference: Section 2816, Business and Professions Code.

History

1. New section filed 3-9-87; effective thirtieth day thereafter (Register 87, No. 11).
2. Renumbering and amendment of former title 17, section 4502 to new title 16, section 1492 and amendment of Notefiled 1-26-96; operative 2-28-96. Submitted to OAL for printing only (Register 96, No. 5).
3. Amendment of subsection (a), repealer of subsections (b) and (f)-(f)(3), subsection relettering, amendment of newly designated subsections (b) and (d)and amendment of Note filed 9-2-98; operative 10-2-98 (Register 98, No. 36).

§ 1493. Issuance of Certificate.

(a) The Board shall provide written notification to the applicant within 30 calendar days of receipt of an application and fee for a Public Health Nurse Certificate that:

(1) The application is complete and accepted for processing; or

(2) The application is deficient and what specific information, documentation, or fee is required to complete the application.

(b) The Board's time periods for processing an initial application for Public Health Nurse Certificate are as follows:

(1) The median time for processing an initial application is 42 calendar days.

(2) The minimum time for processing an initial application is 14 calendar days.

(3) The maximum time for processing an initial application is 365 calendar days.

(c) Written notification by the Board shall be deemed to have occurred on the date such notification is deposited in the U.S. mail.

(d) If an applicant fails to respond within a period of one year to a written request by the Board for additional information, documentation, or fees, the application shall be deemed to have been abandoned by the applicant.

(e) An applicant whose application was deemed abandoned pursuant to subdivision (d) may reapply by submitting a complete new application, fee, and documentation to meet all current requirements.

Authority cited: Section 2715, Business and Professions Code. Reference: Section 2818, Business and Professions Code.

History

1. New section filed 3-9-87; effective thirtieth day thereafter (Register 87, No. 11).

2. Renumbering and amendment of former title 17, section 4503 to new title 16, section 1493 and amendment of Notefiled 1-26-96; operative 2-28-96. Submitted to OAL for printing only (Register 96, No. 5).

3. Editorial correction of subsection (a)(2) (Register 98, No. 36).

4. Amendment of section heading, section and Note filed 9-2-98; operative 10-2-98 (Register 98, No. 36).

ARTICLE 10
SPONSORED FREE HEALTH CARE EVENTS—REQUIREMENTS FOR EXEMPTION [REPEALED]

Section

1495. Definitions. [Repealed]
1495.1. Sponsoring Entity Registration and Recordkeeping Requirements. [Repealed]
1495.2. Out–of–State Practitioner Authorization to Participate in Sponsored Event. [Repealed]
1495.3. Termination of Authorization and Appeal. [Repealed]
1495.4. Disclosure Requirements; Name and License Status. [Repealed]

§ 1495. Definitions. [Repealed]

Authority cited: Sections 901 and 2715, Business and Professions Code. Reference: Section 901, Business and Professions Code.

History

1. New article 10 (sections 1495-1495.4) and section filed 11-27-2012; operative 11-27-2012 pursuant to Government Code section 11343.4 (Register 2012, No. 48).

2. Change without regulatory effect repealing article 10 (sections 1495-1495.4) and section filed 7-20-2020 pursuant to section 100, title 1, California Code of Regulations (Register 2020, No. 30).

§ 1495.1. Sponsoring Entity Registration and Recordkeeping Requirements. [Repealed]

Authority cited: Sections 901 and 2715, Business and Professions Code. Reference: Section 901, Business and Professions Code.

History

1. New section filed 11-27-2012; operative 11-27-2012 pursuant to Government Code section 11343.4 (Register 2012, No. 48).

2. Change without regulatory effect amending subsections (a)-(b) filed 4-24-2014 pursuant to section 100, title 1, California Code of Regulations (Register 2014, No. 17).

3. Change without regulatory effect amending Form 901-A (incorporated by reference) and subsections (a) and (b) filed 8-22-2016 pursuant to section 100, title 1, California Code of Regulations (Register 2016, No. 35).

4. Change without regulatory effect repealing section filed 7-20-2020 pursuant to section 100, title 1, California Code of Regulations (Register 2020, No. 30).

§ 1495.2. Out–of–State Practitioner Authorization to Participate in Sponsored Event. [Repealed]

Authority cited: Sections 901 and 2715, Business and Professions Code. Reference: Sections 144 and 901, Business and Professions Code.

History

1. New section filed 11-27-2012; operative 11-27-2012 pursuant to Government Code section 11343.4 (Register 2012, No. 48).

2. Change without regulatory effect amending subsection (d) filed 2-7-2013 pursuant to section 100, title 1, California Code of Regulations (Register 2013, No. 6).

3. Change without regulatory effect amending subsection (a) filed 4-24-2014 pursuant to section 100, title 1, California Code of Regulations (Register 2014, No. 17).

4. Change without regulatory effect repealing section filed 7-20-2020 pursuant to section 100, title 1, California Code of Regulations (Register 2020, No. 30).

§ 1495.3. Termination of Authorization and Appeal. [Repealed]

Authority cited: Sections 901 and 2715, Business and Professions Code. Reference: Section 901, Business and Professions Code.

History

1. New section filed 11-27-2012; operative 11-27-2012 pursuant to Government Code section 11343.4 (Register 2012, No. 48).

2. Change without regulatory effect repealing section filed 7-20-2020 pursuant to section 100, title 1, California Code of Regulations (Register 2020, No. 30).

§ 1495.4. Disclosure Requirements; Name and License Status. [Repealed]

Authority cited: Sections 680, 901 and 2715, Business and Professions Code. Reference: Sections 680 and 901, Business and Professions Code.

History

1. New section filed 11-27-2012; operative 11-27-2012 pursuant to Government Code section 11343.4 (Register 2012, No. 48).

2. Change without regulatory effect repealing section filed 7-20-2020 pursuant to section 100, title 1, California Code of Regulations (Register 2020, No. 30).

EXTRACTED FROM
BUSINESS & PROFESSIONS CODE

General Provisions.
Division
1. Department of Consumer Affairs.
1.5. Denial, Suspension and Revocation of Licenses.
2. Healing Arts.
7. General Business Regulations.

GENERAL PROVISIONS

Section
7.5. "Conviction"; When action by board following establishment of conviction may be taken; Prohibition against denial of licensure; Application of section.
12.5. Violation of regulation adopted pursuant to code provision; Issuance of citation.
14.1. Legislative intent.
22. "Board".
23. "Department".
23.5. "Director".
23.6. "Appointing power".
23.7. "License".
29.5. Additional qualifications for licensure.
30. Provision of federal employer identification number or social security number by licensee.
31. Compliance with judgment or order for support upon issuance or renewal of license.
32. Legislative findings; AIDS training for health care professionals.

Bus & Prof

HISTORY: Enacted Stats 1937 ch 399.

§ 7.5. "Conviction"; When action by board following establishment of conviction may be taken; Prohibition against denial of licensure; Application of section

(a) A conviction within the meaning of this code means a judgment following a plea or verdict of guilty or a plea of nolo contendere or finding of guilt. Any action which a board is permitted to take following the establishment of a conviction may be taken when the time for appeal has elapsed, or the judgment of conviction has been affirmed on appeal or when an order granting probation is made suspending the imposition of sentence. However, a board may not deny a license to an applicant who is otherwise qualified pursuant to subdivision (b) or (c) of Section 480.

(b)(1) Nothing in this section shall apply to the licensure of persons pursuant to Chapter 4 (commencing with Section 6000) of Division 3.

(2) This section does not in any way modify or otherwise affect the existing authority of the following entities in regard to licensure:

(A) The State Athletic Commission.

(B) The Bureau for Private Postsecondary Education.

(C) The California Horse Racing Board.

(c) Except as provided in subdivision (b), this section controls over and supersedes the definition of conviction contained within individual practice acts under this code.

(d) This section shall become operative on July 1, 2020.

HISTORY:

Added Stats 2018 ch 995 § 2 (AB 2138), effective January 1, 2019, operative July 1, 2020.

§ 12.5. Violation of regulation adopted pursuant to code provision; Issuance of citation

Whenever in any provision of this code authority is granted to issue a citation for a violation of any provision of this code, that authority also includes the authority to issue a citation for the violation of any regulation adopted pursuant to any provision of this code.

HISTORY:

Added Stats 1986 ch 1379 § 1.

§ 14.1. Legislative intent

The Legislature hereby declares its intent that the terms "man" or "men" where appropriate shall be deemed "person" or "persons" and any references to the terms "man" or "men" in sections of this code be changed to "person" or "persons" when such code sections are being amended for any purpose. This act is declaratory and not amendatory of existing law.

HISTORY:

Added Stats 1976 ch 1171 § 1.

§ 22. "Board"

"Board," as used in any provision of this code, refers to the board in which the administration of the provision is vested, and unless otherwise expressly provided, shall include "bureau," "commission," "committee," "department," "division," "examining committee," "program," and "agency."

HISTORY:

Enacted Stats 1937. Amended Stats 1947 ch 1350 § 1; Stats 1980 ch 676 § 1; Stats 1991 ch 654 § 1 (AB 1893); Stats 1999 ch 656 § 1 (SB 1306); Stats 2004 ch 33 § 1 (AB 1467), effective April 13, 2004; Stats 2010 ch 670 § 1 (AB 2130), effective January 1, 2011.

§ 23. "Department"

"Department," unless otherwise defined, refers to the Department of Consumer Affairs.

Wherever the laws of this state refer to the Department of Professional and Vocational Standards, the reference shall be construed to be to the Department of Consumer Affairs.

HISTORY:

Enacted Stats 1937. Amended Stats 1971 ch 716 § 1.

§ 23.5. "Director"

"Director," unless otherwise defined, refers to the Director of Consumer Affairs.

Wherever the laws of this state refer to the Director of Professional and Vocational Standards, the reference shall be construed to be to the Director of Consumer Affairs.

HISTORY:
Added Stats 1939 ch 30 § 2. Amended Stats 1971 ch 716 § 2.

§ 23.6. "Appointing power"

"Appointing power," unless otherwise defined, refers to the Director of Consumer Affairs.

HISTORY:
Added Stats 1945 ch 1276 § 1. Amended Stats 1971 ch 716 § 3.

§ 23.7. "License"

Unless otherwise expressly provided, "license" means license, certificate, registration, or other means to engage in a business or profession regulated by this code or referred to in Section 1000 or 3600.

HISTORY:
Added Stats 1994 ch 26 § 1 (AB 1807), effective March 30, 1994.

§ 29.5. Additional qualifications for licensure

In addition to other qualifications for licensure prescribed by the various acts of boards under the department, applicants for licensure and licensees renewing their licenses shall also comply with Section 17520 of the Family Code.

HISTORY:
Added Stats 1991 ch 542 § 1 (SB 1161). Amended Stats 2003 ch 607 § 1 (SB 1077).

§ 30. Provision of federal employer identification number or social security number by licensee

(a)(1) Notwithstanding any other law, any board, as defined in Section 22, the State Bar of California, and the Department of Real Estate shall, at the time of issuance of the license, require that the applicant provide its federal employer identification number, if the applicant is a partnership, or the applicant's social security number for all other applicants.

(2)(A) In accordance with Section 135.5, a board, as defined in Section 22, the State Bar of California, and the Department of Real Estate shall require either the individual taxpayer identification number or social security number if the applicant is an individual for a license or certificate, as defined in subparagraph (2) of subdivision (e), and for purposes of this subdivision.

(B) In implementing the requirements of subparagraph (A), a licensing board shall not require an individual to disclose either citizenship status or immigration status for purposes of licensure.

(C) A licensing board shall not deny licensure to an otherwise qualified and eligible individual based solely on the individual's citizenship status or immigration status.

(D) The Legislature finds and declares that the requirements of this subdivision are consistent with subsection (d) of Section 1621 of Title 8 of the United States Code.

(b) A licensee failing to provide the federal employer identification number, or the individual taxpayer identification number or social security number shall be reported by the licensing board to the Franchise Tax Board. If the licensee fails to provide that information after notification pursuant to paragraph (1) of subdivision (b) of Section 19528 of the Revenue and Taxation Code, the licensee shall be subject to the penalty provided in paragraph (2) of subdivision (b) of Section 19528 of the Revenue and Taxation Code.

(c) In addition to the penalty specified in subdivision (b), a licensing board shall not process an application for an initial license unless the applicant provides its federal employer identification number, or individual taxpayer identification number or social security number where requested on the application.

(d) A licensing board shall, upon request of the Franchise Tax Board or the Employment Development Department, furnish to the board or the department, as applicable, the following information with respect to every licensee:

(1) Name.

(2) Address or addresses of record.

(3) Federal employer identification number if the licensee is a partnership, or the licensee's individual taxpayer identification number or social security number for all other licensees.

(4) Type of license.

(5) Effective date of license or a renewal.

(6) Expiration date of license.

(7) Whether license is active or inactive, if known.

(8) Whether license is new or a renewal.

(e) For the purposes of this section:

(1) "Licensee" means a person or entity, other than a corporation, authorized by a license, certificate, registration, or other means to engage in a business or profession regulated by this code or referred to in Section 1000 or 3600.

(2) "License" includes a certificate, registration, or any other authorization needed to engage in a business or profession regulated by this code or referred to in Section 1000 or 3600.

(3) "Licensing board" means any board, as defined in Section 22, the State Bar of California, and the Department of Real Estate.

(f) The reports required under this section shall be filed on magnetic media or in other machine-readable form, according to standards furnished by the Franchise Tax Board or the Employment Development Department, as applicable.

(g) Licensing boards shall provide to the Franchise Tax Board or the Employment Development Department the information required by this section at a time that the board or the department, as applicable, may require.

(h) Notwithstanding Division 10 (commencing with Section 7920.000) of Title 1 of the Government Code, a federal employer identification number, individual taxpayer identification number, or social security number furnished pursuant to this section shall not be deemed to be a public record and shall not be open to the public for inspection.

(i) A deputy, agent, clerk, officer, or employee of a licensing board described in subdivision (a), or any former officer or employee or other individual who, in the course of their employment or duty, has or has had access to the information required to be furnished under this section, shall not disclose or make known in any manner that information, except as provided pursuant to this section, to the Franchise Tax Board, the Employment Development Department, the Office of the Chancellor of the California Community Colleges, a collections agency contracted to collect funds owed to the State Bar by licensees pursuant to Sections 6086.10 and 6140.5, or as provided in subdivisions (j) and (k).

(j) It is the intent of the Legislature in enacting this section to utilize the federal employer identification number, individual taxpayer identification number, or social security number for the purpose of establishing the identification of persons affected by state tax laws, for purposes of compliance with Section 17520 of the Family Code, for purposes of measuring employment outcomes of students who participate in career technical education programs offered by the California Community Colleges, and for purposes of collecting funds owed to the State Bar by licensees pursuant to Section 6086.10 and Section 6140.5 and, to that end, the information furnished pursuant to this section shall be used exclusively for those purposes.

(k) If the board utilizes a national examination to issue a license, and if a reciprocity agreement or comity exists between the State of California and the state requesting release of the individual taxpayer identification number or social security number, any deputy, agent, clerk, officer, or employee of any licensing board described in subdivision (a) may release an individual taxpayer identification number or social security number to an examination or licensing entity, only for the purpose of verification of licensure or examination status.

(*l*) For the purposes of enforcement of Section 17520 of the Family Code, and notwithstanding any other law, a board, as defined in Section 22, the State Bar of California, and the Department of Real Estate shall at the time of issuance of the license require that each licensee provide the individual taxpayer identification number or social security number of each individual listed on the license and any person who qualifies for the license. For the purposes of this subdivision, "licensee" means an entity that is issued a license by any board, as defined in Section 22, the State Bar of California, the Department of Real Estate, and the Department of Motor Vehicles.

(m) The department shall, upon request by the Office of the Chancellor of the California Community Colleges, furnish to the chancellor's office, as applicable, the following information with respect to every licensee:

(1) Name.

(2) Federal employer identification number if the licensee is a partnership, or the licensee's individual taxpayer identification number or social security number for all other licensees.

(3) Date of birth.

(4) Type of license.

(5) Effective date of license or a renewal.

(6) Expiration date of license.

(n) The department shall make available information pursuant to subdivision (m) only to allow the chancellor's office to measure employment outcomes of students who participate in career technical education programs offered by the California Community Colleges and recommend how these programs may be improved. Licensure information made available by the department pursuant to this section shall not be used for any other purpose.

(o) The department may make available information pursuant to subdivision (m) only to the extent that making the information available complies with state and federal privacy laws.

(p) The department may, by agreement, condition or limit the availability of licensure information pursuant to subdivision (m) in order to ensure the security of the information and to protect the privacy rights of the individuals to whom the information pertains.

(q) All of the following apply to the licensure information made available pursuant to subdivision (m):

(1) It shall be limited to only the information necessary to accomplish the purpose authorized in subdivision (n).

(2) It shall not be used in a manner that permits third parties to personally identify the individual or individuals to whom the information pertains.

(3) Except as provided in subdivision (n), it shall not be shared with or transmitted to any other party or entity without the consent of the individual or individuals to whom the information pertains.

(4) It shall be protected by reasonable security procedures and practices appropriate to the nature of the information to protect that information from unauthorized access, destruction, use, modification, or disclosure.

(5) It shall be immediately and securely destroyed when no longer needed for the purpose authorized in subdivision (n).

(r) The department or the chancellor's office may share licensure information with a third party who contracts to perform the function described in subdivision (n), if the third party is required by contract to follow the requirements of this section.

HISTORY:

Added Stats 2017 ch 828 § 2 (SB 173), effective January 1, 2018, operative July 1, 2018. Amended Stats 2018 ch 659 § 1 (AB 3249), effective January 1, 2019; Stats 2018 ch 838 § 2.5 (SB 695), effective January 1, 2019 (ch 838 prevails); Stats 2019 ch 351 § 6 (AB 496), effective January 1, 2020; Stats 2021 ch 615 § 2 (AB 474), effective January 1, 2022.

§ 31. Compliance with judgment or order for support upon issuance or renewal of license

(a) As used in this section, "board" means any entity listed in Section 101, the entities referred to in Sections 1000 and 3600, the State Bar, the Department of Real Estate, and any other state agency that issues a license, certificate, or registration authorizing a person to engage in a business or profession.

(b) Each applicant for the issuance or renewal of a license, certificate, registration, or other means to engage in a business or profession regulated by a board who is not in compliance with a judgment or order for support shall be subject to Section 17520 of the Family Code.

(c) "Compliance with a judgment or order for support" has the meaning given in paragraph (4) of subdivision (a) of Section 17520 of the Family Code.

(d) Each licensee or applicant whose name appears on a list of the 500 largest tax delinquencies pursuant to Section 7063 or 19195 of the Revenue and Taxation Code shall be subject to Section 494.5.

(e) Each application for a new license or renewal of a license shall indicate on the application that the law allows the California Department of Tax and

Fee Administration and the Franchise Tax Board to share taxpayer information with a board and requires the licensee to pay the licensee's state tax obligation and that the licensee's license may be suspended if the state tax obligation is not paid.

(f) For purposes of this section, "tax obligation" means the tax imposed under, or in accordance with, Part 1 (commencing with Section 6001), Part 1.5 (commencing with Section 7200), Part 1.6 (commencing with Section 7251), Part 1.7 (commencing with Section 7280), Part 10 (commencing with Section 17001), or Part 11 (commencing with Section 23001) of Division 2 of the Revenue and Taxation Code.

HISTORY:

Added Stats 1991 ch 110 § 4 (SB 101). Amended Stats 1991 ch 542 § 3 (SB 1161); Stats 2010 ch 328 § 1 (SB 1330), effective January 1, 2011; Stats 2011 ch 455 § 1 (AB 1424), effective January 1, 2012; Stats 2013 ch 352 § 2 (AB 1317), effective September 26, 2013, operative July 1, 2013; Stats 2019 ch 351 § 7 (AB 496), effective January 1, 2020.

§ 32. Legislative findings; AIDS training for health care professionals

(a) The Legislature finds that there is a need to ensure that professionals of the healing arts who have or intend to have significant contact with patients who have, or are at risk to be exposed to, acquired immune deficiency syndrome (AIDS) are provided with training in the form of continuing education regarding the characteristics and methods of assessment and treatment of the condition.

(b) A board vested with the responsibility of regulating the following licensees shall consider including training regarding the characteristics and method of assessment and treatment of acquired immune deficiency syndrome (AIDS) in any continuing education or training requirements for those licensees: chiropractors, medical laboratory technicians, dentists, dental hygienists, dental assistants, physicians and surgeons, podiatrists, registered nurses, licensed vocational nurses, psychologists, physician assistants, respiratory therapists, acupuncturists, marriage and family therapists, licensed educational psychologists, clinical social workers, and professional clinical counselors.

HISTORY:

Added Stats 1988 ch 1213 § 1. Amended Stats 1994 ch 26 § 2 (AB 1807), effective March 30, 1994; Stats 2002 ch 1013 § 4 (SB 2026); Stats 2011 ch 381 § 4 (SB 146), effective January 1, 2012.

DIVISION 1

DEPARTMENT OF CONSUMER AFFAIRS

Chapter

1. The Department.
1.5. Unlicensed Activity Enforcement.
2. The Director of Consumer Affairs.
3. Funds of the Department.
4. Consumer Affairs.
6. Public Members.
7. Licensee.

BOARD OF REGISTERED NURSING

HISTORY: Enacted Stats 1937 ch 399. The heading of Division 1, amended to read as above by Stats 1973 ch 77 § 1.

CHAPTER 1
THE DEPARTMENT

Bus & Prof

Section
100. Establishment.
101. Composition of department.
101.6. Purpose.
103. Compensation and reimbursement for expenses.
104. Display of licenses or registrations.
105. Oath of office.
105.5. Tenure of members of boards, etc., within department.
106. Removal of board members.
106.5. Removal of member of licensing board for disclosure of examination information.
107. Executive officers.
107.5. Official seals.
108. Status and powers of boards.
108.5. Witness fees and expenses.
109. Review of decisions; Investigations.
110. Records and property.
111. Commissioners on examination.
112. Publication and sale of directories of authorized persons.
113. Conferences; Traveling expenses.
114. Reinstatement of expired license of licensee serving in military.
114.3. Waiver of fees and requirements for active duty members of armed forces and national guard.
114.5. Military service; Posting of information on Web site about application of military experience and training towards licensure.
115. Applicability of Section 114.
115.4. Licensure process expedited for honorably discharged veterans of Armed Forces.
115.5. Board required to expedite licensure process for certain applicants; Adoption of regulations [Repealed].
115.5. Board required to expedite licensure process for certain applicants; Adoption of regulations.
115.6. Temporary licensure process for spouses of active duty members of Armed Forces [Repealed effective July 1, 2023].
115.6. Temporary licensure process for spouses of active duty members of Armed Forces [Operative July 1, 2023].
115.8. Annual report on military, veteran, and spouse licensure.
115.9. Publishing information on licensing options available to military spouses.
116. Audit and review of disciplinary proceedings; Report to Legislature.
118. Effect of withdrawal of application; Effect of suspension, forfeiture, etc., of license.
119. Misdemeanors pertaining to use of licenses.
121. Practice during period between renewal and receipt of evidence of renewal.
122. Fee for issuance of duplicate certificate.
123. Conduct constituting subversion of licensing examination; Penalties and damages.
123.5. Enjoining violations.
124. Manner of notice.
125. Misdemeanor offenses by licensees.
125.3. Direction to licensee violating licensing act to pay costs of investigation and enforcement.
125.5. Enjoining violations; Restitution orders.
125.6. Unlawful discrimination by licensees.
125.7. Restraining orders.
125.8. Temporary order restraining licensee engaged or about to engage in violation of law.
125.9. System for issuance of citations to licensees; Contents; Fines.
126. Submission of reports to Governor.
127. Submission of reports to director.
128. Sale of equipment, supplies, or services for use in violation of licensing requirements.

Section
128.5. Reduction of license fees in event of surplus funds.
129. Handling of complaints; Reports to Legislature.
130. Terms of office of agency members.
131. Maximum number of terms.
132. Requirements for institution or joinder of legal action by state agency against other state or federal agency.
134. Proration of license fees.
135. Reexamination of applicants.
135.4. Refugees, asylees, and special immigrant visa holders; professional licensing; initial licensure process.
135.5. Licensure and citizenship or immigration status.
136. Notification of change of address; Punishment for failure to comply.
137. Regulations requiring inclusion of license numbers in advertising, etc.
138. Notice that practitioner is licensed; Evaluation of licensing examination.
139. Policy for examination development and validation, and occupational analysis.
139.5. Quarterly internet website posting requirements.
140. Disciplinary action; Licensee's failure to record cash transactions in payment of employee wages.
141. Disciplinary action by foreign jurisdiction; Grounds for disciplinary action by state licensing board.
142. Authority to synchronize renewal dates of licenses; Abandonment date for application; Delinquency fee.
143. Proof of license as condition of bringing action for collection of compensation.
143.5. Provision in agreements to settle certain causes of action prohibited; Adoption of regulations; Exemptions.
144. Requirement of fingerprints for criminal record checks; Applicability.
144.5. Board authority.

HISTORY: Enacted Stats 1937 ch 399.

§ 100. Establishment

There is in the state government, in the Business, Consumer Services, and Housing Agency, a Department of Consumer Affairs.

HISTORY:

Enacted Stats 1937. Amended Stats 1969 ch 138 § 5; Stats 1971 ch 716 § 4; Stats 1984 ch 144 § 1. See this section as modified in Governor's Reorganization Plan No. 2 § 1 of 2012; Amended Stats 2012 ch 147 § 1 (SB 1039), effective January 1, 2013, operative July 1, 2013 (ch 147 prevails).

§ 101. Composition of department

The department is comprised of the following:

(a) The Dental Board of California.
(b) The Medical Board of California.
(c) The California State Board of Optometry.
(d) The California State Board of Pharmacy.
(e) The Veterinary Medical Board.
(f) The California Board of Accountancy.
(g) The California Architects Board.
(h) The State Board of Barbering and Cosmetology.
(i) The Board for Professional Engineers, Land Surveyors, and Geologists.
(j) The Contractors State License Board.
(k) The Bureau for Private Postsecondary Education.
(*l*) The Bureau of Household Goods and Services.
(m) The Board of Registered Nursing.

(n) The Board of Behavioral Sciences.
(o) The State Athletic Commission.
(p) The Cemetery and Funeral Bureau.
(q) The Bureau of Security and Investigative Services.
(r) The Court Reporters Board of California.
(s) The Board of Vocational Nursing and Psychiatric Technicians.
(t) The Landscape Architects Technical Committee.
(u) The Division of Investigation.
(v) The Bureau of Automotive Repair.
(w) The Respiratory Care Board of California.
(x) The Acupuncture Board.
(y) The Board of Psychology.
(z) The Podiatric Medical Board of California.
(aa) The Physical Therapy Board of California.
(ab) The Arbitration Review Program.
(ac) The Physician Assistant Board.
(ad) The Speech-Language Pathology and Audiology and Hearing Aid Dispensers Board.
(ae) The California Board of Occupational Therapy.
(af) The Osteopathic Medical Board of California.
(ag) The California Board of Naturopathic Medicine.
(ah) The Dental Hygiene Board of California.
(ai) The Professional Fiduciaries Bureau.
(aj) The State Board of Chiropractic Examiners.
(ak) The Bureau of Real Estate Appraisers.
(a*l*) The Structural Pest Control Board.
(am) Any other boards, offices, or officers subject to its jurisdiction by law.

HISTORY:

Added Stats 2017 ch 823 § 4 (SB 173), effective January 1, 2018, operative July 1, 2018. Amended Stats 2018 ch 578 § 2 (SB 1483), effective January 1, 2019; Stats 2018 ch 858 § 1.5 (SB 1482), effective January 1, 2019 (ch 858 prevails); Stats 2019 ch 351 § 8 (AB 496), effective January 1, 2020; Stats 2020 ch 312 § 2 (SB 1474), effective January 1, 2021; Stats 2021 ch 70 § 2 (AB 141), effective July 12, 2021; Stats 2021 ch 630 § 2 (AB 1534), effective January 1, 2022; Stats 2022 ch 414 § 1 (AB 2685), effective January 1, 2023.

§ 101.6. Purpose

The boards, bureaus, and commissions in the department are established for the purpose of ensuring that those private businesses and professions deemed to engage in activities which have potential impact upon the public health, safety, and welfare are adequately regulated in order to protect the people of California.

To this end, they establish minimum qualifications and levels of competency and license persons desiring to engage in the occupations they regulate upon determining that such persons possess the requisite skills and qualifications necessary to provide safe and effective services to the public, or register or otherwise certify persons in order to identify practitioners and ensure performance according to set and accepted professional standards. They provide a means for redress of grievances by investigating allegations of unprofessional conduct, incompetence, fraudulent action, or unlawful activity brought to their attention by members of the public and institute disciplinary action against persons licensed or registered under the provisions of this code when such action is warranted. In addition, they conduct periodic checks of licensees, registrants, or otherwise certified persons in order to ensure compliance with the relevant sections of this code.

HISTORY:
Added Stats 1980 ch 375 § 1.

§ 103. Compensation and reimbursement for expenses

Each member of a board, commission, or committee created in the various chapters of Division 2 (commencing with Section 500) and Division 3 (commencing with Section 5000), and in Chapter 2 (commencing with Section 18600) and Chapter 3 (commencing with Section 19000) of Division 8, shall receive the moneys specified in this section when authorized by the respective provisions.

Each such member shall receive a per diem of one hundred dollars ($100) for each day actually spent in the discharge of official duties, and shall be reimbursed for traveling and other expenses necessarily incurred in the performance of official duties.

The payments in each instance shall be made only from the fund from which the expenses of the agency are paid and shall be subject to the availability of money.

Notwithstanding any other provision of law, no public officer or employee shall receive per diem salary compensation for serving on those boards, commissions, or committees on any day when the officer or employee also received compensation for the officer or employee's regular public employment.

HISTORY:
Added Stats 1959 ch 1645 § 1. Amended Stats 1978 ch 1141 § 1; Stats 1985 ch 502 § 1; Stats 1987 ch 850 § 1; Stats 1993 ch 1264 § 1 (SB 574); Stats 2019 ch 351 § 11 (AB 496), effective January 1, 2020.

§ 104. Display of licenses or registrations

All boards or other regulatory entities within the department's jurisdiction that the department determines to be health-related may adopt regulations to require licensees to display their licenses or registrations in the locality in which they are treating patients, and to inform patients as to the identity of the regulatory agency they may contact if they have any questions or complaints regarding the licensee. In complying with this requirement, those boards may take into consideration the particular settings in which licensees practice, or other circumstances which may make the displaying or providing of information to the consumer extremely difficult for the licensee in their particular type of practice.

HISTORY:
Added Stats 1998 ch 991 § 1 (SB1980).

§ 105. Oath of office

Members of boards in the department shall take an oath of office as provided in the Constitution and the Government Code.

HISTORY:
Added Stats 1949 ch 829 § 1.

§ 105.5. Tenure of members of boards, etc., within department

Notwithstanding any other provision of this code, each member of a board, commission, examining committee, or other similarly constituted agency within the department shall hold office until the appointment and qualification of that member's successor or until one year shall have elapsed since the expiration of the term for which the member was appointed, whichever first occurs.

HISTORY:

Added Stats 1967 ch 524 § 1. Amended Stats 2019 ch 351 § 12 (AB 496), effective January 1, 2020.

§ 106. Removal of board members

The appointing authority has power to remove from office at any time any member of any board appointed by the appointing authority for continued neglect of duties required by law, or for incompetence, or unprofessional or dishonorable conduct. Nothing in this section shall be construed as a limitation or restriction on the power of the appointing authority conferred on the appointing authority by any other provision of law to remove any member of any board.

HISTORY:

Enacted Stats 1937. Amended Stats 1945 ch 1276 § 3; Stats 2019 ch 351 § 13 (AB 496), effective January 1, 2020.

§ 106.5. Removal of member of licensing board for disclosure of examination information

Notwithstanding any other provision of law, the Governor may remove from office a member of a board or other licensing entity in the department if it is shown that such member has knowledge of the specific questions to be asked on the licensing entity's next examination and directly or indirectly discloses any such question or questions in advance of or during the examination to any applicant for that examination.

The proceedings for removal shall be conducted in accordance with the provisions of Chapter 5 of Part 1 of Division 3 of Title 2 of the Government Code, and the Governor shall have all the powers granted therein.

HISTORY:

Added Stats 1977 ch 482 § 1.

§ 107. Executive officers

Pursuant to subdivision (e) of Section 4 of Article VII of the California Constitution, each board may appoint a person exempt from civil service, who shall be designated as an executive officer unless the licensing act of the particular board designates the person as a registrar, and may fix that person's salary, with the approval of the Department of Human Resources pursuant to Section 19825 of the Government Code.

HISTORY:

Enacted Stats 1937. Amended Stats 1984 ch 47 § 2, effective March 21, 1984; Stats 1987 ch 850 § 2. See this section as modified in Governor's Reorganization Plan No. 1 § 1 of 2011; Amended Stats 2012 ch 665 § 1 (SB 1308), effective January 1, 2013; Stats 2019 ch 351 § 14 (AB 496), effective January 1, 2020; Stats 2020 ch 370 § 1 (SB 1371), effective January 1, 2021.

§ 107.5. Official seals

If any board in the department uses an official seal pursuant to any provision of this code, the seal shall contain the words "State of California" and "Department of Consumer Affairs" in addition to the title of the board, and shall be in a form approved by the director.

HISTORY:

Added Stats 1967 ch 1272 § 1. Amended Stats 1971 ch 716 § 7.

§ 108. Status and powers of boards

Each of the boards comprising the department exists as a separate unit, and has the functions of setting standards, holding meetings, and setting dates thereof, preparing and conducting examinations, passing upon applicants, conducting investigations of violations of laws under its jurisdiction, issuing citations and holding hearings for the revocation of licenses, and the imposing of penalties following those hearings, insofar as these powers are given by statute to each respective board.

HISTORY:

Enacted Stats 1937. Amended Stats 2008 ch 179 § 1 (SB 1498), effective January 1, 2009.

§ 108.5. Witness fees and expenses

In any investigation, proceeding, or hearing that any board, commission, or officer in the department is empowered to institute, conduct, or hold, any witness appearing at the investigation, proceeding, or hearing whether upon a subpoena or voluntarily, may be paid the sum of twelve dollars ($12) per day for every day in actual attendance at the investigation, proceeding, or hearing and for the witness's actual, necessary, and reasonable expenses and those sums shall be a legal charge against the funds of the respective board, commission, or officer; provided further, that no witness appearing other than at the instance of the board, commission, or officer may be compensated out of the fund.

The board, commission, or officer shall determine the sums due to any witness and enter the amount on its minutes.

HISTORY:

Added Stats 1943 ch 1035 § 1. Amended Stats 1957 ch 1908 § 6; Stats 1970 ch 1061 § 1; Stats 2019 ch 351 § 15 (AB 496), effective January 1, 2020.

§ 109. Review of decisions; Investigations

(a) The decisions of any of the boards comprising the department with respect to setting standards, conducting examinations, passing candidates, and revoking licenses, are not subject to review by the director, but are final within the limits provided by this code which are applicable to the particular board, except as provided in this section.

(b) The director may initiate an investigation of any allegations of misconduct in the preparation, administration, or scoring of an examination which is administered by a board, or in the review of qualifications which are a part of the licensing process of any board. A request for investigation shall be made by the director to the Division of Investigation through the chief of the division or to any law enforcement agency in the jurisdiction where the alleged misconduct occurred.

(c) The director may intervene in any matter of any board where an investigation by the Division of Investigation discloses probable cause to believe that the conduct or activity of a board, or its members or employees constitutes a violation of criminal law.

The term "intervene," as used in paragraph (c) of this section may include, but is not limited to, an application for a restraining order or injunctive relief as specified in Section 123.5, or a referral or request for criminal prosecution. For purposes of this section, the director shall be deemed to have standing under Section 123.5 and shall seek representation of the Attorney General, or other appropriate counsel in the event of a conflict in pursuing that action.

HISTORY:

Enacted Stats 1937. Amended Stats 1991 ch 1013 § 1 (SB 961).

§ 110. Records and property

The department shall have possession and control of all records, books, papers, offices, equipment, supplies, funds, appropriations, land and other property—real or personal—now or hereafter held for the benefit or use of all of the bodies, offices or officers comprising the department. The title to all property held by any of these bodies, offices or officers for the use and benefit of the state, is vested in the State of California to be held in the possession of the department. Except as authorized by a board, the department shall not have the possession and control of examination questions prior to submission to applicants at scheduled examinations.

HISTORY:

Enacted Stats 1937. Amended Stats 1996 ch 829 § 1 (AB 3473).

§ 111. Commissioners on examination

Unless otherwise expressly provided, any board may, with the approval of the appointing power, appoint qualified persons, who shall be designated as commissioners on examination, to give the whole or any portion of any examination. A commissioner on examination need not be a member of the board but shall have the same qualifications as one and shall be subject to the same rules.

HISTORY:

Added Stats 1937 ch 474. Amended Stats 1947 ch 1350 § 3; Stats 1978 ch 1161 § 1; Stats 2019 ch 351 § 16 (AB 496), effective January 1, 2020.

§ 112. Publication and sale of directories of authorized persons

Notwithstanding any other provision of this code, no agency in the department, with the exception of the Board for Professional Engineers and Land Surveyors, shall be required to compile, publish, sell, or otherwise distribute a directory. When an agency deems it necessary to compile and publish a directory, the agency shall cooperate with the director in determining its form and content, the time and frequency of its publication, the persons to whom it is to be sold or otherwise distributed, and its price if it is sold. Any agency that requires the approval of the director for the compilation, publication, or distribution of a directory, under the law in effect at the time the amendment made to this section at the 1970 Regular Session of the Legislature becomes effective, shall continue to require that approval. As used in this section, "directory" means a directory, roster, register, or similar compilation of the names of persons who hold a license, certificate, permit, registration, or similar indicia of authority from the agency.

HISTORY:

Added Stats 1937 ch 474. Amended Stats 1968 ch 1345 § 1; Stats 1970 ch 475 § 1; Stats 1998 ch 59 § 3 (AB 969).

§ 113. Conferences; Traveling expenses

Upon recommendation of the director, officers, and employees of the department, and the officers, members, and employees of the boards, committees, and commissions comprising it or subject to its jurisdiction may confer, in this state or elsewhere, with officers or employees of this state, its political subdivisions, other states, or the United States, or with other persons, associations, or organizations as may be of assistance to the department, board, committee, or commission in the conduct of its work. The officers, members, and employees shall be entitled to their actual traveling expenses incurred in pursuance hereof, but when these expenses are incurred with respect to travel outside of the state, they shall be subject to the approval of the Governor and the Director of Finance.

HISTORY:

Added Stats 1937 ch 474. Amended Stats 1941 ch 885 § 1; Stats 2000 ch 277 § 1 (AB 2697); Stats 2001 ch 159 § 2 (SB 662).

§ 114. Reinstatement of expired license of licensee serving in military

(a) Notwithstanding any other provision of this code, any licensee or registrant of any board, commission, or bureau within the department whose license expired while the licensee or registrant was on active duty as a member of the California National Guard or the United States Armed Forces, may, upon application, reinstate their license or registration without examination or penalty, provided that all of the following requirements are satisfied:

(1) The licensee or registrant's license or registration was valid at the time they entered the California National Guard or the United States Armed Forces.

(2) The application for reinstatement is made while serving in the California National Guard or the United States Armed Forces, or not later than one year from the date of discharge from active service or return to inactive military status.

(3) The application for reinstatement is accompanied by an affidavit showing the date of entrance into the service, whether still in the service, or date of discharge, and the renewal fee for the current renewal period in which the application is filed is paid.

(b) If application for reinstatement is filed more than one year after discharge or return to inactive status, the applicant, in the discretion of the licensing agency, may be required to pass an examination.

(c) If application for reinstatement is filed and the licensing agency determines that the applicant has not actively engaged in the practice of the applicant's profession while on active duty, then the licensing agency may require the applicant to pass an examination.

(d) Unless otherwise specifically provided in this code, any licensee or registrant who, either part time or full time, practices in this state the profession or vocation for which the licensee or registrant is licensed or registered shall be required to maintain their license in good standing even though the licensee or registrant is in military service.

For the purposes in this section, time spent by a licensee in receiving treatment or hospitalization in any veterans' facility during which the licensee is prevented from practicing the licensee's profession or vocation shall be excluded from said period of one year.

HISTORY:

Added Stats 1951 ch 185 § 2. Amended Stats 1953 ch 423 § 1; Stats 1961 ch 1253 § 1; Stats 2010 ch 389 § 1 (AB 2500), effective January 1, 2011; Stats 2011 ch 296 § 1 (AB 1023), effective January 1, 2012; Stats 2019 ch 351 § 17 (AB 496), effective January 1, 2020.

§ 114.3. Waiver of fees and requirements for active duty members of armed forces and national guard

(a) Notwithstanding any other law, every board, as defined in Section 22, within the department shall waive the renewal fees, continuing education requirements, and other renewal requirements as determined by the board, if any are applicable, for a licensee or registrant called to active duty as a member of the United States Armed Forces or the California National Guard if all of the following requirements are met:

(1) The licensee or registrant possessed a current and valid license with the board at the time the licensee or registrant was called to active duty.

(2) The renewal requirements are waived only for the period during which the licensee or registrant is on active duty service.

(3) Written documentation that substantiates the licensee or registrant's active duty service is provided to the board.

(b) For purposes of this section, the phrase "called to active duty" shall have the same meaning as "active duty" as defined in Section 101 of Title 10 of the United States Code and shall additionally include individuals who are on active duty in the California National Guard, whether due to proclamation of a state of insurrection pursuant to Section 143 of the Military and Veterans Code or due to a proclamation of a state extreme emergency or when the California National Guard is otherwise on active duty pursuant to Section 146 of the Military and Veterans Code.

(c)(1) Except as specified in paragraph (2), the licensee or registrant shall not engage in any activities requiring a license during the period that the waivers provided by this section are in effect.

(2) If the licensee or registrant will provide services for which the licensee or registrant is licensed while on active duty, the board shall convert the license status to military active and no private practice of any type shall be permitted.

(d) In order to engage in any activities for which the licensee or registrant is licensed once discharged from active duty, the licensee or registrant shall meet all necessary renewal requirements as determined by the board within six months from the licensee's or registrant's date of discharge from active duty service.

(e) After a licensee or registrant receives notice of the licensee or registrant's discharge date, the licensee or registrant shall notify the board of their discharge from active duty within 60 days of receiving their notice of discharge.

(f) A board may adopt regulations to carry out the provisions of this section.

(g) This section shall not apply to any board that has a similar license renewal waiver process statutorily authorized for that board.

HISTORY:

Added Stats 2012 ch 742 § 1 (AB 1588), effective January 1, 2013. Amended Stats 2019 ch 351 § 18 (AB 496), effective January 1, 2020; Stats 2022 ch 386 § 1 (SB 1237), effective January 1, 2023.

§ 114.5. Military service; Posting of information on Web site about application of military experience and training towards licensure

(a) Each board shall inquire in every application for licensure if the individual applying for licensure is serving in, or has previously served in, the military.

(b) If a board's governing law authorizes veterans to apply military experience and training towards licensure requirements, that board shall post information on the board's Internet Web site about the ability of veteran applicants to apply military experience and training towards licensure requirements.

HISTORY:

Added Stats 2013 ch 693 § 1 (AB 1057), effective January 1, 2014. Amended Stats 2016 ch 174 § 1 (SB 1348), effective January 1, 2017.

§ 115. Applicability of Section 114

The provisions of Section 114 of this code are also applicable to a licensee or registrant whose license or registration was obtained while in the armed services.

HISTORY:

Added Stats 1951 ch 1577 § 1.

§ 115.4. Licensure process expedited for honorably discharged veterans of Armed Forces

(a) Notwithstanding any other law, on and after July 1, 2016, a board within the department shall expedite, and may assist, the initial licensure process for an applicant who supplies satisfactory evidence to the board that the applicant has served as an active duty member of the Armed Forces of the United States and was honorably discharged.

(b) A board may adopt regulations necessary to administer this section.

HISTORY:

Added Stats 2014 ch 657 § 1 (SB 1226), effective January 1, 2015.

§ 115.5. Board required to expedite licensure process for certain applicants; Adoption of regulations [Repealed]

HISTORY:

Added Stats 2012 ch 399 § 1 (AB 1904), effective January 1, 2013. Amended Stats 2019 ch 351 § 19

(AB 496), effective January 1, 2020; Stats 2021 ch 367 § 1 (SB 607), effective January 1, 2022, repealed July 1, 2022.

§ 115.5. Board required to expedite licensure process for certain applicants; Adoption of regulations

(a) A board within the department shall expedite the licensure process and waive the licensure application fee and the initial or original license fee charged by the board for an applicant who meets both of the following requirements:

(1) Supplies evidence satisfactory to the board that the applicant is married to, or in a domestic partnership or other legal union with, an active duty member of the Armed Forces of the United States who is assigned to a duty station in this state under official active duty military orders.

(2) Holds a current license in another state, district, or territory of the United States in the profession or vocation for which the applicant seeks a license from the board.

(b) A board may adopt regulations necessary to administer this section.

(c) This section shall become operative on July 1, 2022.

HISTORY:

Added Stats 2021 ch 367 § 2 (SB 607), effective January 1, 2022, operative July 1, 2022.

§ 115.6. Temporary licensure process for spouses of active duty members of Armed Forces [Repealed effective July 1, 2023]

(a) A board within the department shall, after appropriate investigation, issue the following eligible temporary licenses to an applicant if the applicant meets the requirements set forth in subdivision (c):

(1) Registered nurse license by the Board of Registered Nursing.

(2) Vocational nurse license issued by the Board of Vocational Nursing and Psychiatric Technicians of the State of California.

(3) Psychiatric technician license issued by the Board of Vocational Nursing and Psychiatric Technicians of the State of California.

(4) Speech-language pathologist license issued by the Speech-Language Pathology and Audiology and Hearing Aid Dispensers Board.

(5) Audiologist license issued by the Speech-Language Pathology and Audiology and Hearing Aid Dispensers Board.

(6) Veterinarian license issued by the Veterinary Medical Board.

(7) All licenses issued by the Board for Professional Engineers, Land Surveyors, and Geologists.

(8) All licenses issued by the Medical Board of California.

(9) All licenses issued by the Podiatric Medical Board of California.

(b) The board may conduct an investigation of an applicant for purposes of denying or revoking a temporary license issued pursuant to this section. This investigation may include a criminal background check.

(c) An applicant seeking a temporary license pursuant to this section shall meet the following requirements:

(1) The applicant shall supply evidence satisfactory to the board that the applicant is married to, or in a domestic partnership or other legal union with, an active duty member of the Armed Forces of the United States who

is assigned to a duty station in this state under official active duty military orders.

(2) The applicant shall hold a current, active, and unrestricted license that confers upon the applicant the authority to practice, in another state, district, or territory of the United States, the profession or vocation for which the applicant seeks a temporary license from the board.

(3) The applicant shall submit an application to the board that shall include a signed affidavit attesting to the fact that the applicant meets all of the requirements for the temporary license and that the information submitted in the application is accurate, to the best of the applicant's knowledge. The application shall also include written verification from the applicant's original licensing jurisdiction stating that the applicant's license is in good standing in that jurisdiction.

(4) The applicant shall not have committed an act in any jurisdiction that would have constituted grounds for denial, suspension, or revocation of the license under this code at the time the act was committed. A violation of this paragraph may be grounds for the denial or revocation of a temporary license issued by the board.

(5) The applicant shall not have been disciplined by a licensing entity in another jurisdiction and shall not be the subject of an unresolved complaint, review procedure, or disciplinary proceeding conducted by a licensing entity in another jurisdiction.

(6) The applicant shall, upon request by a board, furnish a full set of fingerprints for purposes of conducting a criminal background check.

(d) A board may adopt regulations necessary to administer this section.

(e) A temporary license issued pursuant to this section may be immediately terminated upon a finding that the temporary licenseholder failed to meet any of the requirements described in subdivision (c) or provided substantively inaccurate information that would affect the person's eligibility for temporary licensure. Upon termination of the temporary license, the board shall issue a notice of termination that shall require the temporary licenseholder to immediately cease the practice of the licensed profession upon receipt.

(f) An applicant seeking a temporary license as a civil engineer, geotechnical engineer, structural engineer, land surveyor, professional geologist, professional geophysicist, certified engineering geologist, or certified hydrogeologist pursuant to this section shall successfully pass the appropriate California-specific examination or examinations required for licensure in those respective professions by the Board for Professional Engineers, Land Surveyors, and Geologists.

(g) A temporary license issued pursuant to this section shall expire 12 months after issuance, upon issuance of an expedited license pursuant to Section 115.5, or upon denial of the application for expedited licensure by the board, whichever occurs first.

(h) This section shall remain in effect only until July 1, 2023, and as of that date is repealed.

HISTORY:

Added Stats 2014 ch 640 § 1 (AB 186), effective January 1, 2015. Amended Stats 2017 ch 775 § 2 (SB 798), effective January 1, 2018; Stats 2019 ch 351 § 20 (AB 496), effective January 1, 2020; Stats 2021 ch 693 § 1 (AB 107), effective January 1, 2022, repealed July 1, 2023.

§ 115.6. Temporary licensure process for spouses of active duty members of Armed Forces [Operative July 1, 2023]

(a)(1) Except as provided in subdivision (j), a board within the department shall, after appropriate investigation, issue a temporary license to practice a profession or vocation to an applicant who meets the requirements set forth in subdivisions (c) and (d).

(2) Revenues from fees for temporary licenses issued by the California Board of Accountancy shall be credited to the Accountancy Fund in accordance with Section 5132.

(b) The board may conduct an investigation of an applicant for purposes of denying or revoking a temporary license issued pursuant to this section. This investigation may include a criminal background check.

(c) An applicant seeking a temporary license pursuant to this section shall meet the following requirements:

(1) The applicant shall supply evidence satisfactory to the board that the applicant is married to, or in a domestic partnership or other legal union with, an active duty member of the Armed Forces of the United States who is assigned to a duty station in this state under official active duty military orders.

(2) The applicant shall hold a current, active, and unrestricted license that confers upon the applicant the authority to practice, in another state, district, or territory of the United States, the profession or vocation within the same scope for which the applicant seeks a temporary license from the board.

(3) The applicant shall submit an application to the board that shall include a signed affidavit attesting to the fact that the applicant meets all of the requirements for the temporary license, and that the information submitted in the application is accurate, to the best of the applicant's knowledge. The application shall also include written verification from the applicant's original licensing jurisdiction stating that the applicant's license is in good standing in that jurisdiction.

(4) The applicant shall not have committed an act in any jurisdiction that would have constituted grounds for denial, suspension, or revocation of the license under this code at the time the act was committed. A violation of this paragraph may be grounds for the denial or revocation of a temporary license issued by the board.

(5) The applicant shall not have been disciplined by a licensing entity in another jurisdiction and shall not be the subject of an unresolved complaint, review procedure, or disciplinary proceeding conducted by a licensing entity in another jurisdiction.

(6)(A) The applicant shall, upon request by a board, furnish a full set of fingerprints for purposes of conducting a criminal background check.

(B) The board shall request a fingerprint-based criminal history information check from the Department of Justice in accordance with subdivision (u) of Section 11105 of the Penal Code and the Department of Justice shall furnish state or federal criminal history information in accordance with subdivision (p) of Section 11105 of the Penal Code.

(d) The applicant shall pass a California law and ethics examination if otherwise required by the board for the profession or vocation for which the applicant seeks licensure.

(e) Except as specified in subdivision (g), a board shall issue a temporary license pursuant to this section within 30 days of receiving documentation that the applicant has met the requirements specified in subdivisions (c) and (d) if the results of the criminal background check do not show grounds for denial.

(f)(1) A temporary license issued pursuant to this section may be immediately terminated upon a finding that the temporary licenseholder failed to meet any of the requirements described in subdivision (c) or (d) or provided substantively inaccurate information that would affect the person's eligibility for temporary licensure. Upon termination of the temporary license, the board shall issue a notice of termination that shall require the temporary licenseholder to immediately cease the practice of the licensed profession upon receipt.

(2) Notwithstanding any other law, if, after notice and an opportunity to be heard, a board finds that a temporary licenseholder engaged in unprofessional conduct or any other act that is a cause for discipline by the board, the board shall revoke the temporary license.

(g) An applicant seeking a temporary license as a civil engineer, geotechnical engineer, structural engineer, land surveyor, professional geologist, professional geophysicist, certified engineering geologist, or certified hydrogeologist pursuant to this section shall successfully pass the appropriate California-specific examination or examinations required for licensure in those respective professions by the Board for Professional Engineers, Land Surveyors, and Geologists. The board shall issue a temporary license pursuant to this subdivision within 30 days of receiving documentation that the applicant has met the requirements specified in this subdivision and subdivisions (c) and (d) if the results of the criminal background check do not show grounds for denial.

(h) A temporary license issued pursuant to this section is nonrenewable and shall expire 12 months after issuance, upon issuance or denial of a standard license, upon issuance or denial of a license by endorsement, or upon issuance or denial of an expedited license pursuant to Section 115.5, whichever occurs first.

(i) A board shall submit to the department for approval, if necessary to implement this section, draft regulations necessary to administer this section. These regulations shall be adopted pursuant to the Administrative Procedure Act (Chapter 3.5 (commencing with Section 11340) of Part 1 of Division 3 of Title 2 of the Government Code).

(j)(1) This section shall not apply to a board that has a process in place by which an out-of-state licensed applicant in good standing who is married to, or in a domestic partnership or other legal union with, an active duty member of the Armed Forces of the United States is able to receive expedited, temporary authorization to practice while meeting state-specific requirements for a period of at least one year or is able to receive an expedited license by endorsement with no additional requirements superseding those described in subdivisions (c) and (d).

(2) This section shall apply only to the extent that it does not amend an initiative or violate constitutional requirements.

(k) This section shall become operative on July 1, 2023.

HISTORY:

Added Stats 2021 ch 693 § 2 (AB 107), effective January 1, 2022, operative July 1, 2023.

§ 115.8. Annual report on military, veteran, and spouse licensure

The Department of Consumer Affairs shall compile information on military, veteran, and spouse licensure into an annual report for the Legislature, which shall be submitted in conformance with Section 9795 of the Government Code. The report shall include all of the following:

(a) The number of applications for a temporary license submitted by active duty servicemembers, veterans, or military spouses per calendar year, pursuant to Section 115.6.

(b) The number of applications for expedited licenses submitted by veterans and active duty spouses pursuant to Sections 115.4 and 115.5.

(c) The number of licenses issued and denied per calendar year pursuant to Sections 115.4, 115.5, and 115.6.

(d) The number of licenses issued pursuant to Section 115.6 that were suspended or revoked per calendar year.

(e) The number of applications for waived renewal fees received and granted pursuant to Section 114.3 per calendar year.

(f) The average length of time between application and issuance of licenses pursuant to Sections 115.4, 115.5, and 115.6 per board and occupation.

HISTORY:

Added Stats 2021 ch 693 § 3 (AB 107), effective January 1, 2022.

§ 115.9. Publishing information on licensing options available to military spouses

The department and each board within the department shall publish information pertinent to all licensing options available to military spouses on the home page of the internet website of the department or board, as applicable, including, but not limited to, the following:

(a) The process for expediting applications for military spouses.

(b) The availability of temporary licensure, the requirements for obtaining a temporary license, and length of time a temporary license is active.

(c) The requirements for full, permanent licensure by endorsement or credential for out-of-state applicants.

HISTORY:

Added Stats 2021 ch 693 § 4 (AB 107), effective January 1, 2022.

§ 116. Audit and review of disciplinary proceedings; Report to Legislature

(a) The director may audit and review, upon the director's own initiative, or upon the request of a consumer or licensee, inquiries and complaints regarding licensees, dismissals of disciplinary cases, the opening, conduct, or closure of investigations, informal conferences, and discipline short of formal accusation by the Medical Board of California, the allied health professional boards, and the Podiatric Medical Board of California. The director may make recommendations for changes to the disciplinary system to the appropriate board, the Legislature, or both.

(b) The director shall report to the Chairpersons of the Senate Business, Professions and Economic Development Committee and the Assembly Business and Professions Committee annually, commencing March 1, 1995, regarding the director's findings from any audit, review, or monitoring and evaluation conducted pursuant to this section.

HISTORY:

Added Stats 1993 ch 1267 § 1 (SB 916). Amended Stats 2019 ch 351 § 21 (AB 496), effective January 1, 2020.

§ 118. Effect of withdrawal of application; Effect of suspension, forfeiture, etc., of license

(a) The withdrawal of an application for a license after it has been filed with a board in the department shall not, unless the board has consented in writing to such withdrawal, deprive the board of its authority to institute or continue a proceeding against the applicant for the denial of the license upon any ground provided by law or to enter an order denying the license upon any such ground.

(b) The suspension, expiration, or forfeiture by operation of law of a license issued by a board in the department, or its suspension, forfeiture, or cancellation by order of the board or by order of a court of law, or its surrender without the written consent of the board, shall not, during any period in which it may be renewed, restored, reissued, or reinstated, deprive the board of its authority to institute or continue a disciplinary proceeding against the licensee upon any ground provided by law or to enter an order suspending or revoking the license or otherwise taking disciplinary action against the licensee on any such ground.

(c) As used in this section, "board" includes an individual who is authorized by any provision of this code to issue, suspend, or revoke a license, and "license" includes "certificate," "registration," and "permit."

HISTORY:

Added Stats 1961 ch 1079 § 1.

§ 119. Misdemeanors pertaining to use of licenses

Any person who does any of the following is guilty of a misdemeanor:

(a) Displays or causes or permits to be displayed or has in the person's possession either of the following:

(1) A canceled, revoked, suspended, or fraudulently altered license.

(2) A fictitious license or any document simulating a license or purporting to be or have been issued as a license.

(b) Lends the person's license to any other person or knowingly permits the use thereof by another.

(c) Displays or represents any license not issued to the person as being the person's license.

(d) Fails or refuses to surrender to the issuing authority upon its lawful written demand any license, registration, permit, or certificate which has been suspended, revoked, or canceled.

(e) Knowingly permits any unlawful use of a license issued to the person.

(f) Photographs, photostats, duplicates, manufactures, or in any way reproduces any license or facsimile thereof in a manner that it could be mistaken for a valid license, or displays or has in the person's possession any such photograph, photostat, duplicate, reproduction, or facsimile unless authorized by this code.

(g) Buys or receives a fraudulent, forged, or counterfeited license knowing that it is fraudulent, forged, or counterfeited. For purposes of this subdivision, "fraudulent" means containing any misrepresentation of fact.

As used in this section, "license" includes "certificate," "permit," "authority," and "registration" or any other indicia giving authorization to engage in a business or profession regulated by this code or referred to in Section 1000 or 3600.

HISTORY:

Added Stats 1965 ch 1083 § 1. Amended Stats 1990 ch 350 § 1 (SB 2084) (ch 1207 prevails), ch 1207 § 1 (AB 3242); Stats 1994 ch 1206 § 1 (SB 1775); Stats 2000 ch 568 § 1 (AB 2888); Stats 2019 ch 351 § 22 (AB 496), effective January 1, 2020.

§ 121. Practice during period between renewal and receipt of evidence of renewal

No licensee who has complied with the provisions of this code relating to the renewal of the licensee's license prior to expiration of such license shall be deemed to be engaged illegally in the practice of the licensee's business or profession during any period between such renewal and receipt of evidence of such renewal which may occur due to delay not the fault of the applicant.

As used in this section, "license" includes "certificate," "permit," "authorization," and "registration," or any other indicia giving authorization, by any agency, board, bureau, commission, committee, or entity within the Department of Consumer Affairs, to engage in a business or profession regulated by this code or by the board referred to in the Chiropractic Act or the Osteopathic Act.

HISTORY:

Added Stats 1979 ch 77 § 1. Amended Stats 2019 ch 351 § 24 (AB 496), effective January 1, 2020.

§ 122. Fee for issuance of duplicate certificate

Except as otherwise provided by law, the department and each of the boards, bureaus, committees, and commissions within the department may charge a fee for the processing and issuance of a duplicate copy of any certificate of licensure or other form evidencing licensure or renewal of licensure. The fee shall be in an amount sufficient to cover all costs incident to the issuance of the duplicate certificate or other form but shall not exceed twenty-five dollars ($25).

HISTORY:

Added Stats 1986 ch 951 § 1.

§ 123. Conduct constituting subversion of licensing examination; Penalties and damages

It is a misdemeanor for any person to engage in any conduct which subverts or attempts to subvert any licensing examination or the administration of an examination, including, but not limited to:

(a) Conduct which violates the security of the examination materials; removing from the examination room any examination materials without authorization; the unauthorized reproduction by any means of any portion of the actual licensing examination; aiding by any means the unauthorized reproduction of any portion of the actual licensing examination; paying or using professional or paid examination-takers for the purpose of reconstructing any portion of the licensing examination; obtaining examination questions or other examination material, except by specific authorization either before, during, or after an examination; or using or purporting to use any examination questions or materials which were improperly removed or taken from any examination for the purpose of instructing or preparing any applicant for examination; or selling, distributing, buying, receiving, or having unauthorized possession of any portion of a future, current, or previously administered licensing examination.

(b) Communicating with any other examinee during the administration of a licensing examination; copying answers from another examinee or permitting one's answers to be copied by another examinee; having in one's possession during the administration of the licensing examination any books, equipment, notes, written or printed materials, or data of any kind, other than the examination materials distributed, or otherwise authorized to be in one's possession during the examination; or impersonating any examinee or having an impersonator take the licensing examination on one's behalf.

Nothing in this section shall preclude prosecution under the authority provided for in any other provision of law.

In addition to any other penalties, a person found guilty of violating this section, shall be liable for the actual damages sustained by the agency administering the examination not to exceed ten thousand dollars ($10,000) and the costs of litigation.

(c) If any provision of this section or the application thereof to any person or circumstances is held invalid, that invalidity shall not affect other provisions or applications of the section that can be given effect without the invalid provision or application, and to this end the provisions of this section are severable.

HISTORY:

Added Stats 1989 ch 1022 § 1. Amended Stats 1991 ch 647 § 1 (SB 879).

§ 123.5. Enjoining violations

Whenever any person has engaged, or is about to engage, in any acts or practices which constitute, or will constitute, a violation of Section 123, the superior court in and for the county wherein the acts or practices take place, or are about to take place, may issue an injunction, or other appropriate order, restraining such conduct on application of a board, the Attorney General or the district attorney of the county.

The proceedings under this section shall be governed by Chapter 3 (commencing with Section 525) of Title 7 of Part 2 of the Code of Civil Procedure.

The remedy provided for by this section shall be in addition to, and not a limitation on, the authority provided for in any other provision of law.

HISTORY:

Added Stats 1983 ch 95 § 2, as B & P C § 497. Amended and renumbered by Stats 1989 ch 1022 § 4.

§ 124. Manner of notice

Notwithstanding subdivision (c) of Section 11505 of the Government Code, whenever written notice, including a notice, order, or document served pursuant to Chapter 3.5 (commencing with Section 11340), Chapter 4 (commencing with Section 11370), or Chapter 5 (commencing with Section 11500), of Part 1 of Division 3 of Title 2 of the Government Code, is required to be given by any board in the department, the notice may be given by regular mail addressed to the last known address of the licensee or by personal service, at the option of the board.

HISTORY:

Added Stats 1961 ch 1253 § 2. Amended Stats 1994 ch 26 § 4 (AB 1807), effective March 30, 1994; Stats 1995 ch 938 § 1 (SB 523), operative July 1, 1997; Stats 2019 ch 351 § 25 (AB 496), effective January 1, 2020.

Bus & Prof

§ 125. Misdemeanor offenses by licensees

Any person, licensed under Division 1 (commencing with Section 100), Division 2 (commencing with Section 500), or Division 3 (commencing with Section 5000) is guilty of a misdemeanor and subject to the disciplinary provisions of this code applicable to them, who conspires with a person not so licensed to violate any provision of this code, or who, with intent to aid or assist that person in violating those provisions does either of the following:

(a) Allows their license to be used by that person.

(b) Acts as their agent or partner.

HISTORY:

Added Stats 1949 ch 308 § 1. Amended Stats 1994 ch 1206 § 2 (SB 1775); Stats 2019 ch 351 § 26 (AB 496), effective January 1, 2020.

§ 125.3. Direction to licensee violating licensing act to pay costs of investigation and enforcement

(a) Except as otherwise provided by law, in any order issued in resolution of a disciplinary proceeding before any board within the department or before the Osteopathic Medical Board, upon request of the entity bringing the proceeding, the administrative law judge may direct a licensee found to have committed a violation or violations of the licensing act to pay a sum not to exceed the reasonable costs of the investigation and enforcement of the case.

(b) In the case of a disciplined licensee that is a corporation or a partnership, the order may be made against the licensed corporate entity or licensed partnership.

(c) A certified copy of the actual costs, or a good faith estimate of costs where actual costs are not available, signed by the entity bringing the proceeding or its designated representative shall be prima facie evidence of reasonable costs of investigation and prosecution of the case. The costs shall include the amount of investigative and enforcement costs up to the date of the hearing, including, but not limited to, charges imposed by the Attorney General.

(d) The administrative law judge shall make a proposed finding of the amount of reasonable costs of investigation and prosecution of the case when requested pursuant to subdivision (a). The finding of the administrative law judge with regard to costs shall not be reviewable by the board to increase the cost award. The board may reduce or eliminate the cost award, or remand to the administrative law judge if the proposed decision fails to make a finding on costs requested pursuant to subdivision (a).

(e) If an order for recovery of costs is made and timely payment is not made as directed in the board's decision, the board may enforce the order for repayment in any appropriate court. This right of enforcement shall be in addition to any other rights the board may have as to any licensee to pay costs.

(f) In any action for recovery of costs, proof of the board's decision shall be conclusive proof of the validity of the order of payment and the terms for payment.

(g)(1) Except as provided in paragraph (2), the board shall not renew or reinstate the license of any licensee who has failed to pay all of the costs ordered under this section.

(2) Notwithstanding paragraph (1), the board may, in its discretion, conditionally renew or reinstate for a maximum of one year the license of any licensee who demonstrates financial hardship and who enters into a formal agreement with the board to reimburse the board within that one-year period for the unpaid costs.

(h) All costs recovered under this section shall be considered a reimbursement for costs incurred and shall be deposited in the fund of the board recovering the costs to be available upon appropriation by the Legislature.

(i) Nothing in this section shall preclude a board from including the recovery of the costs of investigation and enforcement of a case in any stipulated settlement.

(j) This section does not apply to any board if a specific statutory provision in that board's licensing act provides for recovery of costs in an administrative disciplinary proceeding.

HISTORY:

Added Stats 1992 ch 1289 § 1 (AB 2743), effective January 1, 1993. Amended Stats 2001 ch 728 § 1 (SB 724); Stats 2005 ch 674 § 2 (SB 231), effective January 1, 2006; Stats 2006 ch 223 § 2 (SB 1438), effective January 1, 2007; Stats 2019 ch 351 § 27 (AB 496), effective January 1, 2020; Stats 2021 ch 649 § 1 (SB 806), effective January 1, 2022.

§ 125.5. Enjoining violations; Restitution orders

(a) The superior court for the county in which any person has engaged or is about to engage in any act which constitutes a violation of a chapter of this code administered or enforced by a board within the department may, upon a petition filed by the board with the approval of the director, issue an injunction or other appropriate order restraining such conduct. The proceedings under this section shall be governed by Chapter 3 (commencing with Section 525) of Title 7 of Part 2 of the Code of Civil Procedure. As used in this section, "board" includes commission, bureau, division, agency and a medical quality review committee.

(b) The superior court for the county in which any person has engaged in any act which constitutes a violation of a chapter of this code administered or enforced by a board within the department may, upon a petition filed by the board with the approval of the director, order such person to make restitution to persons injured as a result of such violation.

(c) The court may order a person subject to an injunction or restraining order, provided for in subdivision (a) of this section, or subject to an order requiring restitution pursuant to subdivision (b), to reimburse the petitioning board for expenses incurred by the board in its investigation related to its petition.

(d) The remedy provided for by this section shall be in addition to, and not a limitation on, the authority provided for in any other section of this code.

HISTORY:

Added Stats 1972 ch 1238 § 1. Amended Stats 1973 ch 632 § 1; Stats 1975 2d Ex Sess ch 1 § 2; Stats 1982 ch 517 § 1.

§ 125.6. Unlawful discrimination by licensees

(a)(1) With regard to an applicant, every person who holds a license under the provisions of this code is subject to disciplinary action under the disciplinary provisions of this code applicable to that person if, because of any characteristic listed or defined in subdivision (b) or (e) of Section 51 of the Civil Code, the person refuses to perform the licensed activity or aids or incites the refusal to perform that licensed activity by another licensee, or if, because of any characteristic listed or defined in subdivision (b) or (e) of Section 51 of the Civil Code, the person makes any discrimination, or restriction in the performance of the licensed activity.

(2) Nothing in this section shall be interpreted to prevent a physician or health care professional licensed pursuant to Division 2 (commencing with Section 500) from considering any of the characteristics of a patient listed in subdivision (b) or (e) of Section 51 of the Civil Code if that consideration is medically necessary and for the sole purpose of determining the appropriate diagnosis or treatment of the patient.

(3) Nothing in this section shall be interpreted to apply to discrimination by employers with regard to employees or prospective employees, nor shall this section authorize action against any club license issued pursuant to Article 4 (commencing with Section 23425) of Chapter 3 of Division 9 because of discriminatory membership policy.

(4) The presence of architectural barriers to an individual with physical disabilities that conform to applicable state or local building codes and regulations shall not constitute discrimination under this section.

(b)(1) Nothing in this section requires a person licensed pursuant to Division 2 (commencing with Section 500) to permit an individual to participate in, or benefit from, the licensed activity of the licensee where that individual poses a direct threat to the health or safety of others. For this purpose, the term "direct threat" means a significant risk to the health or safety of others that cannot be eliminated by a modification of policies, practices, or procedures or by the provision of auxiliary aids and services.

(2) Nothing in this section requires a person licensed pursuant to Division 2 (commencing with Section 500) to perform a licensed activity for which the person is not qualified to perform.

(c)(1) "Applicant," as used in this section, means a person applying for licensed services provided by a person licensed under this code.

(2) "License," as used in this section, includes "certificate," "permit," "authority," and "registration" or any other indicia giving authorization to engage in a business or profession regulated by this code.

HISTORY:
Added Stats 1974 ch 1350 § 1. Amended Stats 1977 ch 293 § 1; Stats 1980 ch 191 § 1; Stats 1992 ch 913 § 2 (AB 1077); Stats 2007 ch 568 § 2 (AB 14), effective January 1, 2008; Stats 2019 ch 351 § 28 (AB 496), effective January 1, 2020.

§ 125.7. Restraining orders

In addition to the remedy provided for in Section 125.5, the superior court for the county in which any licensee licensed under Division 2 (commencing with Section 500), or any initiative act referred to in that division, has engaged or is about to engage in any act that constitutes a violation of a chapter of this code administered or enforced by a board referred to in Division 2 (commencing with Section 500), may, upon a petition filed by the board and accompanied by an affidavit or affidavits in support thereof and a memorandum of points and authorities, issue a temporary restraining order or other appropriate order restraining the licensee from engaging in the business or profession for which the person is licensed or from any part thereof, in accordance with this section.

(a) If the affidavits in support of the petition show that the licensee has engaged or is about to engage in acts or omissions constituting a violation of a chapter of this code and if the court is satisfied that permitting the licensee to continue to engage in the business or profession for which the license was issued will endanger the public health, safety, or welfare, the court may issue an order temporarily restraining the licensee from engaging in the profession for which he or she is licensed.

(b) The order may not be issued without notice to the licensee unless it appears from facts shown by the affidavits that serious injury would result to the public before the matter can be heard on notice.

(c) Except as otherwise specifically provided by this section, proceedings under this section shall be governed by Chapter 3 (commencing with Section 525) of Title 7 of Part 2 of the Code of Civil Procedure.

(d) When a restraining order is issued pursuant to this section, or within a time to be allowed by the superior court, but in any case not more than 30 days after the restraining order is issued, an accusation shall be filed with the board pursuant to Section 11503 of the Government Code or, in the case of a licensee of the State Department of Health Services, with that department pursuant to Section 100171 of the Health and Safety Code. The accusation shall be served upon the licensee as provided by Section 11505 of the Government Code. The licensee shall have all of the rights and privileges available as specified in Chapter 5 (commencing with Section 11500) of Part 1 of Division 3 of Title 2 of the Government Code. However, if the licensee requests a hearing on the accusation, the board shall provide the licensee with a hearing within 30 days of the request and a decision within 15 days of the date the decision is received from the administrative law judge, or the court may nullify the restraining order previously issued. Any restraining order issued pursuant to this section shall be dissolved by operation of law at the time the board's decision is subject to judicial review pursuant to Section 1094.5 of the Code of Civil Procedure.

(e) The remedy provided for in this section shall be in addition to, and not a limitation upon, the authority provided by any other provision of this code.

HISTORY:
Added Stats 1977 ch 292 § 1. Amended Stats 1982 ch 517 § 2; Stats 1994 ch 1206 § 3 (SB 1775); Stats 1997 ch 220 § 1 (SB 68), effective August 4, 1997; Stats 1998 ch 878 § 1.5 (SB 2239).

§ 125.8. Temporary order restraining licensee engaged or about to engage in violation of law

In addition to the remedy provided for in Section 125.5, the superior court for the county in which any licensee licensed under Division 3 (commencing with Section 5000) or Chapter 2 (commencing with Section 18600) or Chapter 3 (commencing with Section 19000) of Division 8 has engaged or is about to engage in any act which constitutes a violation of a chapter of this code administered or enforced by a board referred to in Division 3 (commencing with Section 5000) or Chapter 2 (commencing with Section 18600) or Chapter 3 (commencing with Section 19000) of Division 8 may, upon a petition filed by the board and accompanied by an affidavit or affidavits in support thereof and a memorandum of points and authorities, issue a temporary restraining order or other appropriate order restraining the licensee from engaging in the business or profession for which the person is licensed or from any part thereof, in accordance with the provisions of this section.

(a) If the affidavits in support of the petition show that the licensee has engaged or is about to engage in acts or omissions constituting a violation of a chapter of this code and if the court is satisfied that permitting the licensee to continue to engage in the business or profession for which the license was issued will endanger the public health, safety, or welfare, the court may issue an order temporarily restraining the licensee from engaging in the profession for which he is licensed.

(b) Such order may not be issued without notice to the licensee unless it appears from facts shown by the affidavits that serious injury would result to the public before the matter can be heard on notice.

(c) Except as otherwise specifically provided by this section, proceedings under this section shall be governed by Chapter 3 (commencing with Section 525) of Title 7 of Part 2 of the Code of Civil Procedure.

(d) When a restraining order is issued pursuant to this section, or within a time to be allowed by the superior court, but in any case not more than 30 days after the restraining order is issued, an accusation shall be filed with the board pursuant to Section 11503 of the Government Code. The accusation shall be served upon the licensee as provided by Section 11505 of the Government Code. The licensee shall have all of the rights and privileges available as specified in Chapter 5 (commencing with Section 11500) of Part 1 of Division 3 of Title 2 of the Government Code; however, if the licensee requests a hearing on the accusation, the board must provide the licensee with a hearing within 30 days of the request and a decision within 15 days of the date of the conclusion of the hearing, or the court may nullify the restraining order previously issued. Any restraining order issued pursuant to this section shall be dissolved by operation of law at such time the board's decision is subject to judicial review pursuant to Section 1094.5 of the Code of Civil Procedure.

HISTORY:

Added Stats 1977 ch 443 § 1. Amended Stats 1982 ch 517 § 3.

§ 125.9. System for issuance of citations to licensees; Contents; Fines

(a) Except with respect to persons regulated under Chapter 11 (commencing with Section 7500), any board, bureau, or commission within the department, the State Board of Chiropractic Examiners, and the Osteopathic Medical Board of California, may establish, by regulation, a system for the issuance to a licensee of a citation which may contain an order of abatement or an order to pay an administrative fine assessed by the board, bureau, or commission where the licensee is in violation of the applicable licensing act or any regulation adopted pursuant thereto.

(b) The system shall contain the following provisions:

(1) Citations shall be in writing and shall describe with particularity the nature of the violation, including specific reference to the provision of law determined to have been violated.

(2) Whenever appropriate, the citation shall contain an order of abatement fixing a reasonable time for abatement of the violation.

(3) In no event shall the administrative fine assessed by the board, bureau, or commission exceed five thousand dollars ($5,000) for each inspection or each investigation made with respect to the violation, or five thousand dollars ($5,000) for each violation or count if the violation involves fraudulent billing submitted to an insurance company, the Medi-Cal program, or Medicare. In assessing a fine, the board, bureau, or commission shall give due consideration to the appropriateness of the amount of the fine with respect to factors such as the gravity of the violation, the good faith of the licensee, and the history of previous violations.

(4) A citation or fine assessment issued pursuant to a citation shall inform the licensee that if the licensee desires a hearing to contest the finding of a violation, that hearing shall be requested by written notice to the board, bureau, or commission within 30 days of the date of issuance of the citation or assessment. If a hearing is not requested pursuant to this section, payment of any fine shall not constitute an admission of the violation charged. Hearings shall be held pursuant to Chapter 5 (commencing with Section 11500) of Part 1 of Division 3 of Title 2 of the Government Code.

(5) Failure of a licensee to pay a fine or comply with an order of abatement, or both, within 30 days of the date of assessment or order, unless the citation is being appealed, may result in disciplinary action being taken by the board, bureau, or commission. Where a citation is not contested and a fine is not paid, the full amount of the assessed fine shall be added to the fee for renewal of the license. A license shall not be renewed without payment of the renewal fee and fine.

(c) The system may contain the following provisions:

(1) A citation may be issued without the assessment of an administrative fine.

(2) Assessment of administrative fines may be limited to only particular violations of the applicable licensing act.

(d) Notwithstanding any other provision of law, if a fine is paid to satisfy an assessment based on the finding of a violation, payment of the fine and compliance with the order of abatement, if applicable, shall be represented as satisfactory resolution of the matter for purposes of public disclosure.

(e) Administrative fines collected pursuant to this section shall be deposited in the special fund of the particular board, bureau, or commission.

HISTORY:

Added Stats 1986 ch 1379 § 2. Amended Stats 1987 ch 1088 § 1; Stats 1991 ch 521 § 1 (SB 650); Stats 1995 ch 381 § 4 (AB 910), effective August 4, 1995, ch 708 § 1 (SB 609); Stats 2000 ch 197 § 1

(SB 1636); Stats 2001 ch 309 § 1 (AB 761), ch 728 § 1.2 (SB 724); Stats 2003 ch 788 § 1 (SB 362); Stats 2012 ch 291 § 1 (SB 1077), effective January 1, 2013; Stats 2019 ch 351 § 29 (AB 496), effective January 1, 2020; Stats 2020 ch 312 § 3 (SB 1474), effective January 1, 2021.

§ 126. Submission of reports to Governor

Notwithstanding any other provision of this code, any board, commission, examining committee, or other similarly constituted agency within the department required prior to the effective date of this section to submit reports to the Governor under any provision of this code shall not be required to submit such reports.

HISTORY:

Added Stats 1967 ch 660 § 1.

§ 127. Submission of reports to director

Notwithstanding any other provision of this code, the director may require such reports from any board, commission, examining committee, or other similarly constituted agency within the department as the director deems reasonably necessary on any phase of their operations.

HISTORY:

Added Stats 1967 ch 660 § 2. Amended Stats 2019 ch 351 § 30 (AB 496), effective January 1, 2020.

§ 128. Sale of equipment, supplies, or services for use in violation of licensing requirements

Notwithstanding any other provision of law, it is a misdemeanor to sell equipment, supplies, or services to any person with knowledge that the equipment, supplies, or services are to be used in the performance of a service or contract in violation of the licensing requirements of this code.

The provisions of this section shall not be applicable to cash sales of less than one hundred dollars ($100).

For the purposes of this section, "person" includes, but is not limited to, a company, partnership, limited liability company, firm, or corporation.

For the purposes of this section, "license" includes certificate or registration.

A violation of this section shall be punishable by a fine of not less than one thousand dollars ($1,000) and by imprisonment in the county jail not exceeding six months.

HISTORY:

Added Stats 1971 ch 1052 § 1. Amended Stats 1994 ch 1010 § 1 (SB 2053).

§ 128.5. Reduction of license fees in event of surplus funds

(a) Notwithstanding any other provision of law, if at the end of any fiscal year, an agency within the Department of Consumer Affairs, except the agencies referred to in subdivision (b), has unencumbered funds in an amount that equals or is more than the agency's operating budget for the next two fiscal years, the agency shall reduce license or other fees, whether the license or other fees be fixed by statute or may be determined by the agency within limits fixed by statute, during the following fiscal year in an amount that will reduce any surplus funds of the agency to an amount less than the agency's operating budget for the next two fiscal years.

(b) Notwithstanding any other provision of law, if at the end of any fiscal year, the California Architects Board, the Board of Behavioral Sciences, the Veterinary Medical Board, the Court Reporters Board of California, the Medical Board of California, the Board of Vocational Nursing and Psychiatric Technicians, or the Bureau of Security and Investigative Services has unencumbered funds in an amount that equals or is more than the agency's operating budget for the next two fiscal years, the agency shall reduce license or other fees, whether the license or other fees be fixed by statute or may be determined by the agency within limits fixed by statute, during the following fiscal year in an amount that will reduce any surplus funds of the agency to an amount less than the agency's operating budget for the next two fiscal years.

HISTORY:

Added Stats 1972 ch 938 § 2, effective August 16, 1972, as B & P C § 128. Amended Stats 1973 ch 863 § 3. Amended and renumbered by Stats 1978 ch 1161 § 4. Amended Stats 1987 ch 850 § 3; Stats 1989 ch 886 § 2; Stats 1993 ch 1263 § 2 (AB 936); Stats 1994 ch 26 § 5 (AB 1807), effective March 30, 1994; Stats 1995 ch 60 § 2 (SB 42), effective July 6, 1995; Stats 1997 ch 759 § 2 (SB 827); Stats 2000 ch 1054 § 1 (SB 1863); Stats 2009 ch 308 § 3 (SB 819), effective January 1, 2010.

§ 129. Handling of complaints; Reports to Legislature

(a) As used in this section, "board" means every board, bureau, commission, committee, and similarly constituted agency in the department that issues licenses.

(b) Each board shall, upon receipt of any complaint respecting an individual licensed by the board, notify the complainant of the initial administrative action taken on the complainant's complaint within 10 days of receipt. Each board shall notify the complainant of the final action taken on the complainant's complaint. There shall be a notification made in every case in which the complainant is known. If the complaint is not within the jurisdiction of the board or if the board is unable to dispose satisfactorily of the complaint, the board shall transmit the complaint together with any evidence or information it has concerning the complaint to the agency, public or private, whose authority in the opinion of the board will provide the most effective means to secure the relief sought. The board shall notify the complainant of this action and of any other means that may be available to the complainant to secure relief.

(c) The board shall, when the board deems it appropriate, notify the person against whom the complaint is made of the nature of the complaint, may request appropriate relief for the complainant, and may meet and confer with the complainant and the licensee in order to mediate the complaint. Nothing in this subdivision shall be construed as authorizing or requiring any board to set or to modify any fee charged by a licensee.

(d) It shall be the continuing duty of the board to ascertain patterns of complaints and to report on all actions taken with respect to those patterns of complaints to the director and to the Legislature at least once per year. The board shall evaluate those complaints dismissed for lack of jurisdiction or no violation and recommend to the director and to the Legislature at least once per year the statutory changes it deems necessary to implement the board's functions and responsibilities under this section.

(e) It shall be the continuing duty of the board to take whatever action it deems necessary, with the approval of the director, to inform the public of its functions under this section.

(f) Notwithstanding any other law, upon receipt of a child custody evaluation report submitted to a court pursuant to Chapter 6 (commencing with Section 3110) of Part 2 of Division 8 of the Family Code, the board shall notify the noncomplaining party in the underlying custody dispute, who is a subject of that report, of the pending investigation.

HISTORY:

Added Stats 1972 ch 1041 § 1. Amended Stats 2014 ch 283 § 1 (AB 1843), effective January 1, 2015; Stats 2019 ch 351 § 31 (AB 496), effective January 1, 2020.

§ 130. Terms of office of agency members

(a) Notwithstanding any other law, the term of office of any member of an agency designated in subdivision (b) shall be for a term of four years expiring on June 1.

(b) Subdivision (a) applies to the following boards or committees:

(1) The Medical Board of California.

(2) The Podiatric Medical Board of California.

(3) The Physical Therapy Board of California.

(4) The Board of Registered Nursing, except as provided in subdivision (c) of Section 2703.

(5) The Board of Vocational Nursing and Psychiatric Technicians.

(6) The California State Board of Optometry.

(7) The California State Board of Pharmacy.

(8) The Veterinary Medical Board.

(9) The California Architects Board.

(10) The Landscape Architect Technical Committee.

(11) The Board for Professional Engineers and Land Surveyors.

(12) The Contractors State License Board.

(13) The Board of Behavioral Sciences.

(14) The Court Reporters Board of California.

(15) The State Athletic Commission.

(16) The Osteopathic Medical Board of California.

(17) The Respiratory Care Board of California.

(18) The Acupuncture Board.

(19) The Board of Psychology.

(20) The Structural Pest Control Board.

HISTORY:

Added Stats 1969 ch 465 § 1. Amended Stats 1971 ch 716 § 8; Stats 1978 ch 1161 § 5; Stats 1983 ch 150 § 2; Stats 1986 ch 655 § 1; Stats 1987 ch 850 § 4; Stats 1989 ch 886 § 3; Stats 1990 ch 1256 § 2 (AB 2649); Stats 1991 ch 359 § 2 (AB 1332); Stats 1994 ch 26 § 6 (AB 1807), effective March 30, 1994, ch 1274 § 1.3 (SB 2039); Stats 1995 ch 60 § 3 (SB 42), effective July 6, 1995; Stats 1997 ch 759 § 3 (SB 827); Stats 1998 ch 59 § 4 (AB 969), ch 970 § 1 (AB 2802), ch 971 § 1 (AB 2721); Stats 2000 ch 1054 § 2 (SB 1863); Stats 2001 ch 159 § 3 (SB 662); Stats 2009–2010 4th Ex Sess ch 18 § 2 (ABX4 20), effective October 23, 2009; Stats 2012 ch 4 § 1 (SB 98), effective February 14, 2012. See this section as modified in Governor's Reorganization Plan No. 2 § 3 of 2012; Amended Stats 2013 ch 352 § 4 (AB 1317), effective September 26, 2013, operative July 1, 2013; Stats 2019 ch 351 § 32 (AB 496), effective January 1, 2020; Stats 2020 ch 312 § 4 (SB 1474), effective January 1, 2021; Stats 2021 ch 630 § 3 (AB 1534), effective January 1, 2022.

§ 131. Maximum number of terms

Notwithstanding any other provision of law, no member of an agency designated in subdivision (b) of Section 130 or member of a board, commission, committee, or similarly constituted agency in the department shall serve more than two consecutive full terms.

HISTORY:

Added Stats 1970 ch 1394 § 1, operative July 1, 1971. Amended Stats 1987 ch 850 § 5.

§ 132. Requirements for institution or joinder of legal action by state agency against other state or federal agency

No board, commission, examining committee, or any other agency within the department may institute or join any legal action against any other agency within the state or federal government without the permission of the director.

Prior to instituting or joining in a legal action against an agency of the state or federal government, a board, commission, examining committee, or any other agency within the department shall present a written request to the director to do so.

Within 30 days of receipt of the request, the director shall communicate the director's approval or denial of the request and the director's reasons for approval or denial to the requesting agency in writing. If the director does not act within 30 days, the request shall be deemed approved.

A requesting agency within the department may override the director's denial of its request to institute or join a legal action against a state or federal agency by a two-thirds vote of the members of the board, commission, examining committee, or other agency, which vote shall include the vote of at least one public member of that board, commission, examining committee, or other agency.

HISTORY:

Added Stats 1990 ch 285 § 1 (AB 2984). Amended Stats 2019 ch 351 § 33 (AB 496), effective January 1, 2020.

§ 134. Proration of license fees

When the term of any license issued by any agency in the department exceeds one year, initial license fees for licenses which are issued during a current license term shall be prorated on a yearly basis.

HISTORY:

Added Stats 1974 ch 743 § 1. Amended Stats 1978 ch 1161 § 6.

§ 135. Reexamination of applicants

No agency in the department shall, on the basis of an applicant's failure to successfully complete prior examinations, impose any additional limitations, restrictions, prerequisites, or requirements on any applicant who wishes to participate in subsequent examinations except that any examining agency which allows an applicant conditional credit for successfully completing a divisible part of an examination may require that an applicant be reexamined in those parts successfully completed if such applicant has not successfully completed all parts of the examination within a required period of time established by the examining agency. Nothing in this section, however, requires the exemption of such applicant from the regular fees and requirements normally associated with examinations.

HISTORY:
Added Stats 1974 ch 743 § 2.

§ 135.4. Refugees, asylees, and special immigrant visa holders; professional licensing; initial licensure process

(a) Notwithstanding any other law, a board within the department shall expedite, and may assist, the initial licensure process for an applicant who supplies satisfactory evidence to the board that they have been admitted to the United States as a refugee under Section 1157 of Title 8 of the United States Code, have been granted asylum by the Secretary of Homeland Security or the Attorney General of the United States pursuant to Section 1158 of Title 8 of the United States Code, or they have a special immigrant visa (SIV) that has been granted a status under Section 1244 of Public Law 110-181, under Public Law 109-163, or under Section 602(b) of Title VI of Division F of Public Law 111-8.

(b) Nothing in this section shall be construed as changing existing licensure requirements. A person applying for expedited licensure under subdivision (a) shall meet all applicable statutory and regulatory licensure requirements.

(c) A board may adopt regulations necessary to administer this section.

HISTORY:
Added Stats 2020 ch 186 § 1 (AB 2113), effective January 1, 2021.

§ 135.5. Licensure and citizenship or immigration status

(a) The Legislature finds and declares that it is in the best interests of the State of California to provide persons who are not lawfully present in the United States with the state benefits provided by all licensing acts of entities within the department, and therefore enacts this section pursuant to subsection (d) of Section 1621 of Title 8 of the United States Code.

(b) Notwithstanding subdivision (a) of Section 30, and except as required by subdivision (e) of Section 7583.23, no entity within the department shall deny licensure to an applicant based on his or her citizenship status or immigration status.

(c) Every board within the department shall implement all required regulatory or procedural changes necessary to implement this section no later than January 1, 2016. A board may implement the provisions of this section at any time prior to January 1, 2016.

HISTORY:
Added Stats 2014 ch 752 § 2 (SB 1159), effective January 1, 2015.

§ 136. Notification of change of address; Punishment for failure to comply

(a) Each person holding a license, certificate, registration, permit, or other authority to engage in a profession or occupation issued by a board within the department shall notify the issuing board at its principal office of any change in the person's mailing address within 30 days after the change, unless the board has specified by regulations a shorter time period.

(b) Except as otherwise provided by law, failure of a licensee to comply with the requirement in subdivision (a) constitutes grounds for the issuance of a citation and administrative fine, if the board has the authority to issue citations and administrative fines.

HISTORY:

Added Stats 1994 ch 26 § 7 (AB 1807), effective March 30, 1994. Amended Stats 2019 ch 351 § 34 (AB 496), effective January 1, 2020.

§ 137. Regulations requiring inclusion of license numbers in advertising, etc.

Any agency within the department may promulgate regulations requiring licensees to include their license numbers in any advertising, soliciting, or other presentments to the public.

However, nothing in this section shall be construed to authorize regulation of any person not a licensee who engages in advertising, solicitation, or who makes any other presentment to the public on behalf of a licensee. Such a person shall incur no liability pursuant to this section for communicating in any advertising, soliciting, or other presentment to the public a licensee's license number exactly as provided by the licensee or for failure to communicate such number if none is provided by the licensee.

HISTORY:

Added Stats 1974 ch 743 § 3. Amended Stats 2019 ch 351 § 35 (AB 496), effective January 1, 2020.

§ 138. Notice that practitioner is licensed; Evaluation of licensing examination

Every board in the department, as defined in Section 22, shall initiate the process of adopting regulations on or before June 30, 1999, to require its licensees, as defined in Section 23.8, to provide notice to their clients or customers that the practitioner is licensed by this state. A board shall be exempt from the requirement to adopt regulations pursuant to this section if the board has in place, in statute or regulation, a requirement that provides for consumer notice of a practitioner's status as a licensee of this state.

HISTORY:

Added Stats 1998 ch 879 § 1 (SB 2238). Amended Stats 1999 ch 67 § 1 (AB 1105), effective July 6, 1999; Stats 2019 ch 351 § 36 (AB 496), effective January 1, 2020.

§ 139. Policy for examination development and validation, and occupational analysis

(a) The Legislature finds and declares that occupational analyses and examination validation studies are fundamental components of licensure programs. It is the intent of the Legislature that the policy developed by the department pursuant to subdivision (b) be used by the fiscal, policy, and sunset review committees of the Legislature in their annual reviews of these boards, programs, and bureaus.

(b) Notwithstanding any other provision of law, the department shall develop, in consultation with the boards, programs, bureaus, and divisions under its jurisdiction, and the Osteopathic Medical Board of California and the State Board of Chiropractic Examiners, a policy regarding examination development and validation, and occupational analysis. The department shall finalize and distribute this policy by September 30, 1999, to each of the boards, programs, bureaus, and divisions under its jurisdiction and to the Osteopathic Medical Board of California and the State Board of Chiropractic Examiners. This policy shall be submitted in draft form at least 30 days prior to that date to the appropriate fiscal, policy, and sunset review committees of the Legislature for review. This policy shall address, but shall not be limited to, the following issues:

(1) An appropriate schedule for examination validation and occupational analyses, and circumstances under which more frequent reviews are appropriate.

(2) Minimum requirements for psychometrically sound examination validation, examination development, and occupational analyses, including standards for sufficient number of test items.

(3) Standards for review of state and national examinations.

(4) Setting of passing standards.

(5) Appropriate funding sources for examination validations and occupational analyses.

(6) Conditions under which boards, programs, and bureaus should use internal and external entities to conduct these reviews.

(7) Standards for determining appropriate costs of reviews of different types of examinations, measured in terms of hours required.

(8) Conditions under which it is appropriate to fund permanent and limited term positions within a board, program, or bureau to manage these reviews.

(c) Every regulatory board and bureau, as defined in Section 22, and every program and bureau administered by the department, the Osteopathic Medical Board of California, and the State Board of Chiropractic Examiners, shall submit to the director on or before December 1, 1999, and on or before December 1 of each subsequent year, its method for ensuring that every licensing examination administered by or pursuant to contract with the board is subject to periodic evaluation. The evaluation shall include (1) a description of the occupational analysis serving as the basis for the examination; (2) sufficient item analysis data to permit a psychometric evaluation of the items; (3) an assessment of the appropriateness of prerequisites for admittance to the examination; and (4) an estimate of the costs and personnel required to perform these functions. The evaluation shall be revised and a new evaluation submitted to the director whenever, in the judgment of the board, program, or bureau, there is a substantial change in the examination or the prerequisites for admittance to the examination.

(d) The evaluation may be conducted by the board, program, or bureau, the Office of Professional Examination Services of the department, the Osteopathic Medical Board of California, or the State Board of Chiropractic Examiners or pursuant to a contract with a qualified private testing firm. A board, program, or bureau that provides for development or administration of a licensing examination pursuant to contract with a public or private entity may rely on an occupational analysis or item analysis conducted by that entity. The department shall compile this information, along with a schedule specifying when examination validations and occupational analyses shall be performed, and submit it to the appropriate fiscal, policy, and sunset review committees of the Legislature by September 30 of each year. It is the intent of the Legislature that the method specified in this report be consistent with the policy developed by the department pursuant to subdivision (b).

HISTORY:

Added Stats 1999 ch 67 § 2 (AB 1105), effective July 6, 1999. Amended Stats 2009 ch 307 § 1 (SB 821), effective January 1, 2010.

§ 139.5. Quarterly internet website posting requirements

Beginning July 1, 2021, each board, as defined in Section 22, within the department that issues a license shall do both of the following on at least a quarterly basis:

(a) Prominently display on its internet website one of the following:

(1) The current average timeframes for processing initial and renewal license applications.

(2) The combined current average timeframe for processing both initial and renewal license applications.

(b) Prominently display on its internet website one of the following:

(1) The current average timeframes for processing each license type that the board administers.

(2) The combined current average timeframe for processing all license types that the board administers.

HISTORY:

Added Stats 2020 ch 131 § 1 (SB 878), effective January 1, 2021.

§ 140. Disciplinary action; Licensee's failure to record cash transactions in payment of employee wages

Any board, as defined in Section 22, which is authorized under this code to take disciplinary action against a person who holds a license may take disciplinary action upon the ground that the licensee has failed to record and preserve for not less than three years, any and all cash transactions involved in the payment of employee wages by a licensee. Failure to make these records available to an authorized representative of the board may be made grounds for disciplinary action. In any action brought and sustained by the board which involves a violation of this section and any regulation adopted thereto, the board may assess the licensee with the actual investigative costs incurred, not to exceed two thousand five hundred dollars ($2,500). Failure to pay those costs may result in revocation of the license. Any moneys collected pursuant to this section shall be deposited in the respective fund of the board.

HISTORY:

Added Stats 1984 ch 1490 § 2, effective September 27, 1984.

§ 141. Disciplinary action by foreign jurisdiction; Grounds for disciplinary action by state licensing board

(a) For any licensee holding a license issued by a board under the jurisdiction of the department, a disciplinary action taken by another state, by any agency of the federal government, or by another country for any act substantially related to the practice regulated by the California license, may be a ground for disciplinary action by the respective state licensing board. A certified copy of the record of the disciplinary action taken against the licensee by another state, an agency of the federal government, or another country shall be conclusive evidence of the events related therein.

(b) Nothing in this section shall preclude a board from applying a specific statutory provision in the licensing act administered by that board that provides for discipline based upon a disciplinary action taken against the licensee by another state, an agency of the federal government, or another country.

HISTORY:

Added Stats 1994 ch 1275 § 2 (SB 2101).

§ 142. Authority to synchronize renewal dates of licenses; Abandonment date for application; Delinquency fee

This section shall apply to the bureaus and programs under the direct authority of the director, and to any board that, with the prior approval of the director, elects to have the department administer one or more of the licensing services set forth in this section.

(a) Notwithstanding any other provision of law, each bureau and program may synchronize the renewal dates of licenses granted to applicants with more than one license issued by the bureau or program. To the extent practicable, fees shall be prorated or adjusted so that no applicant shall be required to pay a greater or lesser fee than he or she would have been required to pay if the change in renewal dates had not occurred.

(b) Notwithstanding any other provision of law, the abandonment date for an application that has been returned to the applicant as incomplete shall be 12 months from the date of returning the application.

(c) Notwithstanding any other provision of law, a delinquency, penalty, or late fee shall be assessed if the renewal fee is not postmarked by the renewal expiration date.

HISTORY:

Added Stats 1998 ch 970 § 2 (AB 2802).

§ 143. Proof of license as condition of bringing action for collection of compensation

(a) No person engaged in any business or profession for which a license is required under this code governing the department or any board, bureau, commission, committee, or program within the department, may bring or maintain any action, or recover in law or equity in any action, in any court of this state for the collection of compensation for the performance of any act or contract for which a license is required without alleging and proving that he or she was duly licensed at all times during the performance of that act or contract, regardless of the merits of the cause of action brought by the person.

(b) The judicial doctrine of substantial compliance shall not apply to this section.

(c) This section shall not apply to an act or contract that is considered to qualify as lawful practice of a licensed occupation or profession pursuant to Section 121.

HISTORY:

Added Stats 1990 ch 1207 § 1.5 (AB 3242).

§ 143.5. Provision in agreements to settle certain causes of action prohibited; Adoption of regulations; Exemptions

(a) No licensee who is regulated by a board, bureau, or program within the Department of Consumer Affairs, nor an entity or person acting as an authorized agent of a licensee, shall include or permit to be included a provision in an agreement to settle a civil dispute, whether the agreement is made before or after the commencement of a civil action, that prohibits the other party in that dispute from contacting, filing a complaint with, or cooperating with the department, board, bureau, or program within the Department of Consumer Affairs that regulates the licensee or that requires the other party to withdraw a complaint from the department, board, bureau, or program within the Department of Consumer Affairs that regulates the licensee. A provision of that nature is void as against public policy, and any licensee who includes or permits to be included a provision of that nature in a settlement agreement is subject to disciplinary action by the board, bureau, or program.

(b) Any board, bureau, or program within the Department of Consumer Affairs that takes disciplinary action against a licensee or licensees based on a complaint or report that has also been the subject of a civil action and that has been settled for monetary damages providing for full and final satisfaction of the parties may not require its licensee or licensees to pay any additional sums to the benefit of any plaintiff in the civil action.

(c) As used in this section, "board" shall have the same meaning as defined in Section 22, and "licensee" means a person who has been granted a license, as that term is defined in Section 23.7.

(d) Notwithstanding any other law, upon granting a petition filed by a licensee or authorized agent of a licensee pursuant to Section 11340.6 of the Government Code, a board, bureau, or program within the Department of Consumer Affairs may, based upon evidence and legal authorities cited in the petition, adopt a regulation that does both of the following:

(1) Identifies a code section or jury instruction in a civil cause of action that has no relevance to the board's, bureau's, or program's enforcement responsibilities such that an agreement to settle such a cause of action based on that code section or jury instruction otherwise prohibited under subdivision (a) will not impair the board's, bureau's, or program's duty to protect the public.

(2) Exempts agreements to settle such a cause of action from the requirements of subdivision (a).

(e) This section shall not apply to a licensee subject to Section 2220.7.

HISTORY:

Added Stats 2012 ch 561 § 1 (AB 2570), effective January 1, 2013.

§ 144. Requirement of fingerprints for criminal record checks; Applicability

(a) Notwithstanding any other law, an agency designated in subdivision (b) shall require an applicant to furnish to the agency a full set of fingerprints for purposes of conducting criminal history record checks. Any agency designated in subdivision (b) may obtain and receive, at its discretion, criminal history information from the Department of Justice and the United States Federal Bureau of Investigation.

(b) Subdivision (a) applies to the following:

(1) California Board of Accountancy.

(2) State Athletic Commission.

(3) Board of Behavioral Sciences.

(4) Court Reporters Board of California.

(5) Dental Board of California.

(6) California State Board of Pharmacy.

(7) Board of Registered Nursing.

(8) Veterinary Medical Board.

(9) Board of Vocational Nursing and Psychiatric Technicians of the State of California.

(10) Respiratory Care Board of California.

(11) Physical Therapy Board of California.

(12) Physician Assistant Board.

(13) Speech-Language Pathology and Audiology and Hearing Aid Dispensers Board.

(14) Medical Board of California.

(15) California State Board of Optometry.

(16) Acupuncture Board.

(17) Cemetery and Funeral Bureau.

(18) Bureau of Security and Investigative Services.

(19) Division of Investigation.

(20) Board of Psychology.

(21) California Board of Occupational Therapy.

(22) Structural Pest Control Board.

(23) Contractors State License Board.

(24) Naturopathic Medicine Committee.

(25) Professional Fiduciaries Bureau.

(26) Board for Professional Engineers, Land Surveyors, and Geologists.

(27) Podiatric Medical Board of California.

(28) Osteopathic Medical Board of California.

(29) California Architects Board, beginning January 1, 2021.

(30) Landscape Architects Technical Committee, beginning January 1, 2022.

(31) Bureau of Household Goods and Services with respect to household movers as described in Chapter 3.1 (commencing with Section 19225) of Division 8.

(c) For purposes of paragraph (26) of subdivision (b), the term "applicant" shall be limited to an initial applicant who has never been registered or licensed by the board or to an applicant for a new licensure or registration category.

HISTORY:

Added Stats 1997 ch 758 § 2 (SB 1346). Amended Stats 2000 ch 697 § 1.2 (SB 1046), operative January 1, 2001; Stats 2001 ch 159 § 4 (SB 662), Stats 2001 ch 687 § 2 (AB 1409) (ch 687 prevails); Stats 2002 ch 744 § 1 (SB 1953), Stats 2002 ch 825 § 1 (SB 1952); Stats 2003 ch 485 § 2 (SB 907), Stats 2003 ch 789 § 1 (SB 364), Stats 2003 ch 874 § 1 (SB 363); Stats 2004 ch 909 § 1.2 (SB 136), effective September 30, 2004; Stats 2009 ch 308 § 4 (SB 819), effective January 1, 2010; Stats 2011 ch 448 § 1 (SB 543), effective January 1, 2012; Stats 2015 ch 719 § 1 (SB 643), effective January 1, 2016; Stats

2016 ch 32 § 3 (SB 837), effective June 27, 2016; Stats 2017 ch 775 § 3 (SB 798), effective January 1, 2018; Stats 2018 ch 6 § 1 (AB 106), effective March 13, 2018; Stats 2019 ch 351 § 37 (AB 496), effective January 1, 2020; Stats 2019 ch 376 § 1 (SB 608), effective January 1, 2020; Stats 2019 ch 865 § 1.3 (AB 1519), effective January 1, 2020 (ch 865 prevails); Stats 2020 ch 312 § 5 (SB 1474), effective January 1, 2021; Stats 2021 ch 70 § 3 (AB 141), effective July 12, 2021; Stats 2021 ch 188 § 2 (SB 826), effective January 1, 2022; Stats 2021 ch 630 § 4.5 (AB 1534), effective January 1, 2022 (ch 630 prevails).

§ 144.5. Board authority

Notwithstanding any other law, a board described in Section 144 may request, and is authorized to receive, from a local or state agency certified records of all arrests and convictions, certified records regarding probation, and any and all other related documentation needed to complete an applicant or licensee investigation. A local or state agency may provide those records to the board upon request.

HISTORY:
Added Stats 2013 ch 516 § 1 (SB 305), effective January 1, 2014.

CHAPTER 1.5

UNLICENSED ACTIVITY ENFORCEMENT

Section
145. Legislative findings and declarations.
146. Violations of specified authorization statutes as infractions; Punishment.
147. Authority to issue written notice to appear in court.
148. Establishment of administrative citation system.
149. Notice to cease advertising in telephone directory; Contest and hearing; Disconnection of service.

HISTORY: Added Stats 1992 ch 1135 § 2.

§ 145. Legislative findings and declarations

The Legislature finds and declares that:

(a) Unlicensed activity in the professions and vocations regulated by the Department of Consumer Affairs is a threat to the health, welfare, and safety of the people of the State of California.

(b) The law enforcement agencies of the state should have sufficient, effective, and responsible means available to enforce the licensing laws of the state.

(c) The criminal sanction for unlicensed activity should be swift, effective, appropriate, and create a strong incentive to obtain a license.

HISTORY:
Added Stats 1992 ch 1135 § 2 (SB 2044).

§ 146. Violations of specified authorization statutes as infractions; Punishment

(a) Notwithstanding any other provision of law, a violation of any code section listed in subdivision (c) is an infraction subject to the procedures described in Sections 19.6 and 19.7 of the Penal Code when either of the following applies:

(1) A complaint or a written notice to appear in court pursuant to Chapter 5C (commencing with Section 853.5) of Title 3 of Part 2 of the Penal Code is filed in court charging the offense as an infraction unless the defendant, at the time he or she is arraigned, after being advised of his or her rights, elects to have the case proceed as a misdemeanor.

(2) The court, with the consent of the defendant and the prosecution, determines that the offense is an infraction in which event the case shall proceed as if the defendant has been arraigned on an infraction complaint.

(b) Subdivision (a) does not apply to a violation of the code sections listed in subdivision (c) if the defendant has had his or her license, registration, or certificate previously revoked or suspended.

(c) The following sections require registration, licensure, certification, or other authorization in order to engage in certain businesses or professions regulated by this code:

(1) Section 2474.
(2) Sections 2052 and 2054.
(3) Section 2570.3.
(4) Section 2630.
(5) Section 2903.
(6) Section 3575.
(7) Section 3660.
(8) Sections 3760 and 3761.
(9) Section 4080.
(10) Section 4825.
(11) Section 4935.
(12) Section 4980.
(13) Section 4989.50.
(14) Section 4996.
(15) Section 4999.30.
(16) Section 5536.
(17) Section 6704.
(18) Section 6980.10.
(19) Section 7317.
(20) Section 7502 or 7592.
(21) Section 7520.
(22) Section 7617 or 7641.
(23) Subdivision (a) of Section 7872.
(24) Section 8016.
(25) Section 8505.
(26) Section 8725.
(27) Section 9681.
(28) Section 9840.
(29) Subdivision (c) of Section 9891.24.
(30) Section 19049.

(d) Notwithstanding any other law, a violation of any of the sections listed in subdivision (c), which is an infraction, is punishable by a fine of not less than two hundred fifty dollars ($250) and not more than one thousand dollars

($1,000). No portion of the minimum fine may be suspended by the court unless as a condition of that suspension the defendant is required to submit proof of a current valid license, registration, or certificate for the profession or vocation that was the basis for his or her conviction.

HISTORY:

Added Stats 1992 ch 1135 § 2 (SB 2044). Amended Stats 1993 ch 1264 § 2 (SB 574), ch 1267 § 2.5 (SB 916); Stats 1994 ch 26 § 8 (AB 1807), effective March 30, 1994; Stats 1997 ch 78 § 2 (AB 71); Stats 2001 ch 357 § 1 (AB 1560); Stats 2003 ch 485 § 3 (SB 907); Stats 2009 ch 308 § 5 (SB 819), effective January 1, 2010, Stats 2009 ch 310 § 3.5 (AB 48), effective January 1, 2010; Stats 2015 ch 426 § 2 (SB 800), effective January 1, 2016; Stats 2017 ch 454 § 1 (AB 1706), effective January 1, 2018; Stats 2017 ch 775 § 4.5 (SB 798), effective January 1, 2018 (ch 775 prevails).

§ 147. Authority to issue written notice to appear in court

(a) Any employee designated by the director shall have the authority to issue a written notice to appear in court pursuant to Chapter 5c (commencing with Section 853.5) of Title 3 of Part 2 of the Penal Code. Employees so designated are not peace officers and are not entitled to safety member retirement benefits, as a result of such designation. The employee's authority is limited to the issuance of written notices to appear for infraction violations of provisions of this code and only when the violation is committed in the presence of the employee.

(b) There shall be no civil liability on the part of, and no cause of action shall arise against, any person, acting pursuant to subdivision (a) and within the scope of his or her authority, for false arrest or false imprisonment arising out of any arrest which is lawful or which the person, at the time of such arrest, had reasonable cause to believe was lawful.

HISTORY:

Added Stats 1992 ch 1135 § 2 (SB 2044).

§ 148. Establishment of administrative citation system

Any board, bureau, or commission within the department may, in addition to the administrative citation system authorized by Section 125.9, also establish, by regulation, a similar system for the issuance of an administrative citation to an unlicensed person who is acting in the capacity of a licensee or registrant under the jurisdiction of that board, bureau, or commission. The administrative citation system authorized by this section shall meet the requirements of Section 125.9 and may not be applied to an unlicensed person who is otherwise exempted from the provisions of the applicable licensing act. The establishment of an administrative citation system for unlicensed activity does not preclude the use of other enforcement statutes for unlicensed activities at the discretion of the board, bureau, or commission.

HISTORY:

Added Stats 1992 ch 1135 § 2 (SB 2044).

§ 149. Notice to cease advertising in telephone directory; Contest and hearing; Disconnection of service

(a) If, upon investigation, an agency designated in Section 101 has probable cause to believe that a person is advertising with respect to the offering or performance of services, without being properly licensed by or registered with the agency to offer or perform those services, the agency may issue a citation under Section 148 containing an order of correction that requires the violator to do both of the following:

(1) Cease the unlawful advertising.

(2) Notify the telephone company furnishing services to the violator to disconnect the telephone service furnished to any telephone number contained in the unlawful advertising.

(b) This action is stayed if the person to whom a citation is issued under subdivision (a) notifies the agency in writing that he or she intends to contest the citation. The agency shall afford an opportunity for a hearing, as specified in Section 125.9.

(c) If the person to whom a citation and order of correction is issued under subdivision (a) fails to comply with the order of correction after that order is final, the agency shall inform the Public Utilities Commission of the violation and the Public Utilities Commission shall require the telephone corporation furnishing services to that person to disconnect the telephone service furnished to any telephone number contained in the unlawful advertising.

(d) The good faith compliance by a telephone corporation with an order of the Public Utilities Commission to terminate service issued pursuant to this section shall constitute a complete defense to any civil or criminal action brought against the telephone corporation arising from the termination of service.

HISTORY:

Added Stats 1992 ch 1135 § 2 (SB 2044). Amended Stats 1993 ch 1263 § 3 (AB 936); Stats 1994 ch 26 § 9 (AB 1807), effective March 30, 1994, ch 1274 § 1.5 (SB 2039); Stats 1995 ch 60 § 4 (SB 42), effective July 6, 1995; Stats 1998 ch 59 § 5 (AB 969); Stats 2000 ch 1054 § 3 (SB 1863), ch 1055 § 2 (AB 2889), effective September 30, 2000, ch 1055 § 2.5 (AB 2889), effective September 30, 2000; Stats 2003 ch 485 § 4 (SB 907); Stats 2009–2010 4th Ex Sess ch 18 § 3 (ABX4 20), effective October 23, 2009; Stats 2009 ch 308 § 6 (SB 819), effective January 1, 2010, ch 309 § 2 (AB 1535), effective January 1, 2010, ch 310 § 4.7 (AB 48), effective January 1, 2010. See this section as modified in Governor's Reorganization Plan No. 2 § 4 of 2012; Amended Stats 2013 ch 352 § 5 (AB 1317), effective September 26, 2013, operative July 1, 2013, ch 436 § 1 (SB 269), effective January 1, 2014; Stats 2014 ch 395 § 2 (SB 1243), effective January 1, 2015.

CHAPTER 2

THE DIRECTOR OF CONSUMER AFFAIRS

Section

150. Designation.
151. Appointment and tenure; Salary and traveling expenses.
152. Departmental organization.
152.5. Extension of renewal dates.
152.6. Establishment of license periods and renewal dates.
153. Investigations.
154. Matters relating to employees of boards.
154.5. Legal assistance for experts aiding in investigations of licensees.
155. Employment of investigators; Inspectors as employees or under contract.
156.1. Retention of records by providers of services related to treatment of alcohol or drug impairment.
156.5. Leases for examination or meeting purposes.
157. Expenses in criminal prosecutions and unprofessional conduct proceedings.

Section
158. Refunds to applicants.
159. Administration of oaths.
159.5. Division of Investigation; Appointments; Health Quality Investigation Unit.
160. Division of Investigation of the department and Dental Board of California.
161. Availability of public records at charge sufficient to pay costs.
162. Evidentiary effect of certificate of records officer as to license, etc.
163. Fee for certification of records, etc.
164. Form and content of license, certificate, permit, or similar indicia of authority.
165. Prohibition against submission of fiscal impact analysis relating to pending legislation without prior submission to director for comment.
166. Development of guidelines for mandatory continuing education programs.

HISTORY: Enacted Stats 1937 ch 399. The heading of Chapter 2, amended to read as above by Stats 1973 ch 77 § 2.

§ 150. Designation

The department is under the control of a civil executive officer who is known as the Director of Consumer Affairs.

HISTORY:
Enacted Stats 1937. Amended Stats 1971 ch 716 § 9.

§ 151. Appointment and tenure; Salary and traveling expenses

The director is appointed by the Governor and holds office at the Governor's pleasure. The director shall receive the annual salary provided for by Chapter 6 (commencing with Section 11550) of Part 1 of Division 3 of Title 2 of the Government Code, and the director's necessary traveling expenses.

HISTORY:
Enacted Stats 1937. Amended Stats 1943 ch 1029 § 1; Stats 1945 ch 1185 § 2; Stats 1947 ch 1442 § 1; Stats 1951 ch 1613 § 14; Stats 1984 ch 144 § 2, ch 268 § 0.1, effective June 30, 1984; Stats 1985 ch 106 § 1; Stats 2019 ch 351 § 38 (AB 496), effective January 1, 2020.

§ 152. Departmental organization

For the purpose of administration, the reregistration and clerical work of the department is organized by the director, subject to the approval of the Governor, in such manner as the director deems necessary to properly segregate and conduct the work of the department.

HISTORY:
Enacted Stats 1937. Amended Stats 2019 ch 351 § 39 (AB 496), effective January 1, 2020; Stats 2020 ch 370 § 2 (SB 1371), effective January 1, 2021.

§ 152.5. Extension of renewal dates

For purposes of distributing the reregistration work of the department uniformly throughout the year as nearly as practicable, the boards in the department may, with the approval of the director, extend by not more than six months the date fixed by law for the renewal of any license, certificate or permit issued by them, except that in such event any renewal fee which may be involved shall be prorated in such manner that no person shall be required to pay a greater or lesser fee than would have been required had the change in renewal dates not occurred.

HISTORY:
Added Stats 1959 ch 1707 § 1.

§ 152.6. Establishment of license periods and renewal dates

Notwithstanding any other provision of this code, each board within the department shall, in cooperation with the director, establish such license periods and renewal dates for all licenses in such manner as best to distribute the renewal work of all boards throughout each year and permit the most efficient, and economical use of personnel and equipment. To the extent practicable, provision shall be made for the proration or other adjustment of fees in such manner that no person shall be required to pay a greater or lesser fee than the person would have been required to pay if the change in license periods or renewal dates had not occurred.

As used in this section "license" includes "certificate," "permit," "authority," "registration," and similar indicia of authority to engage in a business or profession, and "board" includes "board," "bureau," "commission," "committee," and an individual who is authorized to renew a license.

HISTORY:
Added Stats 1968 ch 1248 § 1. Amended Stats 2019 ch 351 § 40 (AB 496), effective January 1, 2020.

§ 153. Investigations

The director may investigate the work of the boards in the department and may obtain a copy of all records and full and complete data in all official matters in possession of the boards and their members, officers, or employees, other than examination questions prior to submission to applicants at scheduled examinations.

HISTORY:
Enacted Stats 1937. Amended Stats 2019 ch 351 § 41 (AB 496), effective January 1, 2020.

§ 154. Matters relating to employees of boards

Any and all matters relating to employment, tenure or discipline of employees of any board, agency or commission, shall be initiated by said board, agency or commission, but all such actions shall, before reference to the State Personnel Board, receive the approval of the appointing power.

To effect the purposes of Division 1 of this code and each agency of the department, employment of all personnel shall be in accord with Article XXIV of the Constitution, the law and rules and regulations of the State Personnel Board. Each board, agency or commission, shall select its employees from a list of eligibles obtained by the appointing power from the State Personnel Board. The person selected by the board, agency or commission to fill any position or vacancy shall thereafter be reported by the board, agency or commission, to the appointing power.

HISTORY:
Enacted Stats 1937. Amended Stats 1945 ch 1276 § 4.

§ 154.5. Legal assistance for experts aiding in investigations of licensees

If a person, not a regular employee of a board under this code, including the Board of Chiropractic Examiners and the Osteopathic Medical Board of

California, is hired or under contract to provide expertise to the board in the evaluation of an applicant or the conduct of a licensee, and that person is named as a defendant in a civil action arising out of the evaluation or any opinions rendered, statements made, or testimony given to the board or its representatives, the board shall provide for representation required to defend the defendant in that civil action. The board shall not be liable for any judgment rendered against the person. The Attorney General shall be utilized in the action and his or her services shall be a charge against the board.

HISTORY:

Added Stats 1986 ch 1205 § 1, as B & P C § 483. Amended and renumbered by Stats 1987 ch 850 § 8; Amended Stats 1991 ch 359 § 3 (AB 1332).

§ 155. Employment of investigators; Inspectors as employees or under contract

(a) In accordance with Section 159.5, the director may employ such investigators, inspectors, and deputies as are necessary properly to investigate and prosecute all violations of any law, the enforcement of which is charged to the department or to any board, agency, or commission in the department.

(b) It is the intent of the Legislature that inspectors used by boards, bureaus, or commissions in the department shall not be required to be employees of the Division of Investigation, but may either be employees of, or under contract to, the boards, bureaus, or commissions. Contracts for services shall be consistent with Article 4.5 (commencing with Section 19130) of Chapter 6 of Part 2 of Division 5 of Title 2 of the Government Code. All civil service employees currently employed as inspectors whose functions are transferred as a result of this section shall retain their positions, status, and rights in accordance with Section 19994.10 of the Government Code and the State Civil Service Act (Part 2 (commencing with Section 18500) of Division 5 of Title 2 of the Government Code).

(c) Nothing in this section limits the authority of, or prohibits, investigators in the Division of Investigation in the conduct of inspections or investigations of any licensee, or in the conduct of investigations of any officer or employee of a board or the department at the specific request of the director or his or her designee.

HISTORY:

Enacted Stats 1937. Amended Stats 1945 ch 1276 § 5; Stats 1971 ch 716 § 10; Stats 1985 ch 1382 § 1.

§ 156.1. Retention of records by providers of services related to treatment of alcohol or drug impairment

(a) Notwithstanding any other law, individuals or entities contracting with the department or any board within the department for the provision of services relating to the treatment and rehabilitation of licensees impaired by alcohol or dangerous drugs shall retain all records and documents pertaining to those services until such time as these records and documents have been reviewed for audit by the department. These records and documents shall be retained for three years from the date of the last treatment or service rendered to that licensee, after which time the records and documents may be purged and destroyed by the contract vendor. This provision shall supersede any other law relating to the purging or destruction of records pertaining to those treatment and rehabilitation programs.

(b) Unless otherwise expressly provided by statute or regulation, all records and documents pertaining to services for the treatment and rehabilitation of licensees impaired by alcohol or dangerous drugs provided by any contract vendor to the department or to any board within the department shall be kept confidential and are not subject to discovery or subpoena.

(c) With respect to all other contracts for services with the department, or any board within the department other than those set forth in subdivision (a), the director or chief deputy director may request an examination and audit by the department's internal auditor of all performance under the contract. For this purpose, all documents and records of the contract vendor in connection with such performance shall be retained by the vendor for a period of three years after final payment under the contract. Nothing in this section shall affect the authority of the State Auditor to conduct any examination or audit under the terms of Section 8546.7 of the Government Code.

HISTORY:

Added Stats 1991 ch 654 § 3 (AB 1893). Amended Stats 2003 ch 107 § 1 (AB 569); Stats 2010 ch 517 § 1 (SB 1172), effective January 1, 2011; Stats 2019 ch 351 § 42 (AB 496), effective January 1, 2020.

§ 156.5. Leases for examination or meeting purposes

The director may negotiate and execute for the department and for its component agencies, rental agreements for short-term hiring of space and furnishings for examination or meeting purposes. The director may, in his or her discretion, negotiate and execute contracts for that space which include provisions which hold harmless the provider of the space where liability resulting from use of the space under the contract is traceable to the state or its officers, agents, or employees. Notwithstanding any other provision of law, the director may, in his or her discretion, advance payments as deposits to reserve and hold examination or meeting space. Any such agreement is subject to the approval of the legal office of the Department of General Services.

HISTORY:

Added Stats 1967 ch 1235 § 1. Amended Stats 1988 ch 1448 § 1.5.

§ 157. Expenses in criminal prosecutions and unprofessional conduct proceedings

Expenses incurred by any board or on behalf of any board in any criminal prosecution or unprofessional conduct proceeding constitute proper charges against the funds of the board.

HISTORY:

Added Stats 1937 ch 474.

§ 158. Refunds to applicants

With the approval of the Director of Consumer Affairs, the boards and commissions comprising the department or subject to its jurisdiction may make refunds to applicants who are found ineligible to take the examinations or whose credentials are insufficient to entitle them to certificates or licenses.

Notwithstanding any other law, any application fees, license fees, or penalties imposed and collected illegally, by mistake, inadvertence, or error shall be refunded. Claims authorized by the department shall be filed with the State Controller, and the Controller shall draw a warrant against the fund of the agency in payment of the refund.

HISTORY:
Added Stats 1937 ch 474. Amended Stats 1945 ch 1378 § 1; Stats 1971 ch 716 § 11; Stats 2019 ch 351 § 43 (AB 496), effective January 1, 2020.

§ 159. Administration of oaths

The members and the executive officer of each board, agency, bureau, division, or commission have power to administer oaths and affirmations in the performance of any business of the board, and to certify to official acts.

HISTORY:
Added Stats 1947 ch 1350 § 5.

§ 159.5. Division of Investigation; Appointments; Health Quality Investigation Unit

(a)(1) There is in the department the Division of Investigation. The division is in the charge of a person with the title of chief of the division.

(2) Except as provided in Section 160, investigators who have the authority of peace officers, as specified in subdivision (a) of Section 160 and in subdivision (a) of Section 830.3 of the Penal Code, shall be in the division and shall be appointed by the director.

(b)(1) There is in the Division of Investigation the Health Quality Investigation Unit. The primary responsibility of the unit is to investigate violations of law or regulation within the jurisdiction of the Medical Board of California, the Podiatric Medical Board of California, the Board of Psychology, the Osteopathic Medical Board of California, the Physician Assistant Board, or any entities under the jurisdiction of the Medical Board of California.

(2) The Medical Board of California shall not be charged an hourly rate for the performance of investigations by the unit.

HISTORY:
Added Stats 1971 ch 716 § 12. Amended Stats 1985 ch 1382 § 2; Stats 2010 ch 719 § 2 (SB 856), effective October 19, 2010; Stats 2013 ch 515 § 1 (SB 304), effective January 1, 2014; Stats 2019 ch 351 § 44 (AB 496), effective January 1, 2020.

§ 160. Division of Investigation of the department and Dental Board of California

(a) The chief and all investigators of the Division of Investigation of the department and all investigators of the Dental Board of California have the authority of peace officers while engaged in exercising the powers granted or performing the duties imposed upon them or the division in investigating the laws administered by the various boards comprising the department or commencing directly or indirectly any criminal prosecution arising from any investigation conducted under these laws. All persons herein referred to shall be deemed to be acting within the scope of employment with respect to all acts and matters set forth in this section.

(b) The Division of Investigation of the department and the Dental Board of California may employ individuals, who are not peace officers, to provide investigative services.

(c) This section shall become operative on July 1, 2014.

HISTORY:

Added Stats 2013 ch 515 § 3 (SB 304), effective January 1, 2014, operative July 1, 2014.

§ 161. Availability of public records at charge sufficient to pay costs

The department, or any board in the department, may, in accordance with the California Public Records Act (Division 10 (commencing with Section 7920.000) of Title 1 of the Government Code) and the Information Practices Act of 1977 (Chapter 1 (commencing with Section 1798) of Title 1.8 of Part 4 of Division 3 of the Civil Code), make available to the public copies of any part of its respective public records, or compilations, extracts, or summaries of information contained in its public records, at a charge sufficient to pay the actual cost thereof. That charge shall be determined by the director with the approval of the Department of General Services.

HISTORY:

Added Stats 1949 ch 704 § 1. Amended Stats 1963 ch 590 § 1; Stats 1965 ch 371 § 9; Stats 2019 ch 351 § 45 (AB 496), effective January 1, 2020; Stats 2021 ch 615 § 3 (AB 474), effective January 1, 2022.

§ 162. Evidentiary effect of certificate of records officer as to license, etc.

The certificate of the officer in charge of the records of any board in the department that any person was or was not on a specified date, or during a specified period of time, licensed, certified or registered under the provisions of law administered by the board, or that the license, certificate or registration of any person was revoked or under suspension, shall be admitted in any court as prima facie evidence of the facts therein recited.

HISTORY:

Added Stats 1949 ch 355 § 1.

§ 163. Fee for certification of records, etc.

Except as otherwise expressly provided by law, the department and each board in the department shall charge a fee of two dollars ($2) for the certification of a copy of any record, document, or paper in its custody or for the certification of any document evidencing the content of any such record, document or paper.

HISTORY:

Added Stats 1961 ch 1858 § 1. Amended Stats 1963 ch 590 § 2.

§ 164. Form and content of license, certificate, permit, or similar indicia of authority

The form and content of any license, certificate, permit, or similar indicia of authority issued by any agency in the department, including any document evidencing renewal of a license, certificate, permit, or similar indicia of authority, shall be determined by the director after consultation with and consideration of the views of the agency concerned.

HISTORY:

Added Stats 1971 ch 716 § 15. Amended Stats 1987 ch 850 § 6.

§ 165. Prohibition against submission of fiscal impact analysis relating to pending legislation without prior submission to director for comment

Notwithstanding any other provision of law, no board, bureau, committee, commission, or program in the Department of Consumer Affairs shall submit to the Legislature any fiscal impact analysis relating to legislation pending before the Legislature until the analysis has been submitted to the Director of Consumer Affairs, or his or her designee, for review and comment. The boards, bureaus, committees, commissions, and programs shall include the comments of the director when submitting any fiscal impact analysis to the Legislature. This section shall not be construed to prohibit boards, bureaus, committees, commissions, and programs from responding to direct requests for fiscal data from Members of the Legislature or their staffs. In those instances it shall be the responsibility of boards, bureaus, committees, commissions, and programs to also transmit that information to the director, or his or her designee, within five working days.

HISTORY:

Added Stats 1984 ch 268 § 0.2, effective June 30, 1984.

§ 166. Development of guidelines for mandatory continuing education programs

The director shall, by regulation, develop guidelines to prescribe components for mandatory continuing education programs administered by any board within the department.

(a) The guidelines shall be developed to ensure that mandatory continuing education is used as a means to create a more competent licensing population, thereby enhancing public protection. The guidelines shall require mandatory continuing education programs to address, at least, the following:

(1) Course validity.
(2) Occupational relevancy.
(3) Effective presentation.
(4) Actual attendance.
(5) Material assimilation.
(6) Potential for application.

(b) The director shall consider educational principles, and the guidelines shall prescribe mandatory continuing education program formats to include, but not be limited to, the following:

(1) The specified audience.
(2) Identification of what is to be learned.
(3) Clear goals and objectives.

(4) Relevant learning methods (participatory, hands-on, or clinical setting).

(5) Evaluation, focused on the learner and the assessment of the intended learning outcomes (goals and objectives).

(c) Any board within the department that, after January 1, 1993, proposes a mandatory continuing education program for its licensees shall submit the proposed program to the director for review to assure that the program contains all the elements set forth in this section and complies with the guidelines developed by the director.

(d) Any board administering a mandatory continuing education program that proposes to amend its current program shall do so in a manner consistent with this section.

(e) Any board currently administering a mandatory continuing education program shall review the components and requirements of the program to determine the extent to which they are consistent with the guidelines developed under this section. The board shall submit a report of their findings to the director. The report shall identify the similarities and differences of its mandatory continuing education program. The report shall include any board-specific needs to explain the variation from the director's guidelines.

(f) Any board administering a mandatory continuing education program, when accepting hours for credit which are obtained out of state, shall ensure that the course for which credit is given is administered in accordance with the guidelines addressed in subdivision (a).

(g) Nothing in this section or in the guidelines adopted by the director shall be construed to repeal any requirements for continuing education programs set forth in any other provision of this code.

HISTORY:

Added Stats 1992 ch 1135 § 2.2 (SB 2044). Amended Stats 1994 ch 146 § 1 (AB 3601).

CHAPTER 3
FUNDS OF THE DEPARTMENT

Section
201. Levy for administrative expenses.
205. Professions and Vocations Fund [Repealed].
205. Professions and Vocations Fund.
206. Dishonored check tendered for payment of fine, fee, or penalty.

HISTORY: Enacted Stats 1937 ch 399.

§ 201. Levy for administrative expenses

(a)(1) A charge for the estimated administrative expenses of the department, not to exceed the available balance in any appropriation for any one fiscal year, may be levied in advance on a pro rata share basis against any of the boards, bureaus, commissions, divisions, and agencies, at the discretion of the director and with the approval of the Department of Finance.

(2) The department shall submit a report of the accounting of the pro rata calculation of administrative expenses to the appropriate policy committees of the Legislature on or before July 1, 2015, and on or before July 1 of each subsequent year.

(b) The department shall conduct a one-time study of its current system for prorating administrative expenses to determine if that system is the most productive, efficient, and cost-effective manner for the department and the agencies comprising the department. The study shall include consideration of whether some of the administrative services offered by the department should be outsourced or charged on an as-needed basis and whether the agencies should be permitted to elect not to receive and be charged for certain administrative services. The department shall include the findings in its report pursuant to paragraph (2) of subdivision (a) that it is required to submit on or before July 1, 2015.

HISTORY:

Enacted Stats 1937. Amended Stats 1947 ch 1350 § 4; Stats 1965 ch 371 § 10; Stats 1974 ch 1221 § 1; Stats 2014 ch 395 § 4 (SB 1243), effective January 1, 2015.

§ 205. Professions and Vocations Fund [Repealed]

HISTORY:

Added Stats 2015 ch 510 § 2.3 (AB 179), effective January 1, 2016, operative July 1, 2016. Amended Stats 2016 ch 800 § 1 (SB 1196), effective January 1, 2017; Stats 2017 ch 421 § 6 (SB 19), effective January 1, 2018, operative July 1, 2018; Stats 2017 ch 669 § 3.5 (AB 1705), effective January 1, 2018, operative July 1, 2018 (ch 669 prevails); Stats 2019 ch 865 § 2 (AB 1519), effective January 1, 2020, repealed July 1, 2022; Stats 2020 ch 312 § 7 (SB 1474), effective January 1, 2021, repealed July 1, 2022.

§ 205. Professions and Vocations Fund

(a) There is in the State Treasury the Professions and Vocations Fund. The fund shall consist of the following special funds:

(1) Accountancy Fund.
(2) California Architects Board Fund.
(3) Athletic Commission Fund.
(4) Barbering and Cosmetology Contingent Fund.
(5) Cemetery and Funeral Fund.
(6) Contractors License Fund.
(7) State Dentistry Fund.
(8) Home Furnishings and Thermal Insulation Fund.
(9) California Architects Board-Landscape Architects Fund.
(10) Contingent Fund of the Medical Board of California.
(11) Optometry Fund.
(12) Pharmacy Board Contingent Fund.
(13) Physical Therapy Fund.
(14) Private Security Services Fund.
(15) Professional Engineer's, Land Surveyor's, and Geologist's Fund.
(16) Consumer Affairs Fund.
(17) Behavioral Sciences Fund.
(18) Licensed Midwifery Fund.
(19) Court Reporters' Fund.

(20) Veterinary Medical Board Contingent Fund.
(21) Vocational Nursing and Psychiatric Technicians Fund.
(22) Electronic and Appliance Repair Fund.
(23) Acupuncture Fund.
(24) Physician Assistant Fund.
(25) Board of Podiatric Medicine Fund.
(26) Psychology Fund.
(27) Respiratory Care Fund.
(28) Speech-Language Pathology and Audiology and Hearing Aid Dispensers Fund.
(29) Board of Registered Nursing Fund.
(30) Animal Health Technician Examining Committee Fund.
(31) State Dental Hygiene Fund.
(32) Structural Pest Control Fund.
(33) Structural Pest Control Education and Enforcement Fund.
(34) Structural Pest Control Research Fund.
(35) Household Movers Fund.

(b) For accounting and recordkeeping purposes, the Professions and Vocations Fund shall be deemed to be a single special fund, and each of the several special funds therein shall constitute and be deemed to be a separate account in the Professions and Vocations Fund. Each account or fund shall be available for expenditure only for the purposes as are now or may hereafter be provided by law.

HISTORY:

Added Stats 2019 ch 865 § 3 (AB 1519), effective January 1, 2020, operative July 1, 2022. Amended Stats 2020 ch 121 § 1 (AB 896), effective September 24, 2020, operative July 1, 2022; Stats 2020 ch 312 § 8.5 (SB 1474), effective January 1, 2021, operative July 1, 2022; Stats 2022 ch 511 § 1 (SB 1495), effective January 1, 2023.

§ 206. Dishonored check tendered for payment of fine, fee, or penalty

Notwithstanding any other provision of law, any person tendering a check for payment of a fee, fine, or penalty that was subsequently dishonored, shall not be granted a license, or other authority that they were seeking, until the applicant pays the amount outstanding from the dishonored payment together with the applicable fee, including any delinquency fee. The board may require the person whose check was returned unpaid to make payment of all fees by cashier's check or money order.

HISTORY:

Added Stats 1994 ch 26 § 12 (AB 1807), effective March 30, 1994.

CHAPTER 4

CONSUMER AFFAIRS

Article

3. Powers and Duties.
3.6. Uniform Standards Regarding Substance-Abusing Healing Arts Licensees.
4. Representation of Consumers.

Article
5. Consumer Complaints.

HISTORY: Added Stats 1970 ch 1394 § 3, operative July 1, 1971.

ARTICLE 3
POWERS AND DUTIES

Section
310. Director's powers and duties.
312. Report to Governor and Legislature.
313.1. Compliance with section as requirement for effectiveness of specified rules or regulations; Submission of records; Authority for disapproval.
313.2. Adoption of regulations in conformance with Americans with Disabilities Act.

HISTORY: Added Stats 1970 ch 1394 § 3, operative July 1, 1971.

§ 310. Director's powers and duties

The director shall have the following powers and it shall be his duty to:

(a) Recommend and propose the enactment of such legislation as necessary to protect and promote the interests of consumers.

(b) Represent the consumer's interests before federal and state legislative hearings and executive commissions.

(c) Assist, advise, and cooperate with federal, state, and local agencies and officials to protect and promote the interests of consumers.

(d) Study, investigate, research, and analyze matters affecting the interests of consumers.

(e) Hold public hearings, subpoena witnesses, take testimony, compel the production of books, papers, documents, and other evidence, and call upon other state agencies for information.

(f) Propose and assist in the creation and development of consumer education programs.

(g) Promote ethical standards of conduct for business and consumers and undertake activities to encourage public responsibility in the production, promotion, sale and lease of consumer goods and services.

(h) Advise the Governor and Legislature on all matters affecting the interests of consumers.

(i) Exercise and perform such other functions, powers and duties as may be deemed appropriate to protect and promote the interests of consumers as directed by the Governor or the Legislature.

(j) Maintain contact and liaison with consumer groups in California and nationally.

HISTORY:
Added Stats 1970 ch 1394 § 3, operative July 1, 1971. Amended Stats 1975 ch 1262 § 4.

§ 312. Report to Governor and Legislature

(a) The director shall submit to the Governor and the Legislature on or before January 1, 2003, and annually thereafter, a report of programmatic and statistical information regarding the activities of the department and its constituent entities for the previous fiscal year. The report shall include information concerning the director's activities pursuant to Section 326, including the number and general patterns of consumer complaints and the action taken on those complaints.

(b) The report shall include information relative to the performance of each constituent entity, including, but not limited to, length of time for a constituent entity to reach each of the following milestones in the enforcement process:

(1) Average number of days from when a constituent entity receives a complaint until the constituent entity assigns an investigator to the complaint.

(2) Average number of days from a constituent entity opening an investigation conducted by the constituent entity staff or the Division of Investigation to closing the investigation regardless of outcome.

(3) Average number of days from a constituent entity closing an investigation to imposing formal discipline.

(c) A report submitted pursuant to subdivision (a) shall be submitted in compliance with Section 9795 of the Government Code.

HISTORY:

Added Stats 1970 ch 1394 § 3, operative July 1, 1971. Amended Stats 1975 ch 1262 § 5; Stats 1998 ch 829 § 1 SB 1652; Stats 2002 ch 405 § 3 (AB 2973); Stats 2014 ch 395 § 6 (SB 1243), effective January 1, 2015.

§ 313.1. Compliance with section as requirement for effectiveness of specified rules or regulations; Submission of records; Authority for disapproval

(a) Notwithstanding any other provision of law to the contrary, no rule or regulation, except those relating to examinations and qualifications for licensure, and no fee change proposed or promulgated by any of the boards, commissions, or committees within the department, shall take effect pending compliance with this section.

(b) The director shall be formally notified of and shall be provided a full opportunity to review, in accordance with the requirements of Article 5 (commencing with Section 11346) of Chapter 3.5 of Part 1 of Division 3 of Title 2 of the Government Code, and this section, all of the following:

(1) All notices of proposed action, any modifications and supplements thereto, and the text of proposed regulations.

(2) Any notices of sufficiently related changes to regulations previously noticed to the public, and the text of proposed regulations showing modifications to the text.

(3) Final rulemaking records.

(c) The submission of all notices and final rulemaking records to the director and the completion of the director's review, as authorized by this section, shall be a precondition to the filing of any rule or regulation with the Office of Administrative Law. The Office of Administrative Law shall have no jurisdiction to review a rule or regulation subject to this section until after the completion of the director's review and only then if the director has not disapproved it. The filing of any document with the Office of Administrative

Law shall be accompanied by a certification that the board, commission, or committee has complied with the requirements of this section.

(d) Following the receipt of any final rulemaking record subject to subdivision (a), the director shall have the authority for a period of 30 days to disapprove a proposed rule or regulation on the ground that it is injurious to the public health, safety, or welfare.

(e) Final rulemaking records shall be filed with the director within the one-year notice period specified in Section 11346.4 of the Government Code. If necessary for compliance with this section, the one-year notice period may be extended, as specified by this subdivision.

(1) In the event that the one-year notice period lapses during the director's 30-day review period, or within 60 days following the notice of the director's disapproval, it may be extended for a maximum of 90 days.

(2) If the director approves the final rulemaking record or declines to take action on it within 30 days, the board, commission, or committee shall have five days from the receipt of the record from the director within which to file it with the Office of Administrative Law.

(3) If the director disapproves a rule or regulation, it shall have no force or effect unless, within 60 days of the notice of disapproval, (A) the disapproval is overridden by a unanimous vote of the members of the board, commission, or committee, and (B) the board, commission, or committee files the final rulemaking record with the Office of Administrative Law in compliance with this section and the procedures required by Chapter 3.5 (commencing with Section 11340) of Part 1 of Division 3 of Title 2 of the Government Code.

(f) Nothing in this section shall be construed to prohibit the director from affirmatively approving a proposed rule, regulation, or fee change at any time within the 30-day period after it has been submitted to him or her, in which event it shall become effective upon compliance with this section and the procedures required by Chapter 3.5 (commencing with Section 11340) of Part 1 of Division 3 of Title 2 of the Government Code.

HISTORY:

Added Stats 1972 ch 1251 § 1, as B & P C § 313. Amended and renumbered by Stats 1973 ch 40 § 1, effective May 10, 1973; Amended Stats 1984 ch 144 § 4; Stats 1991 ch 654 § 4 (AB 1893); Stats 1992 ch 1289 § 2 (AB 2743); Stats 1994 ch 26 § 13 (AB 1807), effective March 30, 1994.

§ 313.2. Adoption of regulations in conformance with Americans with Disabilities Act

The director shall adopt regulations to implement, interpret, and make specific the provisions of the Americans with Disabilities Act (P.L. 101–336), as they relate to the examination process for professional licensing and certification programs under the purview of the department.

HISTORY:

Added Stats 1992 ch 1289 § 3 (AB 2743).

ARTICLE 3.6

UNIFORM STANDARDS REGARDING SUBSTANCE-ABUSING HEALING ARTS LICENSEES

Section

315. Establishment of Substance Abuse Coordination Committee; Members; Duties.
315.2. Cease practice order.
315.4. Cease practice order for violation of probation or diversion program.

HISTORY: Added Stats 2008 ch 548 § 3, effective January 1, 2009.

§ 315. Establishment of Substance Abuse Coordination Committee; Members; Duties

(a) For the purpose of determining uniform standards that will be used by healing arts boards in dealing with substance-abusing licensees, there is established in the Department of Consumer Affairs the Substance Abuse Coordination Committee. The committee shall be comprised of the executive officers of the department's healing arts boards established pursuant to Division 2 (commencing with Section 500), the State Board of Chiropractic Examiners, the Osteopathic Medical Board of California, and a designee of the State Department of Health Care Services. The Director of Consumer Affairs shall chair the committee and may invite individuals or stakeholders who have particular expertise in the area of substance abuse to advise the committee.

(b) The committee shall be subject to the Bagley-Keene Open Meeting Act (Article 9 (commencing with Section 11120) of Division 3 of Title 2 of the Government Code).

(c) By January 1, 2010, the committee shall formulate uniform and specific standards in each of the following areas that each healing arts board shall use in dealing with substance-abusing licensees, whether or not a board chooses to have a formal diversion program:

(1) Specific requirements for a clinical diagnostic evaluation of the licensee, including, but not limited to, required qualifications for the providers evaluating the licensee.

(2) Specific requirements for the temporary removal of the licensee from practice, in order to enable the licensee to undergo the clinical diagnostic evaluation described in paragraph (1) and any treatment recommended by the evaluator described in paragraph (1) and approved by the board, and specific criteria that the licensee must meet before being permitted to return to practice on a full-time or part-time basis.

(3) Specific requirements that govern the ability of the licensing board to communicate with the licensee's employer about the licensee's status and condition.

(4) Standards governing all aspects of required testing, including, but not limited to, frequency of testing, randomness, method of notice to the licensee, number of hours between the provision of notice and the test, standards for specimen collectors, procedures used by specimen collectors, the permissible locations of testing, whether the collection process must be observed by the

collector, backup testing requirements when the licensee is on vacation or otherwise unavailable for local testing, requirements for the laboratory that analyzes the specimens, and the required maximum timeframe from the test to the receipt of the result of the test.

(5) Standards governing all aspects of group meeting attendance requirements, including, but not limited to, required qualifications for group meeting facilitators, frequency of required meeting attendance, and methods of documenting and reporting attendance or nonattendance by licensees.

(6) Standards used in determining whether inpatient, outpatient, or other type of treatment is necessary.

(7) Worksite monitoring requirements and standards, including, but not limited to, required qualifications of worksite monitors, required methods of monitoring by worksite monitors, and required reporting by worksite monitors.

(8) Procedures to be followed when a licensee tests positive for a banned substance.

(9) Procedures to be followed when a licensee is confirmed to have ingested a banned substance.

(10) Specific consequences for major violations and minor violations. In particular, the committee shall consider the use of a "deferred prosecution" stipulation similar to the stipulation described in Section 1000 of the Penal Code, in which the licensee admits to self-abuse of drugs or alcohol and surrenders his or her license. That agreement is deferred by the agency unless or until the licensee commits a major violation, in which case it is revived and the license is surrendered.

(11) Criteria that a licensee must meet in order to petition for return to practice on a full-time basis.

(12) Criteria that a licensee must meet in order to petition for reinstatement of a full and unrestricted license.

(13) If a board uses a private-sector vendor that provides diversion services, standards for immediate reporting by the vendor to the board of any and all noncompliance with any term of the diversion contract or probation; standards for the vendor's approval process for providers or contractors that provide diversion services, including, but not limited to, specimen collectors, group meeting facilitators, and worksite monitors; standards requiring the vendor to disapprove and discontinue the use of providers or contractors that fail to provide effective or timely diversion services; and standards for a licensee's termination from the program and referral to enforcement.

(14) If a board uses a private-sector vendor that provides diversion services, the extent to which licensee participation in that program shall be kept confidential from the public.

(15) If a board uses a private-sector vendor that provides diversion services, a schedule for external independent audits of the vendor's performance in adhering to the standards adopted by the committee.

(16) Measurable criteria and standards to determine whether each board's method of dealing with substance-abusing licensees protects patients from harm and is effective in assisting its licensees in recovering from substance abuse in the long term.

(d) Notwithstanding any other law, by January 1, 2019, the committee shall review the existing criteria for Uniform Standard #4 established pursuant to paragraph (4) of subdivision (c). The committee's review and findings shall determine whether the existing criteria for Uniform Standard #4 should be updated to reflect recent developments in testing research and technology. The committee shall consider information from, but not limited to, the American Society of Addiction Medicine, and other sources of best practices.

HISTORY:

Added Stats 2008 ch 548 § 3 (SB 1441), effective January 1, 2009. Amended Stats 2009 ch 140 § 1 (AB 1164), effective January 1, 2010; Stats 2013 ch 22 § 1 (AB 75), effective June 27, 2013, operative July 1, 2013; Stats 2017 ch 600 § 1 (SB 796), effective January 1, 2018.

§ 315.2. Cease practice order

(a) A board, as described in Section 315, shall order a licensee of the board to cease practice if the licensee tests positive for any substance that is prohibited under the terms of the licensee's probation or diversion program.

(b) An order to cease practice under this section shall not be governed by the provisions of Chapter 5 (commencing with Section 11500) of Part 1 of Division 3 of Title 2 of the Government Code.

(c) A cease practice order under this section shall not constitute disciplinary action.

(d) This section shall have no effect on the Board of Registered Nursing pursuant to Article 3.1 (commencing with Section 2770) of Chapter 6 of Division 2.

HISTORY:

Added Stats 2010 ch 517 § 2 (SB 1172), effective January 1, 2011.

§ 315.4. Cease practice order for violation of probation or diversion program

(a) A board, as described in Section 315, may adopt regulations authorizing the board to order a licensee on probation or in a diversion program to cease practice for major violations and when the board orders a licensee to undergo a clinical diagnostic evaluation pursuant to the uniform and specific standards adopted and authorized under Section 315.

(b) An order to cease practice under this section shall not be governed by the provisions of Chapter 5 (commencing with Section 11500) of Part 1 of Division 3 of Title 2 of the Government Code.

(c) A cease practice order under this section shall not constitute disciplinary action.

(d) This section shall have no effect on the Board of Registered Nursing pursuant to Article 3.1 (commencing with Section 2770) of Chapter 6 of Division 2.

HISTORY:

Added Stats 2010 ch 517 § 3 (SB 1172), effective January 1, 2011.

ARTICLE 4
REPRESENTATION OF CONSUMERS

Section

320. Intervention in administrative or judicial proceedings.

Section
321. Commencement of legal proceedings.

HISTORY: Added Stats 1970 ch 1394 § 3, operative July 1, 1971.

§ 320. Intervention in administrative or judicial proceedings

Whenever there is pending before any state commission, regulatory agency, department, or other state agency, or any state or federal court or agency, any matter or proceeding which the director finds may affect substantially the interests of consumers within California, the director, or the Attorney General, may intervene in such matter or proceeding in any appropriate manner to represent the interests of consumers. The director, or any officer or employee designated by the director for that purpose, or the Attorney General, may thereafter present to such agency, court, or department, in conformity with the rules of practice and procedure thereof, such evidence and argument as he shall determine to be necessary, for the effective protection of the interests of consumers.

HISTORY:
Added Stats 1970 ch 1394 § 3, operative July 1, 1971. Amended Stats 1975 ch 1262 § 8.

§ 321. Commencement of legal proceedings

Whenever it appears to the director that the interests of the consumers of this state are being damaged, or may be damaged, by any person who engaged in, or intends to engage in, any acts or practices in violation of any law of this state, or any federal law, the director or any officer or employee designated by the director, or the Attorney General, may commence legal proceedings in the appropriate forum to enjoin such acts or practices and may seek other appropriate relief on behalf of such consumers.

HISTORY:
Added Stats 1975 ch 1262 § 9.

ARTICLE 5
CONSUMER COMPLAINTS

Section
325. Actionable complaints.
326. Proceedings on receipt of complaint.
328. Implementation of Complaint Prioritization Guidelines.

HISTORY: Added Stats 1970 ch 1394 § 3, operative July 1, 1971.

§ 325. Actionable complaints

It shall be the duty of the director to receive complaints from consumers concerning (a) unfair methods of competition and unfair or deceptive acts or practices undertaken by any person in the conduct of any trade or commerce; (b) the production, distribution, sale, and lease of any goods and services undertaken by any person which may endanger the public health, safety, or welfare; (c) violations of provisions of this code relating to businesses and professions licensed by any agency of the department, and regulations promulgated pursuant thereto; (d) student concerns related to the Bureau for Private Postsecondary Education's performance of its responsibilities, including concerns that arise re- lated to the Bureau for Private Postsecondary Education's handling of a complaint or its administration of the Student Tuition Recovery Fund, established in Article 14 (commencing with Section 94923) of Chapter 8 of Part 59 of Division 10 of Title 3 of the Education Code; and (e) other matters consistent with the purposes of this chapter, whenever appropriate.

HISTORY:

Added Stats 1970 ch 1394 § 3, operative July 1, 1971. Amended Stats 2016 ch 593 § 1 (SB 1192), effective January 1, 2017.

§ 326. Proceedings on receipt of complaint

(a) Upon receipt of any complaint pursuant to Section 325, the director may notify the person against whom the complaint is made of the nature of the complaint and may request appropriate relief for the consumer.

(b) The director shall also transmit any valid complaint to the local, state or federal agency whose authority provides the most effective means to secure the relief.

The director shall, if appropriate, advise the consumer of the action taken on the complaint and of any other means which may be available to the consumer to secure relief.

(c) If the director receives a complaint or receives information from any source indicating a probable violation of any law, rule, or order of any regulatory agency of the state, or if a pattern of complaints from consumers develops, the director shall transmit any complaint he or she considers to be valid to any appropriate law enforcement or regulatory agency and any evidence or information he or she may have concerning the probable violation or pattern of complaints or request the Attorney General to undertake appropriate legal action. It shall be the continuing duty of the director to discern patterns of complaints and to ascertain the nature and extent of action taken with respect to the probable violations or pattern of complaints.

HISTORY:

Added Stats 1970 ch 1394 § 3, operative July 1, 1971. Amended Stats 1978 ch 1161 § 8; Stats 1989 ch 1360 § 1.

§ 328. Implementation of Complaint Prioritization Guidelines

(a) In order to implement the Consumer Protection Enforcement Initiative of 2010, the director, through the Division of Investigation, shall implement "Complaint Prioritization Guidelines" for boards to utilize in prioritizing their respective complaint and investigative workloads. The guidelines shall be used to determine the referral of complaints to the division and those that are retained by the health care boards for investigation.

(b) Neither the Medical Board of California nor the Podiatric Medical Board of California shall be required to utilize the guidelines implemented pursuant to subdivision (a).

(c) On or before July 1, 2019, the director shall amend the guidelines implemented pursuant to subdivision (a) to include the category of "allegations of serious harm to a minor" under the "urgent" or "highest priority" level.

HISTORY:
Added Stats 2015 ch 656 § 2 (SB 467), effective January 1, 2016. Amended Stats 2017 ch 775 § 5 (SB 798), effective January 1, 2018; Stats 2018 ch 571 § 2 (SB 1480), effective January 1, 2019; Stats 2019 ch 351 § 47 (AB 496), effective January 1, 2020.

CHAPTER 6

PUBLIC MEMBERS

Section
450. Qualifications generally.
450.2. Avoiding conflict of interest.
450.3. Conflicting pecuniary interests.
450.5. Prior industrial and professional pursuits.
450.6. Age.
451. Delegation of duties.
452. "Board".
453. Training and orientation program for new board members.

HISTORY: Added Stats 1961 ch 2232 § 2.

§ 450. Qualifications generally

In addition to the qualifications provided in the respective chapters of this code, a public member or a lay member of any board shall not be, nor shall they have been within the period of five years immediately preceding their appointment, any of the following:

(a) An employer, or an officer, director, or substantially full-time representative of an employer or group of employers, of any licensee of a board, except that this subdivision shall not preclude the appointment of a person who maintains infrequent employer status with a licensee, or maintains a client, patient, or customer relationship with a licensee that does not constitute more than 2 percent of the practice or business of the licensee.

(b) A person maintaining a contractual relationship with a licensee of a board that would constitute more than 2 percent of the practice or business of the licensee, or an officer, director, or substantially full-time representative of that person or group of persons.

(c) An employee of a licensee of a board, or a representative of the employee, except that this subdivision shall not preclude the appointment of a person who maintains an infrequent employee relationship or renders professional or related services to a licensee if the employment or service does not constitute more than 2 percent of the employment or practice of the member of the board.

HISTORY:
Added Stats 1961 ch 2232 § 2. Amended Stats 2019 ch 351 § 48 (AB 496), effective January 1, 2020.

§ 450.2. Avoiding conflict of interest

In order to avoid a potential for a conflict of interest, a public member of a board shall not:

(a) Be a current or past licensee of that board.

(b) Be a close family member of a licensee of that board.

HISTORY:
Added Stats 2002 ch 1150 § 1.2 (SB 1955).

§ 450.3. Conflicting pecuniary interests

No public member shall either at the time of their appointment or during their tenure in office have any financial interest in any organization subject to regulation by the board, commission, or committee of which they are a member.

HISTORY:
Added Stats 1972 ch 1032 § 1. Amended Stats 2019 ch 351 § 49 (AB 496), effective January 1, 2020.

§ 450.5. Prior industrial and professional pursuits

A public member, or a lay member, at any time within five years immediately preceding his or her appointment, shall not have been engaged in pursuits which lie within the field of the industry or profession, or have provided representation to the industry or profession, regulated by the board of which he or she is a member, nor shall he or she engage in those pursuits or provide that representation during his or her term of office.

HISTORY:
Added Stats 1961 ch 2232 § 2. Amended Stats 2003 ch 563 § 2 (AB 827).

§ 450.6. Age

Notwithstanding any other section of law, a public member may be appointed without regard to age so long as the public member has reached the age of majority prior to appointment.

HISTORY:
Added Stats 1976 ch 1188 § 1.3.

§ 451. Delegation of duties

If any board shall as a part of its functions delegate any duty or responsibility to be performed by a single member of such board, such delegation shall not be made solely to any public member or any lay member of the board in any of the following instances:

(a) The actual preparation of, the administration of, and the grading of, examinations.

(b) The inspection or investigation of licentiates, the manner or method of practice or doing business, or their place of practice or business.

Nothing in this section shall be construed as precluding a public member or a lay member from participating in the formation of policy relating to the scope of the activities set forth in subdivisions (a) and (b) or in the approval, disapproval or modification of the action of its individual members, nor preclude such member from participating as a member of a subcommittee consisting of more than one member of the board in the performance of any duty.

HISTORY:
Added Stats 1961 ch 2232 § 2.

§ 452. "Board"

"Board," as used in this chapter, includes a board, advisory board, commission, examining committee, committee or other similarly constituted body exercising powers under this code.

HISTORY:
Added Stats 1961 ch 2232 § 2. Amended Stats 1976 ch 1188 § 1.5.

§ 453. Training and orientation program for new board members

Every newly appointed board member shall, within one year of assuming office, complete a training and orientation program offered by the department regarding, among other things, his or her functions, responsibilities, and obligations as a member of a board. The department shall adopt regulations necessary to establish this training and orientation program and its content.

HISTORY:
Added Stats 2002 ch 1150 § 1.4 (SB 1955).

CHAPTER 7
LICENSEE

Section
460. Powers of local governmental entities.
461. Asking applicant to reveal arrest record prohibited.
462. Inactive category of licensure.
464. Retired category of licensure.

HISTORY: Added Stats 1967 ch 1095 § 1.

§ 460. Powers of local governmental entities

(a) No city, county, or city and county shall prohibit a person or group of persons, authorized by one of the agencies in the Department of Consumer Affairs or an entity established pursuant to this code by a license, certificate, or other means to engage in a particular business, from engaging in that business, occupation, or profession or any portion of that business, occupation, or profession.

(b)(1) No city, county, or city and county shall prohibit a healing arts professional licensed with the state under Division 2 (commencing with Section 500) or licensed or certified by an entity established pursuant to this code from engaging in any act or performing any procedure that falls within the professionally recognized scope of practice of that licensee.

(2) This subdivision shall not be construed to prohibit the enforcement of a local ordinance in effect prior to January 1, 2010, related to any act or procedure that falls within the professionally recognized scope of practice of a healing arts professional licensed under Division 2 (commencing with Section 500).

(c) This section shall not be construed to prevent a city, county, or city and county from adopting or enforcing any local ordinance governing zoning, business licensing, or reasonable health and safety requirements for establishments or businesses of a healing arts professional licensed under Division 2 (commencing with Section 500) or licensed or certified by an entity established under this code or a person or group of persons described in subdivision (a).

(d) Nothing in this section shall prohibit any city, county, or city and county from levying a business license tax solely for revenue purposes, nor any city or county from levying a license tax solely for the purpose of covering the cost of regulation.

HISTORY:

Added Stats 1967 ch 1095 § 1. Amended Stats 1971 ch 716 § 24; Stats 2009 ch 16 § 1 (SB 762), effective January 1, 2010; Stats 2014 ch 406 § 1 (AB 1147), effective January 1, 2015.

§ 461. Asking applicant to reveal arrest record prohibited

No public agency, state or local, shall, on an initial application form for any license, certificate or registration, ask for or require the applicant to reveal a record of arrest that did not result in a conviction or a plea of nolo contendere. A violation of this section is a misdemeanor.

This section shall apply in the case of any license, certificate or registration provided for by any law of this state or local government, including, but not limited to, this code, the Corporations Code, the Education Code, and the Insurance Code.

HISTORY:

Added Stats 1975 ch 883 § 1.

§ 462. Inactive category of licensure

(a) Any of the boards, bureaus, commissions, or programs within the department may establish, by regulation, a system for an inactive category of licensure for persons who are not actively engaged in the practice of their profession or vocation.

(b) The regulation shall contain the following provisions:

(1) The holder of an inactive license issued pursuant to this section shall not engage in any activity for which a license is required.

(2) An inactive license issued pursuant to this section shall be renewed during the same time period in which an active license is renewed. The holder of an inactive license need not comply with any continuing education requirement for renewal of an active license.

(3) The renewal fee for a license in an active status shall apply also for a renewal of a license in an inactive status, unless a lesser renewal fee is specified by the board.

(4) In order for the holder of an inactive license issued pursuant to this section to restore his or her license to an active status, the holder of an inactive license shall comply with all the following:

(A) Pay the renewal fee.

(B) If the board requires completion of continuing education for renewal of an active license, complete continuing education equivalent to that required for renewal of an active license, unless a different requirement is specified by the board.

(c) This section shall not apply to any healing arts board as specified in Section 701.

HISTORY:
Added Stats 1994 ch 26 § 14 (AB 1807), effective March 30, 1994.

§ 464. Retired category of licensure

(a) Any of the boards within the department may establish, by regulation, a system for a retired category of licensure for persons who are not actively engaged in the practice of their profession or vocation.

(b) The regulation shall contain the following:

(1) A retired license shall be issued to a person with either an active license or an inactive license that was not placed on inactive status for disciplinary reasons.

(2) The holder of a retired license issued pursuant to this section shall not engage in any activity for which a license is required, unless the board, by regulation, specifies the criteria for a retired licensee to practice his or her profession or vocation.

(3) The holder of a retired license shall not be required to renew that license.

(4) The board shall establish an appropriate application fee for a retired license to cover the reasonable regulatory cost of issuing a retired license.

(5) In order for the holder of a retired license issued pursuant to this section to restore his or her license to an active status, the holder of that license shall meet all the following:

(A) Pay a fee established by statute or regulation.

(B) Certify, in a manner satisfactory to the board, that he or she has not committed an act or crime constituting grounds for denial of licensure.

(C) Comply with the fingerprint submission requirements established by regulation.

(D) If the board requires completion of continuing education for renewal of an active license, complete continuing education equivalent to that required for renewal of an active license, unless a different requirement is specified by the board.

(E) Complete any other requirements as specified by the board by regulation.

(c) A board may upon its own determination, and shall upon receipt of a complaint from any person, investigate the actions of any licensee, including a person with a license that either restricts or prohibits the practice of that person in his or her profession or vocation, including, but not limited to, a license that is retired, inactive, canceled, revoked, or suspended.

(d) Subdivisions (a) and (b) shall not apply to a board that has other statutory authority to establish a retired license.

HISTORY:
Added Stats 2016 ch 473 § 1 (AB 2859), effective January 1, 2017.

DIVISION 1.5

DENIAL, SUSPENSION AND REVOCATION OF LICENSES

Chapter
1. General Provisions.

Chapter
2. Denial of Licenses.
3. Suspension and Revocation of Licenses.
4. Public Reprovals.
5. Examination Security.

HISTORY: Added Stats 1972 ch 903 § 1.

CHAPTER 1
GENERAL PROVISIONS

Section
475. Applicability of division.
476. Exemptions.
477. "Board"; "License".
478. "Application"; "Material".

Bus & Prof

HISTORY: Added Stats 1972 ch 903 § 1.

§ 475. Applicability of division

(a) Notwithstanding any other provisions of this code, the provisions of this division shall govern the denial of licenses on the grounds of:

(1) Knowingly making a false statement of material fact, or knowingly omitting to state a material fact, in an application for a license.

(2) Conviction of a crime.

(3) Commission of any act involving dishonesty, fraud or deceit with the intent to substantially benefit himself or another, or substantially injure another.

(4) Commission of any act which, if done by a licentiate of the business or profession in question, would be grounds for suspension or revocation of license.

(b) Notwithstanding any other provisions of this code, the provisions of this division shall govern the suspension and revocation of licenses on grounds specified in paragraphs (1) and (2) of subdivision (a).

(c) A license shall not be denied, suspended, or revoked on the grounds of a lack of good moral character or any similar ground relating to an applicant's character, reputation, personality, or habits.

HISTORY:

Added Stats 1972 ch 903 § 1. Amended Stats 1974 ch 1321 § 1; Stats 1992 ch 1289 § 5 (AB 2743).

§ 476. Exemptions

(a) Except as provided in subdivision (b), nothing in this division shall apply to the licensure or registration of persons pursuant to Chapter 4 (commencing with Section 6000) of Division 3, or pursuant to Division 9 (commencing with Section 23000) or pursuant to Chapter 5 (commencing with Section 19800) of Division 8.

(b) Section 494.5 shall apply to the licensure of persons authorized to practice law pursuant to Chapter 4 (commencing with Section 6000) of Division 3, and the licensure or registration of persons pursuant to Chapter 5 (commencing with Section 19800) of Division 8 or pursuant to Division 9 (commencing with Section 23000).

HISTORY:
Added Stats 1972 ch 903 § 1. Amended Stats 1983 ch 721 § 1; Stats 2011 ch 455 § 2 (AB 1424), effective January 1, 2012.

§ 477. "Board"; "License"

As used in this division:

(a) "Board" includes "bureau," "commission," "committee," "department," "division," "examining committee," "program," and "agency."

(b) "License" includes certificate, registration or other means to engage in a business or profession regulated by this code.

HISTORY:
Added Stats 1972 ch 903 § 1. Amended Stats 1974 ch 1321 § 2; Stats 1983 ch 95 § 1; Stats 1991 ch 654 § 5 (AB 1893).

§ 478. "Application"; "Material"

(a) As used in this division, "application" includes the original documents or writings filed and any other supporting documents or writings including supporting documents provided or filed contemporaneously, or later, in support of the application whether provided or filed by the applicant or by any other person in support of the application.

(b) As used in this division, "material" includes a statement or omission substantially related to the qualifications, functions, or duties of the business or profession.

HISTORY:
Added Stats 1992 ch 1289 § 6 (AB 2743).

CHAPTER 2

DENIAL OF LICENSES

Section
480. Grounds for denial; Effect of obtaining certificate of rehabilitation [Repealed].
480. Grounds for denial by board; Effect of obtaining certificate of rehabilitation.
480.5. Completion of licensure requirements while incarcerated.
481. Crime and job-fitness criteria [Repealed].
481. Crime and job-fitness criteria.
482. Rehabilitation criteria [Repealed].
482. Rehabilitation criteria.
484. Attestation to good moral character of applicant.
485. Procedure upon denial.
486. Contents of decision or notice.
487. Hearing; Time.
488. Hearing request [Repealed].
488. Hearing request.
489. Denial of application without a hearing.

HISTORY: Added Stats 1972 ch 903 § 1.

§ 480. Grounds for denial; Effect of obtaining certificate of rehabilitation [Repealed]

HISTORY:

Added Stats 1974 ch 1321 § 4. Amended Stats 1976 ch 947 § 1; Stats 1979 ch 876 § 2; Stats 2008 ch 179 § 2 (SB 1498), effective January 1, 2009; Stats 2014 ch 737 § 1 (AB 2396), effective January 1, 2015; Stats 2018 ch 995 § 3 (AB 2138), effective January 1, 2019, inoperative July 1, 2020, repealed January 1, 2021; Stats 2019 ch 578 § 1 (AB 1076), effective January 1, 2020, inoperative July 1, 2020, repealed January 1, 2021.

§ 480. Grounds for denial by board; Effect of obtaining certificate of rehabilitation

(a) Notwithstanding any other provision of this code, a board may deny a license regulated by this code on the grounds that the applicant has been convicted of a crime or has been subject to formal discipline only if either of the following conditions are met:

(1) The applicant has been convicted of a crime within the preceding seven years from the date of application that is substantially related to the qualifications, functions, or duties of the business or profession for which the application is made, regardless of whether the applicant was incarcerated for that crime, or the applicant has been convicted of a crime that is substantially related to the qualifications, functions, or duties of the business or profession for which the application is made and for which the applicant is presently incarcerated or for which the applicant was released from incarceration within the preceding seven years from the date of application. However, the preceding seven-year limitation shall not apply in either of the following situations:

(A) The applicant was convicted of a serious felony, as defined in Section 1192.7 of the Penal Code or a crime for which registration is required pursuant to paragraph (2) or (3) of subdivision (d) of Section 290 of the Penal Code.

(B) The applicant was convicted of a financial crime currently classified as a felony that is directly and adversely related to the fiduciary qualifications, functions, or duties of the business or profession for which the application is made, pursuant to regulations adopted by the board, and for which the applicant is seeking licensure under any of the following:

(i) Chapter 6 (commencing with Section 6500) of Division 3.

(ii) Chapter 9 (commencing with Section 7000) of Division 3.

(iii) Chapter 11.3 (commencing with Section 7512) of Division 3.

(iv) Licensure as a funeral director or cemetery manager under Chapter 12 (commencing with Section 7600) of Division 3.

(v) Division 4 (commencing with Section 10000).

(2) The applicant has been subjected to formal discipline by a licensing board in or outside California within the preceding seven years from the date of application based on professional misconduct that would have been cause for discipline before the board for which the present application is made and that is substantially related to the qualifications, functions, or duties of the business or profession for which the present application is made. However,

prior disciplinary action by a licensing board within the preceding seven years shall not be the basis for denial of a license if the basis for that disciplinary action was a conviction that has been dismissed pursuant to Section 1203.4, 1203.4a, 1203.41, 1203.42, or 1203.425 of the Penal Code or a comparable dismissal or expungement. Formal discipline that occurred earlier than seven years preceding the date of application may be grounds for denial of a license only if the formal discipline was for conduct that, if committed in this state by a physician and surgeon licensed pursuant to Chapter 5 (commencing with Section 2000) of Division 2, would have constituted an act of sexual abuse, misconduct, or relations with a patient pursuant to Section 726 or sexual exploitation as defined in subdivision (a) of Section 729.

(b) Notwithstanding any other provision of this code, a person shall not be denied a license on the basis that the person has been convicted of a crime, or on the basis of acts underlying a conviction for a crime, if that person has obtained a certificate of rehabilitation under Chapter 3.5 (commencing with Section 4852.01) of Title 6 of Part 3 of the Penal Code, has been granted clemency or a pardon by a state or federal executive, or has made a showing of rehabilitation pursuant to Section 482.

(c) Notwithstanding any other provision of this code, a person shall not be denied a license on the basis of any conviction, or on the basis of the acts underlying the conviction, that has been dismissed pursuant to Section 1203.4, 1203.4a, 1203.41, 1203.42, or 1203.425 of the Penal Code, or a comparable dismissal or expungement. An applicant who has a conviction that has been dismissed pursuant to Section 1203.4, 1203.4a, 1203.41, or 1203.42 of the Penal Code shall provide proof of the dismissal if it is not reflected on the report furnished by the Department of Justice.

(d) Notwithstanding any other provision of this code, a board shall not deny a license on the basis of an arrest that resulted in a disposition other than a conviction, including an arrest that resulted in an infraction, citation, or a juvenile adjudication.

(e) A board may deny a license regulated by this code on the ground that the applicant knowingly made a false statement of fact that is required to be revealed in the application for the license. A board shall not deny a license based solely on an applicant's failure to disclose a fact that would not have been cause for denial of the license had it been disclosed.

(f) A board shall follow the following procedures in requesting or acting on an applicant's criminal history information:

(1) A board issuing a license pursuant to Chapter 3 (commencing with Section 5500), Chapter 3.5 (commencing with Section 5615), Chapter 10 (commencing with Section 7301), Chapter 20 (commencing with Section 9800), or Chapter 20.3 (commencing with Section 9880), of Division 3, or Chapter 3 (commencing with Section 19000) or Chapter 3.1 (commencing with Section 19225) of Division 8 may require applicants for licensure under those chapters to disclose criminal conviction history on an application for licensure.

(2) Except as provided in paragraph (1), a board shall not require an applicant for licensure to disclose any information or documentation regarding the applicant's criminal history. However, a board may request mitigat-

ing information from an applicant regarding the applicant's criminal history for purposes of determining substantial relation or demonstrating evidence of rehabilitation, provided that the applicant is informed that disclosure is voluntary and that the applicant's decision not to disclose any information shall not be a factor in a board's decision to grant or deny an application for licensure.

(3) If a board decides to deny an application for licensure based solely or in part on the applicant's conviction history, the board shall notify the applicant in writing of all of the following:

(A) The denial or disqualification of licensure.

(B) Any existing procedure the board has for the applicant to challenge the decision or to request reconsideration.

(C) That the applicant has the right to appeal the board's decision.

(D) The processes for the applicant to request a copy of the applicant's complete conviction history and question the accuracy or completeness of the record pursuant to Sections 11122 to 11127 of the Penal Code.

(g)(1) For a minimum of three years, each board under this code shall retain application forms and other documents submitted by an applicant, any notice provided to an applicant, all other communications received from and provided to an applicant, and criminal history reports of an applicant.

(2) Each board under this code shall retain the number of applications received for each license and the number of applications requiring inquiries regarding criminal history. In addition, each licensing authority shall retain all of the following information:

(A) The number of applicants with a criminal record who received notice of denial or disqualification of licensure.

(B) The number of applicants with a criminal record who provided evidence of mitigation or rehabilitation.

(C) The number of applicants with a criminal record who appealed any denial or disqualification of licensure.

(D) The final disposition and demographic information, consisting of voluntarily provided information on race or gender, of any applicant described in subparagraph (A), (B), or (C).

(3)(A) Each board under this code shall annually make available to the public through the board's internet website and through a report submitted to the appropriate policy committees of the Legislature deidentified information collected pursuant to this subdivision. Each board shall ensure confidentiality of the individual applicants.

(B) A report pursuant to subparagraph (A) shall be submitted in compliance with Section 9795 of the Government Code.

(h) "Conviction" as used in this section shall have the same meaning as defined in Section 7.5.

(i) This section does not in any way modify or otherwise affect the existing authority of the following entities in regard to licensure:

(1) The State Athletic Commission.

(2) The Bureau for Private Postsecondary Education.

(3) The California Horse Racing Board.

HISTORY:

Added Stats 2018 ch 995 § 4 (AB 2138), effective January 1, 2019, operative July 1, 2020. Amended Stats 2019 ch 359 § 1 (AB 1521), effective January 1, 2020, operative July 1, 2020; Stats 2019 ch 578

§ 2.5 (AB 1076), effective January 1, 2020, operative July 1, 2020 (ch 578 prevails); Stats 2022 ch 453 § 1 (AB 1636), effective January 1, 2023.

§ 480.5. Completion of licensure requirements while incarcerated

(a) An individual who has satisfied any of the requirements needed to obtain a license regulated under this division while incarcerated, who applies for that license upon release from incarceration, and who is otherwise eligible for the license shall not be subject to a delay in processing his or her application or a denial of the license solely on the basis that some or all of the licensure requirements were completed while the individual was incarcerated.

(b) Nothing in this section shall be construed to apply to a petition for reinstatement of a license or to limit the ability of a board to deny a license pursuant to Section 480.

(c) This section shall not apply to the licensure of individuals under the initiative act referred to in Chapter 2 (commencing with Section 1000) of Division 2.

HISTORY:

Added Stats 2014 ch 410 § 1 (AB 1702), effective January 1, 2015.

§ 481. Crime and job-fitness criteria [Repealed]

HISTORY:

Added Stats 1974 ch 1321 § 6. Amended Stats 2018 ch 995 § 6 (AB 2138), effective January 1, 2019, inoperative July 1, 2020, repealed January 1, 2021.

§ 481. Crime and job-fitness criteria

(a) Each board under this code shall develop criteria to aid it, when considering the denial, suspension, or revocation of a license, to determine whether a crime is substantially related to the qualifications, functions, or duties of the business or profession it regulates.

(b) Criteria for determining whether a crime is substantially related to the qualifications, functions, or duties of the business or profession a board regulates shall include all of the following:

(1) The nature and gravity of the offense.

(2) The number of years elapsed since the date of the offense.

(3) The nature and duties of the profession in which the applicant seeks licensure or in which the licensee is licensed.

(c) A board shall not deny a license based in whole or in part on a conviction without considering evidence of rehabilitation submitted by an applicant pursuant to any process established in the practice act or regulations of the particular board and as directed by Section 482.

(d) Each board shall post on its Internet Web site a summary of the criteria used to consider whether a crime is considered to be substantially related to the qualifications, functions, or duties of the business or profession it regulates consistent with this section.

(e) This section does not in any way modify or otherwise affect the existing authority of the following entities in regard to licensure:

(1) The State Athletic Commission.

(2) The Bureau for Private Postsecondary Education.

(3) The California Horse Racing Board.

(f) This section shall become operative on July 1, 2020.

HISTORY:

Added Stats 2018 ch 995 § 7 (AB 2138), effective January 1, 2019, operative July 1, 2020.

§ 482. Rehabilitation criteria [Repealed]

HISTORY:

Added Stats 1972 ch 903 § 1. Amended Stats 1974 ch 1321 § 7; Stats 2018 ch 995 § 8 (AB 2138), effective January 1, 2019, inoperative July 1, 2020, repealed January 1, 2021.

§ 482. Rehabilitation criteria

(a) Each board under this code shall develop criteria to evaluate the rehabilitation of a person when doing either of the following:

(1) Considering the denial of a license by the board under Section 480.

(2) Considering suspension or revocation of a license under Section 490.

(b) Each board shall consider whether an applicant or licensee has made a showing of rehabilitation if either of the following are met:

(1) The applicant or licensee has completed the criminal sentence at issue without a violation of parole or probation.

(2) The board, applying its criteria for rehabilitation, finds that the applicant is rehabilitated.

(c) This section does not in any way modify or otherwise affect the existing authority of the following entities in regard to licensure:

(1) The State Athletic Commission.

(2) The Bureau for Private Postsecondary Education.

(3) The California Horse Racing Board.

(d) This section shall become operative on July 1, 2020.

HISTORY:

Added Stats 2018 ch 995 § 9 (AB 2138), effective January 1, 2019, operative July 1, 2020.

§ 484. Attestation to good moral character of applicant

No person applying for licensure under this code shall be required to submit to any licensing board any attestation by other persons to his good moral character.

HISTORY:

Added Stats 1972 ch 903 § 1. Amended Stats 1974 ch 1321 § 9.

§ 485. Procedure upon denial

Upon denial of an application for a license under this chapter or Section 496, the board shall do either of the following:

(a) File and serve a statement of issues in accordance with Chapter 5 (commencing with Section 11500) of Part 1 of Division 3 of Title 2 of the Government Code.

(b) Notify the applicant that the application is denied, stating (1) the reason for the denial, and (2) that the applicant has the right to a hearing under Chapter 5 (commencing with Section 11500) of Part 1 of Division 3 of Title 2 of the Government Code if written request for hearing is made within

60 days after service of the notice of denial. Unless written request for hearing is made within the 60-day period, the applicant's right to a hearing is deemed waived.

Service of the notice of denial may be made in the manner authorized for service of summons in civil actions, or by registered mail addressed to the applicant at the latest address filed by the applicant in writing with the board in his or her application or otherwise. Service by mail is complete on the date of mailing.

HISTORY:

Added Stats 1972 ch 903 § 1. Amended Stats 1997 ch 758 § 2.3 (SB 1346).

§ 486. Contents of decision or notice

Where the board has denied an application for a license under this chapter or Section 496, it shall, in its decision, or in its notice under subdivision (b) of Section 485, inform the applicant of the following:

(a) The earliest date on which the applicant may reapply for a license which shall be one year from the effective date of the decision, or service of the notice under subdivision (b) of Section 485, unless the board prescribes an earlier date or a later date is prescribed by another statute.

(b) That all competent evidence of rehabilitation presented will be considered upon a reapplication.

Along with the decision, or the notice under subdivision (b) of Section 485, the board shall serve a copy of the criteria relating to rehabilitation formulated under Section 482.

HISTORY:

Added Stats 1972 ch 903 § 1. Amended Stats 1974 ch 1321 § 9.5; Stats 1997 ch 758 § 2.4 (SB 1346).

§ 487. Hearing; Time

If a hearing is requested by the applicant, the board shall conduct such hearing within 90 days from the date the hearing is requested unless the applicant shall request or agree in writing to a postponement or continuance of the hearing. Notwithstanding the above, the Office of Administrative Hearings may order, or on a showing of good cause, grant a request for, up to 45 additional days within which to conduct a hearing, except in cases involving alleged examination or licensing fraud, in which cases the period may be up to 180 days. In no case shall more than two such orders be made or requests be granted.

HISTORY:

Added Stats 1972 ch 903 § 1. Amended Stats 1974 ch 1321 § 10; Stats 1986 ch 220 § 1, effective June 30, 1986.

§ 488. Hearing request [Repealed]

HISTORY:

Added Stats 2000 ch 568 § 2 (AB 2888). Amended Stats 2018 ch 995 § 10 (AB 2138), effective January 1, 2019, inoperative July 1, 2020, repealed January 1, 2021.

§ 488. Hearing request

(a) Except as otherwise provided by law, following a hearing requested by an applicant pursuant to subdivision (b) of Section 485, the board may take any of the following actions:

(1) Grant the license effective upon completion of all licensing requirements by the applicant.

(2) Grant the license effective upon completion of all licensing requirements by the applicant, immediately revoke the license, stay the revocation, and impose probationary conditions on the license, which may include suspension.

(3) Deny the license.

(4) Take other action in relation to denying or granting the license as the board in its discretion may deem proper.

(b) This section does not in any way modify or otherwise affect the existing authority of the following entities in regard to licensure:

(1) The State Athletic Commission.

(2) The Bureau for Private Postsecondary Education.

(3) The California Horse Racing Board.

(c) This section shall become operative on July 1, 2020.

HISTORY:

Added Stats 2018 ch 995 § 11 (AB 2138), effective January 1, 2019, operative July 1, 2020.

§ 489. Denial of application without a hearing

Any agency in the department which is authorized by law to deny an application for a license upon the grounds specified in Section 480 or 496, may without a hearing deny an application upon any of those grounds, if within one year previously, and after proceedings conducted in accordance with Chapter 5 (commencing with Section 11500) of Part 1 of Division 3 of Title 2 of the Government Code, that agency has denied an application from the same applicant upon the same ground.

HISTORY:

Added Stats 1955 ch 1151 § 1, as B & P C § 116. Amended Stats 1978 ch 1161 § 2. Renumbered by Stats 1989 ch 1104 § 1. Amended Stats 1997 ch 758 § 2.5 (SB 1346).

CHAPTER 3
SUSPENSION AND REVOCATION OF LICENSES

Section

490. Grounds for suspension or revocation; Discipline for substantially related crimes; Conviction; Legislative findings.
490.5. Suspension of license for failure to comply with child support order.
491. Procedure upon suspension or revocation.
492. Effect of completion of drug diversion program on disciplinary action or denial of license.
493. Evidentiary effect of record of conviction of crime substantially related to licensee's qualifications, functions, and duties [Repealed].
493. Evidentiary effect of record of conviction of crime substantially related to licensee's qualifications, functions, and duties.
494. Interim suspension or restriction order.
494.5. Agency actions when licensee is on certified list; Definitions; Collection and distribution of certified list information; Timing; Notices; Challenges by applicants and licensees; Release forms; Interagency agreements; Fees; Remedies; Inquiries and disclosure of information; Severability.

Section
494.6. Suspension under Labor Code Section 244.

HISTORY: Added Stats 1972 ch 903 § 1.

§ 490. Grounds for suspension or revocation; Discipline for substantially related crimes; Conviction; Legislative findings

(a) In addition to any other action that a board is permitted to take against a licensee, a board may suspend or revoke a license on the ground that the licensee has been convicted of a crime, if the crime is substantially related to the qualifications, functions, or duties of the business or profession for which the license was issued.

(b) Notwithstanding any other provision of law, a board may exercise any authority to discipline a licensee for conviction of a crime that is independent of the authority granted under subdivision (a) only if the crime is substantially related to the qualifications, functions, or duties of the business or profession for which the licensee's license was issued.

(c) A conviction within the meaning of this section means a plea or verdict of guilty or a conviction following a plea of nolo contendere. An action that a board is permitted to take following the establishment of a conviction may be taken when the time for appeal has elapsed, or the judgment of conviction has been affirmed on appeal, or when an order granting probation is made suspending the imposition of sentence, irrespective of a subsequent order under Section 1203.4 of the Penal Code.

(d) The Legislature hereby finds and declares that the application of this section has been made unclear by the holding in Petropoulos v. Department of Real Estate (2006) 142 Cal.App.4th 554, and that the holding in that case has placed a significant number of statutes and regulations in question, resulting in potential harm to the consumers of California from licensees who have been convicted of crimes. Therefore, the Legislature finds and declares that this section establishes an independent basis for a board to impose discipline upon a licensee, and that the amendments to this section made by Chapter 33 of the Statutes of 2008 do not constitute a change to, but rather are declaratory of, existing law.

HISTORY:
Added Stats 1974 ch 1321 § 13. Amended Stats 1979 ch 876 § 3; Stats 1980 ch 548 § 1; Stats 1992 ch 1289 § 7 (AB 2743); Stats 2008 ch 33 § 2 (SB 797) (ch 33 prevails), effective June 23, 2008, ch 179 § 3 (SB 1498), effective January 1, 2009; Stats 2010 ch 328 § 2 (SB 1330), effective January 1, 2011.

§ 490.5. Suspension of license for failure to comply with child support order

A board may suspend a license pursuant to Section 17520 of the Family Code if a licensee is not in compliance with a child support order or judgment.

HISTORY:
Added Stats 1994 ch 906 § 1 (AB 923), operative January 1, 1996. Amended Stats 2010 ch 328 § 3 (SB 1330), effective January 1, 2011.

§ 491. Procedure upon suspension or revocation

Upon suspension or revocation of a license by a board on one or more of the grounds specified in Section 490, the board shall:

(a) Send a copy of the provisions of Section 11522 of the Government Code to the ex-licensee.

(b) Send a copy of the criteria relating to rehabilitation formulated under Section 482 to the ex-licensee.

HISTORY:

Added Stats 1972 ch 903 § 1. Amended Stats 1974 ch 1321 § 14; Stats 1975 ch 678 § 1.

§ 492. Effect of completion of drug diversion program on disciplinary action or denial of license

Notwithstanding any other provision of law, successful completion of any diversion program under the Penal Code, or successful completion of an alcohol and drug problem assessment program under Article 5 (commencing with Section 23249.50) of Chapter 12 of Division 11 of the Vehicle Code, shall not prohibit any agency established under Division 2 (commencing with Section 500) of this code, or any initiative act referred to in that division, from taking disciplinary action against a licensee or from denying a license for professional misconduct, notwithstanding that evidence of that misconduct may be recorded in a record pertaining to an arrest.

This section shall not be construed to apply to any drug diversion program operated by any agency established under Division 2 (commencing with Section 500) of this code, or any initiative act referred to in that division.

HISTORY:

Added Stats 1987 ch 1183 § 1. Amended Stats 1994 ch 26 § 15 (AB 1807), effective March 30, 1994.

§ 493. Evidentiary effect of record of conviction of crime substantially related to licensee's qualifications, functions, and duties [Repealed]

HISTORY:

Added Stats 1961 ch 934 § 1, as B & P C § 117. Amended Stats 1978 ch 1161 § 3. Renumbered by Stats 1989 ch 1104 § 1.3. Amended Stats 2018 ch 995 § 12 (AB 2138), effective January 1, 2019, inoperative July 1, 2020, repealed January 1, 2021.

§ 493. Evidentiary effect of record of conviction of crime substantially related to licensee's qualifications, functions, and duties

(a) Notwithstanding any other law, in a proceeding conducted by a board within the department pursuant to law to deny an application for a license or to suspend or revoke a license or otherwise take disciplinary action against a person who holds a license, upon the ground that the applicant or the licensee has been convicted of a crime substantially related to the qualifications, functions, and duties of the licensee in question, the record of conviction of the crime shall be conclusive evidence of the fact that the conviction occurred, but only of that fact.

(b)(1) Criteria for determining whether a crime is substantially related to the qualifications, functions, or duties of the business or profession the board regulates shall include all of the following:

(A) The nature and gravity of the offense.

(B) The number of years elapsed since the date of the offense.

(C) The nature and duties of the profession.

(2) A board shall not categorically bar an applicant based solely on the type of conviction without considering evidence of rehabilitation.

(c) As used in this section, "license" includes "certificate," "permit," "authority," and "registration."

(d) This section does not in any way modify or otherwise affect the existing authority of the following entities in regard to licensure:

(1) The State Athletic Commission.

(2) The Bureau for Private Postsecondary Education.

(3) The California Horse Racing Board.

(e) This section shall become operative on July 1, 2020.

HISTORY:

Added Stats 2018 ch 995 § 13 (AB 2138), effective January 1, 2019, operative July 1, 2020.

§ 494. Interim suspension or restriction order

(a) A board or an administrative law judge sitting alone, as provided in subdivision (h), may, upon petition, issue an interim order suspending any licentiate or imposing license restrictions, including, but not limited to, mandatory biological fluid testing, supervision, or remedial training. The petition shall include affidavits that demonstrate, to the satisfaction of the board, both of the following:

(1) The licentiate has engaged in acts or omissions constituting a violation of this code or has been convicted of a crime substantially related to the licensed activity.

(2) Permitting the licentiate to continue to engage in the licensed activity, or permitting the licentiate to continue in the licensed activity without restrictions, would endanger the public health, safety, or welfare.

(b) No interim order provided for in this section shall be issued without notice to the licentiate unless it appears from the petition and supporting documents that serious injury would result to the public before the matter could be heard on notice.

(c) Except as provided in subdivision (b), the licentiate shall be given at least 15 days' notice of the hearing on the petition for an interim order. The notice shall include documents submitted to the board in support of the petition. If the order was initially issued without notice as provided in subdivision (b), the licentiate shall be entitled to a hearing on the petition within 20 days of the issuance of the interim order without notice. The licentiate shall be given notice of the hearing within two days after issuance of the initial interim order, and shall receive all documents in support of the petition. The failure of the board to provide a hearing within 20 days following the issuance of the interim order without notice, unless the licentiate waives his or her right to the hearing, shall result in the dissolution of the interim order by operation of law.

(d) At the hearing on the petition for an interim order, the licentiate may:

(1) Be represented by counsel.

(2) Have a record made of the proceedings, copies of which shall be available to the licentiate upon payment of costs computed in accordance with the provisions for transcript costs for judicial review contained in Section 11523 of the Government Code.

(3) Present affidavits and other documentary evidence.

(4) Present oral argument.

(e) The board, or an administrative law judge sitting alone as provided in subdivision (h), shall issue a decision on the petition for interim order within five business days following submission of the matter. The standard of proof required to obtain an interim order pursuant to this section shall be a preponderance of the evidence standard. If the interim order was previously issued without notice, the board shall determine whether the order shall remain in effect, be dissolved, or modified.

(f) The board shall file an accusation within 15 days of the issuance of an interim order. In the case of an interim order issued without notice, the time shall run from the date of the order issued after the noticed hearing. If the licentiate files a Notice of Defense, the hearing shall be held within 30 days of the agency's receipt of the Notice of Defense. A decision shall be rendered on the accusation no later than 30 days after submission of the matter. Failure to comply with any of the requirements in this subdivision shall dissolve the interim order by operation of law.

(g) Interim orders shall be subject to judicial review pursuant to Section 1094.5 of the Code of Civil Procedure and shall be heard only in the superior court in and for the Counties of Sacramento, San Francisco, Los Angeles, or San Diego. The review of an interim order shall be limited to a determination of whether the board abused its discretion in the issuance of the interim order. Abuse of discretion is established if the respondent board has not proceeded in the manner required by law, or if the court determines that the interim order is not supported by substantial evidence in light of the whole record.

(h) The board may, in its sole discretion, delegate the hearing on any petition for an interim order to an administrative law judge in the Office of Administrative Hearings. If the board hears the noticed petition itself, an administrative law judge shall preside at the hearing, rule on the admission and exclusion of evidence, and advise the board on matters of law. The board shall exercise all other powers relating to the conduct of the hearing but may delegate any or all of them to the administrative law judge. When the petition has been delegated to an administrative law judge, he or she shall sit alone and exercise all of the powers of the board relating to the conduct of the hearing. A decision issued by an administrative law judge sitting alone shall be final when it is filed with the board. If the administrative law judge issues an interim order without notice, he or she shall preside at the noticed hearing, unless unavailable, in which case another administrative law judge may hear the matter. The decision of the administrative law judge sitting alone on the petition for an interim order is final, subject only to judicial review in accordance with subdivision (g).

(i) Failure to comply with an interim order issued pursuant to subdivision (a) or (b) shall constitute a separate cause for disciplinary action against any licentiate, and may be heard at, and as a part of, the noticed hearing provided for in subdivision (f). Allegations of noncompliance with the interim order may be filed at any time prior to the rendering of a decision on the accusation. Violation of the interim order is established upon proof that the licentiate was on notice of the interim order and its terms, and that the order was in effect at the time of the violation. The finding of a violation of an interim order made at the hearing on the accusation shall be reviewed as a part of any review of a final decision of the agency.

If the interim order issued by the agency provides for anything less than a complete suspension of the licentiate from his or her business or profession, and the licentiate violates the interim order prior to the hearing on the accusation provided for in subdivision (f), the agency may, upon notice to the licentiate and proof of violation, modify or expand the interim order.

(j) A plea or verdict of guilty or a conviction after a plea of nolo contendere is deemed to be a conviction within the meaning of this section. A certified record of the conviction shall be conclusive evidence of the fact that the conviction occurred. A board may take action under this section notwithstanding the fact that an appeal of the conviction may be taken.

(k) The interim orders provided for by this section shall be in addition to, and not a limitation on, the authority to seek injunctive relief provided in any other provision of law.

(*l*) In the case of a board, a petition for an interim order may be filed by the executive officer. In the case of a bureau or program, a petition may be filed by the chief or program administrator, as the case may be.

(m) "Board," as used in this section, shall include any agency described in Section 22, and any allied health agency within the jurisdiction of the Medical Board of California. Board shall also include the Osteopathic Medical Board of California and the State Board of Chiropractic Examiners. The provisions of this section shall not be applicable to the Medical Board of California, the Board of Podiatric Medicine, or the State Athletic Commission.

HISTORY:

Added Stats 1993 ch 840 § 1 (SB 842). Amended Stats 1994 ch 1275 § 4 (SB 2101).

§ 494.5. Agency actions when licensee is on certified list; Definitions; Collection and distribution of certified list information; Timing; Notices; Challenges by applicants and licensees; Release forms; Interagency agreements; Fees; Remedies; Inquiries and disclosure of information; Severability

(a)(1) Except as provided in paragraphs (2), (3), and (4), a state governmental licensing entity shall refuse to issue, reactivate, reinstate, or renew a license and shall suspend a license if a licensee's name is included on a certified list.

(2) The Department of Motor Vehicles shall suspend a license if a licensee's name is included on a certified list. Any reference in this section to the issuance, reactivation, reinstatement, renewal, or denial of a license shall not apply to the Department of Motor Vehicles.

(3) The State Bar of California may recommend to refuse to issue, reactivate, reinstate, or renew a license and may recommend to suspend a license if a licensee's name is included on a certified list. The word "may" shall be substituted for the word "shall" relating to the issuance of a temporary license, refusal to issue, reactivate, reinstate, renew, or suspend a license in this section for licenses under the jurisdiction of the California Supreme Court.

(4) The Department of Alcoholic Beverage Control may refuse to issue, reactivate, reinstate, or renew a license, and may suspend a license, if a licensee's name is included on a certified list.

(b) For purposes of this section:

(1) "Certified list" means either the list provided by the State Board of Equalization or the list provided by the Franchise Tax Board of persons whose names appear on the lists of the 500 largest tax delinquencies pursuant to Section 7063 or 19195 of the Revenue and Taxation Code, as applicable.

(2) "License" includes a certificate, registration, or any other authorization to engage in a profession or occupation issued by a state governmental licensing entity. "License" includes a driver's license issued pursuant to Chapter 1 (commencing with Section 12500) of Division 6 of the Vehicle Code. "License" excludes a vehicle registration issued pursuant to Division 3 (commencing with Section 4000) of the Vehicle Code.

(3) "Licensee" means an individual authorized by a license to drive a motor vehicle or authorized by a license, certificate, registration, or other authorization to engage in a profession or occupation issued by a state governmental licensing entity.

(4) "State governmental licensing entity" means any entity listed in Section 101, 1000, or 19420, the office of the Attorney General, the Department of Insurance, the Department of Motor Vehicles, the State Bar of California, the Department of Real Estate, and any other state agency, board, or commission that issues a license, certificate, or registration authorizing an individual to engage in a profession or occupation, including any certificate, business or occupational license, or permit or license issued by the Department of Motor Vehicles or the Department of the California Highway Patrol. "State governmental licensing entity" shall not include the Contractors State License Board.

(c) The State Board of Equalization and the Franchise Tax Board shall each submit its respective certified list to every state governmental licensing entity. The certified lists shall include the name, social security number or taxpayer identification number, and the last known address of the persons identified on the certified lists.

(d) Notwithstanding any other law, each state governmental licensing entity shall collect the social security number or the federal taxpayer identification number from all applicants for the purposes of matching the names of the certified lists provided by the State Board of Equalization and the Franchise Tax Board to applicants and licensees.

(e)(1) Each state governmental licensing entity shall determine whether an applicant or licensee is on the most recent certified list provided by the State Board of Equalization and the Franchise Tax Board.

(2) If an applicant or licensee is on either of the certified lists, the state governmental licensing entity shall immediately provide a preliminary notice to the applicant or licensee of the entity's intent to suspend or withhold issuance or renewal of the license. The preliminary notice shall be delivered personally or by mail to the applicant's or licensee's last known mailing address on file with the state governmental licensing entity within 30 days of receipt of the certified list. Service by mail shall be completed in accordance with Section 1013 of the Code of Civil Procedure.

(A) The state governmental licensing entity shall issue a temporary license valid for a period of 90 days to any applicant whose name is on a certified list if the applicant is otherwise eligible for a license.

(B) The 90-day time period for a temporary license shall not be extended. Only one temporary license shall be issued during a regular license term and the term of the temporary license shall coincide with the first 90 days of the regular license term. A license for the full term or the remainder of the license term may be issued or renewed only upon compliance with this section.

(C) In the event that a license is suspended or an application for a license or the renewal of a license is denied pursuant to this section, any funds paid by the applicant or licensee shall not be refunded by the state governmental licensing entity.

(f)(1) A state governmental licensing entity shall refuse to issue or shall suspend a license pursuant to this section no sooner than 90 days and no later than 120 days of the mailing of the preliminary notice described in paragraph (2) of subdivision (e), unless the state governmental licensing entity has received a release pursuant to subdivision (h). The procedures in the administrative adjudication provisions of the Administrative Procedure Act (Chapter 4.5 (commencing with Section 11400) and Chapter 5 (commencing with Section 11500) of Part 1 of Division 3 of Title 2 of the Government Code) shall not apply to the denial or suspension of, or refusal to renew, a license or the issuance of a temporary license pursuant to this section.

(2) Notwithstanding any other law, if a board, bureau, or commission listed in Section 101, other than the Contractors State License Board, fails to take action in accordance with this section, the Department of Consumer Affairs shall issue a temporary license or suspend or refuse to issue, reactivate, reinstate, or renew a license, as appropriate.

(g) Notices shall be developed by each state governmental licensing entity. For an applicant or licensee on the State Board of Equalization's certified list, the notice shall include the address and telephone number of the State Board of Equalization, and shall emphasize the necessity of obtaining a release from the State Board of Equalization as a condition for the issuance, renewal, or continued valid status of a license or licenses. For an applicant or licensee on the Franchise Tax Board's certified list, the notice shall include the address and telephone number of the Franchise Tax Board, and shall emphasize the necessity of obtaining a release from the Franchise Tax Board as a condition for the issuance, renewal, or continued valid status of a license or licenses.

(1) The notice shall inform the applicant that the state governmental licensing entity shall issue a temporary license, as provided in subparagraph (A) of paragraph (2) of subdivision (e), for 90 calendar days if the applicant is otherwise eligible and that upon expiration of that time period, the license will be denied unless the state governmental licensing entity has received a release from the State Board of Equalization or the Franchise Tax Board, whichever is applicable.

(2) The notice shall inform the licensee that any license suspended under this section will remain suspended until the state governmental licensing entity receives a release along with applications and fees, if applicable, to reinstate the license.

(3) The notice shall also inform the applicant or licensee that if an application is denied or a license is suspended pursuant to this section, any moneys paid by the applicant or licensee shall not be refunded by the state

governmental licensing entity. The state governmental licensing entity shall also develop a form that the applicant or licensee shall use to request a release by the State Board of Equalization or the Franchise Tax Board. A copy of this form shall be included with every notice sent pursuant to this subdivision.

(h) If the applicant or licensee wishes to challenge the submission of their name on a certified list, the applicant or licensee shall make a timely written request for release to the State Board of Equalization or the Franchise Tax Board, whichever is applicable. The State Board of Equalization or the Franchise Tax Board shall immediately send a release to the appropriate state governmental licensing entity and the applicant or licensee, if any of the following conditions are met:

(1) The applicant or licensee has complied with the tax obligation, either by payment of the unpaid taxes or entry into an installment payment agreement, as described in Section 6832 or 19008 of the Revenue and Taxation Code, to satisfy the unpaid taxes.

(2) The applicant or licensee has submitted a request for release not later than 45 days after the applicant's or licensee's receipt of a preliminary notice described in paragraph (2) of subdivision (e), but the State Board of Equalization or the Franchise Tax Board, whichever is applicable, will be unable to complete the release review and send notice of its findings to the applicant or licensee and state governmental licensing entity within 45 days after the State Board of Equalization's or the Franchise Tax Board's receipt of the applicant's or licensee's request for release. Whenever a release is granted under this paragraph, and, notwithstanding that release, the applicable license or licenses have been suspended erroneously, the state governmental licensing entity shall reinstate the applicable licenses with retroactive effect back to the date of the erroneous suspension and that suspension shall not be reflected on any license record.

(3) The applicant or licensee is unable to pay the outstanding tax obligation due to a current financial hardship. "Financial hardship" means financial hardship as determined by the State Board of Equalization or the Franchise Tax Board, whichever is applicable, where the applicant or licensee is unable to pay any part of the outstanding liability and the applicant or licensee is unable to qualify for an installment payment arrangement as provided for by Section 6832 or Section 19008 of the Revenue and Taxation Code. In order to establish the existence of a financial hardship, the applicant or licensee shall submit any information, including information related to reasonable business and personal expenses, requested by the State Board of Equalization or the Franchise Tax Board, whichever is applicable, for purposes of making that determination.

(i) An applicant or licensee is required to act with diligence in responding to notices from the state governmental licensing entity and the State Board of Equalization or the Franchise Tax Board with the recognition that the temporary license will lapse or the license suspension will go into effect after 90 days and that the State Board of Equalization or the Franchise Tax Board must have time to act within that period. An applicant's or licensee's delay in acting, without good cause, which directly results in the inability of the State Board of Equalization or the Franchise Tax Board, whichever is applicable, to complete a review of the applicant's or licensee's request for release shall not constitute the diligence required under this section which would justify the issuance of a release. An applicant or licensee shall have the burden of establishing that they diligently responded to notices from the state governmental licensing entity or the State Board of Equalization or the Franchise Tax Board and that any delay was not without good cause.

(j) The State Board of Equalization or the Franchise Tax Board shall create release forms for use pursuant to this section. When the applicant or licensee has complied with the tax obligation by payment of the unpaid taxes, or entry into an installment payment agreement, or establishing the existence of a current financial hardship as defined in paragraph (3) of subdivision (h), the State Board of Equalization or the Franchise Tax Board, whichever is applicable, shall mail a release form to the applicant or licensee and provide a release to the appropriate state governmental licensing entity. Any state governmental licensing entity that has received a release from the State Board of Equalization and the Franchise Tax Board pursuant to this subdivision shall process the release within five business days of its receipt. If the State Board of Equalization or the Franchise Tax Board determines subsequent to the issuance of a release that the licensee has not complied with their installment payment agreement, the State Board of Equalization or the Franchise Tax Board, whichever is applicable, shall notify the state governmental licensing entity and the licensee in a format prescribed by the State Board of Equalization or the Franchise Tax Board, whichever is applicable, that the licensee is not in compliance and the release shall be rescinded. The State Board of Equalization and the Franchise Tax Board may, when it is economically feasible for the state governmental licensing entity to develop an automated process for complying with this subdivision, notify the state governmental licensing entity in a manner prescribed by the State Board of Equalization or the Franchise Tax Board, whichever is applicable, that the licensee has not complied with the installment payment agreement. Upon receipt of this notice, the state governmental licensing entity shall immediately notify the licensee on a form prescribed by the state governmental licensing entity that the licensee's license will be suspended on a specific date, and this date shall be no longer than 30 days from the date the form is mailed. The licensee shall be further notified that the license will remain suspended until a new release is issued in accordance with this subdivision.

(k) The State Board of Equalization and the Franchise Tax Board may enter into interagency agreements with the state governmental licensing entities necessary to implement this section.

(*l*) Notwithstanding any other law, a state governmental licensing entity, with the approval of the appropriate department director or governing body, may impose a fee on a licensee whose license has been suspended pursuant to this section. The fee shall not exceed the amount necessary for the state governmental licensing entity to cover its costs in carrying out the provisions of this section. Fees imposed pursuant to this section shall be deposited in the fund in which other fees imposed by the state governmental licensing entity are deposited and shall be available to that entity upon appropriation in the annual Budget Act.

(m) The process described in subdivision (h) shall constitute the sole administrative remedy for contesting the issuance of a temporary license or the denial or suspension of a license under this section.

(n) Any state governmental licensing entity receiving an inquiry as to the licensed status of an applicant or licensee who has had a license denied or suspended under this section or who has been granted a temporary license under this section shall respond that the license was denied or suspended or the temporary license was issued only because the licensee appeared on a list of the 500 largest tax delinquencies pursuant to Section 7063 or 19195 of the Revenue and Taxation Code. Information collected pursuant to this section by any state agency, board, or department shall be subject to the Information Practices Act of 1977 (Chapter 1 (commencing with Section 1798) of Title 1.8 of Part 4 of Division 3 of the Civil Code). Any state governmental licensing entity that discloses on its internet website or other publication that the licensee has had a license denied or suspended under this section or has been granted a temporary license under this section shall prominently disclose, in bold and adjacent to the information regarding the status of the license, that the only reason the license was denied, suspended, or temporarily issued is because the licensee failed to pay taxes.

(o) Any rules and regulations issued pursuant to this section by any state agency, board, or department may be adopted as emergency regulations in accordance with the rulemaking provisions of the Administrative Procedure Act (Chapter 3.5 (commencing with Section 11340) of Part 1 of Division 3 of Title 2 of the Government Code). The adoption of these regulations shall be deemed an emergency and necessary for the immediate preservation of the public peace, health, and safety, or general welfare. The regulations shall become effective immediately upon filing with the Secretary of State.

(p) The State Board of Equalization, the Franchise Tax Board, and state governmental licensing entities, as appropriate, shall adopt regulations as necessary to implement this section.

(q)(1) Neither the state governmental licensing entity, nor any officer, employee, or agent, or former officer, employee, or agent of a state governmental licensing entity, may disclose or use any information obtained from the State Board of Equalization or the Franchise Tax Board, pursuant to this section, except to inform the public of the denial, refusal to renew, or suspension of a license or the issuance of a temporary license pursuant to this section. The release or other use of information received by a state governmental licensing entity pursuant to this section, except as authorized by this section, is punishable as a misdemeanor. This subdivision may not be interpreted to prevent the State Bar of California from filing a request with the Supreme Court of California to suspend a member of the bar pursuant to this section.

(2) A suspension of, or refusal to renew, a license or issuance of a temporary license pursuant to this section does not constitute denial or discipline of a licensee for purposes of any reporting requirements to the National Practitioner Data Bank and shall not be reported to the National Practitioner Data Bank or the Healthcare Integrity and Protection Data Bank.

(3) Upon release from the certified list, the suspension or revocation of the applicant's or licensee's license shall be purged from the state governmental

licensing entity's internet website or other publication within three business days. This paragraph shall not apply to the State Bar of California.

(r) If any provision of this section or the application thereof to any person or circumstance is held invalid, that invalidity shall not affect other provisions or applications of this section that can be given effect without the invalid provision or application, and to this end the provisions of this section are severable.

(s) All rights to review afforded by this section to an applicant shall also be afforded to a licensee.

(t) Unless otherwise provided in this section, the policies, practices, and procedures of a state governmental licensing entity with respect to license suspensions under this section shall be the same as those applicable with respect to suspensions pursuant to Section 17520 of the Family Code.

(u) No provision of this section shall be interpreted to allow a court to review and prevent the collection of taxes prior to the payment of those taxes in violation of the California Constitution.

(v) This section shall apply to any licensee whose name appears on a list of the 500 largest tax delinquencies pursuant to Section 7063 or 19195 of the Revenue and Taxation Code on or after July 1, 2012.

HISTORY:

Added Stats 2011 ch 455 § 3 (AB 1424), effective January 1, 2012. Amended Stats 2012 ch 327 § 1 (SB 937), effective January 1, 2013; Stats 2020 ch 312 § 9 (SB 1474), effective January 1, 2021.

§ 494.6. Suspension under Labor Code Section 244

(a) A business license regulated by this code may be subject to suspension or revocation if the licensee has been determined by the Labor Commissioner or the court to have violated subdivision (b) of Section 244 of the Labor Code and the court or Labor Commissioner has taken into consideration any harm such a suspension or revocation would cause to employees of the licensee, as well as the good faith efforts of the licensee to resolve any alleged violations after receiving notice.

(b) Notwithstanding subdivision (a), a licensee of an agency within the Department of Consumer Affairs who has been found by the Labor Commissioner or the court to have violated subdivision (b) of Section 244 of the Labor Code may be subject to disciplinary action by his or her respective licensing agency.

(c) An employer shall not be subject to suspension or revocation under this section for requiring a prospective or current employee to submit, within three business days of the first day of work for pay, an I-9 Employment Eligibility Verification form.

HISTORY:

Added Stats 2013 ch 577 § 1 (SB 666), effective January 1, 2014. Amended Stats 2014 ch 71 § 1 (SB 1304), effective January 1, 2015.

CHAPTER 4
PUBLIC REPROVALS

Section

495. Public reproval of licentiate or certificate holder for act constituting grounds for suspension or revocation of license or certificate; Proceedings.

HISTORY: Added Stats 1977 ch 886 § 1.

§ 495. Public reproval of licentiate or certificate holder for act constituting grounds for suspension or revocation of license or certificate; Proceedings

Notwithstanding any other provision of law, any entity authorized to issue a license or certificate pursuant to this code may publicly reprove a licentiate or certificate holder thereof, for any act that would constitute grounds to suspend or revoke a license or certificate. Any proceedings for public reproval, public reproval and suspension, or public reproval and revocation shall be conducted in accordance with Chapter 5 (commencing with Section 11500) of Part 1 of Division 3 of Title 2 of the Government Code, or, in the case of a licensee or certificate holder under the jurisdiction of the State Department of Health Services, in accordance with Section 100171 of the Health and Safety Code.

HISTORY:
Added Stats 1977 ch 886 § 1. Amended Stats 1997 ch 220 § 2 (SB 68), effective August 4, 1997.

CHAPTER 5

EXAMINATION SECURITY

Section

496. Grounds for denial, suspension, or revocation of license.
498. Fraud, deceit or misrepresentation as grounds for action against license.
499. Action against license based on licentiate's actions regarding application of another.

HISTORY: Added Stats 1983 ch 95 § 2.

§ 496. Grounds for denial, suspension, or revocation of license

A board may deny, suspend, revoke, or otherwise restrict a license on the ground that an applicant or licensee has violated Section 123 pertaining to subversion of licensing examinations.

HISTORY:
Added Stats 1989 ch 1022 § 3.

§ 498. Fraud, deceit or misrepresentation as grounds for action against license

A board may revoke, suspend, or otherwise restrict a license on the ground that the licensee secured the license by fraud, deceit, or knowing misrepresentation of a material fact or by knowingly omitting to state a material fact.

HISTORY:
Added Stats 1992 ch 1289 § 8 (AB 2743).

§ 499. Action against license based on licentiate's actions regarding application of another

A board may revoke, suspend, or otherwise restrict a license on the ground that the licensee, in support of another person's application for license, knowingly made a false statement of a material fact or knowingly omitted to state a material fact to the board regarding the application.

HISTORY:
Added Stats 1992 ch 1289 § 9 (AB 2743).

DIVISION 2
HEALING ARTS

Chapter
1. General Provisions.
1.5. Exemption from Licensure.
3. Clinical Laboratory Technology.
5. Medicine.
6.6. Psychologists.
9. Pharmacy.
15. Telephone Medical Advice Services.

CHAPTER 1
GENERAL PROVISIONS

Article
1.5. Advocacy for Appropriate Health Care.
4. Frauds of Medical Records.
7. Nursing.
7.5. Health Care Practitioners.
10. Federal Personnel and Tribal Health Programs.
10.5. Unprofessional Conduct.
11. Professional Reporting.
12. Insurance Fraud.
12.5. Mental Illness or Physical Illness.

HISTORY: Enacted Stats 1937 ch 399.

ARTICLE 1.5
ADVOCACY FOR APPROPRIATE HEALTH CARE

Section
510. Protection against retaliation for physicians who "advocate for medically appropriate health care".

HISTORY: Added Stats 1994 ch 1119 § 1.

§ 510. Protection against retaliation for physicians who "advocate for medically appropriate health care"

(a) The purpose of this section is to provide protection against retaliation for health care practitioners who advocate for appropriate health care for their patients pursuant to Wickline v. State of California 192 Cal. App. 3d 1630.

(b) It is the public policy of the State of California that a health care practitioner be encouraged to advocate for appropriate health care for his or her patients. For purposes of this section, "to advocate for appropriate health care" means to appeal a payer's decision to deny payment for a service pursuant to the reasonable grievance or appeal procedure established by a medical group, independent practice association, preferred provider organization, foundation, hospital medical staff and governing body, or payer, or to protest a decision, policy, or practice that the health care practitioner, consistent with that degree of learning and skill ordinarily possessed by reputable health care practitioners with the same license or certification and practicing according to the applicable legal standard of care, reasonably believes impairs the health care practitioner's ability to provide appropriate health care to his or her patients.

(c) The application and rendering by any individual, partnership, corporation, or other organization of a decision to terminate an employment or other contractual relationship with or otherwise penalize a health care practitioner principally for advocating for appropriate health care consistent with that degree of learning and skill ordinarily possessed by reputable health care practitioners with the same license or certification and practicing according to the applicable legal standard of care violates the public policy of this state.

(d) This section shall not be construed to prohibit a payer from making a determination not to pay for a particular medical treatment or service, or the services of a type of health care practitioner, or to prohibit a medical group, independent practice association, preferred provider organization, foundation, hospital medical staff, hospital governing body acting pursuant to Section 809.05, or payer from enforcing reasonable peer review or utilization review protocols or determining whether a health care practitioner has complied with those protocols.

(e)(1) Except as provided in paragraph (2), appropriate health care in a hospital licensed pursuant to Section 1250 of the Health and Safety Code shall be defined by the appropriate hospital committee and approved by the hospital medical staff and the governing body, consistent with that degree of learning and skill ordinarily possessed by reputable health care practitioners with the same license or certification and practicing according to the applicable legal standard of care.

(2) To the extent the issue is under the jurisdiction of the medical staff and its committees, appropriate health care in a hospital licensed pursuant to Section 1250 of the Health and Safety Code shall be defined by the hospital medical staff and approved by the governing body, consistent with that degree of learning and skill ordinarily possessed by reputable health care practitioners with the same license or certification and practicing according to the applicable legal standard of care.

(f) Nothing in this section shall be construed to prohibit the governing body of a hospital from taking disciplinary actions against a health care practitioner as authorized by Sections 809.05, 809.4, and 809.5.

(g) Nothing in this section shall be construed to prohibit the appropriate licensing authority from taking disciplinary actions against a health care practitioner.

(h) For purposes of this section, "health care practitioner" means a person who is described in subdivision (f) of Section 900 and who is either (1) a licentiate as defined in Section 805, or (2) a party to a contract with a payer whose decision, policy, or practice is subject to the advocacy described in subdivision (b), or (3) an individual designated in a contract with a payer whose decision, policy, or practice is subject to the advocacy described in subdivision (b), where the individual is granted the right to appeal denials of payment or authorization for treatment under the contract.

(i) Nothing in this section shall be construed to revise or expand the scope of practice of any health care practitioner, or to revise or expand the types of health care practitioners who are authorized to obtain medical staff privileges or to submit claims for reimbursement to payers.

(j) The protections afforded health care practitioners by this section shall be in addition to the protections available under any other law of this state.

HISTORY:
Added Stats 1994 ch 1119 § 1 (AB 3390).

ARTICLE 4
FRAUDS OF MEDICAL RECORDS

Section
580. Sale or barter of degree, certificate, or transcript.
581. Purchase or fraudulent alteration of diplomas or other writings.
582. Use of illegally obtained, altered, or counterfeit diploma, certificate, or transcript.
583. False statements in documents or writings.
584. Violation of examination security; Impersonation.
585. Punishment.

HISTORY: Enacted Stats 1937 ch 399.

§ 580. Sale or barter of degree, certificate, or transcript

No person, company, or association shall sell or barter or offer to sell or barter any medical degree, podiatric degree, or osteopathic degree, or chiropractic degree, or any other degree which is required for licensure, certification, or registration under this division, or any degree, certificate, transcript, or any other writing, made or purporting to be made pursuant to any laws regulating the licensing and registration or issuing of a certificate to physicians and surgeons, podiatrists, osteopathic physicians, chiropractors, persons lawfully engaged in any other system or mode of treating the sick or afflicted, or to any other person licensed, certified, or registered under this division.

HISTORY:
Enacted Stats 1937. Amended Stats 1939 ch 269 § 1; Stats 1961 ch 215 § 1; Stats 1986 ch 220 § 2, effective June 30, 1986.

§ 581. Purchase or fraudulent alteration of diplomas or other writings

No person, company, or association shall purchase or procure by barter or by any unlawful means or method, or have in possession any diploma, certificate, transcript, or any other writing with intent that it shall be used as evidence of the holder's qualifications to practice as a physician and surgeon, osteopathic physician, podiatrist, any other system or mode of treating the sick or afflicted, as provided in the Medical Practice Act, Chapter 5 (commencing with Section 2000), or to practice as any other licentiate under this division or in any fraud of the law regulating this practice or, shall with fraudulent intent, alter in a material regard, any such diploma, certificate, transcript, or any other writing.

HISTORY:

Enacted Stats 1937. Amended Stats 1937 ch 446; Stats 1961 ch 215 § 1.5; Stats 1984 ch 144 § 5; Stats 1986 ch 220 § 3, effective June 30, 1986.

§ 582. Use of illegally obtained, altered, or counterfeit diploma, certificate, or transcript

No person, company, or association shall use or attempt to use any diploma, certificate, transcript, or any other writing which has been purchased, fraudulently issued, illegally obtained, counterfeited, or materially altered, either as a certificate or as to character or color of certificate, to practice as a physician and surgeon, podiatrist, osteopathic physician, or a chiropractor, or to practice any other system or mode of treating the sick or afflicted, as provided in the Medical Practice Act, Chapter 5 (commencing with Section 2000) or to practice as any other licentiate under this division.

HISTORY:

Enacted Stats 1937. Amended Stats 1961 ch 215 § 2; Stats 1984 ch 144 § 6; Stats 1986 ch 220 § 4, effective June 30, 1986.

§ 583. False statements in documents or writings

No person shall in any document or writing required of an applicant for examination, license, certificate, or registration under this division, the Osteopathic Initiative Act, or the Chiropractic Initiative Act, willfully make a false statement in a material regard.

HISTORY:

Enacted Stats 1937. Amended Stats 1984 ch 144 § 7; Stats 1986 ch 220 § 5, effective June 30, 1986.

§ 584. Violation of examination security; Impersonation

No person shall violate the security of any examination, as defined in subdivision (a) of Section 123, or impersonate, attempt to impersonate, or solicit the impersonation of, another in any examination for a license, certificate, or registration to practice as provided in this division, the Osteopathic Initiative Act, or the Chiropractic Initiative Act, or under any other law providing for the regulation of any other system or method of treating the sick or afflicted in this state.

HISTORY:

Enacted Stats 1937. Amended Stats 1984 ch 144 § 8; Stats 1986 ch 220 § 6, effective June 30, 1986; Stats 1989 ch 1022 § 5.

§ 585. Punishment

Any person, company, or association violating the provisions of this article is guilty of a felony and upon conviction thereof shall be punishable by a fine of not less than two thousand dollars ($2,000) nor more than six thousand dollars

($6,000), or by imprisonment pursuant to subdivision (h) of Section 1170 of the Penal Code. The enforcement remedies provided under this article are not exclusive and shall not preclude the use of any other criminal, civil, or administrative remedy.

HISTORY:
Enacted Stats 1937. Amended Stats 1976 ch 1139 § 1, operative July 1, 1977; Stats 1983 ch 1092 § 2, effective September 27, 1983, operative January 1, 1984; Stats 1986 ch 220 § 7, effective June 30, 1986; Stats 2011 ch 15 § 2 (AB 109), effective April 4, 2011, operative October 1, 2011.

ARTICLE 7
NURSING

Section
675. Unaccredited instructional courses.
676. Applicability of article.
677. Inspection of records.
678. Failure to give notice as voiding contract.
679. Violations.

HISTORY: Added Stats 1959 ch 1490 § 1.

§ 675. Unaccredited instructional courses

Every person, firm, association, partnership, or corporation offering a course of instruction in any type of nursing, including vocational nursing or practical nursing, which course of instruction is not accredited by the Board of Registered Nursing or by the Board of Vocational Nursing and Psychiatric Technicians and completion of which will not qualify a person to take any examination given by either board shall notify an applicant for admission thereto that the course of instruction is not accredited by either board and that completion thereof will not qualify the person to take any examination given by either board.

The notice required by this section shall be in writing in at least 12-point boldface type, and in no event less than two points larger than the type in any other portion of the notice or contract, and shall be given to an applicant prior to the signing of any contract by the applicant or, if no contract is signed, prior to the making of any deposit or other payment by the applicant.

If an applicant is required to sign a contract in order to enroll in the course of instruction, the notice required by this section shall be contained in the contract directly above the place for the applicant's signature.

HISTORY:
Added Stats 1959 ch 1490 § 1. Amended Stats 1978 ch 1161 § 20; Stats 1997 ch 759 § 8 (SB 827).

§ 676. Applicability of article

The provisions contained in this article shall not apply to inservice training programs given in institutions for the purpose of qualifying persons to work therein, to public schools, to private schools or institutions offering advanced nursing education to registered nurses or vocational nurses licensed in the United States, or to schools conducted by any recognized church or denomination for the purpose of training the adherents of such church or denomination in the care of the sick in accordance with its religious tenets.

HISTORY:
Added Stats 1959 ch 1490 § 1.

§ 677. Inspection of records

Every person, firm, association, partnership, or corporation subject to the provisions of this article shall maintain records for at least three years, which records shall be open to inspection by investigators of the Division of Investigation of the department and by peace officers acting in their official capacity.

The records shall include the names and address of the persons admitted to the course of instruction and a copy of any written contract signed by such a person or, if no contract is signed, a copy of the written notice given to such person.

A correspondence school whose home office is located outside of this state need maintain the foregoing records only for persons residing in this state.

HISTORY:
Added Stats 1959 ch 1490 § 1. Amended Stats 1971 ch 716 § 26.

§ 678. Failure to give notice as voiding contract

The failure to give the notice required by this article shall make any contract entered into between the parties null and void.

HISTORY:
Added Stats 1959 ch 1490 § 1.

§ 679. Violations

Any person, firm, association, partnership, or corporation who violates this article is guilty of a misdemeanor.

HISTORY:
Added Stats 1959 ch 1490 § 1.

ARTICLE 7.5
HEALTH CARE PRACTITIONERS

Section
680. Health care practitioner's disclosure of name and license status.
681. Securing specimens; Marking containers; Violations; "Locked container".
683. Reporting name and license number of licensee prohibited from practicing.
684. Notice of practice of stem cell therapy not approved by FDA.
685. Citation of health care practitioner in default of education loan [Repealed].
686. Providing services via telehealth.

HISTORY: Added Stats 1998 ch 1013 § 1.

§ 680. Health care practitioner's disclosure of name and license status

(a) Except as otherwise provided in this section, a health care practitioner shall disclose, while working, his or her name and practitioner's license status, as granted by this state, on a name tag in at least 18-point type. A health care practitioner in a practice or an office, whose license is prominently displayed, may opt to not wear a name tag. If a health care practitioner or a licensed clinical social worker is working in a psychiatric setting or in a setting that is not licensed by the state, the employing entity or agency shall have the discretion to make an exception from the name tag requirement for individual safety or therapeutic concerns. In the interest of public safety and consumer awareness, it shall be unlawful for any person to use the title "nurse" in reference to himself or herself and in any capacity, except for an individual who is a registered nurse or a licensed vocational nurse, or as otherwise provided in Section 2800. Nothing in this section shall prohibit a certified nurse assistant from using his or her title.

(b) Facilities licensed by the State Department of Social Services, the State Department of Public Health, or the State Department of Health Care Services shall develop and implement policies to ensure that health care practitioners providing care in those facilities are in compliance with subdivision (a). The State Department of Social Services, the State Department of Public Health, and the State Department of Health Care Services shall verify through periodic inspections that the policies required pursuant to subdivision (a) have been developed and implemented by the respective licensed facilities.

(c) For purposes of this article, "health care practitioner" means any person who engages in acts that are the subject of licensure or regulation under this division or under any initiative act referred to in this division.

HISTORY:

Added Stats 1998 ch 1013 § 1 (AB 1439). Amended Stats 1999 ch 411 § 1 (AB 1433); Stats 2000 ch 135 § 2 (AB 2539); Stats 2012 ch 34 § 2 (SB 1009), effective June 27, 2012; Stats 2013 ch 23 § 1 (AB 82), effective June 27, 2013.

§ 681. Securing specimens; Marking containers; Violations; "Locked container"

(a) Commencing July 1, 2000, every person licensed pursuant to this division who collects human biological specimens for clinical testing or examination, shall secure, or ensure that his or her employees, agents, or contractors secure, those specimens in a locked container when those specimens are placed in a public location outside of the custodial control of the licensee, or his or her employees, agents, or contractors.

(b) Containers used for human biological specimens put into use on or after January 1, 2001, shall be marked "Caution: Biohazardous Material – Please Do Not Touch or Handle," or words of similar meaning.

(c) This section shall not apply where the biological specimens have been placed in the mail in compliance with all applicable laws and regulations.

(d) The licensing board having jurisdiction of the licensee may impose appropriate sanctions for violations of this section, including, if otherwise authorized by the licensing act, the imposition of a fine not to exceed one thousand dollars ($1,000).

(e) As used in this section, "locked container" means a secure container that is fully enclosed and locked by a padlock, key lock, combination lock, or similar locking device.

HISTORY:
Added Stats 1999 ch 748 § 1 (SB 765).

§ 683. Reporting name and license number of licensee prohibited from practicing

(a) A board shall report, within 10 working days, to the State Department of Health Care Services the name and license number of a person whose license has been revoked, suspended, surrendered, made inactive by the licensee, or placed in another category that prohibits the licensee from practicing their profession. The purpose of the reporting requirement is to prevent reimbursement by the state for Medi-Cal and Denti-Cal services provided after the cancellation of a provider's professional license.

(b) "Board," as used in this section, means the Dental Board of California, the Medical Board of California, the Board of Psychology, the California State Board of Optometry, the California State Board of Pharmacy, the Osteopathic Medical Board of California, the State Board of Chiropractic Examiners, the Board of Behavioral Sciences, the California Board of Podiatric Medicine, and the California Board of Occupational Therapy.

(c) This section shall become operative on January 1, 2015.

HISTORY:
Added Stats 2012 ch 154 § 2 (AB 367), effective January 1, 2013, operative January 1, 2015. Amended Stats 2017 ch 775 § 8 (SB 798), effective January 1, 2018; Stats 2021 ch 630 § 13 (AB 1534), effective January 1, 2022.

§ 684. Notice of practice of stem cell therapy not approved by FDA

(a) For the purpose of this section:

(1) "FDA" means the United States Food and Drug Administration.

(2) "HCT/Ps" means human cells, tissues, or cellular or tissue-based products, as defined in Section 1271.3 of Title 21 of the Code of Federal Regulations, as amended August 31, 2016, as published in the Federal Register (81 Fed. Reg. 60223).

(3) "Stem cell therapy" means a therapy involving the use of HCT/Ps, but shall not include a therapy involving HCT/Ps that meets the criteria set out in Section 1271.10 of Title 21 of the Code of Federal Regulations, as amended May 25, 2004, as published in the Federal Register (69 Fed. Reg. 29829), or that qualifies for any of the exceptions described in Section 1271.15 of Title 21 of the Code of Federal Regulations, as amended May 25, 2004, as published in the Federal Register (69 Fed. Reg. 29829).

(b)(1) A health care practitioner licensed under this division who performs a stem cell therapy that is subject to FDA regulation, but is not FDA-approved, shall communicate to a patient seeking stem cell therapy the following information in English:

THIS NOTICE MUST BE PROVIDED TO YOU UNDER CALIFORNIA LAW. This health care practitioner performs one or more stem cell therapies that have not been approved by the United States Food and Drug Administration. You are encouraged to consult with your primary care physician prior to undergoing a stem cell therapy.

(2) The information in paragraph (1) shall be communicated to the patient in all of the following ways:

(A) In a prominent display in an area visible to patients in the health care practitioner's office and posted conspicuously in the entrance of the health care practitioner's office. These notices shall be at least eight and one-half inches by 11 inches and written in no less than 40-point type.

(B) Prior to providing the initial stem cell therapy, a health care practitioner shall provide the patient with the notice described in paragraph (1) in writing. The notice shall be at least eight and one-half inches by 11 inches and written in no less than 40-point type.

(c) This section does not apply to a health care practitioner licensed under this division who has obtained approval or clearance for an investigational new drug, or an investigational device exemption, from the FDA for the use of HCT/Ps.

(d)(1) The licensing board having jurisdiction of the health care practitioner may cite and fine the health care practitioner, not to exceed one thousand dollars ($1,000) per violation of this section.

(2) No citation shall be issued and no fine shall be assessed upon the first complaint against a health care practitioner who violates this section.

(3) Upon a second or subsequent violation of this section, a citation and administrative fine not to exceed one thousand dollars ($1,000) per violation may be assessed.

(e) The Medical Board of California shall indicate in its annual report, commencing with the 2018-19 annual report, all of the following with regard to licensees who provide stem cell therapies:

(1) The number of complaints received.

(2) Any disciplinary actions taken.

(3) Any administrative actions taken.

HISTORY:

Added Stats 2017 ch 428 § 1 (SB 512), effective January 1, 2018. Amended Stats 2018 ch 424 § 1 (SB 1495), effective January 1, 2019.

§ 685. Citation of health care practitioner in default of education loan [Repealed]

HISTORY:

Added Stats 2002 ch 683 § 1 (SB 2019), effective January 1, 2003, operative July 1, 2003. Repealed Stats 2017 ch 195 § 1 (AB 508), effective January 1, 2018.

§ 686. Providing services via telehealth

A health care practitioner licensed under Division 2 (commencing with Section 500) providing services via telehealth shall be subject to the requirements and definitions set forth in Section 2290.5, to the practice act relating to his or her licensed profession, and to the regulations adopted by a board pursuant to that practice act.

HISTORY:

Added Stats 2012 ch 782 § 1 (AB 1733), effective January 1, 2013.

ARTICLE 10

FEDERAL PERSONNEL AND TRIBAL HEALTH PROGRAMS

Section

715. Licenses to practice in state.
716. Denial of license; Disciplinary action against holder of state license.
717. Construction of article.
719. Employment of health care practitioner licensed in another state by tribal health program (First of two).
719. Certain persons employed by a tribal health program exempt from licensing requirement (Second of two).

HISTORY: Added Stats 1969 ch 1592 § 1. Heading amended Stats 1983 ch 239 § 1. The heading of Article 10, which formerly read "Federal Personnel," amended to read as above by Stats 2012 ch 119 § 1 (AB 1896), effective January 1, 2013.

§ 715. Licenses to practice in state

Unless otherwise required by federal law or regulation, no board under this division which licenses dentists, physicians and surgeons, podiatrists, or nurses may require a person to obtain or maintain any license to practice a profession or render services in the State of California if one of the following applies:

(a) The person practicing a profession or rendering services does so exclusively as an employee of a department, bureau, office, division, or similarly constituted agency of the federal government, and provides medical services exclusively on a federal reservation or at any facility wholly supported by and maintained by the United States government.

(b) The person practicing a profession or rendering services does so solely pursuant to a contract with the federal government on a federal reservation or at any facility wholly supported and maintained by the United States government.

(c) The person practicing a profession or rendering services does so pursuant to, or as a part of a program or project conducted or administered by a department, bureau, office, division, or similarly constituted agency of the federal government which by federal statute expressly exempts persons practicing a profession or rendering services as part of the program or project from state laws requiring licensure.

HISTORY:

Added Stats 1983 ch 239 § 2. Amended Stats 1986 ch 220 § 7.5, effective June 30, 1986.

§ 716. Denial of license; Disciplinary action against holder of state license

Notwithstanding any other provision of law, a board under this division may deny issuance of a license to an applicant or take disciplinary action against the holder of a California license for acts or omissions committed by the applicant or licensee in the course of professional practice or rendering services described in Section 715 if both of the following apply:

(a) The acts or omissions committed by the applicant or licensee constituted grounds for denial or discipline pursuant to the laws of this state governing licensees or applicants for licensure for the profession or vocation in question.

(b) The acts or omissions constituting the basis for denial or discipline by the agency were not authorized, exempted or rendered inconsistent by federal statute.

HISTORY:

Added Stats 1983 ch 239 § 3.

§ 717. Construction of article

This article is not intended to address the scope of practice of a dentist, physician and surgeon, or nurse licensed under this division, and nothing in this article shall be construed to restrict, expand, alter, or modify the existing scope of practice established by federal statute or regulation.

HISTORY:

Added Stats 1983 ch 239 § 4.

§ 719. Employment of health care practitioner licensed in another state by tribal health program (First of two)

(a) A person who is licensed as a health care practitioner in any other state and is employed by a tribal health program, as defined in Section 1603 of Title 25 of the United States Code, shall be exempt from any licensing requirement described in this division with respect to acts authorized under the person's license where the tribal health program performs the services described in the contract or compact of the tribal health program under the Indian Self-Determination and Education Assistance Act (25 U.S.C. Sec. 450 et seq.).

(b) For purposes of this section, "health care practitioner" means any person who engages in acts that are the subject of licensure or regulation under the law of any other state.

HISTORY:

Added Stats 2012 ch 119 § 2 (AB 1896), effective January 1, 2013.

§ 719. Certain persons employed by a tribal health program exempt from licensing requirement (Second of two)

(a) A person who possesses a current, valid license as a health care practitioner in any other state and is employed by a tribal health program, as defined in Section 1603 of Title 25 of the United States Code, shall be exempt from any licensing requirement described in this division with respect to acts authorized under the person's license where the tribal health program performs the services described in the contract or compact of the tribal health program under the Indian Self-Determination and Education Assistance Act (25 U.S.C. Sec. 450 et seq.).

(b) For purposes of this section, "health care practitioner" means any person who engages in acts that are the subject of licensure or regulation under the law of any other state.

HISTORY:
Added Stats 2012 ch 799 § 1 (SB 1575), effective January 1, 2013.

ARTICLE 10.5
UNPROFESSIONAL CONDUCT

Section
726. Commission of act of sexual abuse or misconduct with patient or client.
730.5. Acupuncture without license.

HISTORY: Added Stats 1979 ch 348 § 2.

§ 726. Commission of act of sexual abuse or misconduct with patient or client

(a) The commission of any act of sexual abuse, misconduct, or relations with a patient, client, or customer constitutes unprofessional conduct and grounds for disciplinary action for any person licensed under this division or under any initiative act referred to in this division.

(b) This section shall not apply to consensual sexual contact between a licensee and his or her spouse or person in an equivalent domestic relationship when that licensee provides medical treatment, other than psychotherapeutic treatment, to his or her spouse or person in an equivalent domestic relationship.

HISTORY:
Added Stats 1979 ch 955 § 1, as B & P C § 730. Renumbered by Stats 1981 ch 714 § 3. Amended Stats 1983 ch 928 § 1; Stats 1993 ch 1072 § 1 (SB 743); Stats 2015 ch 510 § 3 (AB 179), effective January 1, 2016.

§ 730.5. Acupuncture without license

(a) It is unprofessional conduct and a crime, as provided in Section 4935, for a physician and surgeon, osteopathic physician, dentist, or podiatrist to direct or supervise the performance of acupuncture involving the application of a needle to the body of a human being by a person licensed under this division who is not licensed pursuant to the Acupuncture Licensure Act established by Chapter 12 (commencing with Section 4925).

(b) It is unprofessional conduct and a crime, as provided in Section 4935, for a person licensed under this division who is not licensed pursuant to the Acupuncture Licensure Act established by Chapter 12 (commencing with Section 4925) to perform acupuncture involving the application of a needle to the body of a human being at the direction or under the supervision of a physician and surgeon, osteopathic physician, dentist, or podiatrist.

HISTORY:
Added Stats 1997 ch 400 § 1 (AB 174), as B & P C § 730. Amended and renumbered by Stats 1999 ch 83 § 1 (SB 966).

ARTICLE 11
PROFESSIONAL REPORTING

Section

800. Central files of licensees' individual historical records.
801. Insurers' reports of malpractice settlements or arbitration awards; Insured's written consent to settlement.
801.01. Report of settlement of arbitration award over a specified amount in case of alleged negligence, error, or omission in practice or the licensee's rendering of unauthorized professional services; Procedure.
801.1. Report of settlement or arbitration award where state or local government acts as self-insurer in cases of negligence, error, omission in practice, or rendering of unauthorized services resulting in death or personal injury.
802. Reports of malpractice settlements or arbitration awards involving uninsured licensees; Penalties for noncompliance.
803. Report of crime or liability for death or injury on part of specified licensees to licensing agency.
804. Form and content of reports.
806. Statistical reports and recommendations to Legislature.

HISTORY: Added Stats 2d Ex Sess 1975 ch 1 § 2.3. Former Article 11, consisting of §§ 800–803, relating to reporting of malpractice actions, was added Stats 1970 ch 1111 § 1, operative January 1, 1971, and repealed Stats 2d Ex Sess 1975 ch 1 § 2.2.

§ 800. Central files of licensees' individual historical records

(a) The Medical Board of California, the Podiatric Medical Board of California, the Board of Psychology, the Dental Board of California, the Dental Hygiene Board of California, the Osteopathic Medical Board of California, the State Board of Chiropractic Examiners, the Board of Registered Nursing, the Board of Vocational Nursing and Psychiatric Technicians of the State of California, the California State Board of Optometry, the Veterinary Medical Board, the Board of Behavioral Sciences, the Physical Therapy Board of California, the California State Board of Pharmacy, the Speech-Language Pathology and Audiology and Hearing Aid Dispensers Board, the California Board of Occupational Therapy, the Acupuncture Board, and the Physician Assistant Board shall each separately create and maintain a central file of the names of all persons who hold a license, certificate, or similar authority from that board. Each central file shall be created and maintained to provide an individual historical record for each licensee with respect to the following information:

(1) Any conviction of a crime in this or any other state that constitutes unprofessional conduct pursuant to the reporting requirements of Section 803.

(2) Any judgment or settlement requiring the licensee or the licensee's insurer to pay any amount of damages in excess of three thousand dollars ($3,000) for any claim that injury or death was proximately caused by the licensee's negligence, error, or omission in practice, or by rendering unauthorized professional services, pursuant to the reporting requirements of Section 801 or 802.

(3) Any public complaints for which provision is made pursuant to subdivision (b).

(4) Disciplinary information reported pursuant to Section 805, including any additional exculpatory or explanatory statements submitted by the licentiate pursuant to subdivision (f) of Section 805. If a court finds, in a final judgment, that the peer review resulting in the 805 report was conducted in bad faith and the licensee who is the subject of the report notifies the board of that finding, the board shall include that finding in the central file. For purposes of this paragraph, "peer review" has the same meaning as defined in Section 805.

(5) Information reported pursuant to Section 805.01, including any explanatory or exculpatory information submitted by the licensee pursuant to subdivision (b) of that section.

(b)(1) Each board shall prescribe and promulgate forms on which members of the public and other licensees or certificate holders may file written complaints to the board alleging any act of misconduct in, or connected with, the performance of professional services by the licensee.

(2) If a board, or division thereof, a committee, or a panel has failed to act upon a complaint or report within five years, or has found that the complaint or report is without merit, the central file shall be purged of information relating to the complaint or report.

(3) Notwithstanding this subdivision, the Board of Psychology, the Board of Behavioral Sciences, and the Respiratory Care Board of California shall maintain complaints or reports as long as each board deems necessary.

(c)(1) The contents of any central file that are not public records under any other provision of law shall be confidential except that the licensee involved, or the licensee's counsel or representative, may inspect and have copies made of the licensee's complete file except for the provision that may disclose the identity of an information source. For the purposes of this section, a board may protect an information source by providing a copy of the material with only those deletions necessary to protect the identity of the source or by providing a summary of the substance of the material. Whichever method is used, the board shall ensure that full disclosure is made to the subject of any personal information that could reasonably in any way reflect or convey anything detrimental, disparaging, or threatening to a licensee's reputation, rights, benefits, privileges, or qualifications, or be used by a board to make a determination that would affect a licensee's rights, benefits, privileges, or qualifications. The information required to be disclosed pursuant to Section 803.1 shall not be considered among the contents of a central file for the purposes of this subdivision.

(2) The licensee may, but is not required to, submit any additional exculpatory or explanatory statement or other information that the board shall include in the central file.

(3) Each board may permit any law enforcement or regulatory agency when required for an investigation of unlawful activity or for licensing, certification, or regulatory purposes to inspect and have copies made of that licensee's file, unless the disclosure is otherwise prohibited by law.

(4) These disclosures shall effect no change in the confidential status of these records.

HISTORY:

Added Stats 1975 2d Ex Sess ch 1 § 2.3. Amended Stats 1975 2d Ex Sess ch 2 § 1.005, effective September 24, 1975, operative December 12, 1975; Stats 1976 ch 1185 § 1; Stats 1980 ch 1313 § 1;

Stats 1987 ch 721 § 1; Stats 1989 ch 354 § 1, ch 886 § 10 (ch 354 prevails); Stats 1991 ch 359 § 5 (AB 1332), ch 1091 § 1 (AB 1487) (ch 359 prevails); Stats 1994 ch 26 § 15.5 (AB 1807), effective March 30, 1994; Stats 1995 ch 60 § 6 (SB 42), effective July 6, 1995, and ch 5 § 1 (SB 158), ch 708 § 1.5 (SB 609), ch 796 § 1 (SB 45) (ch 708 prevails), effective January 1, 1996; Stats 1997 ch 759 § 9 (SB 827); Stats 1999 ch 252 § 1 (AB 352), ch 655 § 2 (SB 1308); Stats 2002 ch 1085 § 1 (SB 1950), ch 1150 § 2.5 (SB 1955); Stats 2006 ch 659 § 2 (SB 1475), effective January 1, 2007; Stats 2009 ch 308 § 9 (SB 819), effective January 1, 2010; Stats 2010 ch 505 § 1 (SB 700), effective January 1, 2011; Stats 2012 ch 332 § 1 (SB 1236), effective January 1, 2013; Stats 2015 ch 426 § 5 (SB 800), effective January 1, 2016; Stats 2017 ch 775 § 9 (SB 798), effective January 1, 2018; Stats 2018 ch 858 § 2 (SB 1482), effective January 1, 2019; Stats 2019 ch 849 § 1 (SB 425), effective January 1, 2020; Stats 2021 ch 630 § 14 (AB 1534), effective January 1, 2022.

§ 801. Insurers' reports of malpractice settlements or arbitration awards; Insured's written consent to settlement

(a) Except as provided in Section 801.01 and subdivisions (b), (c), (d), and (e) of this section, every insurer providing professional liability insurance to a person who holds a license, certificate, or similar authority from or under any agency specified in subdivision (a) of Section 800 shall send a complete report to that agency as to any settlement or arbitration award over three thousand dollars ($3,000) of a claim or action for damages for death or personal injury caused by that person's negligence, error, or omission in practice, or by his or her rendering of unauthorized professional services. The report shall be sent within 30 days after the written settlement agreement has been reduced to writing and signed by all parties thereto or within 30 days after service of the arbitration award on the parties.

(b) Every insurer providing professional liability insurance to a person licensed pursuant to Chapter 13 (commencing with Section 4980), Chapter 14 (commencing with Section 4990), or Chapter 16 (commencing with Section 4999.10) shall send a complete report to the Board of Behavioral Sciences as to any settlement or arbitration award over ten thousand dollars ($10,000) of a claim or action for damages for death or personal injury caused by that person's negligence, error, or omission in practice, or by his or her rendering of unauthorized professional services. The report shall be sent within 30 days after the written settlement agreement has been reduced to writing and signed by all parties thereto or within 30 days after service of the arbitration award on the parties.

(c) Every insurer providing professional liability insurance to a dentist licensed pursuant to Chapter 4 (commencing with Section 1600) shall send a complete report to the Dental Board of California as to any settlement or arbitration award over ten thousand dollars ($10,000) of a claim or action for damages for death or personal injury caused by that person's negligence, error, or omission in practice, or rendering of unauthorized professional services. The report shall be sent within 30 days after the written settlement agreement has been reduced to writing and signed by all parties thereto or within 30 days after service of the arbitration award on the parties.

(d) Every insurer providing liability insurance to a veterinarian licensed pursuant to Chapter 11 (commencing with Section 4800) shall send a complete report to the Veterinary Medical Board of any settlement or arbitration award over ten thousand dollars ($10,000) of a claim or action for damages for death or injury caused by that person's negligence, error, or omission in practice, or rendering of unauthorized professional service. The report shall be sent within

30 days after the written settlement agreement has been reduced to writing and signed by all parties thereto or within 30 days after service of the arbitration award on the parties.

(e) Every insurer providing professional liability insurance to a person licensed pursuant to Chapter 6 (commencing with Section 2700) shall send a complete report to the Board of Registered Nursing as to any settlement or arbitration award over ten thousand dollars ($10,000) of a claim or action for damages for death or personal injury caused by that person's negligence, error, or omission in practice, or by his or her rendering of unauthorized professional services. The report shall be sent within 30 days after the written settlement agreement has been reduced to writing and signed by all parties thereto or within 30 days after service of the arbitration award on the parties.

(f) The insurer shall notify the claimant, or if the claimant is represented by counsel, the insurer shall notify the claimant's attorney, that the report required by subdivision (a), (b), or (c) has been sent to the agency. If the attorney has not received this notice within 45 days after the settlement was reduced to writing and signed by all of the parties, the arbitration award was served on the parties, or the date of entry of the civil judgment, the attorney shall make the report to the agency.

(g) Notwithstanding any other provision of law, no insurer shall enter into a settlement without the written consent of the insured, except that this prohibition shall not void any settlement entered into without that written consent. The requirement of written consent shall only be waived by both the insured and the insurer.

(h) For purposes of this section, "insurer" means the following:

(1) The insurer providing professional liability insurance to the licensee.

(2) The licensee, or his or her counsel, if the licensee does not possess professional liability insurance.

(3) A state or local governmental agency, including, but not limited to, a joint powers authority, that self-insures the licensee. As used in this paragraph, "state governmental agency" includes, but is not limited to, the University of California.

HISTORY:

Added Stats 1975 2d Ex Sess ch 1 § 2.3. Amended Stats 1979 ch 923 § 1; Stats 1989 ch 398 § 1, ch 886 § 11 (ch 398 prevails); Stats 1991 ch 359 § 6 (AB 1332), ch 1091 § 2 (AB 1487) (ch 359 prevails); Stats 1994 ch 468 § 1 (AB 559), ch 1206 § 8 (SB 1775); Stats 1995 ch 5 § 2 (SB 158); Stats 1997 ch 359 § 1 (AB 103); Stats 2002 ch 1085 § 2 (SB 1950); Stats 2004 ch 467 § 1 (SB 1548); Stats 2006 ch 223 § 3 (SB 1438) (ch 223 prevails), effective January 1, 2007, ch 538 § 2 (SB 1852); Stats 2009 ch 308 § 10 (SB 819), effective January 1, 2010; Stats 2011 ch 381 § 6 (SB 146), effective January 1, 2012; Stats 2017 ch 520 § 1 (SB 799), effective January 1, 2018.

§ 801.01. Report of settlement of arbitration award over a specified amount in case of alleged negligence, error, or omission in practice or the licensee's rendering of unauthorized professional services; Procedure

The Legislature finds and declares that the filing of reports with the applicable state agencies required under this section is essential for the protection of the public. It is the intent of the Legislature that the reporting requirements set forth in this section be interpreted broadly in order to expand reporting obligations.

(a) A complete report shall be sent to the Medical Board of California, the Osteopathic Medical Board of California, the California Board of Podiatric Medicine, or the Physician Assistant Board with respect to a licensee of the board as to the following:

(1) A settlement over thirty thousand dollars ($30,000) or arbitration award of any amount or a civil judgment of any amount, whether or not vacated by a settlement after entry of the judgment, that was not reversed on appeal, of a claim or action for damages for death or personal injury caused by the licensee's alleged negligence, error, or omission in practice, or by the licensee's rendering of unauthorized professional services.

(2) A settlement over thirty thousand dollars ($30,000), if the settlement is based on the licensee's alleged negligence, error, or omission in practice, or on the licensee's rendering of unauthorized professional services, and a party to the settlement is a corporation, medical group, partnership, or other corporate entity in which the licensee has an ownership interest or that employs or contracts with the licensee.

(b) The report shall be sent by any of the following:

(1) The insurer providing professional liability insurance to the licensee.

(2) The licensee, or the licensee's counsel.

(3) A state or local governmental agency that self-insures the licensee. For purposes of this section, "state governmental agency" includes, but is not limited to, the University of California.

(c) The entity, person, or licensee obligated to report pursuant to subdivision (b) shall send the complete report if the judgment, settlement agreement, or arbitration award is entered against or paid by the employer of the licensee and not entered against or paid by the licensee. "Employer," as used in this paragraph, means a professional corporation, a group practice, a health care facility or clinic licensed or exempt from licensure under the Health and Safety Code, a licensed health care service plan, a medical care foundation, an educational institution, a professional institution, a professional school or college, a general law corporation, a public entity, or a nonprofit organization that employs, retains, or contracts with a licensee referred to in this section. Nothing in this paragraph shall be construed to authorize the employment of, or contracting with, any licensee in violation of Section 2400.

(d) The report shall be sent to the Medical Board of California, the Osteopathic Medical Board of California, the California Board of Podiatric Medicine, or the Physician Assistant Board as appropriate, within 30 days after the written settlement agreement has been reduced to writing and signed by all parties thereto, within 30 days after service of the arbitration award on the parties, or within 30 days after the date of entry of the civil judgment.

(e) The entity, person, or licensee required to report under subdivision (b) shall notify the claimant or the claimant's counsel, if the claimant is represented by counsel, that the report has been sent to the Medical Board of California, the Osteopathic Medical Board of California, the California Board of Podiatric Medicine, or the Physician Assistant Board. If the claimant or the claimant's counsel has not received this notice within 45 days after the settlement was reduced to writing and signed by all of the parties or the arbitration award was served on the parties or the date of entry of the civil judgment, the claimant or the claimant's counsel shall make the report to the appropriate board.

(f) Failure to substantially comply with this section is a public offense punishable by a fine of not less than five hundred dollars ($500) and not more than five thousand dollars ($5,000).

(g)(1) The Medical Board of California, the Osteopathic Medical Board of California, the California Board of Podiatric Medicine, and the Physician Assistant Board may develop a prescribed form for the report.

(2) The report shall be deemed complete only if it includes the following information:

(A) The name and last known business and residential addresses of every plaintiff or claimant involved in the matter, whether or not the person received an award under the settlement, arbitration, or judgment.

(B) The name and last known business and residential addresses of every licensee who was alleged to have acted improperly, whether or not that person was a named defendant in the action and whether or not that person was required to pay any damages pursuant to the settlement, arbitration award, or judgment.

(C) The name, address, and principal place of business of every insurer providing professional liability insurance to any person described in subparagraph (B), and the insured's policy number.

(D) The name of the court in which the action or any part of the action was filed, and the date of filing and case number of each action.

(E) A description or summary of the facts of each claim, charge, or allegation, including the date of occurrence and the licensee's role in the care or professional services provided to the patient with respect to those services at issue in the claim or action.

(F) The name and last known business address of each attorney who represented a party in the settlement, arbitration, or civil action, including the name of the client the attorney represented.

(G) The amount of the judgment, the date of its entry, and a copy of the judgment; the amount of the arbitration award, the date of its service on the parties, and a copy of the award document; or the amount of the settlement and the date it was reduced to writing and signed by all parties and a copy of the settlement agreement. If an otherwise reportable settlement is entered into after a reportable judgment or arbitration award is issued, the report shall include both a copy of the settlement agreement and a copy of the judgment or award.

(H) The specialty or subspecialty of the licensee who was the subject of the claim or action.

(I) Any other information the Medical Board of California, the Osteopathic Medical Board of California, the California Board of Podiatric Medicine, or the Physician Assistant Board may, by regulation, require.

(3) Every professional liability insurer, self-insured governmental agency, or licensee or the licensee's counsel that makes a report under this section and has received a copy of any written or electronic patient medical

or hospital records prepared by the treating physician and surgeon, podiatrist, or physician assistant, or the staff of the treating physician and surgeon, podiatrist, or hospital, describing the medical condition, history, care, or treatment of the person whose death or injury is the subject of the report, or a copy of any deposition in the matter that discusses the care, treatment, or medical condition of the person, shall include with the report, copies of the records and depositions, subject to reasonable costs to be paid by the Medical Board of California, the Osteopathic Medical Board of California, the California Board of Podiatric Medicine, or the Physician Assistant Board. If confidentiality is required by court order and, as a result, the reporter is unable to provide the records and depositions, documentation to that effect shall accompany the original report. The applicable board may, upon prior notification of the parties to the action, petition the appropriate court for modification of any protective order to permit disclosure to the board. A professional liability insurer, self-insured governmental agency, or licensee or the licensee's counsel shall maintain the records and depositions referred to in this paragraph for at least one year from the date of filing of the report required by this section.

(h) If the board, within 60 days of its receipt of a report filed under this section, notifies a person named in the report, that person shall maintain for the period of three years from the date of filing of the report any records that person has as to the matter in question and shall make those records available upon request to the board to which the report was sent.

(i) Notwithstanding any other provision of law, no insurer shall enter into a settlement without the written consent of the insured, except that this prohibition shall not void any settlement entered into without that written consent. The requirement of written consent shall only be waived by both the insured and the insurer.

(j)(1) A state or local governmental agency that self-insures licensees shall, prior to sending a report pursuant to this section, do all of the following with respect to each licensee who will be identified in the report:

(A) Before deciding that a licensee will be identified, provide written notice to the licensee that the agency intends to submit a report in which the licensee may be identified, based on the licensee's role in the care or professional services provided to the patient that were at issue in the claim or action. This notice shall describe the reasons for notifying the licensee. The agency shall include with this notice a reasonable opportunity for the licensee to review a copy of records to be used by the agency in deciding whether to identify the licensee in the report.

(B) Provide the licensee with a reasonable opportunity to provide a written response to the agency and written materials in support of the licensee's position. If the licensee is identified in the report, the agency shall include this response and materials in the report submitted to a board under this section if requested by the licensee.

(C) At least 10 days prior to the expiration of the 30-day reporting requirement under subdivision (d), provide the licensee with the opportunity to present arguments to the body that will make the final decision or to that body's designee. The body shall review the care or professional services provided to the patient with respect to those services at issue in the claim or action and determine the licensee or licensees to be identified in the report and the amount of the settlement to be apportioned to the licensee.

(2) Nothing in this subdivision shall be construed to modify either the content of a report required under this section or the timeframe for filing that report.

(k) For purposes of this section, "licensee" means a licensee of the Medical Board of California, the Osteopathic Medical Board of California, the California Board of Podiatric Medicine, or the Physician Assistant Board.

HISTORY:

Added Stats 2006 ch 223 § 4 (SB 1438), effective January 1, 2007. Amended Stats 2009 ch 505 § 1 (AB 1070), effective January 1, 2010; Stats 2012 ch 332 § 2 (SB 1236), effective January 1, 2013; Stats 2021 ch 649 § 2 (SB 806), effective January 1, 2022.

§ 801.1. Report of settlement or arbitration award where state or local government acts as self-insurer in cases of negligence, error, omission in practice, or rendering of unauthorized services resulting in death or personal injury

(a) Every state or local governmental agency that self-insures a person who holds a license, certificate, or similar authority from or under any agency specified in subdivision (a) of Section 800 (except a person licensed pursuant to Chapter 3 (commencing with Section 1200) or Chapter 5 (commencing with Section 2000) or the Osteopathic Initiative Act) shall send a complete report to that agency as to any settlement or arbitration award over three thousand dollars ($3,000) of a claim or action for damages for death or personal injury caused by that person's negligence, error, or omission in practice, or rendering of unauthorized professional services. The report shall be sent within 30 days after the written settlement agreement has been reduced to writing and signed by all parties thereto or within 30 days after service of the arbitration award on the parties.

(b) Every state or local governmental agency that self-insures a person licensed pursuant to Chapter 13 (commencing with Section 4980), Chapter 14 (commencing with Section 4990), or Chapter 16 (commencing with Section 4999.10) shall send a complete report to the Board of Behavioral Science Examiners as to any settlement or arbitration award over ten thousand dollars ($10,000) of a claim or action for damages for death or personal injury caused by that person's negligence, error, or omission in practice, or rendering of unauthorized professional services. The report shall be sent within 30 days after the written settlement agreement has been reduced to writing and signed by all parties thereto or within 30 days after service of the arbitration award on the parties.

HISTORY:

Added Stats 1995 ch 708 § 2 (SB 609). Amended Stats 2002 ch 1085 § 3 (SB 1950); Stats 2006 ch 223 § 5 (SB 1438), effective January 1, 2007; Stats 2011 ch 381 § 7 (SB 146), effective January 1, 2012.

§ 802. Reports of malpractice settlements or arbitration awards involving uninsured licensees; Penalties for noncompliance

(a) Every settlement, judgment, or arbitration award over three thousand dollars ($3,000) of a claim or action for damages for death or personal injury caused by negligence, error or omission in practice, or by the unauthorized rendering of professional services, by a person who holds a license, certificate, or other similar authority from an agency specified in subdivision (a) of Section 800 (except a person licensed pursuant to Chapter 3 (commencing with Section 1200) or Chapter 5 (commencing with Section 2000) or the Osteopathic Initiative Act) who does not possess professional liability insurance as to that claim shall, within 30 days after the written settlement agreement has been reduced to writing and signed by all the parties thereto or 30 days after service of the judgment or arbitration award on the parties, be reported to the agency that issued the license, certificate, or similar authority. A complete report shall be made by appropriate means by the person or his or her counsel, with a copy of the communication to be sent to the claimant through his or her counsel if the person is so represented, or directly if he or she is not. If, within 45 days of the conclusion of the written settlement agreement or service of the judgment or arbitration award on the parties, counsel for the claimant (or if the claimant is not represented by counsel, the claimant himself or herself) has not received a copy of the report, he or she shall himself or herself make the complete report. Failure of the licensee or claimant (or, if represented by counsel, their counsel) to comply with this section is a public offense punishable by a fine of not less than fifty dollars ($50) or more than five hundred dollars ($500). Knowing and intentional failure to comply with this section or conspiracy or collusion not to comply with this section, or to hinder or impede any other person in the compliance, is a public offense punishable by a fine of not less than five thousand dollars ($5,000) nor more than fifty thousand dollars ($50,000).

(b) Every settlement, judgment, or arbitration award over ten thousand dollars ($10,000) of a claim or action for damages for death or personal injury caused by negligence, error or omission in practice, or by the unauthorized rendering of professional services, by a marriage and family therapist, a clinical social worker, or a professional clinical counselor licensed pursuant to Chapter 13 (commencing with Section 4980), Chapter 14 (commencing with Section 4990), or Chapter 16 (commencing with Section 4999.10), respectively, who does not possess professional liability insurance as to that claim shall within 30 days after the written settlement agreement has been reduced to writing and signed by all the parties thereto or 30 days after service of the judgment or arbitration award on the parties be reported to the agency that issued the license, certificate, or similar authority. A complete report shall be made by appropriate means by the person or his or her counsel, with a copy of the communication to be sent to the claimant through his or her counsel if he or she is so represented, or directly if he or she is not. If, within 45 days of the conclusion of the written settlement agreement or service of the judgment or arbitration award on the parties, counsel for the claimant (or if he or she is not represented by counsel, the claimant himself or herself) has not received a copy of the report, he or she shall himself or herself make a complete report. Failure of the marriage and family therapist, clinical social worker, or professional clinical counselor or claimant (or, if represented by counsel, his or her counsel) to comply with this section is a public offense punishable by a fine of not less than fifty dollars ($50) nor more than five hundred dollars ($500). Knowing and intentional failure to comply with this section, or conspiracy or collusion not to comply with this section or to hinder or impede any other person in that compliance, is a public offense punishable by a fine of not less than five thousand dollars ($5,000) nor more than fifty thousand dollars ($50,000).

HISTORY:

Added Stats 1975 2d Ex Sess ch 1 § 2.3. Amended Stats 1979 ch 923 § 2; Stats 1989 ch 398 § 2; Stats 1997 ch 359 § 2 (AB 103); Stats 2001 ch 728 § 1.5 (SB 724); Stats 2002 ch 1085 § 4 (SB 1950); Stats 2005 ch 674 § 4 (SB 231), effective January 1, 2006; Stats 2006 ch 223 § 6 (SB 1438), effective January 1, 2007; Stats 2011 ch 381 § 8 (SB 146), effective January 1, 2012.

§ 803. Report of crime or liability for death or injury on part of specified licensees to licensing agency

(a) Except as provided in subdivision (b), within 10 days after a judgment by a court of this state that a person who holds a license, certificate, or other similar authority from the Board of Behavioral Sciences or from an agency mentioned in subdivision (a) of Section 800 (except a person licensed pursuant to Chapter 3 (commencing with Section 1200)) has committed a crime, or is liable for any death or personal injury resulting in a judgment for an amount in excess of thirty thousand dollars ($30,000) caused by his or her negligence, error or omission in practice, or his or her rendering unauthorized professional services, the clerk of the court that rendered the judgment shall report that fact to the agency that issued the license, certificate, or other similar authority.

(b) For purposes of a physician and surgeon, osteopathic physician and surgeon, doctor of podiatric medicine, or physician assistant, who is liable for any death or personal injury resulting in a judgment of any amount caused by his or her negligence, error or omission in practice, or his or her rendering unauthorized professional services, the clerk of the court that rendered the judgment shall report that fact to the agency that issued the license.

HISTORY:

Added Stats 1993 ch 1267 § 4 (SB 916). Amended Stats 1995 ch 708 § 4 (SB 609); Stats 1997 ch 359 § 3 (AB 103); Stats 2001 ch 728 § 2 (SB 724); Stats 2005 ch 216 § 3 (AB 268), effective January 1, 2006; Stats 2006 ch 223 § 9 (SB 1438), effective January 1, 2007; Stats 2009 ch 308 § 11 (SB 819), effective January 1, 2010; Stats 2012 ch 332 § 5 (SB 1236), effective January 1, 2013.

§ 804. Form and content of reports

(a) Any agency to whom reports are to be sent under Section 801, 801.1, 802, or 803, may develop a prescribed form for the making of the reports, usage of which it may, but need not, by regulation, require in all cases.

(b) A report required to be made by Sections 801, 801.1, or 802 shall be deemed complete only if it includes the following information: (1) the name and last known business and residential addresses of every plaintiff or claimant involved in the matter, whether or not each plaintiff or claimant recovered anything; (2) the name and last known business and residential addresses of every physician or provider of health care services who was claimed or alleged to have acted improperly, whether or not that person was a named defendant and whether or not any recovery or judgment was had against that person; (3) the name, address, and principal place of business of every insurer providing professional liability insurance as to any person named in (2), and the insured's policy number; (4) the name of the court in which the action or any part of the action was filed along with the date of filing and docket number of each action; (5) a brief description or summary of the facts upon which each claim, charge or judgment rested including the date of occurrence; (6) the names and last known business and residential addresses of every person who acted as counsel for any party in the litigation or negotiations, along with an identification of the party whom said person represented; (7) the date and amount of final judgment or settlement; and (8) any other information the agency to whom the reports are to be sent may, by regulation, require.

(c) Every person named in the report, who is notified by the board within 60 days of the filing of the report, shall maintain for the period of three years from the filing of the report any records he or she has as to the matter in question and shall make those available upon request to the agency with which the report was filed.

HISTORY:
Added Stats 2d Ex Sess 1975 ch 1 § 2.3. Amended Stats 2d Ex Sess 1975 ch 2 § 1.01, effective September 24, 1975, operative December 12, 1975; Stats 1994 ch 1206 § 13 (SB 1775); Stats 1995 ch 708 § 7 (SB 609); Stats 2006 ch 223 § 14 (SB 1438), effective January 1, 2007.

§ 806. Statistical reports and recommendations to Legislature

Each agency in the department receiving reports pursuant to the preceding sections shall prepare a statistical report based upon these records for presentation to the Legislature not later than 30 days after the commencement of each regular session of the Legislature, including by the type of peer review body, and, where applicable, type of health care facility, the number of reports received and a summary of administrative and disciplinary action taken with respect to these reports and any recommendations for corrective legislation if the agency considers legislation to be necessary.

HISTORY:
Added Stats 2d Ex Sess 1975 ch 1 § 2.3. Amended Stats 2001 ch 614 § 8 (SB 16).

ARTICLE 12
INSURANCE FRAUD

Section
810. Grounds for disciplinary action against health care professional.

HISTORY: Added Stats 1978 ch 174 § 1, effective May 31, 1978.

§ 810. Grounds for disciplinary action against health care professional

(a) It shall constitute unprofessional conduct and grounds for disciplinary action, including suspension or revocation of a license or certificate, for a health care professional to do any of the following in connection with their professional activities:

(1) Knowingly present or cause to be presented any false or fraudulent claim for the payment of a loss under a contract of insurance.

(2) Knowingly prepare, make, or subscribe any writing, with intent to present or use the same, or to allow it to be presented or used in support of any false or fraudulent claim.

(b) It shall constitute cause for revocation or suspension of a license or certificate for a health care professional to engage in any conduct prohibited under Section 1871.4 of the Insurance Code or Section 549 or 550 of the Penal Code.

(c)(1) It shall constitute cause for automatic suspension of a license or certificate issued pursuant to Chapter 4 (commencing with Section 1600), Chapter 5 (commencing with Section 2000), Chapter 6.6 (commencing with Section 2900), Chapter 7 (commencing with Section 3000), or Chapter 9 (commencing with Section 4000), or pursuant to the Chiropractic Act or the Osteopathic Act, if a licensee or certificate holder has been convicted of any felony involving fraud committed by the licensee or certificate holder in conjunction with providing benefits covered by worker's compensation insurance, or has been convicted of any felony involving Medi-Cal fraud committed by the licensee or certificate holder in conjunction with the Medi-Cal program, including the Denti-Cal element of the Medi-Cal program, pursuant to Chapter 7 (commencing with Section 14000), or Chapter 8 (commencing with Section 14200), of Part 3 of Division 9 of the Welfare and Institutions Code. The board shall convene a disciplinary hearing to determine whether or not the license or certificate shall be suspended, revoked, or some other disposition shall be considered, including, but not limited to, revocation with the opportunity to petition for reinstatement, suspension, or other limitations on the license or certificate as the board deems appropriate.

(2) It shall constitute cause for automatic suspension and for revocation of a license or certificate issued pursuant to Chapter 4 (commencing with Section 1600), Chapter 5 (commencing with Section 2000), Chapter 6.6 (commencing with Section 2900), Chapter 7 (commencing with Section 3000), or Chapter 9 (commencing with Section 4000), or pursuant to the Chiropractic Act or the Osteopathic Act, if a licensee or certificate holder has more than one conviction of any felony arising out of separate prosecutions involving fraud committed by the licensee or certificate holder in conjunction with providing benefits covered by worker's compensation insurance, or in conjunction with the Medi-Cal program, including the Denti-Cal element of the Medi-Cal program pursuant to Chapter 7 (commencing with Section 14000), or Chapter 8 (commencing with Section 14200), of Part 3 of Division 9 of the Welfare and Institutions Code. The board shall convene a disciplinary hearing to revoke the license or certificate and an order of revocation shall be issued unless the board finds mitigating circumstances to order some other disposition.

(3) It is the intent of the Legislature that paragraph (2) apply to a licensee or certificate holder who has one or more convictions prior to January 1, 2004, as provided in this subdivision.

(4) Nothing in this subdivision shall preclude a board from suspending or revoking a license or certificate pursuant to any other provision of law.

(5) "Board," as used in this subdivision, means the Dental Board of California, the Medical Board of California, the California Board of Podiatric Medicine, the Board of Psychology, the California State Board of Optometry, the California State Board of Pharmacy, the Osteopathic Medical Board of California, and the State Board of Chiropractic Examiners.

(6) "More than one conviction," as used in this subdivision, means that the licensee or certificate holder has one or more convictions prior to January 1,

2004, and at least one conviction on or after that date, or the licensee or certificate holder has two or more convictions on or after January 1, 2004. However, a licensee or certificate holder who has one or more convictions prior to January 1, 2004, but who has no convictions and is currently licensed or holds a certificate after that date, does not have "more than one conviction" for the purposes of this subdivision.

(d) As used in this section, health care professional means any person licensed or certified pursuant to this division, or licensed pursuant to the Osteopathic Initiative Act, or the Chiropractic Initiative Act.

HISTORY:
Added Stats 1978 ch 174 § 1, effective May 31, 1978. Amended Stats 1991 ch 116 § 1 (SB 1218); Stats 1997 ch 758 § 2.6 (SB 1346); Stats 2003 ch 595 § 1 (SB 359), ch 659 § 1.5 (AB 747); Stats 2004 ch 333 § 1 (AB 2835); Stats 2017 ch 775 § 16 (SB 798), effective January 1, 2018; Stats 2021 ch 630 § 15 (AB 1534), effective January 1, 2022.

ARTICLE 12.5
MENTAL ILLNESS OR PHYSICAL ILLNESS

Section
820. Examination of licentiate for mental illness or physical illness affecting competency.
821. Effect of licentiate's failure to comply with order for examination.
822. Action by licensing agency.
823. Reinstatement of licentiate.
824. Options open to licensing agency when proceeding against licentiate.
825. "Licensing agency".
826. Format of proceedings under Sections 821 and 822; Rights and powers.
827. Authority of licensing agency to convene in closed session.
828. Determination of insufficient evidence to bring action against licentiate; Effect on records of proceedings.

HISTORY: Added Stats 1982 ch 1183 § 1.

§ 820. Examination of licentiate for mental illness or physical illness affecting competency

Whenever it appears that any person holding a license, certificate or permit under this division or under any initiative act referred to in this division may be unable to practice his or her profession safely because the licentiate's ability to practice is impaired due to mental illness, or physical illness affecting competency, the licensing agency may order the licentiate to be examined by one or more physicians and surgeons or psychologists designated by the agency. The report of the examiners shall be made available to the licentiate and may be received as direct evidence in proceedings conducted pursuant to Section 822.

HISTORY:
Added Stats 1982 ch 1183 § 1. Amended Stats 1989 ch 1104 § 1.7.

§ 821. Effect of licentiate's failure to comply with order for examination

The licentiate's failure to comply with an order issued under Section 820 shall constitute grounds for the suspension or revocation of the licentiate's certificate or license.

HISTORY:
Added Stats 1982 ch 1183 § 1.

§ 822. Action by licensing agency

If a licensing agency determines that its licentiate's ability to practice his or her profession safely is impaired because the licentiate is mentally ill, or physically ill affecting competency, the licensing agency may take action by any one of the following methods:

(a) Revoking the licentiate's certificate or license.

(b) Suspending the licentiate's right to practice.

(c) Placing the licentiate on probation.

(d) Taking such other action in relation to the licentiate as the licensing agency in its discretion deems proper.

The licensing agency shall not reinstate a revoked or suspended certificate or license until it has received competent evidence of the absence or control of the condition which caused its action and until it is satisfied that with due regard for the public health and safety the person's right to practice his or her profession may be safely reinstated.

HISTORY:
Added Stats 1982 ch 1183 § 1.

§ 823. Reinstatement of licentiate

Notwithstanding any other provisions of law, reinstatement of a licentiate against whom action has been taken pursuant to Section 822 shall be governed by the procedures in this article. In reinstating a certificate or license which has been revoked or suspended under Section 822, the licensing agency may impose terms and conditions to be complied with by the licentiate after the certificate or license has been reinstated. The authority of the licensing agency to impose terms and conditions includes, but is not limited to, the following:

(a) Requiring the licentiate to obtain additional professional training and to pass an examination upon the completion of the training.

(b) Requiring the licentiate to pass an oral, written, practical, or clinical examination, or any combination thereof to determine his or her present fitness to engage in the practice of his or her profession.

(c) Requiring the licentiate to submit to a complete diagnostic examination by one or more physicians and surgeons or psychologists appointed by the licensing agency. If the licensing agency requires the licentiate to submit to such an examination, the licensing agency shall receive and consider any other report of a complete diagnostic examination given by one or more physicians and surgeons or psychologists of the licentiate's choice.

(d) Requiring the licentiate to undergo continuing treatment.

(e) Restricting or limiting the extent, scope or type of practice of the licentiate.

HISTORY:
Added Stats 1982 ch 1183 § 1.

§ 824. Options open to licensing agency when proceeding against licentiate

The licensing agency may proceed against a licentiate under either Section 820, or 822, or under both sections.

HISTORY:
Added Stats 1982 ch 1183 § 1.

§ 825. "Licensing agency"

As used in this article with reference to persons holding licenses as physicians and surgeons, "licensing agency" means a panel of the Division of Medical Quality.

HISTORY:
Added Stats 1982 ch 1183 § 1. Amended Stats 1993 ch 1267 § 9 (SB 916).

§ 826. Format of proceedings under Sections 821 and 822; Rights and powers

The proceedings under Sections 821 and 822 shall be conducted in accordance with Chapter 5 (commencing with Section 11500) of Part 1 of Division 3 of Title 2 of the Government Code, and the licensing agency and the licentiate shall have all the rights and powers granted therein.

HISTORY:
Added Stats 1982 ch 1183 § 1.

§ 827. Authority of licensing agency to convene in closed session

Notwithstanding the provisions of Article 9 (commencing with Section 11120) of Chapter 1 of Part 1 of Division 3 of Title 2 of the Government Code, relating to public meetings, the licensing agency may convene in closed session to consider any evidence relating to the licentiate's mental or physical illness obtained pursuant to the proceedings under Section 820. The licensing agency shall only convene in closed session to the extent that it is necessary to protect the privacy of a licentiate.

HISTORY:
Added Stats 1982 ch 1183 § 1.

§ 828. Determination of insufficient evidence to bring action against licentiate; Effect on records of proceedings

If the licensing agency determines, pursuant to proceedings conducted under Section 820, that there is insufficient evidence to bring an action against the licentiate pursuant to Section 822, then all licensing agency records of the proceedings, including the order for the examination, investigative reports, if any, and the report of the physicians and surgeons or psychologists, shall be kept confidential and are not subject to discovery or subpoena. If no further proceedings are conducted to determine the licentiates fitness to practice during a period of five years from the date of the determination by the licensing agency of the proceeding pursuant to Section 820, then the licensing agency shall purge and destroy all records pertaining to the proceedings. If new proceedings are instituted during the five-year period against the licentiate by the licensing agency, the records, including the report of the physicians and surgeons or psychologists, may be used in the proceedings and shall be available to the respondent pursuant to the provisions of Section 11507.6 of the Government Code.

HISTORY:
Added Stats 1982 ch 1183 § 1.

CHAPTER 1.5
EXEMPTION FROM LICENSURE

Section
900. Requirements for exemption; Immunity from liability.
901. Exemption from licensure requirements for services provided under enumerated circumstances; Prior authorization; Steps necessary for sponsoring entity; Report; List of health care practitioners providing health care services under this section; Compliance [Repealed].

Bus & Prof

HISTORY: Added Stats 1989 ch 97 § 2, effective July 7, 1989. Former Chapter 1.5, entitled "Continuing Education", consisting of §§ 900–905, was added Stats 1971 ch 1516 § 1 and repealed Stats 1974 ch 923 § 1.

§ 900. Requirements for exemption; Immunity from liability

(a) Nothing in this division applies to a health care practitioner licensed in another state or territory of the United States who offers or provides health care for which he or she is licensed, if the health care is provided only during a state of emergency as defined in subdivision (b) of Section 8558 of the Government Code, which emergency overwhelms the response capabilities of California health care practitioners and only upon the request of the Director of the Emergency Medical Services Authority.

(b) The director shall be the medical control and shall designate the licensure and specialty health care practitioners required for the specific emergency and shall designate the areas to which they may be deployed.

(c) Health care practitioners shall provide, upon request, a valid copy of a professional license and a photograph identification issued by the state in which the practitioner holds licensure before being deployed by the director.

(d) Health care practitioners deployed pursuant to this chapter shall provide the appropriate California licensing authority with verification of licensure upon request.

(e) Health care practitioners providing health care pursuant to this chapter shall have immunity from liability for services rendered as specified in Section 8659 of the Government Code.

(f) For the purposes of this section, "health care practitioner" means any person who engages in acts which are the subject of licensure or regulation under this division or under any initiative act referred to in this division.

(g) For purposes of this section, "director" means the Director of the Emergency Medical Services Authority who shall have the powers specified in Division 2.5 (commencing with Section 1797) of the Health and Safety Code.

HISTORY:
Added Stats 1989 ch 97 § 2, effective July 7, 1989. Amended Stats 2010 ch 270 § 1 (AB 2699), effective January 1, 2011.

§ 901. Exemption from licensure requirements for services provided under enumerated circumstances; Prior authorization; Steps necessary for sponsoring entity; Report; List of health care practitioners providing health care services under this section; Compliance [Repealed]

HISTORY:

Added Stats 2010 ch 270 § 2 (AB 2699), effective January 1, 2011, repealed January 1, 2014. Amended Stats 2011 ch 296 § 3 (AB 1023), effective January 1, 2012, repealed January 1, 2014; Stats 2013 ch 111 § 1 (AB 512), effective January 1, 2014. Repealed January 1, 2018, by its own terms.

CHAPTER 3

CLINICAL LABORATORY TECHNOLOGY

Article
3. Application of the Chapter.
3.5. Hemodialysis Training.

HISTORY: Added Stats 1951 ch 1727 § 2, effective January 1, 1952. Former Chapter 3, also entitled "Clinical Laboratory Technology," consisting of §§ 1200–1305, was added Stats 1941 ch 42 § 1 and repealed Stats 1951 ch 1727 § 1, effective January 1, 1952.

ARTICLE 3

APPLICATION OF THE CHAPTER

Section
1242.5. Regulations allowing unlicensed persons to withdraw blood and perform blood tests.
1242.6. Withdrawal of blood by registered or licensed vocational nurse or respiratory care practitioner.
1243. When student authorized to perform arterial puncture, etc.
1245. Authority to perform blood gas analysis; Application to certified respiratory care practitioner.
1246. Authority for unlicensed person to perform venipuncture or skin puncture; Blood collection by certified phlebotomy technician.

HISTORY: Added Stats 1951 ch 1727 § 2, effective January 1, 1952.

§ 1242.5. Regulations allowing unlicensed persons to withdraw blood and perform blood tests

Notwithstanding paragraphs (2) and (3) of subdivision (b) of Section 1241, the department may by regulation authorize laboratory personnel certified pursuant to Section 1246 to perform venipuncture, arterial puncture, or skin puncture for the purposes of withdrawing blood or for clinical laboratory test purposes, as defined by regulations established by the department.

HISTORY:

Added Stats 1979 ch 176 § 1. Amended Stats 1988 ch 1396 § 1, effective September 26, 1988; Stats 1999 ch 695 § 2 (AB 1557).

§ 1242.6. Withdrawal of blood by registered or licensed vocational nurse or respiratory care practitioner

(a) Any registered nurse licensed under the provisions of Chapter 6 (commencing with Section 2700) of Division 2 may perform arterial puncture, venipuncture, or skin puncture for the purposes of withdrawing blood or for test purposes upon authorization from any licensed physician and surgeon or any licensed dentist.

(b) Any licensed vocational nurse licensed under the provisions of Chapter 6.5 (commencing with Section 2840) of Division 2 may perform arterial puncture, venipuncture, or skin puncture for the purposes of withdrawing blood or for test purposes upon authorization from any licensed physician and surgeon, or any licensed dentist if prior thereto the licensed vocational nurse has been instructed by a physician and surgeon and has demonstrated competence to the physician and surgeon in the proper procedure to be employed when withdrawing blood, or has satisfactorily completed a prescribed course of instruction approved by the Board of Vocational Nursing and Psychiatric Technicians or has demonstrated competence to the satisfaction of that board.

(c) Any respiratory care practitioner certified under the provisions of Chapter 8.3 (commencing with Section 3700) of Division 2 may perform arterial puncture, venipuncture, or skin puncture for the purposes of withdrawing blood or for test purposes upon authorization from any licensed physician and surgeon.

HISTORY:

Added Stats 1973 ch 748 § 1. Amended Stats 1974 ch 838 § 1; Stats 1975 ch 629 § 1; Stats 1988 ch 1396 § 1.5, effective September 26, 1988; Stats 1997 ch 759 § 10 (SB 827).

§ 1243. When student authorized to perform arterial puncture, etc.

A student regularly matriculated in any college or university accredited by an accrediting agency acceptable to the department, or in any legally chartered school approved by the department for training purposes may perform arterial puncture, venipuncture, or skin puncture as a part of the necessary training program when done under the direct and responsible supervision of a person licensed to perform tests under the provisions of this chapter or a licensed physician and surgeon.

HISTORY:

Added Stats 1951 ch 1727 § 2, effective January 1, 1952. Amended Stats 1957 ch 1802 § 6; Stats 1963 ch 194 § 1; Stats 1970 ch 1377 § 16.

§ 1245. Authority to perform blood gas analysis; Application to certified respiratory care practitioner

(a) Any individual may perform a blood gas analysis if all the following conditions exist:

(1) He or she has earned a high school diploma or equivalent, as determined by HCFA pursuant to CLIA.

(2) He or she performs the blood gas analysis in a clinic or a general acute care hospital, as defined respectively in Sections 1202 and 1250 of the Health and Safety Code.

(3) He or she has been instructed by a physician and surgeon licensed in this state, who is in charge of a department of pulmonary physiology or clinical pathology in licensed clinics or hospitals, as defined respectively in

Sections 1202 and 1250 of the Health and Safety Code, in the proper procedure to be employed when performing a blood gas analysis.

(4) He or she performs the blood gas analysis under the direction and supervision of the physician and surgeon.

(5) He or she submits the analysis for interpretation to the physician and surgeon under whose direction and supervision he or she performed the analysis.

(b) After September 1, 1997, any person may perform a blood gas analysis classified as of high complexity under CLIA, if, in addition to the requirements of subdivision (a), he or she has earned an associate degree related to pulmonary function from an accredited institution as determined by HCFA pursuant to CLIA.

(c) Nothing contained in this section shall be construed as authorizing any individual, not otherwise authorized, to withdraw blood.

(d) Nothing contained in this section is applicable to a person licensed as a respiratory care practitioner under Chapter 8.3 (commencing with Section 3700). Those persons are authorized to perform those functions set forth in that chapter.

HISTORY:

Added Stats 1979 ch 176 § 2. Amended Stats 1987 ch 839 § 2; Stats 1995 ch 510 § 23 (SB 113).

§ 1246. Authority for unlicensed person to perform venipuncture or skin puncture; Blood collection by certified phlebotomy technician

(a)(1) On and after the effective date of the regulations specified in paragraph (2), any unlicensed person employed by a clinical laboratory performing the duties described in this section shall possess a valid and current certification as a certified phlebotomy technician issued by the department.

(2) The department shall adopt regulations for certification by January 1, 2001, as a certified phlebotomy technician that shall include all of the following:

(A) The applicant shall hold a valid, current certification as a phlebotomist issued by a national accreditation agency approved by the department, and shall submit proof of that certification when applying for certification pursuant to this section.

(B) An applicant with fewer than 1,040 hours of work experience shall complete education, training, and experience requirements as specified by regulations that shall include, but not be limited to, the following:

(i) At least 40 hours of didactic instruction.

(ii) At least 40 hours of practical instruction.

(iii) At least 50 successful venipunctures.

(C)An applicant who has at least 1,040 hours of work experience that includes at least 50 successful venipunctures shall complete at least 20 hours of didactic instruction, as specified in regulations adopted by the department.

(D) Each certified phlebotomy technician shall complete at least three hours per year or six hours every two years of continuing education or training. The department shall consider a variety of programs in determining the programs that meet the continuing education or training requirement.

(E) The applicant has been found to be competent in phlebotomy by a licensed physician and surgeon or person licensed pursuant to this chapter.

(F) The applicant works under the supervision of a licensed physician and surgeon, licensed registered nurse, or person licensed under this chapter, or the designee of a licensed physician and surgeon or the designee of a person licensed under this chapter.

(3) A certified phlebotomy technician may collect blood through a peripheral venous catheter if all of the following are met:

(A) The blood collection procedure is performed in a facility licensed under Division 2 (commencing with Section 1200) of the Health and Safety Code.

(B) The blood collection procedures or protocols are developed and approved by the facility's supervising physician and surgeon or licensed clinical laboratory director and approved by the licensed facility.

(C) The certified phlebotomy technician has received a minimum of three hours of training by the supervising physician and surgeon or their delegate in the proper procedures to be employed when collecting blood through a peripheral venous catheter.

(i) Training in the blood collection procedure through a peripheral venous catheter shall be conducted according to standardized training procedures developed and approved by the facility's supervising physician and surgeon or licensed clinical laboratory director. The facility shall make these standardized procedures available to the department upon request.

(ii) The instructor shall document the certified phlebotomy technician's successful completion of training. The facility shall maintain and make available to the department, upon request, documentation of training completed by a certified phlebotomy technician pursuant to this paragraph.

(D) The certified phlebotomy technician performs the blood collection procedure under the supervision of a physician and surgeon licensed under Chapter 5 (commencing with Section 2000). Notwithstanding subdivision (b), the physician and surgeon may only delegate the supervision duties in this subparagraph to a registered nurse. A physician and surgeon or a registered nurse may restrict or limit a certified phlebotomy technician's ability to collect blood from a patient's peripheral venous catheter.

(E) The certified phlebotomy technician performs the blood collection procedure using a device or devices approved by the licensed facility and the United States Food and Drug Administration.

(F) This paragraph does not authorize the certified phlebotomy technician to manage, stop, or restart a patient's active intravenous infusion or insert or remove a peripheral intravenous catheter.

(4) Paragraph (3) does not authorize a certified phlebotomy technician to withdraw blood through a peripherally inserted central catheter or central venous catheter.

(5) The department shall adopt regulations establishing standards for approving training programs designed to prepare applicants for certification pursuant to this section. The standards shall ensure that these programs

meet the state's minimum education and training requirements for comparable programs.

(6) The department shall adopt regulations establishing standards for approving national accreditation agencies to administer certification examinations and tests pursuant to this section.

(7) The department shall charge fees for application for and renewal of the certificate authorized by this section of no more than one hundred dollars ($100) for a two-year period.

(b)(1)(A) A certified phlebotomy technician may perform venipuncture or skin puncture to obtain a specimen for nondiagnostic tests assessing the health of an individual, for insurance purposes, provided that the technician works under the general supervision of a physician and surgeon licensed under Chapter 5 (commencing with Section 2000). The physician and surgeon may delegate the general supervision duties to a registered nurse or a person licensed under this chapter, but shall remain responsible for ensuring that all those duties and responsibilities are properly performed. The physician and surgeon shall make available to the department, upon request, records maintained documenting when a certified phlebotomy technician has performed venipuncture or skin puncture pursuant to this paragraph.

(B) As used in this paragraph, general supervision requires the supervisor of the technician to determine that the technician is competent to perform venipuncture or skin puncture, or to collect blood, before the technician's first blood withdrawal, and on an annual basis thereafter. The supervisor is also required to determine, on a monthly basis, that the technician complies with appropriate venipuncture, skin puncture, and blood collection policies and procedures approved by the medical director and required by state regulations. The supervisor, or another designated licensed physician and surgeon, registered nurse, or person licensed under this chapter, shall be available for consultation with the technician, either in person or through telephonic or electronic means, at the time of blood withdrawal.

(2)(A) Notwithstanding any other law, a person who has been issued a certified phlebotomy technician certificate pursuant to this section may draw blood following policies and procedures approved by a physician and surgeon licensed under Chapter 5 (commencing with Section 2000), appropriate to the location where the blood is being drawn and in accordance with state regulations. The blood collection shall be done at the request and in the presence of a peace officer for forensic purposes in a jail, law enforcement facility, or medical facility, with general supervision.

(B) As used in this paragraph, "general supervision" means that the supervisor of the technician is licensed under this code as a physician and surgeon, physician assistant, clinical laboratory bioanalyst, registered nurse, or clinical laboratory scientist, and reviews the competency of the technician before the technician may perform blood withdrawals without direct supervision, and on an annual basis thereafter. The supervisor is also required to review the work of the technician at least once a month to ensure compliance with venipuncture policies, procedures, and regulations. The supervisor, or another person licensed under this code as a physician and surgeon, physician assistant, clinical laboratory bioanalyst, registered nurse, or clinical laboratory scientist, shall be accessible to the location where the technician is working to provide onsite, telephone, or electronic consultation, within 30 minutes when needed.

(c) The department may adopt regulations providing for the issuance of a certificate to an unlicensed person employed by a clinical laboratory authorizing only the performance of skin punctures for test purposes.

HISTORY:

Added Stats 1970 ch 1605 § 1. Amended Stats 1971 ch 686 § 1; Stats 1973 ch 142 § 6, effective June 30, 1973, operative July 1, 1973; Stats 1977 ch 635 § 1; Stats 1978 ch 429 § 9, effective July 17, 1978, operative July 1, 1978; Stats 1999 ch 695 § 3 (AB 1557); Stats 2004 ch 14 § 1 (AB 371), effective February 11, 2004, ch 18 § 1.5 (AB 1087), effective February 23, 2004; Stats 2006 ch 14 § 1 (SB 169), effective March 29, 2006; Stats 2007 ch 483 § 2 (SB 1039), effective January 1, 2008; Stats 2009 ch 201 § 3 (SB 744), effective October 11, 2009; Stats 2010 ch 328 § 6 (SB 1330), effective January 1, 2011; Stats 2022 ch 685 § 1 (AB 1120), effective January 1, 2023.

ARTICLE 3.5

HEMODIALYSIS TRAINING

Section

1247.3. Treatment by technician; Administration of medications and anesthetics.

HISTORY: Added Stats 1987 ch 1297 § 4.

§ 1247.3. Treatment by technician; Administration of medications and anesthetics

The treatment of patients by a hemodialysis technician includes performing venipuncture and arterial puncture for the purpose of providing dialysis treatment for a patient. The treatment of patients includes the administration of local anesthetics, heparin, and sodium chloride solutions. The administration of these medications shall be pursuant to protocol established by the medical director of the hemodialysis clinic or unit and shall be under the immediate supervision of a licensed physician and surgeon or a licensed registered nurse. The administration of local anesthetics shall be limited to intradermal, subcutaneous, or topical administration. Hemodialysis technicians who treat patients in the home and are certified by the Board of Nephrology Examination for Nurses and Technicians are exempted from the requirements of immediate supervision until January 1, 1991.

HISTORY:

Added Stats 1987 ch 1297 § 4. Amended Stats 1989 ch 248 § 2, effective July 28, 1989.

CHAPTER 5

MEDICINE

Article

18. Corporations.

HISTORY: Added Stats 1980 ch 1313 § 2. Former Chapter 5, also entitled "Medicine", consisting of §§ 2000–2528.3, was added Stats 1937 ch 414 and repealed Stats 1980 chs 1313, 1314.

ARTICLE 18

CORPORATIONS

Section
2406. Medical or podiatry corporation defined.
2406.5. Disclosure statement for physical therapy referral.

HISTORY: Added Stats 1980 ch 1313 § 2.

§ 2406. Medical or podiatry corporation defined

A medical corporation or podiatry corporation is a corporation that is authorized to render professional services, as defined in Section 13401 of the Corporations Code, so long as that corporation and its shareholders, officers, directors, and employees rendering professional services who are physicians and surgeons, psychologists, registered nurses, optometrists, podiatrists, chiropractors, acupuncturists, naturopathic doctors, physical therapists, occupational therapists, or, in the case of a medical corporation only, physician assistants, marriage and family therapists, clinical counselors, or clinical social workers, are in compliance with the Moscone-Knox Professional Corporation Act, the provisions of this article, and all other statutes and regulations now or hereafter enacted or adopted pertaining to the corporation and the conduct of its affairs.

With respect to a medical corporation or podiatry corporation, the governmental agency referred to in the Moscone-Knox Professional Corporation Act is the board.

HISTORY:
Added Stats 1980 ch 1314 § 4.1. Amended Stats 1981 ch 621 § 1; Stats 1982 ch 1304 § 1; Stats 1994 ch 26 § 24 (AB 1807), effective March 30, 1994; Stats 2013 ch 620 § 2 (AB 1000), effective January 1, 2014.

§ 2406.5. Disclosure statement for physical therapy referral

(a) When a physician and surgeon, podiatrist, or other referring practitioner refers a patient to receive services by a physical therapist employed by a professional corporation as defined in Section 13401 of the Corporations Code, the referring practitioner shall comply with Article 6 (commencing with Section 650) of Chapter 1, and shall provide notice of the following to the patient, orally and in writing, in at least 14-point type and signed by the patient:

(1) That the patient may seek physical therapy treatment services from a physical therapy provider of his or her choice who may not necessarily be employed by the medical or podiatry corporation.

(2) If the patient chooses to be treated by an employed physical therapist, any financial interest the referring practitioner has in the corporation.

(b) This section shall not apply to a physician and surgeon, podiatrist, or other referring practitioner who is in a medical group with which a health care service plan, that is licensed pursuant to the Knox-Keene Health Care Service Plan Act of 1975 (Chapter 2.2 (commencing with Section 1340) of Division 2 of the Health and Safety Code) and is also exempt from federal taxation pursuant to Section 501(c)(3) of the Internal Revenue Code, exclusively contracts to provide professional medical services for its enrollees.

HISTORY:
Added Stats 2013 ch 620 § 3 (AB 1000), effective January 1, 2014.

CHAPTER 6.6
PSYCHOLOGISTS

Article
1. General Provisions.
9. Psychological Corporations.

HISTORY: Added Stats 1967 ch 1677 § 2. Former Chapter 6, also entitled "Pschologists" consisting of §§ 2900–2984, was added Stats 1957 ch 2320 § 1 and repealed Stats 1967 ch 1677 § 1.

ARTICLE 1
GENERAL PROVISIONS

Section
2908. Exemption of other professions.

HISTORY: Added Stats 1967 ch 1677 § 2. Former Article 1, also titled "General Provisions," was Added Stats 1957 ch 2320 § 1 and repealed Stats 1967 ch 1677 § 1.

§ 2908. Exemption of other professions

Nothing in this chapter shall be construed to prevent qualified members of other recognized professional groups licensed to practice in the State of California, such as, but not limited to, physicians, clinical social workers, educational psychologists, marriage and family therapists, licensed professional clinical counselors, optometrists, psychiatric technicians, or registered nurses, or attorneys admitted to the State Bar of California, or persons utilizing hypnotic techniques by referral from persons licensed to practice medicine, dentistry, or psychology, or persons utilizing hypnotic techniques which offer avocational or vocational self-improvement and do not offer therapy for emotional or mental disorders, or duly ordained members of the recognized clergy, or duly ordained religious practitioners from doing work of a psychological nature consistent with the laws governing their respective professions, provided they do not hold themselves out to the public by any title or description of services incorporating the words "psychological," "psychologist," "psychology," "psychometrist," "psychometrics," or "psychometry," or that they do not state or imply that they are licensed to practice psychology; except that persons licensed under Chapter 13.5 (commencing with Section 4989.10) of Division 2 may hold themselves out to the public as licensed educational psychologists.

HISTORY:

Added Stats 1967 ch 1677 § 2. Amended Stats 1973 ch 758 § 3; Stats 1978 ch 1208 § 4; Stats 1980 ch 324 § 1; Stats 1983 ch 928 § 2; Stats 2002 ch 1013 § 10 (SB 2026); Stats 2018 ch 389 § 1 (AB 2296), effective January 1, 2019.

ARTICLE 9
PSYCHOLOGICAL CORPORATIONS

Section
2995. Psychological corporation.

HISTORY: Added Stats 1980 ch 1314 § 15. Former Article 9, also entitled "Psychological Corporations," consisting of §§ 2995–2996.6, was added Stats 1969 ch 1436 § 3 and repealed Stats 1980 ch 1314 § 14.

§ 2995. Psychological corporation

A psychological corporation is a corporation that is authorized to render professional services, as defined in Section 13401 of the Corporations Code, so long as that corporation and its shareholders, officers, directors, and employees rendering professional services who are psychologists, podiatrists, registered nurses, optometrists, marriage and family therapists, licensed professional clinical counselors, licensed clinical social workers, chiropractors, acupuncturists, or physicians are in compliance with the Moscone-Knox Professional Corporation Act, this article, and all other statutes and regulations now or hereafter enacted or adopted pertaining to that corporation and the conduct of its affairs.

HISTORY:

Added Stats 1980 ch 1314 § 15. Amended Stats 1981 ch 621 § 3; Stats 1989 ch 886 § 60 (ch 888 prevails), ch 888 § 45; Stats 1990 ch 622 § 6 (SB 2720); Stats 2000 ch 836 § 23 (SB 1554); Stats 2001 ch 159 § 10 (SB 662); Stats 2018 ch 389 § 2 (AB 2296), effective January 1, 2019.

CHAPTER 9
PHARMACY

Article
4. Requirements for Prescriptions.

HISTORY: Added Stats 1996 ch 890 § 3. Former Chapter 9, also entitled "Pharmacy", consisting of §§ 4000–4480, was added Stats 1955 ch 950 § 3 and repealed Stats 1996 ch 890 § 2. Former Chapter 9, also entitled "Pharmacy", consisting of §§ 4000–4256, was added Stats 1937 ch 425 and repealed Stats 1955 ch 550 § 1.

ARTICLE 4
REQUIREMENTS FOR PRESCRIPTIONS

Section
4072. Oral or electronic transmission of prescription by nurse or other healing arts licentiate at health care facility.

HISTORY: Added Stats 1996 ch 890 § 3 (AB 2802).

§ 4072. Oral or electronic transmission of prescription by nurse or other healing arts licentiate at health care facility

(a) Notwithstanding any other provision of law, a pharmacist, registered nurse, licensed vocational nurse, licensed psychiatric technician, or other healing arts licentiate, if so authorized by administrative regulation, who is employed by or serves as a consultant for a licensed skilled nursing, intermediate care, or other health care facility, may orally or electronically transmit to the furnisher a prescription lawfully ordered by a person authorized to prescribe drugs or devices pursuant to Sections 4040 and 4070. The furnisher shall take appropriate steps to determine that the person who transmits the prescription is authorized to do so and shall record the name of the person who transmits the order. This section shall not apply to orders for Schedule II controlled substances.

(b) In enacting this section, the Legislature recognizes and affirms the role of the State Department of Public Health in regulating drug order processing requirements for licensed health care facilities as set forth in Title 22 of the California Code of Regulations as they may be amended from time to time.

HISTORY:

Added Stats 1996 ch 890 § 3 (AB 2802). Amended Stats 1997 ch 549 § 47 (SB 1349); Stats 2010 ch 653 § 25 (SB 1489), effective January 1, 2011.

CHAPTER 15

TELEPHONE MEDICAL ADVICE SERVICES

Section

4999. "Telephone medical advice service".
4999.1. Application for registration [Repealed].
4999.2. Compliance with professional requirements; Recordkeeping and retention; Information request response.
4999.3. Discipline and denial of application [Repealed].
4999.4. Expiration and renewal of registration [Repealed].
4999.5. Enforcement.
4999.6. Rules and regulations [Repealed].
4999.7. Effect on other practices and provisions.

HISTORY: Added Stats 1999 ch 535 § 1.

§ 4999. "Telephone medical advice service"

"Telephone medical advice service" means any business entity that employs, or contracts or subcontracts, directly or indirectly, with, the full-time equivalent of five or more persons functioning as health care professionals, whose primary function is to provide telephone medical advice, that provides telephone medical advice services to a patient at a California address. "Telephone medical advice service" does not include a medical group that operates in multiple locations in California if no more than five full-time equivalent persons at any one location perform telephone medical advice services and those persons limit the telephone medical advice services to patients being treated at that location.

HISTORY:

Added Stats 1999 ch 535 § 1 (AB 285). Amended Stats 2000 ch 857 § 2.1; Stats 2002 ch 107 § 22 (AB 269); Stats 2006 ch 659 § 29 (SB 1475), effective January 1, 2007; Stats 2016 ch 799 § 28 (SB 1039), effective January 1, 2017.

§ 4999.1. Application for registration [Repealed]

HISTORY:

Added Stats 1999 ch 535 § 1 (AB 285). Amended Stats 2006 ch 659 § 30 (SB 1475), effective January 1, 2007; Stats 2015 ch 426 § 47 (SB 800), effective January 1, 2016. Repealed Stats 2016 ch 799 § 29 (SB 1039), effective January 1, 2017.

§ 4999.2. Compliance with professional requirements; Recordkeeping and retention; Information request response

A telephone medical advice service shall be responsible for complying with the following requirements:

(a)(1) Ensuring that all health care professionals who provide medical advice services are appropriately licensed, certified, or registered as a physician and surgeon pursuant to Chapter 5 (commencing with Section 2000) or the Osteopathic Initiative Act, as a dentist, dental hygienist, dental hygienist in alternative practice, or dental hygienist in extended functions pursuant to Chapter 4 (commencing with Section 1600), as an occupational therapist pursuant to Chapter 5.6 (commencing with Section 2570), as a registered nurse pursuant to Chapter 6 (commencing with Section 2700), as a psychologist pursuant to Chapter 6.6 (commencing with Section 2900), as a naturopathic doctor pursuant to Chapter 8.2 (commencing with Section 3610), as a marriage and family therapist pursuant to Chapter 13 (commencing with Section 4980), as a licensed clinical social worker pursuant to Chapter 14 (commencing with Section 4991), as a licensed professional clinical counselor pursuant to Chapter 16 (commencing with Section 4999.10), as an optometrist pursuant to Chapter 7 (commencing with Section 3000), or as a chiropractor pursuant to the Chiropractic Initiative Act, and operating consistent with the laws governing their respective scopes of practice in the state within which they provide telephone medical advice services, except as provided in subdivision (b).

(2) Ensuring that all health care professionals who provide telephone medical advice services from an out-of-state location, as identified in paragraph (1), are licensed, registered, or certified in the state within which they are providing the telephone medical advice services and are operating consistent with the laws governing their respective licenses and scopes of practice.

(b) Ensuring that the telephone medical advice provided is consistent with good professional practice.

(c) Maintaining records of telephone medical advice services, including records of complaints, provided to patients in California for a period of at least five years.

(d) Ensuring that no staff member uses a title or designation when speaking to an enrollee, subscriber, or consumer that may cause a reasonable person to believe that the staff member is a licensed, certified, or registered health care professional described in paragraph (1) of subdivision (a), unless the staff member is a licensed, certified, or registered professional.

(e) Complying with all directions and requests for information made by the Department of Consumer Affairs and respective healing arts licensing boards.

HISTORY:

Added Stats 1999 ch 535 § 1 (AB 285). Amended Stats 2001 ch 728 § 49 (SB 724); Stats 2002 ch 1013 § 51 (SB 2026); Stats 2003 ch 885 § 1 (SB 969); Stats 2008 ch 31 § 48 (SB 853) (ch 31 prevails), effective January 1, 2009, operative July 1, 2009; Stats 2008, ch 179 § 9, effective January 1, 2009; Stats 2009 ch 307 § 63 (SB 821), effective January 1, 2010; Stats 2010 ch 328 § 12 (SB 1330), effective January 1, 2011; Stats 2015 ch 426 § 48 (SB 800), effective January 1, 2016; Stats 2016 ch 799 § 30 (SB 1039), effective January 1, 2017; Stats 2022 ch 684 § 1 (AB 1102), effective January 1, 2023.

§ 4999.3. Discipline and denial of application [Repealed]

HISTORY:

Added Stats 1999 ch 535 § 1 (AB 285). Amended Stats 2015 ch 426 § 49 (SB 800), effective January 1, 2016. Repealed Stats 2016 ch 799 § 31 (SB 1039), effective January 1, 2017.

§ 4999.4. Expiration and renewal of registration [Repealed]

HISTORY:

Added Stats 1999 ch 535 § 1 (AB 285). Amended Stats 2000 ch 857 § 2.2 (AB 2903); Stats 2006 ch 659 § 31 (SB 1475), effective January 1, 2007; Stats 2015 ch 426 § 50 (SB 800), effective January 1, 2016. Repealed Stats 2016 ch 799§ 32 (SB 1039), effective January 1, 2017.

§ 4999.5. Enforcement

The respective healing arts licensing boards shall be responsible for enforcing this chapter and any other laws and regulations affecting California licensed health care professionals providing telephone medical advice services.

HISTORY:

Added Stats 2016 ch 799 § 34 (SB 1039), effective January 1, 2017.

§ 4999.6. Rules and regulations [Repealed]

HISTORY:

Added Stats 1999 ch 535 § 1 (AB 285). Amended Stats 2000 ch 857 § 2.3. Repealed Stats 2016 ch 799 § 35 (SB 1039), effective January 1, 2017.

§ 4999.7. Effect on other practices and provisions

(a) This section does not limit, preclude, or otherwise interfere with the practices of other persons licensed or otherwise authorized to practice, under any other provision of this division, telephone medical advice services consistent with the laws governing their respective scopes of practice, or licensed under the Osteopathic Initiative Act or the Chiropractic Initiative Act and operating consistent with the laws governing their respective scopes of practice.

(b) For purposes of this chapter, "telephone medical advice" means a telephonic communication between a patient and a health care professional in which the health care professional's primary function is to provide to the patient a telephonic response to the patient's questions regarding his or her or a family member's medical care or treatment. "Telephone medical advice" includes assessment, evaluation, or advice provided to patients or their family members.

(c) For purposes of this chapter, "health care professional" is an employee or independent contractor described in Section 4999.2 who provides medical advice services and is appropriately licensed, certified, or registered as a dentist, dental hygienist, dental hygienist in alternative practice, or dental hygienist in extended functions pursuant to Chapter 4 (commencing with Section 1600), as a physician and surgeon pursuant to Chapter 5 (commencing with Section 2000) or the Osteopathic Initiative Act, as a registered nurse pursuant to Chapter 6 (commencing with Section 2700), as a psychologist pursuant to Chapter 6.6 (commencing with Section 2900), as a naturopathic doctor pursuant to Chapter 8.2 (commencing with Section 3610), as an optometrist pursuant to Chapter 7 (commencing with Section 3000), as a marriage and family therapist pursuant to Chapter 13 (commencing with Section 4980), as a licensed clinical social worker pursuant to Chapter 14 (commencing with Section 4991), as a licensed professional clinical counselor pursuant to Chapter 16 (commencing with Section 4999.10), or as a chiropractor pursuant to the Chiropractic Initiative Act, and who is operating consistent with the laws governing his or her respective scopes of practice in the state in which he or she provides telephone medical advice services.

HISTORY:

Amended Stats 2008 ch 31 § 49 (SB 853) (ch 31 prevails), effective January 1, 2009, operative July 1, 2009, ch 179 § 10, effective January 1, 2009; Stats 2010 ch 328 § 13 (SB 1330), effective January 1, 2011; Stats 2015 ch 426 § 52 (SB 800), effective January 1, 2016.

DIVISION 7

GENERAL BUSINESS REGULATIONS

Part
3. Representations to the Public.

HISTORY: Added Stats 1941 ch 61 § 1.

PART 3

REPRESENTATIONS TO THE PUBLIC

Chapter
1. Advertising.

HISTORY: Added Stats 1941 ch 63 § 1.

CHAPTER 1
ADVERTISING

Article
1. False Advertising in General.

ARTICLE 1
FALSE ADVERTISING IN GENERAL

Section
17500. False or misleading statements generally.
17500.1. Prohibition against enactment of rule, regulation, or code of ethics restricting or prohibiting advertising not violative of law.
17502. Exemption of broadcasting stations and publishers from provisions of article.
17506.5. "Board within the Department of Consumer Affairs"; "Local consumer affairs agency".

§ 17500. False or misleading statements generally

It is unlawful for any person, firm, corporation or association, or any employee thereof with intent directly or indirectly to dispose of real or personal property or to perform services, professional or otherwise, or anything of any nature whatsoever or to induce the public to enter into any obligation relating thereto, to make or disseminate or cause to be made or disseminated before the public in this state, or to make or disseminate or cause to be made or disseminated from this state before the public in any state, in any newspaper or other publication, or any advertising device, or by public outcry or proclamation, or in any other manner or means whatever, including over the Internet, any statement, concerning that real or personal property or those services, professional or otherwise, or concerning any circumstance or matter of fact connected with the proposed performance or disposition thereof, which is untrue or misleading, and which is known, or which by the exercise of reasonable care should be known, to be untrue or misleading, or for any person, firm, or corporation to so make or disseminate or cause to be so made or disseminated any such statement as part of a plan or scheme with the intent not to sell that personal property or those services, professional or otherwise, so advertised at the price stated therein, or as so advertised. Any violation of the provisions of this section is a misdemeanor punishable by imprisonment in the county jail not exceeding six months, or by a fine not exceeding two thousand five hundred dollars ($2,500), or by both that imprisonment and fine.

HISTORY:
Added Stats 1941 ch 63 § 1. Amended Stats 1955 ch 1358 § 1; Stats 1976 ch 1125 § 4; Stats 1979 ch 492 § 1; Stats 1998 ch 599 § 2.5 (SB 597).

§ 17500.1. Prohibition against enactment of rule, regulation, or code of ethics restricting or prohibiting advertising not violative of law

Notwithstanding any other provision of law, no trade or professional association, or state agency, state board, or state commission within the Department of Consumer Affairs shall enact any rule, regulation, or code of professional ethics which shall restrict or prohibit advertising by any commercial or professional person, firm, partnership or corporation which does not violate the provisions of Section 17500 of the Business and Professions Code, or which is not prohibited by other provisions of law.

The provisions of this section shall not apply to any rules or regulations heretofore or hereafter formulated pursuant to Section 6076.

HISTORY:
Added Stats 1949 ch 186 § 1. Amended Stats 1971 ch 716 § 180; Stats 1979 ch 653 § 12.

§ 17502. Exemption of broadcasting stations and publishers from provisions of article

This article does not apply to any visual or sound radio broadcasting station, to any internet service provider or commercial online service, or to any publisher of a newspaper, magazine, or other publication, who broadcasts or publishes, including over the Internet, an advertisement in good faith, without knowledge of its false, deceptive, or misleading character.

HISTORY:
Added Stats 1941 ch 63 § 1. Amended Stats 1951 ch 627 § 1; Stats 1998 ch 599 § 3 (SB 597).

§ 17506.5. "Board within the Department of Consumer Affairs"; "Local consumer affairs agency"

As used in this chapter:

(a) "Board within the Department of Consumer Affairs" includes any commission, bureau, division, or other similarly constituted agency within the Department of Consumer Affairs.

(b) "Local consumer affairs agency" means and includes any city or county body which primarily provides consumer protection services.

HISTORY:
Added Stats 1979 ch 897 § 4.

[illegible] of Consumer Affairs shall [illegible] and [illegible] regulations, the [illegible] [illegible] advertising [illegible] any commercial [illegible] [illegible] violate the [illegible] [illegible] (commencing [illegible]).

[illegible] section shall [illegible] [illegible] or regulations [illegible] to section [illegible].

HISTORY:

[illegible]

§ 17[illegible]. [illegible] of [illegible] and [illegible]

[illegible]

HISTORY:

Added [illegible]

§ 17[illegible]. [illegible] of Consumer Affairs [illegible]

[illegible]

HISTORY:

[illegible]

Bus & Prof

EXTRACTED FROM
CIVIL CODE

Division
1. Persons.

DIVISION 1
PERSONS

Part
2. Personal Rights.

HISTORY: Enacted 1872. Heading amended Stats 1988 ch 160 § 12.

PART 2
PERSONAL RIGHTS

Section
43.8. Immunity as to communication in aid of evaluation of practitioner of healing or veterinary arts.
47. Privileged publication or broadcast.

HISTORY: Enacted 1872.

§ 43.8. Immunity as to communication in aid of evaluation of practitioner of healing or veterinary arts

(a) In addition to the privilege afforded by Section 47, there shall be no monetary liability on the part of, and no cause of action for damages shall arise against, any person on account of the communication of information in the possession of that person to any hospital, hospital medical staff, veterinary hospital staff, professional society, medical, dental, podiatric, psychology, marriage and family therapy, professional clinical counselor, midwifery, or veterinary school, professional licensing board or division, committee or panel of a licensing board, the Senior Assistant Attorney General of the Health Quality Enforcement Section appointed under Section 12529 of the Government Code, peer review committee, quality assurance committees established in compliance with Sections 4070 and 5624 of the Welfare and Institutions Code, or underwriting committee described in Section 43.7 when the communication is intended to aid in the evaluation of the qualifications, fitness, character, or insurability of a practitioner of the healing or veterinary arts.

(b) The immunities afforded by this section and by Section 43.7 shall not affect the availability of any absolute privilege that may be afforded by Section 47.

(c) Nothing in this section is intended in any way to affect the California Supreme Court's decision in Hassan v. Mercy American River Hospital (2003) 31 Cal.4th 709, holding that subdivision (a) provides a qualified privilege.

HISTORY:

Added Stats 1974 ch 1086 § 1. Amended Stats 1975 2d Ex Sess ch 1 § 24.4; Stats 1976 ch 532 § 2; Stats 1977 ch 934 § 2; Stats 1982 ch 234 § 3, effective June 2, 1982, ch 705 § 2; Stats 1983 ch 1081 § 2; Stats 1984 ch 515 § 4; Stats 1983 ch 1081 § 2, operative January 1, 1990; Stats 1990 ch 1597 § 30 (SB 2375); Stats 2002 ch 664 § 31 (AB 3034); Stats 2007 ch 36 § 1 (SB 822), effective January 1, 2008; Stats 2008 ch 23 § 1 (AB 164), effective January 1, 2009; Stats 2011 ch 381 § 15 (SB 146), effective January 1, 2012; Stats 2017 ch 775 § 106 (SB 798), effective January 1, 2018.

§ 47. Privileged publication or broadcast

A privileged publication or broadcast is one made:

(a) In the proper discharge of an official duty.

(b) In any (1) legislative proceeding, (2) judicial proceeding, (3) in any other official proceeding authorized by law, or (4) in the initiation or course of any other proceeding authorized by law and reviewable pursuant to Chapter 2 (commencing with Section 1084) of Title 1 of Part 3 of the Code of Civil Procedure, except as follows:

(1) An allegation or averment contained in any pleading or affidavit filed in an action for marital dissolution or legal separation made of or concerning a person by or against whom no affirmative relief is prayed in the action shall not be a privileged publication or broadcast as to the person making the allegation or averment within the meaning of this section unless the pleading is verified or affidavit sworn to, and is made without malice, by one having reasonable and probable cause for believing the truth of the allegation or averment and unless the allegation or averment is material and relevant to the issues in the action.

(2) This subdivision does not make privileged any communication made in furtherance of an act of intentional destruction or alteration of physical evidence undertaken for the purpose of depriving a party to litigation of the use of that evidence, whether or not the content of the communication is the subject of a subsequent publication or broadcast which is privileged pursuant to this section. As used in this paragraph, "physical evidence" means evidence specified in Section 250 of the Evidence Code or evidence that is property of any type specified in Chapter 14 (commencing with Section 2031.010) of Title 4 of Part 4 of the Code of Civil Procedure.

(3) This subdivision does not make privileged any communication made in a judicial proceeding knowingly concealing the existence of an insurance policy or policies.

(4) A recorded lis pendens is not a privileged publication unless it identifies an action previously filed with a court of competent jurisdiction which affects the title or right of possession of real property, as authorized or required by law.

(5) This subdivision does not make privileged any communication between a person and a law enforcement agency in which the person makes a false report that another person has committed, or is in the act of committing, a criminal act or is engaged in an activity requiring law enforcement intervention, knowing that the report is false, or with reckless disregard for the truth or falsity of the report.

(c) In a communication, without malice, to a person interested therein, (1) by one who is also interested, or (2) by one who stands in such a relation to the person interested as to afford a reasonable ground for supposing the motive for the communication to be innocent, or (3) who is requested by the person interested to give the information. This subdivision applies to and includes a communication concerning the job performance or qualifications of an applicant for employment, based upon credible evidence, made without malice, by a current or former employer of the applicant to, and upon request of, one whom the employer reasonably believes is a prospective employer of the applicant. This subdivision applies to and includes a complaint of sexual harassment by an employee, without malice, to an employer based upon credible evidence and communications between the employer and interested persons, without malice, regarding a complaint of sexual harassment. This subdivision authorizes a current or former employer, or the employer's agent, to answer, without malice, whether or not the employer would rehire a current or former employee and whether the decision to not rehire is based upon the employer's determination that the former employee engaged in sexual harassment. This subdivision does not apply to a communication concerning the speech or activities of an applicant for employment if the speech or activities are constitutionally protected, or otherwise protected by Section 527.3 of the Code of Civil Procedure or any other provision of law.

(d)(1) By a fair and true report in, or a communication to, a public journal, of (A) a judicial, (B) legislative, or (C) other public official proceeding, or (D) of anything said in the course thereof, or (E) of a verified charge or complaint made by any person to a public official, upon which complaint a warrant has been issued.

(2) Paragraph (1) does not make privileged any communication to a public journal that does any of the following:

(A) Violates Rule 5-120 of the State Bar Rules of Professional Conduct.

(B) Breaches a court order.

(C) Violates a requirement of confidentiality imposed by law.

(e) By a fair and true report of (1) the proceedings of a public meeting, if the meeting was lawfully convened for a lawful purpose and open to the public, or (2) the publication of the matter complained of was for the public benefit.

HISTORY:

Enacted 1872. Amended Code Amdts 1873–74 ch 612 § 11; Stats 1895 ch 163 § 1; Stats 1927 ch 866 § 1; Stats 1945 ch 1489 § 3; Stats 1979 ch 184 § 1; Stats 1990 ch 1491 § 1 (AB 3765); Stats 1991 ch 432 § 1 (AB 529); Stats 1992 ch 615 § 1 (SB 1804); Stats 1994 ch 364 § 1 (AB 2778), ch 700 § 2.5 (SB 1457); Stats 1996 ch 1055 § 2 (SB 1540); Stats 2002 ch 1029 § 1 (AB 2868), effective September 28, 2002; Stats 2004 ch 182 § 4 (AB 3081), operative July 1, 2005; Stats 2018 ch 82 § 1 (AB 2770), effective January 1, 2019; Stats 2020 ch 327 § 2 (AB 1775), effective January 1, 2021.

EXTRACTED FROM
CORPORATIONS CODE

Title
1. Corporations.

TITLE 1
CORPORATIONS

Division
3. Corporations for Specific Purposes.

DIVISION 3
CORPORATIONS FOR SPECIFIC PURPOSES

Part
4. Professional Corporations.

PART 4
PROFESSIONAL CORPORATIONS

Section
13401. Definitions.
13401.5. Licensees as shareholders, officers, directors, or employees.

HISTORY: Added Stats 1968 ch 1375 § 9.

§ 13401. Definitions

As used in this part:

(a) "Professional services" means any type of professional services that may be lawfully rendered only pursuant to a license, certification, or registration authorized by the Business and Professions Code, the Chiropractic Act, or the Osteopathic Act.

(b) "Professional corporation" means a corporation organized under the General Corporation Law or pursuant to subdivision (b) of Section 13406 that is engaged in rendering professional services in a single profession, except as otherwise authorized in Section 13401.5, pursuant to a certificate of registration issued by the governmental agency regulating the profession as herein provided and that in its practice or business designates itself as a professional or other corporation as may be required by statute. However, any professional corporation or foreign professional corporation rendering professional services by persons duly licensed by the Medical Board of California or any examining committee under the jurisdiction of the board, the California Board of Podiatric Medicine, the Osteopathic Medical Board of

California, the Dental Board of California, the Dental Hygiene Board of California, the California State Board of Pharmacy, the Veterinary Medical Board, the California Architects Board, the Court Reporters Board of California, the Board of Behavioral Sciences, the Speech-Language Pathology and Audiology Board, the Board of Registered Nursing, the State Board of Optometry, or the California Board of Occupational Therapy shall not be required to obtain a certificate of registration in order to render those professional services.

(c) "Foreign professional corporation" means a corporation organized under the laws of a state of the United States other than this state that is engaged in a profession of a type for which there is authorization in the Business and Professions Code for the performance of professional services by a foreign professional corporation.

(d) "Licensed person" means any natural person who is duly licensed under the provisions of the Business and Professions Code, the Chiropractic Act, or the Osteopathic Act to render the same professional services as are or will be rendered by the professional corporation or foreign professional corporation of which the person is, or intends to become, an officer, director, shareholder, or employee.

(e) "Disqualified person" means a licensed person who for any reason becomes legally disqualified (temporarily or permanently) to render the professional services that the particular professional corporation or foreign professional corporation of which they are an officer, director, shareholder, or employee is or was rendering.

HISTORY:

Added Stats 1968 ch 1375 § 9. Amended Stats 1970 ch 1110 § 3, operative July 1, 1971; Stats 1977 ch 1126 § 3; Stats 1979 ch 472 § 2; Stats 1980 ch 1314 § 16; Stats 1981 ch 383 § 2; Stats 1985 ch 220 § 2, ch 1578 § 2; Stats 1987 ch 571 § 7; Stats 1988 ch 1448 § 28.5; Stats 1989 ch 886 § 82; Stats 1991 ch 566 § 20 (AB 766); Stats 1992 ch 1289 § 50 (AB 2743); Stats 1993 ch 910 § 2 (SB 687), ch 955 § 5.3 (SB 312); Stats 1994 ch 26 § 225 (AB 1807), effective March 30, 1994 (ch 26 prevails), ch 1010 § 66.1 (SB 2053); Stats 1995 ch 60 § 43 (SB 42), effective July 6, 1995; Stats 1997 ch 168 § 8 (AB 348); Stats 1999 ch 657 § 34 (AB 1677); Stats 2000 ch 197 § 4 (SB 1636), ch 836 § 51 (SB 1554); Stats 2004 ch 695 § 51 (SB 1913); Stats 2006 ch 564 § 17 (AB 2256), effective January 1, 2007; Stats 2015 ch 516 § 3 (AB 502), effective January 1, 2016; Stats 2017 ch 775 § 107 (SB 798), effective January 1, 2018; Stats 2018 ch 858 § 61 (SB 1482), effective January 1, 2019; Stats 2022 ch 290 § 6 (AB 2671), effective January 1, 2023.

§ 13401.5. Licensees as shareholders, officers, directors, or employees

Notwithstanding subdivision (d) of Section 13401 and any other provision of law, the following licensed persons may be shareholders, officers, directors, or professional employees of the professional corporations designated in this section so long as the sum of all shares owned by those licensed persons does not exceed 49 percent of the total number of shares of the professional corporation so designated herein, and so long as the number of those licensed persons owning shares in the professional corporation so designated herein does not exceed the number of persons licensed by the governmental agency regulating the designated professional corporation. This section does not limit employment by a professional corporation designated in this section to only those licensed professionals listed under each subdivision. Any person duly licensed under Division 2 (commencing with Section 500) of the Business and

Professions Code, the Chiropractic Act, or the Osteopathic Act may be employed to render professional services by a professional corporation designated in this section.

(a) Medical corporation.

(1) Licensed doctors of podiatric medicine.

(2) Licensed psychologists.

(3) Registered nurses.

(4) Licensed optometrists.

(5) Licensed marriage and family therapists.

(6) Licensed clinical social workers.

(7) Licensed physician assistants.

(8) Licensed chiropractors.

(9) Licensed acupuncturists.

(10) Naturopathic doctors.

(11) Licensed professional clinical counselors.

(12) Licensed physical therapists.

(13) Licensed pharmacists.

(14) Licensed midwives.

(15) Licensed occupational therapists.

(b) Podiatric medical corporation.

(1) Licensed physicians and surgeons.

(2) Licensed psychologists.

(3) Registered nurses.

(4) Licensed optometrists.

(5) Licensed chiropractors.

(6) Licensed acupuncturists.

(7) Naturopathic doctors.

(8) Licensed physical therapists.

(c) Psychological corporation.

(1) Licensed physicians and surgeons.

(2) Licensed doctors of podiatric medicine.

(3) Registered nurses.

(4) Licensed optometrists.

(5) Licensed marriage and family therapists.

(6) Licensed clinical social workers.

(7) Licensed chiropractors.

(8) Licensed acupuncturists.

(9) Naturopathic doctors.

(10) Licensed professional clinical counselors.

(11) Licensed midwives.

(d) Speech-language pathology corporation.

(1) Licensed audiologists.

(e) Audiology corporation.

(1) Licensed speech-language pathologists.

(f) Nursing corporation.

(1) Licensed physicians and surgeons.

(2) Licensed doctors of podiatric medicine.

(3) Licensed psychologists.

(4) Licensed optometrists.

(5) Licensed marriage and family therapists.
(6) Licensed clinical social workers.
(7) Licensed physician assistants.
(8) Licensed chiropractors.
(9) Licensed acupuncturists.
(10) Naturopathic doctors.
(11) Licensed professional clinical counselors.
(12) Licensed midwives.

(g) Marriage and family therapist corporation.
(1) Licensed physicians and surgeons.
(2) Licensed psychologists.
(3) Licensed clinical social workers.
(4) Registered nurses.
(5) Licensed chiropractors.
(6) Licensed acupuncturists.
(7) Naturopathic doctors.
(8) Licensed professional clinical counselors.
(9) Licensed midwives.

(h) Licensed clinical social worker corporation.
(1) Licensed physicians and surgeons.
(2) Licensed psychologists.
(3) Licensed marriage and family therapists.
(4) Registered nurses.
(5) Licensed chiropractors.
(6) Licensed acupuncturists.
(7) Naturopathic doctors.
(8) Licensed professional clinical counselors.

(i) Physician assistants corporation.
(1) Licensed physicians and surgeons.
(2) Registered nurses.
(3) Licensed acupuncturists.
(4) Naturopathic doctors.
(5) Licensed midwives.

(j) Optometric corporation.
(1) Licensed physicians and surgeons.
(2) Licensed doctors of podiatric medicine.
(3) Licensed psychologists.
(4) Registered nurses.
(5) Licensed chiropractors.
(6) Licensed acupuncturists.
(7) Naturopathic doctors.

(k) Chiropractic corporation.
(1) Licensed physicians and surgeons.
(2) Licensed doctors of podiatric medicine.
(3) Licensed psychologists.
(4) Registered nurses.
(5) Licensed optometrists.
(6) Licensed marriage and family therapists.
(7) Licensed clinical social workers.

(8) Licensed acupuncturists.
(9) Naturopathic doctors.
(10) Licensed professional clinical counselors.
(11) Licensed midwives.

(*l*) Acupuncture corporation.
(1) Licensed physicians and surgeons.
(2) Licensed doctors of podiatric medicine.
(3) Licensed psychologists.
(4) Registered nurses.
(5) Licensed optometrists.
(6) Licensed marriage and family therapists.
(7) Licensed clinical social workers.
(8) Licensed physician assistants.
(9) Licensed chiropractors.
(10) Naturopathic doctors.
(11) Licensed professional clinical counselors.
(12) Licensed midwives.

(m) Naturopathic doctor corporation.
(1) Licensed physicians and surgeons.
(2) Licensed psychologists.
(3) Registered nurses.
(4) Licensed physician assistants.
(5) Licensed chiropractors.
(6) Licensed acupuncturists.
(7) Licensed physical therapists.
(8) Licensed doctors of podiatric medicine.
(9) Licensed marriage and family therapists.
(10) Licensed clinical social workers.
(11) Licensed optometrists.
(12) Licensed professional clinical counselors.
(13) Licensed midwives.

(n) Dental corporation.
(1) Licensed physicians and surgeons.
(2) Dental assistants.
(3) Registered dental assistants.
(4) Registered dental assistants in extended functions.
(5) Registered dental hygienists.
(6) Registered dental hygienists in extended functions.
(7) Registered dental hygienists in alternative practice.

(o) Professional clinical counselor corporation.
(1) Licensed physicians and surgeons.
(2) Licensed psychologists.
(3) Licensed clinical social workers.
(4) Licensed marriage and family therapists.
(5) Registered nurses.
(6) Licensed chiropractors.
(7) Licensed acupuncturists.
(8) Naturopathic doctors.
(9) Licensed midwives.

(p) Physical therapy corporation.
(1) Licensed physicians and surgeons.
(2) Licensed doctors of podiatric medicine.
(3) Licensed acupuncturists.
(4) Naturopathic doctors.
(5) Licensed occupational therapists.
(6) Licensed speech-language therapists.
(7) Licensed audiologists.
(8) Registered nurses.
(9) Licensed psychologists.
(10) Licensed physician assistants.
(11) Licensed midwives.
(q) Registered dental hygienist in alternative practice corporation.
(1) Registered dental assistants.
(2) Licensed dentists.
(3) Registered dental hygienists.
(4) Registered dental hygienists in extended functions.
(r) Licensed midwifery corporation.
(1) Licensed physicians and surgeons.
(2) Licensed psychologists.
(3) Registered nurses.
(4) Licensed marriage and family therapists.
(5) Licensed clinical social workers.
(6) Licensed physician assistants.
(7) Licensed chiropractors.
(8) Licensed acupuncturists.
(9) Licensed naturopathic doctors.
(10) Licensed professional clinical counselors.
(11) Licensed physical therapists.
(s) Occupational therapy corporation.
(1) Licensed physicians and surgeons.
(2) Licensed doctors of podiatric medicine.
(3) Licensed acupuncturists.
(4) Naturopathic doctors.
(5) Licensed physical therapists.
(6) Licensed speech-language therapists.
(7) Licensed audiologists.
(8) Registered nurses.
(9) Licensed psychologists.
(10) Licensed physician assistants.
(11) Licensed midwives.
(12) Licensed clinical social workers.
(13) Licensed marriage and family therapists.
(14) Licensed occupational therapy assistants.

HISTORY:

Added Stats 1980 ch 1314 § 17.1. Amended Stats 1981 ch 621 § 5; Stats 1982 ch 1304 § 3, ch 1315 § 1; Stats 1983 ch 1026 § 23, ch 1084 § 1; Stats 1988 ch 507 § 1; Stats 1990 ch 1691 § 1 (AB 3324); Stats 1994 ch 26 § 226 (AB 1807), effective March 30, 1994, ch 815 § 2 (SB 1279); Stats 1997 ch 758 § 84 (SB 1346); Stats 1998 ch 175 § 1 (AB 2120); Stats 2002 ch 1013 § 75 (SB 2026); Stats 2003 ch 485

§ 6 (SB 907), ch 549 § 4 (AB 123); Stats 2004 ch 183 § 50 (AB 3082); Stats 2011 ch 381 § 18 (SB 146), effective January 1, 2012; Stats 2013 ch 620 § 6 (AB 1000), effective January 1, 2014; Stats 2015 ch 516 § 4 (AB 502), effective January 1, 2016; Stats 2016 ch 484 § 53 (SB 1193), effective January 1, 2017; Stats 2017 ch 775 § 108 (SB 798), effective January 1, 2018; Stats 2022 ch 290 § 7 (AB 2671), effective January 1, 2023.

EXTRACTED FROM
EDUCATION CODE

Title
3. Postsecondary Education.

TITLE 3
POSTSECONDARY EDUCATION

Division
5. General Provisions.
8. California State University.

HISTORY: Enacted Stats 1976 ch 1010 § 2, operative April 30, 1977.

DIVISION 5
GENERAL PROVISIONS

Part
40. Donahoe Higher Education Act.

HISTORY: Enacted Stats 1976 ch 1010 § 2, operative April 30, 1977.

PART 40
DONAHOE HIGHER EDUCATION ACT

Chapter
9.2. Student Transfer.

HISTORY: Enacted Stats 1976 ch 1010 § 2, operative April 30, 1977.

CHAPTER 9.2
STUDENT TRANSFER

Article
1.5. Common Course Numbering System.
2. Transfer Functions.

HISTORY: Added Stats 1988 ch 973 § 7, effective January 1, 1989.

ARTICLE 1.5
COMMON COURSE NUMBERING SYSTEM

Section
66725. Legislative intent, findings and declarations.

Section
66725.3. Common course numbering system; Report; Date for incorporation into catalogue.
66725.5. Common course numbering system in California Community Colleges.

HISTORY: Added Stats 2004 ch 737 § 1 (SB 1415), effective January 1, 2005.

§ 66725. Legislative intent, findings and declarations

(a) It is the intent of the Legislature to facilitate articulation and seamless integration of California's postsecondary institutions by facilitating the adoption and integration of a common course numbering system among the public and private postsecondary institutions. The purpose of building and implementing a common course numbering system is to provide for the effective and efficient progression of students within and among the higher education segments and to minimize duplication of coursework.

(b) The Legislature finds and declares both of the following:

(1) Effective transfer programs provide a clear path for obtaining the preparation necessary for upper–division major coursework and graduation at a four–year college or university. The segments have made significant progress in developing articulation agreements that specify required coursework and other academic preparation necessary for transfer students to succeed at a four–year institution. These articulation agreements are essential to provide the basis for a common course numbering system that facilitates transfer student success.

(2) In implementing this article, the public postsecondary educational institutions and other parties involved should assess programs and build upon those proving to be the most effective in communicating articulation, such as the California Articulation Number (CAN) system, the Intersegmental Major Preparation Articulated Curriculum (IMPAC) project, the Intersegmental General Education Transfer Curriculum (IGETC), and the Articulation System Stimulating Interinstitutional Student Transfer (ASSIST).

HISTORY:
Added Stats 2004 ch 737 § 1 (SB 1415).

§ 66725.3. Common course numbering system; Report; Date for incorporation into catalogue

(a) Not later than June 1, 2006, the California Community Colleges and the California State University shall adopt, and the University of California and private postsecondary institutions may adopt, a common course numbering system for the 20 highest–demand majors in the respective segments.

(b) Not later than June 30, 2006, the Board of Governors of the California Community Colleges and the Trustees of the California State University shall, and the Regents of the University of California are requested to, report to the Legislature on the status of the activities of their respective segments as they relate to subdivision (a) and on the plans of their respective segments to implement a common course numbering system for the majors that are not covered by subdivision (a).

(c) Each campus of a public postsecondary educational institution shall incorporate the common course numbering system in its catalogue. This incorporation into a campus catalogue shall occur at the next adoption of a campus catalogue after June 1, 2006.

HISTORY:
Added Stats 2004 ch 737 § 1 (SB 1415).

§ 66725.5. Common course numbering system in California Community Colleges

(a)(1) To streamline transfer from two- to four-year postsecondary educational institutions and reduce excess credit accumulation, on or before July 1, 2024, both of the following shall occur:

(A) The California Community Colleges shall adopt a common course numbering system for all general education requirement courses and transfer pathway courses.

(B) Each community college campus shall incorporate common course numbers from the adopted common course numbering system in its catalog.

(2) The common course numbering system shall be student facing, based on the work of the workgroup established in Item 6870-101-0001 of Section 2.00 of the Budget Act of 2021, and ensure that comparable courses across all community colleges have the same course number.

(3) To support the development and implementation of a common course numbering system for the California Community College system, the workgroup established in Item 6870-101-0001 of Section 2.00 of the Budget Act of 2021 shall consider starting with courses included in the Course Identification Numbering System (C-ID) and expanding to general education requirements and transfer pathway courses pursuant to subdivision (b).

(b) The common course numbering system may have the same alphabetical identifier and same numerical identifier for each course that shares the same C-ID course description, pursuant to both of the following:

(1) For all courses included in the C-ID, the California Community Colleges may adopt the alphabetical and numerical identifier of the C-ID course descriptor as the same common course number at all community colleges.

(2) For all general education requirements and transfer pathway courses that are not included in the C-ID, intersegmental discipline faculty through the C-ID process may develop a C-ID course descriptor for each of these community college courses. Once a C-ID course descriptor is developed, the California Community Colleges may adopt the alphabetical and numerical identifier of the C-ID course descriptor as the same common course number at all community colleges.

HISTORY:
Added Stats 2021 ch 568 § 2 (AB 1111), effective January 1, 2022.

ARTICLE 2
TRANSFER FUNCTIONS

Section
66739.5. Legislative findings and declarations; Legislative intent; Construction; Program with

purpose of enabling community college students to earn baccalaureate degree at a campus of California State University.

HISTORY: Added Stats 1991 ch 1188 § 5 (SB 121), effective January 1, 1992.

§ 66739.5. Legislative findings and declarations; Legislative intent; Construction; Program with purpose of enabling community college students to earn baccalaureate degree at a campus of California State University

(a) The Legislature finds and declares all of the following:

(1) The California Master Plan and supporting statutes place utmost importance on the effective transfer of community college students to the University of California (UC) and the California State University (CSU) as a means of providing access to the baccalaureate degree.

(2) In 2002, CSU enrolled 55,000 transfer students from community colleges.

(3) Two out of three students who earn CSU baccalaureate degrees begin in a community college.

(4) Effective use of state and student time and resources would be maximized by students accruing fewer unrequired units in earning their degrees.

(5) Additional access to community colleges and CSU will be created by higher graduation rates and fewer nonessential units taken.

(6) The state budget situation makes it urgent to streamline the path of the transfer student to the baccalaureate degree.

(b) It is, therefore, the intent of the Legislature to ensure that community college students who wish to earn the baccalaureate degree at CSU are provided with a clear and effective path to this degree.

(c) This section shall not be construed to limit in any way the ability of students to gain admission through alternative paths to transfer, such as the Intersegmental General Education Transfer Curriculum (IGETC) or the California State University General Education-Breadth Requirements.

(d) On or before February 1, 2005, the Chancellor of CSU shall establish transfer student admissions requirements that give highest priority to transfer students who are qualified in accordance with subdivision (f) and paragraph (3) of subdivision (g).

(e)(1) CSU campuses admitting students qualified in accordance with subdivision (f) and paragraph (3) of subdivision (g) will make it possible for these students to complete their baccalaureate degree in the minimum number of remaining units required for that degree major.

(2) For purposes of this subdivision, the "minimum number of remaining units" is the minimum number of units required for a degree major after subtracting the number of fully degree-transferable units earned at the community college.

(f) The Chancellor of CSU, in consultation with the Academic Senate of CSU, shall establish the following components necessary for a clear degree path for transfer students:

(1) On or before June 1, 2005, the Chancellor of CSU, in consultation with the Academic Senate of CSU and with the faculty responsible for each

high-demand baccalaureate degree major program, shall specify for each high-demand baccalaureate program major a systemwide lower division transfer curriculum composed of at least 45 semester course units, or the quarter-unit equivalent, that will be common across all CSU campuses offering specific major programs.

(2)(A) The systemwide lower division transfer curriculum for each high-demand baccalaureate degree major program shall be composed of at least 45 semester units, or the quarter-unit equivalent, and shall include all of the following:

(i) General education courses.

(ii) Any other lower division courses required for graduation.

(iii) Lower division components of the student's declared major.

(iv) Elective units, as appropriate.

(B) The coursework described in subparagraph (A) shall be designated by the CSU faculty responsible for the student's major degree program.

(3) The systemwide lower division transfer curriculum shall be specified in sufficient manner and detail so that existing and future community college lower division courses may be articulated, according to the usual procedures, to the corresponding CSU courses or course descriptions.

(g)(1) On or before June 1, 2006, the Chancellor of CSU and the Chancellor of the California Community Colleges, in consultation with the Academic Senate of the California Community Colleges, shall articulate those lower division, baccalaureate-level courses at each campus of the California Community Colleges that meet for each degree major the systemwide lower division transfer curriculum requirements specified in paragraph (1) of subdivision (f).

(2) To the extent that the goals of efficiency and urgency are advanced, existing articulation procedures such as the California Articulation Number (CAN) program shall be employed.

(3) On or before June 1, 2006, each CSU campus shall have identified any additional specific, nonelective course requirements beyond the systemwide lower division transfer curriculum requirements for each major, up to a maximum of 60 semester units or the quarter-unit equivalent, for the systemwide and campus-specific requirements combined. To the extent these additional course requirements are identified, each CSU campus shall provide that information to all community colleges.

(4) The Chancellor of CSU shall amend CSU's transfer admissions procedures to encourage prospective community college transfer students to identify and, to the extent possible, commit to, a specific CSU transfer destination campus before earning more than 45 semester units, or the quarter-unit equivalent, of lower division, baccalaureate-level courses, as described in subdivision (f).

(h) As allowed by enrollment demand and available space, each CSU campus shall develop a transfer admission agreement with each student who intends to meet the requirements of this section, including the declaration of a major and identification of a choice of a destination campus, before earning more than 45 systemwide semester units, or the quarter-unit equivalent. The transfer admission agreement shall guarantee admission to the campus and major identified in that agreement and transfer of all 60 semester units, or the quarter-unit equivalent, as creditable to the baccalaureate degree, subject to the student's meeting the following conditions:

(1) Completion of the 60 semester units of college-level coursework, or the quarter-unit equivalent, specified for the student's major degree program.

(2) Declaration of a major.

(3) Satisfactory completion of the systemwide lower division transfer curriculum requirements for the student's declared major.

(4) Satisfactory completion of any requirements beyond the systemwide lower division transfer curriculum that are specified by the CSU destination campus.

(5) Any impaction criteria for that campus or major.

(i) A CSU campus shall guarantee that the transfer students admitted under this section will be able to complete the baccalaureate degree in the minimum number of course units required for that degree.

HISTORY:

Added Stats 2004 ch 743 § 1 (SB 1785). Amended Stats 2005 ch 22 § 52 (SB 1108), effective January 1, 2006.

DIVISION 8

CALIFORNIA STATE UNIVERSITY

Part
55. California State University.

HISTORY: Enacted Stats 1976 ch 1010 § 2, operative April 30, 1977. The heading of Division 8, which previously read "California State University and Colleges", was amended to read as above by Stats 1983 ch 143 § 87.

PART 55

CALIFORNIA STATE UNIVERSITY

Chapter
2. Education Programs.

HISTORY: Enacted Stats 1976 ch 1010 § 2, operative April 30, 1977. The heading of Division 8, which previously read "California State University and Colleges", was amended to read as above by Stats 1983 ch 143 § 87.

Misc.

CHAPTER 2

EDUCATION PROGRAMS

Article
8. Entry–Level Master's Nursing Programs (Repealed January 1, 2014).

HISTORY: Enacted Stats 1976 ch 1010 § 2, operative April 30, 1977.

ARTICLE 8

ENTRY-LEVEL MASTER'S NURSING PROGRAMS (REPEALED JANUARY 1, 2014)

HISTORY: Added Stats 2004 ch 718 § 1, repealed January 1, 2014.

Misc.

EXTRACTED FROM
GOVERNMENT CODE

Title
1. General.
2. Government of the State of California.
3. Government of Counties.

TITLE 1
GENERAL

Division
7. Miscellaneous.

DIVISION 7
MISCELLANEOUS

Chapter
3.5. Inspection of Public Records.

CHAPTER 3.5
INSPECTION OF PUBLIC RECORDS

Article
1. General Provisions [Repealed].

HISTORY: Added Stats 1968 ch 1473 § 39. Amended Stats 2021 ch 614 § 1 (AB 473), effective January 1, 2022, repealed January 1, 2023 (repealer added).

ARTICLE 1
GENERAL PROVISIONS [REPEALED]

Section
6250. Legislative finding and declaration [Repealed].
6251. Citation of chapter [Repealed].
6252. Definitions [Repealed].
6252.5. Elected member or officer's access to public records [Repealed].
6252.6. Disclosure of name, date of birth and date of death of minor foster child [Repealed].
6252.7. Discrimination in allowing access of members of legislative body of local agency to writing or portion thereof prohibited [Repealed].
6253. Time for inspection of public records; Unusual circumstances; Posting of public record on internet website [Repealed].
6253.1. Agency to assist in inspection of public record [Repealed].
6253.3. Control of disclosure by another party [Repealed].
6253.31. Contract of state or local agency requiring private entity to review, audit or report on agency [Repealed].

Section
6253.4. Records to be made available.
6254.5. Disclosure of otherwise exempt records; Exceptions.

HISTORY: Heading added Stats 1998 ch 620 § 1. Amended Stats 2021 ch 614 § 1 (AB 473), effective January 1, 2022, repealed January 1, 2023 (repealer added).

§ 6250. Legislative finding and declaration [Repealed]

HISTORY:

Added Stats 1968 ch 1473 § 39. Amended Stats 1970 ch 575 § 1; Stats 2021 ch 614 § 1 (AB 473), effective January 1, 2022, repealed January 1, 2023 (repealer added).

§ 6251. Citation of chapter [Repealed]

HISTORY:

Added Stats 1968 ch 1473 § 39. Amended Stats 2021 ch 614 § 1 (AB 473), effective January 1, 2022, repealed January 1, 2023 (repealer added).

§ 6252. Definitions [Repealed]

HISTORY:

Added Stats 1968 ch 1473 § 39. Amended Stats 1970 ch 575 § 2; Stats 1975 ch 1246 § 2; Stats 1981 ch 968 § 1; Stats 1991 ch 181 § 1 (AB 788); Stats 1994 ch 1010 § 136 (SB 2053); Stats 1998 ch 620 § 2 (SB 143); Stats 2002 ch 945 § 2.5 (AB 1962), ch 1073 § 1.5 (AB 2937); Stats 2004 ch 937 § 1 (AB 1933); Stats 2015 ch 537 § 20 (SB 387), effective January 1, 2016; Stats 2021 ch 614 § 1 (AB 473), effective January 1, 2022, repealed January 1, 2023 (repealer added).

§ 6252.5. Elected member or officer's access to public records [Repealed]

HISTORY:

Added Stats 1998 ch 620 § 3 (SB 143). Amended Stats 2021 ch 614 § 1 (AB 473), effective January 1, 2022, repealed January 1, 2023(repealer added).

§ 6252.6. Disclosure of name, date of birth and date of death of minor foster child [Repealed]

HISTORY:

Added Stats 2003 ch 847 § 3 (AB 1151). Amended Stats 2021 ch 614 § 1 (AB 473), effective January 1, 2022, repealed January 1, 2023 (repealer added).

§ 6252.7. Discrimination in allowing access of members of legislative body of local agency to writing or portion thereof prohibited [Repealed]

Notwithstanding Section 6252.5 or any other provision of law, when the members of a legislative body of a local agency are authorized to access a writing of the body or of the agency as permitted by law in the administration of their duties, the local agency, as defined in Section 54951, shall not discriminate between or among any of those members as to which writing or portion thereof is made available or when it is made available.

HISTORY:

Added Stats 2008 ch 63 § 2 (SB 1732), effective January 1, 2009. Amended Stats 2021 ch 614 § 1 (AB 473), effective January 1, 2022, repealed January 1, 2023 (repealer added).

§ 6253. Time for inspection of public records; Unusual circumstances; Posting of public record on internet website [Repealed]

HISTORY:
Added Stats 1998 ch 620 § 5 (SB 143). Amended Stats 1999 ch 83 § 64 (SB 966); Stats 2000 ch 982 § 1 (AB 2799); Stats 2001 ch 355 § 2 (AB 1014); Stats 2016 ch 275 § 1 (AB 2853), effective January 1, 2017; Stats 2019 ch 695 § 1 (AB 1819), effective January 1, 2020; Stats 2021 ch 614 § 1 (AB 473), effective January 1, 2022, repealed January 1, 2023 (repealer added).

§ 6253.1. Agency to assist in inspection of public record [Repealed]

HISTORY:
Added Stats 2001 ch 355 § 3 (AB 1014). Amended Stats 2021 ch 614 § 1 (AB 473), effective January 1, 2022, repealed January 1, 2023 (repealer added).

§ 6253.3 Control of disclosure by another party [Repealed]

HISTORY:
Added Stats 2008 ch 62 § 1 (SB 1696), effective January 1, 2009. Amended Stats 2021 ch 614 § 1 (AB 473), effective January 1, 2022, repealed January 1, 2023 (repealer added).

§ 6253.31 Contract of state or local agency requiring private entity to review, audit or report on agency [Repealed]

HISTORY:
Added Stats 2008 ch 62 § 2 (SB 1696), effective January 1, 2009. Amended Stats 2021 ch 614 § 1 (AB 473), effective January 1, 2022, repealed January 1, 2023 (repealer added).

§ 6253.4. Records to be made available

(a) Every agency may adopt regulations stating the procedures to be followed when making its records available in accordance with this section.

(b) The following state and local bodies shall establish written guidelines for accessibility of records. A copy of these guidelines shall be posted in a conspicuous public place at the offices of these bodies, and a copy of the guidelines shall be available upon request free of charge to any person requesting that body's records:

(1) Department of Motor Vehicles
(2) Department of Consumer Affairs
(3) Transportation Agency
(4) Bureau of Real Estate
(5) Department of Corrections and Rehabilitation
(6) Division of Juvenile Justice
(7) Department of Justice
(8) Department of Insurance
(9) Department of Financial Protection and Innovation
(10) Department of Managed Health Care
(11) Secretary of State
(12) State Air Resources Board
(13) Department of Water Resources
(14) Department of Parks and Recreation
(15) San Francisco Bay Conservation and Development Commission
(16) State Board of Equalization

(17) State Department of Health Care Services
(18) Employment Development Department
(19) State Department of Public Health
(20) State Department of Social Services
(21) State Department of State Hospitals
(22) State Department of Developmental Services
(23) Public Employees' Retirement System
(24) Teachers' Retirement Board
(25) Department of Industrial Relations
(26) Department of General Services
(27) Department of Veterans Affairs
(28) Public Utilities Commission
(29) California Coastal Commission
(30) State Water Resources Control Board
(31) San Francisco Bay Area Rapid Transit District
(32) All regional water quality control boards
(33) Los Angeles County Air Pollution Control District
(34) Bay Area Air Pollution Control District
(35) Golden Gate Bridge, Highway and Transportation District
(36) Department of Toxic Substances Control
(37) Office of Environmental Health Hazard Assessment

(c) Guidelines and regulations adopted pursuant to this section shall be consistent with all other sections of this chapter and shall reflect the intention of the Legislature to make the records accessible to the public. The guidelines and regulations adopted pursuant to this section shall not operate to limit the hours public records are open for inspection as prescribed in Section 6253.

HISTORY:

Added Stats 1968 ch 1473 § 39, as Gov C § 6253. Amended Stats 1973 ch 664 § 1; Stats 1974 ch 544 § 7; Stats 1975 ch 957 § 6; Stats 1977 ch 1252 § 96, operative July 1, 1978; Stats 1979 ch 373 § 120; Stats 1983 ch 826 § 1; Stats 1988 ch 409 § 1. Supplemented by Governor's Reorganization Plan No. 1 of 1991 § 70, effective July 17, 1991; Amended and renumbered by Stats 1998 ch 620 § 4 (SB 143); Amended Stats 1999 ch 525 § 11 (AB 78); Stats 2000 ch 857 § 9 (AB 2903); Stats 2006 ch 241 § 2 (SB 162), effective January 1, 2007, operative July 1, 2007; Stats 2012 ch 440 § 7 (AB 1488), effective September 22, 2012; Stats 2013 ch 22 § 7 (AB 75), effective June 27, 2013, operative July 1, 2013; Stats 2018 ch 92 § 88 (SB 1289), effective January 1, 2019; Stats 2021 ch 614 § 1 (AB 473), effective January 1, 2022, repealed January 1, 2023 (repealer added); Stats 2022 ch 452 § 169 (SB 1498), effective January 1, 2023.

§ 6254.5. Disclosure of otherwise exempt records; Exceptions

Notwithstanding any other law, if a state or local agency discloses a public record that is otherwise exempt from this chapter, to a member of the public, this disclosure shall constitute a waiver of the exemptions specified in Section 6254 or 6254.7, or other similar provisions of law. For purposes of this section, "agency" includes a member, agent, officer, or employee of the agency acting within the scope of that membership, agency, office, or employment.

This section, however, shall not apply to disclosures:

(a) Made pursuant to the Information Practices Act (Chapter 1 (commencing with Section 1798) of Title 1.8 of Part 4 of Division 3 of the Civil Code) or discovery proceedings.

(b) Made through other legal proceedings or as otherwise required by law.

(c) Within the scope of disclosure of a statute that limits disclosure of specified writings to certain purposes.

(d) Not required by law, and prohibited by formal action of an elected legislative body of the local agency that retains the writings.

(e) Made to a governmental agency that agrees to treat the disclosed material as confidential. Only persons authorized in writing by the person in charge of the agency shall be permitted to obtain the information. Any information obtained by the agency shall only be used for purposes that are consistent with existing law.

(f) Of records relating to a financial institution or an affiliate thereof, if the disclosures are made to the financial institution or affiliate by a state agency responsible for the regulation or supervision of the financial institution or affiliate.

(g) Of records relating to a person who is subject to the jurisdiction of the Department of Business Oversight, if the disclosures are made to the person who is the subject of the records for the purpose of corrective action by that person, or, if a corporation, to an officer, director, or other key personnel of the corporation for the purpose of corrective action, or to any other person to the extent necessary to obtain information from that person for the purpose of an investigation by the Department of Business Oversight.

(h) Made by the Commissioner of Business Oversight under Section 450, 452, 8009, or 18396 of the Financial Code.

(i) Of records relating to a person who is subject to the jurisdiction of the Department of Managed Health Care, if the disclosures are made to the person who is the subject of the records for the purpose of corrective action by that person, or, if a corporation, to an officer, director, or other key personnel of the corporation for the purpose of corrective action, or to any other person to the extent necessary to obtain information from that person for the purpose of an investigation by the Department of Managed Health Care.

(j) A disclosure made through the sharing of information between the Independent System Operator and a state agency.

HISTORY:

Added Stats 1981 ch 968 § 3. Amended Stats 1983 ch 101 § 57; Stats 1987 ch 1453 § 5; Stats 1993 ch 469 § 11 (AB 729); Stats 1995 ch 480 § 199 (AB 1482), effective October 2, 1995, operative October 2, 1995; Stats 1996 ch 1064 § 780 (AB 3351), operative July 1, 1997; Stats 1999 ch 525 § 12 (AB 78) operative July 1, 2000; Stats 2000 ch 857 § 10 (AB 2093); Stats 2008 ch 501 § 23 (AB 2749), effective January 1, 2009; Stats 2014 ch 401 § 35 (AB 2763), effective January 1, 2015; Stats 2015 ch 190 § 59 (AB 1517), effective January 1, 2016; Stats 2016 ch 86 § 151 (SB 1171), effective January 1, 2017; Stats 2021 ch 614 § 1 (AB 473), effective January 1, 2022, repealed January 1, 2023 (repealer added); Stats 2022 ch 251 § 5 (AB 209), effective September 6, 2022; Stats 2022 ch 452 § 170 (SB 1498), effective January 1, 2023 (ch 251 prevails).

TITLE 2

GOVERNMENT OF THE STATE OF CALIFORNIA

Division
3. Executive Department.

DIVISION 3
EXECUTIVE DEPARTMENT

Part
1. State Departments and Agencies.
2.8. CIVIL RIGHTS DEPARTMENT.
5.5. Department of General Services.

HISTORY: Added Stats 1945 ch 111 § 3.

PART 1
STATE DEPARTMENTS AND AGENCIES

Chapter
1. State Agencies.

CHAPTER 1
STATE AGENCIES

Article
9. Meetings.

ARTICLE 9
MEETINGS

Section
11120. Legislative finding and declaration; Open proceedings; Citation of article.
11121. "State body".
11121.9. Providing copy of article to members of state bodies.
11122. "Action taken".
11123. Open meeting requirement for state bodies; Meetings by teleconference; Public reporting requirement for actions at meeting.
11123.5. Teleconference meeting.
11124. Prohibited conditions to attendance.
11124.1. Recording of proceedings; Inspection of recording.
11125. Notice of meeting.
11125.1. Agendas of public meetings and other "writings" as public record; Exemptions; Public inspection; Alternative format requirements; Fee.
11125.2. Public report of action taken regarding public employee.
11125.5. Emergency meetings; Notification of media.
11125.7. Opportunity for public to address state body.
11126. Closed session on issues relating to public employee; Employee's right to public hearing; Closed sessions not prohibited by article; Abrogation of lawyer-client privilege.
11126.1. Minute book of closed session.
11126.2. Closed session for response to final draft audit report.
11126.3. Disclosure of items to be discussed in closed session; Discussion of additional pending litigation matters arising after disclosure.
11126.5. Clearing room when meeting wilfully interrupted.
11126.7. Fees.

Section
11127. State bodies subject to article.
11128. When closed sessions held.
11128.5. Adjournment of meeting; Posting of copy of order or notice of adjournment.
11129. Continuance or recontinuance of hearing.
11130. Action to stop or prevent violations of article; Order for recording of closed sessions; Discovery of recording.
11130.3. Cause of action to void action taken by state agency in violation of open meeting requirements.
11130.5. Costs and attorney fees.
11130.7. Offenses.
11131. Prohibition against use of certain facilities.
11132. Prohibition against closed sessions except as expressly authorized.
11133. Public meetings [Repealed effective July 1, 2023].

HISTORY: Added Stats 1967 ch 1656 § 122.

§ 11120. Legislative finding and declaration; Open proceedings; Citation of article

It is the public policy of this state that public agencies exist to aid in the conduct of the people's business and the proceedings of public agencies be conducted openly so that the public may remain informed.

In enacting this article the Legislature finds and declares that it is the intent of the law that actions of state agencies be taken openly and that their deliberation be conducted openly.

The people of this state do not yield their sovereignty to the agencies which serve them. The people, in delegating authority, do not give their public servants the right to decide what is good for the people to know and what is not good for them to know. The people insist on remaining informed so that they may retain control over the instruments they have created.

This article shall be known and may be cited as the Bagley-Keene Open Meeting Act.

HISTORY:

Added Stats 1967 ch 1656 § 122. Amended Stats 1980 ch 1284 § 4; Stats 1981 ch 968 § 4.

§ 11121. "State body"

As used in this article, "state body" means each of the following:

(a) Every state board, or commission, or similar multimember body of the state that is created by statute or required by law to conduct official meetings and every commission created by executive order.

(b) A board, commission, committee, or similar multimember body that exercises any authority of a state body delegated to it by that state body.

(c) An advisory board, advisory commission, advisory committee, advisory subcommittee, or similar multimember advisory body of a state body, if created by formal action of the state body or of any member of the state body, and if the advisory body so created consists of three or more persons.

(d) A board, commission, committee, or similar multimember body on which a member of a body that is a state body pursuant to this section serves in his or her official capacity as a representative of that state body and that is supported, in whole or in part, by funds provided by the state body, whether the multimember body is organized and operated by the state body or by a private corporation.

(e) Notwithstanding subdivision (a) of Section 11121.1, the State Bar of California, as described in Section 6001 of the Business and Professions Code. This subdivision shall become operative on April 1, 2016.

HISTORY:

Added Stats 1967 ch 1656 § 122. Amended Stats 1980 ch 515 § 1; Stats 1981 ch 968 § 5; Stats 1984 ch 193 § 38; Stats 1996 ch 1023 § 88 (SB 1497), effective September 29, 1996, ch 1064 § 783.1 (AB 3351), operative July 1, 1997; Stats 2001 ch 243 § 1 (AB 192); Stats 2003 ch 62 § 117 (SB 600); Stats 2015 ch 537 § 22 (SB 387), effective January 1, 2016, operative April 1, 2016.

§ 11121.9. Providing copy of article to members of state bodies

Each state body shall provide a copy of this article to each member of the state body upon his or her appointment to membership or assumption of office.

HISTORY:

Added Stats 1980 ch 1284 § 6. Amended Stats 1981 ch 714 § 175, ch 968 § 7.1.

§ 11122. "Action taken"

As used in this article "action taken" means a collective decision made by the members of a state body, a collective commitment or promise by the members of the state body to make a positive or negative decision or an actual vote by the members of a state body when sitting as a body or entity upon a motion, proposal, resolution, order or similar action.

HISTORY:

Added Stats 1967 ch 1656 § 122. Amended Stats 1981 ch 968 § 7.3.

§ 11123. Open meeting requirement for state bodies; Meetings by teleconference; Public reporting requirement for actions at meeting

(a) All meetings of a state body shall be open and public and all persons shall be permitted to attend any meeting of a state body except as otherwise provided in this article.

(b)(1) This article does not prohibit a state body from holding an open or closed meeting by teleconference for the benefit of the public and state body. The meeting or proceeding held by teleconference shall otherwise comply with all applicable requirements or laws relating to a specific type of meeting or proceeding, including the following:

(A) The teleconferencing meeting shall comply with all requirements of this article applicable to other meetings.

(B) The portion of the teleconferenced meeting that is required to be open to the public shall be audible to the public at the location specified in the notice of the meeting.

(C) If the state body elects to conduct a meeting or proceeding by teleconference, it shall post agendas at all teleconference locations and conduct teleconference meetings in a manner that protects the rights of any party or member of the public appearing before the state body. Each teleconference location shall be identified in the notice and agenda of the meeting or proceeding, and each teleconference location shall be accessible to the public. The agenda shall provide an opportunity for members of the public to address the state body directly pursuant to Section 11125.7 at each teleconference location.

(D) All votes taken during a teleconferenced meeting shall be by rollcall.

(E) The portion of the teleconferenced meeting that is closed to the public may not include the consideration of any agenda item being heard pursuant to Section 11125.5.

(F) At least one member of the state body shall be physically present at the location specified in the notice of the meeting.

(2) For the purposes of this subdivision, "teleconference" means a meeting of a state body, the members of which are at different locations, connected by electronic means, through either audio or both audio and video. This section does not prohibit a state body from providing members of the public with additional locations in which the public may observe or address the state body by electronic means, through either audio or both audio and video.

(c) The state body shall publicly report any action taken and the vote or abstention on that action of each member present for the action.

HISTORY:

Added Stats 1967 ch 1656 § 122. Amended Stats 1981 ch 968 § 7.5; Stats 1994 ch 1153 § 1 (AB 3467); Stats 1997 ch 52 § 1 (AB 1097); Stats 2001 ch 243 § 7 (AB 192); Stats 2014 ch 510 § 1 (AB 2720), effective January 1, 2015.

§ 11123.5. Teleconference meeting

(a) In addition to the authorization to hold a meeting by teleconference pursuant to subdivision (b) of Section 11123, any state body that is an advisory board, advisory commission, advisory committee, advisory subcommittee, or similar multimember advisory body may hold an open meeting by teleconference as described in this section, provided the meeting complies with all of the section's requirements and, except as set forth in this section, it also complies with all other applicable requirements of this article.

(b) A member of a state body as described in subdivision (a) who participates in a teleconference meeting from a remote location subject to this section's requirements shall be listed in the minutes of the meeting.

(c) The state body shall provide notice to the public at least 24 hours before the meeting that identifies any member who will participate remotely by posting the notice on its Internet Web site and by emailing notice to any person who has requested notice of meetings of the state body under this article. The location of a member of a state body who will participate remotely is not required to be disclosed in the public notice or email and need not be accessible to the public. The notice of the meeting shall also identify the primary physical meeting location designated pursuant to subdivision (e).

(d) This section does not affect the requirement prescribed by this article that the state body post an agenda of a meeting at least 10 days in advance of the meeting. The agenda shall include information regarding the physical meeting location designated pursuant to subdivision (e), but is not required to disclose information regarding any remote location.

(e) A state body described in subdivision (a) shall designate the primary physical meeting location in the notice of the meeting where members of the public may physically attend the meeting and participate. A quorum of the members of the state body shall be in attendance at the primary physical meeting location, and members of the state body participating remotely shall not count towards establishing a quorum. All decisions taken during a meeting by teleconference shall be by rollcall vote. The state body shall post the agenda at the primary physical meeting location, but need not post the agenda at a remote location.

(f) When a member of a state body described in subdivision (a) participates remotely in a meeting subject to this section's requirements, the state body shall provide a means by which the public may remotely hear audio of the meeting or remotely observe the meeting, including, if available, equal access equivalent to members of the state body participating remotely. The applicable teleconference phone number or Internet Web site, or other information indicating how the public can access the meeting remotely, shall be in the 24-hour notice described in subdivision (a) that is available to the public.

(g) Upon discovering that a means of remote access required by subdivision (f) has failed during a meeting, the state body described in subdivision (a) shall end or adjourn the meeting in accordance with Section 11128.5. In addition to any other requirements that may apply, the state body shall provide notice of the meeting's end or adjournment on its Internet Web site and by email to any person who has requested notice of meetings of the state body under this article. If the meeting will be adjourned and reconvened on the same day, further notice shall be provided by an automated message on a telephone line posted on the state body's agenda, or by a similar means, that will communicate when the state body intends to reconvene the meeting and how a member of the public may hear audio of the meeting or observe the meeting.

(h) For purposes of this section:

(1) "Participate remotely" means participation in a meeting at a location other than the physical location designated in the agenda of the meeting.

(2) "Remote location" means a location other than the primary physical location designated in the agenda of a meeting.

(3) "Teleconference" has the same meaning as in Section 11123.

(i) This section does not limit or affect the ability of a state body to hold a teleconference meeting under another provision of this article.

HISTORY:

Added Stats 2018 ch 881 § 1 (AB 2958), effective January 1, 2019.

§ 11124. Prohibited conditions to attendance

No person shall be required, as a condition to attendance at a meeting of a state body, to register his or her name, to provide other information, to complete a questionnaire, or otherwise to fulfill any condition precedent to his or her attendance.

If an attendance list, register, questionnaire, or other similar document is posted at or near the entrance to the room where the meeting is to be held, or is circulated to persons present during the meeting, it shall state clearly that the signing, registering, or completion of the document is voluntary, and that all persons may attend the meeting regardless of whether a person signs, registers, or completes the document.

HISTORY:

Added Stats 1967 ch 1656 § 122. Amended Stats 1981 ch 968 § 8.

§ 11124.1. Recording of proceedings; Inspection of recording

(a) Any person attending an open and public meeting of the state body shall have the right to record the proceedings with an audio or video recorder or a still or motion picture camera in the absence of a reasonable finding by the state body that the recording cannot continue without noise, illumination, or obstruction of view that constitutes, or would constitute, a persistent disruption of the proceedings.

(b) Any audio or video recording of an open and public meeting made for whatever purpose by or at the direction of the state body shall be subject to inspection pursuant to the California Public Records Act (Division 10 (commencing with Section 7920.000) of Title 1), but may be erased or destroyed 30 days after the recording. Any inspection of an audio or video recording shall be provided without charge on equipment made available by the state body.

(c) No state body shall prohibit or otherwise restrict the broadcast of its open and public meetings in the absence of a reasonable finding that the broadcast cannot be accomplished without noise, illumination, or obstruction of view that would constitute a persistent disruption of the proceedings.

HISTORY:

Added Stats 1980 ch 1284 § 7. Amended Stats 1981 ch 968 § 9; Stats 1997 ch 949 § 2 (SB 95); Stats 2009 ch 88 § 42 (AB 176), effective January 1, 2010; Stats 2021 ch 615 § 161 (AB 474), effective January 1, 2022.

§ 11125. Notice of meeting

(a) The state body shall provide notice of its meeting to any person who requests that notice in writing. Notice shall be given and also made available on the Internet at least 10 days in advance of the meeting, and shall include the name, address, and telephone number of any person who can provide further information prior to the meeting, but need not include a list of witnesses expected to appear at the meeting. The written notice shall additionally include the address of the Internet site where notices required by this article are made available.

(b) The notice of a meeting of a body that is a state body shall include a specific agenda for the meeting, containing a brief description of the items of business to be transacted or discussed in either open or closed session. A brief general description of an item generally need not exceed 20 words. A description of an item to be transacted or discussed in closed session shall include a citation of the specific statutory authority under which a closed session is being held. No item shall be added to the agenda subsequent to the provision of this notice, unless otherwise permitted by this article.

(c) Notice of a meeting of a state body that complies with this section shall also constitute notice of a meeting of an advisory body of that state body, provided that the business to be discussed by the advisory body is covered by the notice of the meeting of the state body, provided that the specific time and place of the advisory body's meeting is announced during the open and public state body's meeting, and provided that the advisory body's meeting is conducted within a reasonable time of, and nearby, the meeting of the state body.

(d) A person may request, and shall be provided, notice pursuant to subdivision (a) for all meetings of a state body or for a specific meeting or meetings. In addition, at the state body's discretion, a person may request, and may be provided, notice of only those meetings of a state body at which a particular subject or subjects specified in the request will be discussed.

(e) A request for notice of more than one meeting of a state body shall be subject to the provisions of Section 14911.

(f) The notice shall be made available in appropriate alternative formats, as required by Section 202 of the Americans with Disabilities Act of 1990 (42 U.S.C. Sec. 12132), and the federal rules and regulations adopted in implementation thereof, upon request by any person with a disability. The notice shall include information regarding how, to whom, and by when a request for any disability-related modification or accommodation, including auxiliary aids or services may be made by a person with a disability who requires these aids or services in order to participate in the public meeting.

HISTORY:

Added Stats 1967 ch 1656 § 122. Amended Stats 1973 ch 1126 § 1; Stats 1975 ch 708 § 1; Stats 1979 ch 284 § 1, effective July 24, 1979; Stats 1981 ch 968 § 10; Stats 1997 ch 949 § 3 (SB 95); Stats 1999 ch 393 § 1 (AB 1234); Stats 2001 ch 243 § 8 (AB 192); Stats 2002 ch 300 § 2 (AB 3035).

§ 11125.1. Agendas of public meetings and other "writings" as public record; Exemptions; Public inspection; Alternative format requirements; Fee

(a) Notwithstanding Section 7922.000 or any other provisions of law, agendas of public meetings and other writings, when distributed to all, or a majority of all, of the members of a state body by any person in connection with a matter subject to discussion or consideration at a public meeting of the body, are disclosable public records under the California Public Records Act (Division 10 (commencing with Section 7920.000) of Title 1), and shall be made available upon request without delay. However, this section shall not include any writing exempt from public disclosure under Section 7924.100, 7924.105, 7924.110, 7924.510, or 7924.700 of this code, any provision listed in Section 7920.505 of this code, or Section 489.1 or 583 of the Public Utilities Code.

(b) Writings that are public records under subdivision (a) and that are distributed to members of the state body prior to or during a meeting, pertaining to any item to be considered during the meeting, shall be made available for public inspection at the meeting if prepared by the state body or a member of the state body, or after the meeting if prepared by some other person. These writings shall be made available in appropriate alternative formats, as required by Section 202 of the Americans with Disabilities Act of 1990 (42 U.S.C. Sec. 12132), and the federal rules and regulations adopted in implementation thereof, upon request by a person with a disability.

(c) In the case of the Franchise Tax Board, prior to that state body taking final action on any item, writings pertaining to that item that are public records under subdivision (a) that are prepared and distributed by the Franchise Tax Board staff or individual members to members of the state body prior to or during a meeting shall be:

(1) Made available for public inspection at that meeting.

(2) Distributed to all persons who request notice in writing pursuant to subdivision (a) of Section 11125.

(3) Made available on the internet.

(d) Prior to the State Board of Equalization taking final action on any item that does not involve a named taxpayer or feepayer, writings pertaining to that item that are public records under subdivision (a) that are prepared and distributed by board staff or individual members to members of the state body prior to or during a meeting shall be:

(1) Made available for public inspection at that meeting.

(2) Distributed to all persons who request or have requested copies of these writings.

(3) Made available on the internet.

(e) Nothing in this section shall be construed to prevent a state body from charging a fee or deposit for a copy of a public record pursuant to Section 7922.530, except that no surcharge shall be imposed on persons with disabilities in violation of Section 202 of the Americans with Disabilities Act of 1990 (42 U.S.C. Sec. 12132), and the federal rules and regulations adopted in implementation thereof. The writings described in subdivision (b) are subject to the requirements of the California Public Records Act (Division 10 (commencing with Section 7920.000) of Title 1), and shall not be construed to limit or delay the public's right to inspect any record required to be disclosed by that act, or to limit the public's right to inspect any record covered by that act. This section shall not be construed to be applicable to any writings solely because they are properly discussed in a closed session of a state body. Nothing in this article shall be construed to require a state body to place any paid advertisement or any other paid notice in any publication.

(f) "Writing" for purposes of this section means "writing" as defined under Section 7920.545.

HISTORY:

Added Stats 1975 ch 959 § 4. Amended Stats 1980 ch 1284 § 8; Stats 1981 ch 968 § 10.1; Stats 1997 ch 949 § 4 (SB 95); Stats 2001 ch 670 § 1 (SB 445); Stats 2002 ch 156 § 1 (AB 1752), ch 300 § 3.5 (AB 3035); Stats 2005 ch 188 § 1 (AB 780), effective January 1, 2006; Stats 2021 ch 615 § 162 (AB 474), effective January 1, 2022.

§ 11125.2. Public report of action taken regarding public employee

Any state body shall report publicly at a subsequent public meeting any action taken, and any rollcall vote thereon, to appoint, employ, or dismiss a public employee arising out of any closed session of the state body.

HISTORY:

Added Stats 1980 ch 1284 § 9. Amended Stats 1981 ch 968 § 10.3.

§ 11125.5. Emergency meetings; Notification of media

(a) In the case of an emergency situation involving matters upon which prompt action is necessary due to the disruption or threatened disruption of public facilities, a state body may hold an emergency meeting without complying with the 10-day notice requirement of Section 11125 or the 48-hour notice requirement of Section 11125.4.

(b) For purposes of this section, "emergency situation" means any of the following, as determined by a majority of the members of the state body during a meeting prior to the emergency meeting, or at the beginning of the emergency meeting:

(1) Work stoppage or other activity that severely impairs public health or safety, or both.

(2) Crippling disaster that severely impairs public health or safety, or both.

(c) However, newspapers of general circulation and radio or television stations that have requested notice of meetings pursuant to Section 11125 shall be notified by the presiding officer of the state body, or a designee thereof, one hour prior to the emergency meeting by telephone. Notice shall also be made available on the Internet as soon as is practicable after the decision to call the emergency meeting has been made. If telephone services are not functioning, the notice requirements of this section shall be deemed waived, and the presiding officer of the state body, or a designee thereof, shall notify those newspapers, radio stations, or television stations of the fact of the holding of the emergency meeting, the purpose of the meeting, and any action taken at the meeting as soon after the meeting as possible.

(d) The minutes of a meeting called pursuant to this section, a list of persons who the presiding officer of the state body, or a designee thereof, notified or attempted to notify, a copy of the rollcall vote, and any action taken at the meeting shall be posted for a minimum of 10 days in a public place, and also made available on the Internet for a minimum of 10 days, as soon after the meeting as possible.

HISTORY:

Added Stats 1981 ch 968 § 11. Amended Stats 1982 ch 1346 § 5.5; Stats 1992 ch 1312 § 11 (AB 2912), effective September 30, 1992; Stats 1997 ch 949 § 6 (SB 95); Stats 1999 ch 393 § 3 (AB 1234), operative July 1, 2001.

§ 11125.7. Opportunity for public to address state body

(a) Except as otherwise provided in this section, the state body shall provide an opportunity for members of the public to directly address the state body on each agenda item before or during the state body's discussion or consideration of the item. This section is not applicable if the agenda item has already been considered by a committee composed exclusively of members of the state body at a public meeting where interested members of the public were afforded the opportunity to address the committee on the item, before or during the committee's consideration of the item, unless the item has been substantially changed since the committee heard the item, as determined by the state body. Every notice for a special meeting at which action is proposed to be taken on an item shall provide an opportunity for members of the public to directly address the state body concerning that item prior to action on the item. In addition, the notice requirement of Section 11125 shall not preclude the acceptance of testimony at meetings, other than emergency meetings, from members of the public if no action is taken by the state body at the same meeting on matters brought before the body by members of the public.

(b) The state body may adopt reasonable regulations to ensure that the intent of subdivision (a) is carried out, including, but not limited to, regulations limiting the total amount of time allocated for public comment on particular issues and for each individual speaker.

(c)(1) Notwithstanding subdivision (b), when a state body limits time for public comment the state body shall provide at least twice the allotted time to a member of the public who utilizes a translator or other translating technology to ensure that non-English speakers receive the same opportunity to directly address the state body.

(2) Paragraph (1) shall not apply if the state body utilizes simultaneous translation equipment in a manner that allows the state body to hear the translated public testimony simultaneously.

(d) The state body shall not prohibit public criticism of the policies, programs, or services of the state body, or of the acts or omissions of the state body. Nothing in this subdivision shall confer any privilege or protection for expression beyond that otherwise provided by law.

(e) This section is not applicable to any of the following:

(1) Closed sessions held pursuant to Section 11126.

(2) Decisions regarding proceedings held pursuant to Chapter 5 (commencing with Section 11500), relating to administrative adjudication, or to the conduct of those proceedings.

(3) Hearings conducted by the California Victim Compensation Board pursuant to Sections 13963 and 13963.1.

(4) Agenda items that involve decisions of the Public Utilities Commission regarding adjudicatory hearings held pursuant to Chapter 9 (commencing with Section 1701) of Part 1 of Division 1 of the Public Utilities Code. For all other agenda items, the commission shall provide members of the public, other than those who have already participated in the proceedings underlying the agenda item, an opportunity to directly address the commission before or during the commission's consideration of the item.

HISTORY:

Added Stats 1993 ch 1289 § 2 (SB 367), operative until July 1, 1997. Amended Stats 1995 ch 938 § 13 (SB 523), operative July 1, 1997; Stats 1997 ch 949 § 7 (SB 95); Stats 2006 ch 538 § 248 (SB 1852), effective January 1, 2007; Stats 2012 ch 551 § 1 (SB 965), effective January 1, 2013; Stats 2016 ch 31 § 71 (SB 836), effective June 27, 2016; Stats 2021 ch 63 § 1 (AB 1291), effective January 1, 2022.

§ 11126. Closed session on issues relating to public employee; Employee's right to public hearing; Closed sessions not prohibited by article; Abrogation of lawyer-client privilege

(a)(1) Nothing in this article shall be construed to prevent a state body from holding closed sessions during a regular or special meeting to consider the appointment, employment, evaluation of performance, or dismissal of a public employee or to hear complaints or charges brought against that employee by another person or employee unless the employee requests a public hearing.

(2) As a condition to holding a closed session on the complaints or charges to consider disciplinary action or to consider dismissal, the employee shall be given written notice of their right to have a public hearing, rather than a closed session, and that notice shall be delivered to the employee personally or by mail at least 24 hours before the time for holding a regular or special meeting. If notice is not given, any disciplinary or other action taken against any employee at the closed session shall be null and void.

(3) The state body also may exclude from any public or closed session, during the examination of a witness, any or all other witnesses in the matter being investigated by the state body.

(4) Following the public hearing or closed session, the body may deliberate on the decision to be reached in a closed session.

(b) For the purposes of this section, "employee" does not include any person who is elected to, or appointed to a public office by, any state body. However, officers of the California State University who receive compensation for their services, other than per diem and ordinary and necessary expenses, shall, when engaged in that capacity, be considered employees. Furthermore, for purposes of this section, the term employee includes a person exempt from civil service pursuant to subdivision (e) of Section 4 of Article VII of the California Constitution.

(c) Nothing in this article shall be construed to do any of the following:

(1) Prevent state bodies that administer the licensing of persons engaging in businesses or professions from holding closed sessions to prepare, approve, grade, or administer examinations.

(2) Prevent an advisory body of a state body that administers the licensing of persons engaged in businesses or professions from conducting a closed session to discuss matters that the advisory body has found would constitute an unwarranted invasion of the privacy of an individual licensee or applicant if discussed in an open meeting, provided the advisory body does not include a quorum of the members of the state body it advises. Those matters may include review of an applicant's qualifications for licensure and an inquiry specifically related to the state body's enforcement program concerning an individual licensee or applicant where the inquiry occurs prior to the filing of a civil, criminal, or administrative disciplinary action against the licensee or applicant by the state body.

(3) Prohibit a state body from holding a closed session to deliberate on a decision to be reached in a proceeding required to be conducted pursuant to Chapter 5 (commencing with Section 11500) or similar provisions of law.

(4) Grant a right to enter any correctional institution or the grounds of a correctional institution where that right is not otherwise granted by law, nor shall anything in this article be construed to prevent a state body from holding a closed session when considering and acting upon the determination of a term, parole, or release of any individual or other disposition of an individual case, or if public disclosure of the subjects under discussion or consideration is expressly prohibited by statute.

(5) Prevent any closed session to consider the conferring of honorary degrees, or gifts, donations, and bequests that the donor or proposed donor has requested in writing to be kept confidential.

(6) Prevent the Alcoholic Beverage Control Appeals Board or the Cannabis Control Appeals Panel from holding a closed session for the purpose of holding a deliberative conference as provided in Section 11125.

(7)(A) Prevent a state body from holding closed sessions with its negotiator prior to the purchase, sale, exchange, or lease of real property by or for the state body to give instructions to its negotiator regarding the price and terms of payment for the purchase, sale, exchange, or lease.

(B) However, prior to the closed session, the state body shall hold an open and public session in which it identifies the real property or real properties that the negotiations may concern and the person or persons with whom its negotiator may negotiate.

(C) For purposes of this paragraph, the negotiator may be a member of the state body.

(D) For purposes of this paragraph, "lease" includes renewal or renegotiation of a lease.

(E) Nothing in this paragraph shall preclude a state body from holding a closed session for discussions regarding eminent domain proceedings pursuant to subdivision (e).

(8) Prevent the California Postsecondary Education Commission from holding closed sessions to consider matters pertaining to the appointment or termination of the Director of the California Postsecondary Education Commission.

(9) Prevent the Council for Private Postsecondary and Vocational Education from holding closed sessions to consider matters pertaining to the appointment or termination of the Executive Director of the Council for Private Postsecondary and Vocational Education.

(10) Prevent the Franchise Tax Board from holding closed sessions for the purpose of discussion of confidential tax returns or information the public disclosure of which is prohibited by law, or from considering matters pertaining to the appointment or removal of the Executive Officer of the Franchise Tax Board.

(11) Require the Franchise Tax Board to notice or disclose any confidential tax information considered in closed sessions, or documents executed in connection therewith, the public disclosure of which is prohibited pursuant to Article 2 (commencing with Section 19542) of Chapter 7 of Part 10.2 of Division 2 of the Revenue and Taxation Code.

(12) Prevent the Corrections Standards Authority from holding closed sessions when considering reports of crime conditions under Section 6027 of the Penal Code.

(13) Prevent the State Air Resources Board from holding closed sessions when considering the proprietary specifications and performance data of manufacturers.

(14) Prevent the State Board of Education or the Superintendent of Public Instruction, or any committee advising the board or the Superintendent, from holding closed sessions on those portions of its review of assessment instruments pursuant to Chapter 5 (commencing with Section 60600) of Part 33 of Division 4 of Title 2 of the Education Code during which actual test content is reviewed and discussed. The purpose of this provision is to maintain the confidentiality of the assessments under review.

(15) Prevent the Department of Resources Recycling and Recovery or its auxiliary committees from holding closed sessions for the purpose of discussing confidential tax returns, discussing trade secrets or confidential or proprietary information in its possession, or discussing other data, the public disclosure of which is prohibited by law.

(16) Prevent a state body that invests retirement, pension, or endowment funds from holding closed sessions when considering investment decisions. For purposes of consideration of shareholder voting on corporate stocks held by the state body, closed sessions for the purposes of voting may be held only with respect to election of corporate directors, election of independent auditors, and other financial issues that could have a material effect on the

net income of the corporation. For the purpose of real property investment decisions that may be considered in a closed session pursuant to this paragraph, a state body shall also be exempt from the provisions of paragraph (7) relating to the identification of real properties prior to the closed session.

(17) Prevent a state body, or boards, commissions, administrative officers, or other representatives that may properly be designated by law or by a state body, from holding closed sessions with its representatives in discharging its responsibilities under Chapter 10 (commencing with Section 3500), Chapter 10.3 (commencing with Section 3512), Chapter 10.5 (commencing with Section 3525), or Chapter 10.7 (commencing with Section 3540) of Division 4 of Title 1 as the sessions relate to salaries, salary schedules, or compensation paid in the form of fringe benefits. For the purposes enumerated in the preceding sentence, a state body may also meet with a state conciliator who has intervened in the proceedings.

(18)(A) Prevent a state body from holding closed sessions to consider matters posing a threat or potential threat of criminal or terrorist activity against the personnel, property, buildings, facilities, or equipment, including electronic data, owned, leased, or controlled by the state body, where disclosure of these considerations could compromise or impede the safety or security of the personnel, property, buildings, facilities, or equipment, including electronic data, owned, leased, or controlled by the state body.

(B) Notwithstanding any other law, a state body, at any regular or special meeting, may meet in a closed session pursuant to subparagraph (A) upon a two-thirds vote of the members present at the meeting.

(C) After meeting in closed session pursuant to subparagraph (A), the state body shall reconvene in open session prior to adjournment and report that a closed session was held pursuant to subparagraph (A), the general nature of the matters considered, and whether any action was taken in closed session.

(D) After meeting in closed session pursuant to subparagraph (A), the state body shall submit to the Legislative Analyst written notification stating that it held this closed session, the general reason or reasons for the closed session, the general nature of the matters considered, and whether any action was taken in closed session. The Legislative Analyst shall retain for no less than four years any written notification received from a state body pursuant to this subparagraph.

(19) Prevent the California Sex Offender Management Board from holding a closed session for the purpose of discussing matters pertaining to the application of a sex offender treatment provider for certification pursuant to Sections 290.09 and 9003 of the Penal Code. Those matters may include review of an applicant's qualifications for certification.

(d)(1) Notwithstanding any other law, any meeting of the Public Utilities Commission at which the rates of entities under the commission's jurisdiction are changed shall be open and public.

(2) Nothing in this article shall be construed to prevent the Public Utilities Commission from holding closed sessions to deliberate on the institution of proceedings, or disciplinary actions against any person or entity under the jurisdiction of the commission.

(e)(1) Nothing in this article shall be construed to prevent a state body, based on the advice of its legal counsel, from holding a closed session to confer with, or receive advice from, its legal counsel regarding pending litigation when discussion in open session concerning those matters would prejudice the position of the state body in the litigation.

(2) For purposes of this article, all expressions of the lawyer-client privilege other than those provided in this subdivision are hereby abrogated. This subdivision is the exclusive expression of the lawyer-client privilege for purposes of conducting closed session meetings pursuant to this article. For purposes of this subdivision, litigation shall be considered pending when any of the following circumstances exist:

(A) An adjudicatory proceeding before a court, an administrative body exercising its adjudicatory authority, a hearing officer, or an arbitrator, to which the state body is a party, has been initiated formally.

(B)(i) A point has been reached where, in the opinion of the state body on the advice of its legal counsel, based on existing facts and circumstances, there is a significant exposure to litigation against the state body.

(ii) Based on existing facts and circumstances, the state body is meeting only to decide whether a closed session is authorized pursuant to clause (i).

(C) Based on existing facts and circumstances, the state body has decided to initiate or is deciding whether to initiate litigation.

(3) The legal counsel of the state body shall prepare and submit to it a memorandum stating the specific reasons and legal authority for the closed session. If the closed session is pursuant to subparagraph (A) of paragraph (2), the memorandum shall include the title of the litigation. If the closed session is pursuant to subparagraph (B) or (C) of paragraph (2), the memorandum shall include the existing facts and circumstances on which it is based. The legal counsel shall submit the memorandum to the state body prior to the closed session, if feasible, and in any case no later than one week after the closed session. The memorandum shall be exempt from disclosure pursuant to Section 7927.205.

(4) For purposes of this subdivision, "litigation" includes any adjudicatory proceeding, including eminent domain, before a court, administrative body exercising its adjudicatory authority, hearing officer, or arbitrator.

(5) Disclosure of a memorandum required under this subdivision shall not be deemed as a waiver of the lawyer-client privilege, as provided for under Article 3 (commencing with Section 950) of Chapter 4 of Division 8 of the Evidence Code.

(f) In addition to subdivisions (a), (b), and (c), nothing in this article shall be construed to do any of the following:

(1) Prevent a state body operating under a joint powers agreement for insurance pooling from holding a closed session to discuss a claim for the payment of tort liability or public liability losses incurred by the state body or any member agency under the joint powers agreement.

(2) Prevent the examining committee established by the State Board of Forestry and Fire Protection, pursuant to Section 763 of the Public Resources Code, from conducting a closed session to consider disciplinary

action against an individual professional forester prior to the filing of an accusation against the forester pursuant to Section 11503.

(3) Prevent the enforcement advisory committee established by the California Board of Accountancy pursuant to Section 5020 of the Business and Professions Code from conducting a closed session to consider disciplinary action against an individual accountant prior to the filing of an accusation against the accountant pursuant to Section 11503. Nothing in this article shall be construed to prevent the qualifications examining committee established by the California Board of Accountancy pursuant to Section 5023 of the Business and Professions Code from conducting a closed hearing to interview an individual applicant or accountant regarding the applicant's qualifications.

(4) Prevent a state body, as defined in subdivision (b) of Section 11121, from conducting a closed session to consider any matter that properly could be considered in closed session by the state body whose authority it exercises.

(5) Prevent a state body, as defined in subdivision (d) of Section 11121, from conducting a closed session to consider any matter that properly could be considered in a closed session by the body defined as a state body pursuant to subdivision (a) or (b) of Section 11121.

(6) Prevent a state body, as defined in subdivision (c) of Section 11121, from conducting a closed session to consider any matter that properly could be considered in a closed session by the state body it advises.

(7) Prevent the State Board of Equalization from holding closed sessions for either of the following:

(A) When considering matters pertaining to the appointment or removal of the Executive Secretary of the State Board of Equalization.

(B) For the purpose of hearing confidential taxpayer appeals or data, the public disclosure of which is prohibited by law.

(8) Require the State Board of Equalization to disclose any action taken in closed session or documents executed in connection with that action, the public disclosure of which is prohibited by law pursuant to Sections 15619 and 15641 of this code and Sections 833, 7056, 8255, 9255, 11655, 30455, 32455, 38705, 38706, 43651, 45982, 46751, 50159, 55381, and 60609 of the Revenue and Taxation Code.

(9) Prevent the California Earthquake Prediction Evaluation Council, or other body appointed to advise the Director of Emergency Services or the Governor concerning matters relating to volcanic or earthquake predictions, from holding closed sessions when considering the evaluation of possible predictions.

(g) This article does not prevent either of the following:

(1) The Teachers' Retirement Board or the Board of Administration of the Public Employees' Retirement System from holding closed sessions when considering matters pertaining to the recruitment, appointment, employment, or removal of the chief executive officer or when considering matters pertaining to the recruitment or removal of the Chief Investment Officer of the State Teachers' Retirement System or the Public Employees' Retirement System.

(2) The Commission on Teacher Credentialing from holding closed ses-

sions when considering matters relating to the recruitment, appointment, or removal of its executive director.

(h) This article does not prevent the Board of Administration of the Public Employees' Retirement System from holding closed sessions when considering matters relating to the development of rates and competitive strategy for plans offered pursuant to Chapter 15 (commencing with Section 21660) of Part 3 of Division 5 of Title 2.

(i) This article does not prevent the Managed Risk Medical Insurance Board from holding closed sessions when considering matters related to the development of rates and contracting strategy for entities contracting or seeking to contract with the board, entities with which the board is considering a contract, or entities with which the board is considering or enters into any other arrangement under which the board provides, receives, or arranges services or reimbursement, pursuant to Part 6.2 (commencing with Section 12693), former Part 6.3 (commencing with Section 12695), former Part 6.4 (commencing with Section 12699.50), former Part 6.5 (commencing with Section 12700), Part 6.6 (commencing with Section 12739.5), or Part 6.7 (commencing with Section 12739.70) of Division 2 of the Insurance Code.

(j) Nothing in this article shall be construed to prevent the board of the State Compensation Insurance Fund from holding closed sessions in the following:

(1) When considering matters related to claims pursuant to Chapter 1 (commencing with Section 3200) of Division 4 of the Labor Code, to the extent that confidential medical information or other individually identifiable information would be disclosed.

(2) To the extent that matters related to audits and investigations that have not been completed would be disclosed.

(3) To the extent that an internal audit containing proprietary information would be disclosed.

(4) To the extent that the session would address the development of rates, contracting strategy, underwriting, or competitive strategy, pursuant to the powers granted to the board in Chapter 4 (commencing with Section 11770) of Part 3 of Division 2 of the Insurance Code, when discussion in open session concerning those matters would prejudice the position of the State Compensation Insurance Fund.

(k) The State Compensation Insurance Fund shall comply with the procedures specified in Section 11125.4 of the Government Code with respect to any closed session or meeting authorized by subdivision (j), and in addition shall provide an opportunity for a member of the public to be heard on the issue of the appropriateness of closing the meeting or session.

HISTORY:

Added Stats 1967 ch 1656 § 122. Amended Stats 1968 ch 1272 § 1; Stats 1970 ch 346 § 5; Stats 1972 ch 431 § 43, ch 1010 § 63, effective August 17, 1972, operative July 1, 1972; Stats 1974 ch 1254 § 1, ch 1539 § 1; Stats 1975 ch 197 § 1, ch 959 § 5; Stats 1977 ch 730 § 5, effective September 12, 1977; Stats 1980 ch 1197 § 1, ch 1284 § 11; Stats 1981 ch 180 § 1, ch 968 § 12; Stats 1982 ch 454 § 40; Stats 1983 ch 143 § 187; Stats 1984 ch 678 § 1, ch 1284 § 4; Stats 1985 ch 186 § 1; Ch 1091 § 1; Stats 1986 ch 575 § 1; Stats 1987 ch 1320 § 2; Stats 1988 ch 1448 § 29; Stats 1989 ch 177 § 2, ch 882 § 2, ch 1360 § 52 (ch 1427 prevails), ch 1427 § 1, effective October 2, 1989, operative January 1, 1990; Stats 1991 ch 788 § 4 (AB 1440); Stats 1992 ch 1050 § 17 (AB 2987); Stats 1994 ch 26 § 230 (AB 1807), effective March 30, 1994, ch 422 § 15.5 (AB 2589), effective September 6, 1994, ch 845 § 1 (SB 1316); Stats 1995 ch 975 § 3 (AB 265); Stats 1996 ch 1041 § 2 (AB 3358); Stats 1997 ch 949 § 8 (SB 95); Stats 1998 ch 210 § 1 (SB 2008), ch 972 § 1 (SB 989); Stats 1999 ch 735 § 9 (SB 366), effective October 10, 1999; Stats

2000 ch 1002 § 1 (SB 1998), ch 1055 § 30 (AB 2889), effective September 30, 2000; Stats 2001 ch 21 § 1 (SB 54), effective June 25, 2001, ch 243 § 10 (AB 192); Stats 2002 ch 664 § 93.7 (AB 3034), ch 2002 ch 1113 § 1 (AB 2072); Stats 2005 ch 288 § 1 (AB 277), effective January 1, 2006; Stats 2007 ch 577 § 4 (AB 1750), effective October 13, 2007; Stats 2008 ch 179 § 91 (SB 1498), effective January 1, 2008, ch 344 § 3 (SB 1145) (ch 344 prevails), effective September 26, 2008; Stats 2010 ch 32 § 2 (AB 1887), effective June 29, 2010, ch 328 § 81 (SB 1330), effective January 1, 2011, ch 618 § 124 (AB 2791) (ch 618 prevails), effective January 1, 2011; Stats 2011 ch 357 § 1 (AB 813), effective January 1, 2012; Stats 2013 ch 352 § 234 (AB 1317), effective September 26, 2013, operative July 1, 2013; Stats 2017 ch 641 § 22 (AB 830), effective January 1, 2018; Stats 2019 ch 40 § 15 (AB 97), effective July 1, 2019; Stats 2021 ch 615 § 163 (AB 474), effective January 1, 2022.

§ 11126.1. Minute book of closed session

The state body shall designate a clerk or other officer or employee of the state body, who shall then attend each closed session of the state body and keep and enter in a minute book a record of topics discussed and decisions made at the meeting. The minute book made pursuant to this section is not a public record subject to inspection pursuant to the California Public Records Act (Division 10 (commencing with Section 7920.000")" of Title 1), and shall be kept confidential. The minute book shall be available to members of the state body or, if a violation of this chapter is alleged to have occurred at a closed session, to a court of general jurisdiction. The minute book may, but need not, consist of a recording of the closed session.

HISTORY:

Added Stats 1980 ch 1284 § 12. Amended Stats 1981 ch 968 § 13; Stats 2021 ch 615 § 164 (AB 474), effective January 1, 2022.

§ 11126.2. Closed session for response to final draft audit report

(a) Nothing in this article shall be construed to prohibit a state body that has received a confidential final draft audit report from the Bureau of State Audits from holding closed sessions to discuss its response to that report.

(b) After the public release of an audit report by the Bureau of State Audits, if a state body meets to discuss the audit report, it shall do so in an open session unless exempted from that requirement by some other provision of law.

HISTORY:

Added Stats 2004 ch 576 § 2 (AB 1827).

§ 11126.3. Disclosure of items to be discussed in closed session; Discussion of additional pending litigation matters arising after disclosure

(a) Prior to holding any closed session, the state body shall disclose, in an open meeting, the general nature of the item or items to be discussed in the closed session. The disclosure may take the form of a reference to the item or items as they are listed by number or letter on the agenda. If the session is closed pursuant to paragraph (2) of subdivision (d) of Section 11126, the state body shall state the title of, or otherwise specifically identify, the proceeding or disciplinary action contemplated. However, should the body determine that to do so would jeopardize the body's ability to effectuate service of process upon one or more unserved parties if the proceeding or disciplinary action is commenced or that to do so would fail to protect the private economic and business reputation of the person or entity if the proceeding or disciplinary action is not commenced, then the state body shall notice that there will be a closed session and describe in general terms the purpose of that session. If the session is closed pursuant to subparagraph (A) of paragraph (2) of subdivision (e) of Section 11126, the state body shall state the title of, or otherwise specifically identify, the litigation to be discussed unless the body states that to do so would jeopardize the body's ability to effectuate service of process upon one or more unserved parties, or that to do so would jeopardize its ability to conclude existing settlement negotiations to its advantage.

(b) In the closed session, the state body may consider only those matters covered in its disclosure.

(c) The disclosure shall be made as part of the notice provided for the meeting pursuant to Section 11125 or pursuant to subdivision (a) of Section 92032 of the Education Code and of any order or notice required by Section 11129.

(d) If, after the agenda has been published in compliance with this article, any pending litigation (under subdivision (e) of Section 11126) matters arise, the postponement of which will prevent the state body from complying with any statutory, court-ordered, or other legally imposed deadline, the state body may proceed to discuss those matters in closed session and shall publicly announce in the meeting the title of, or otherwise specifically identify, the litigation to be discussed, unless the body states that to do so would jeopardize the body's ability to effectuate service of process upon one or more unserved parties, or that to do so would jeopardize its ability to conclude existing settlement negotiations to its advantage. Such an announcement shall be deemed to comply fully with the requirements of this section.

(e) Nothing in this section shall require or authorize a disclosure of names or other information that would constitute an invasion of privacy or otherwise unnecessarily divulge the particular facts concerning the closed session or the disclosure of which is prohibited by state or federal law.

(f) After any closed session, the state body shall reconvene into open session prior to adjournment and shall make any reports, provide any documentation, and make any other disclosures required by Section 11125.2 of action taken in the closed session.

(g) The announcements required to be made in open session pursuant to this section may be made at the location announced in the agenda for the closed session, as long as the public is allowed to be present at that location for the purpose of hearing the announcement.

HISTORY:

Added Stats 1980 ch 1284 § 13. Amended Stats 1981 ch 968 § 14; Stats 1987 ch 1320 § 3; Stats 1997 ch 949 § 10 (SB 95); Stats 1998 ch 210 § 2 (SB 2008); Stats 2001 ch 243 § 11 (AB 192).

§ 11126.5. Clearing room when meeting wilfully interrupted

In the event that any meeting is willfully interrupted by a group or groups of persons so as to render the orderly conduct of such meeting unfeasible and order cannot be restored by the removal of individuals who are willfully interrupting the meeting the state body conducting the meeting may order the meeting room cleared and continue in session. Nothing in this section shall prohibit the state body from establishing a procedure for readmitting an individual or individuals not responsible for willfully disturbing the orderly conduct of the meeting. Notwithstanding any other provision of law, only matters appearing on the agenda may be considered in such a session. Representatives of the press or other news media, except those participating in the disturbance, shall be allowed to attend any session held pursuant to this section.

HISTORY:
Added Stats 1970 ch 1598 § 1. Amended Stats 1981 ch 968 § 15.

§ 11126.7. Fees

No fees may be charged by a state body for providing a notice required by Section 11125 or for carrying out any provision of this article, except as specifically authorized pursuant to this article.

HISTORY:
Added Stats 1980 ch 1284 § 14. Amended Stats 1981 ch 968 § 16.

§ 11127. State bodies subject to article

Each provision of this article shall apply to every state body unless the body is specifically excepted from that provision by law or is covered by any other conflicting provision of law.

HISTORY:
Added Stats 1967 ch 1656 § 122. Amended Stats 1981 ch 968 § 17.

§ 11128. When closed sessions held

Each closed session of a state body shall be held only during a regular or special meeting of the body.

HISTORY:
Added Stats 1967 ch 1656 § 122. Amended Stats 1980 ch 1284 § 15; Stats 1981 ch 968 § 18.

§ 11128.5. Adjournment of meeting; Posting of copy of order or notice of adjournment

The state body may adjourn any regular, adjourned regular, special, or adjourned special meeting to a time and place specified in the order of adjournment. Less than a quorum may so adjourn from time to time. If all members are absent from any regular or adjourned regular meeting, the clerk or secretary of the state body may declare the meeting adjourned to a stated time and place and he or she shall cause a written notice of the adjournment to be given in the same manner as provided in Section 11125.4 for special meetings, unless that notice is waived as provided for special meetings. A copy of the order or notice of adjournment shall be conspicuously posted on or near the door of the place where the regular, adjourned regular, special, or adjourned special meeting was held within 24 hours after the time of the adjournment. When a regular or adjourned regular meeting is adjourned as provided in this section, the resulting adjourned regular meeting is a regular meeting for all purposes. When an order of adjournment of any meeting fails to state the hour at which the adjourned meeting is to be held, it shall be held at the hour specified for regular meetings by law or regulation.

HISTORY:
Added Stats 1997 ch 949 § 11 (SB 95).

§ 11129. Continuance or recontinuance of hearing

Any hearing being held, or noticed or ordered to be held by a state body at any meeting may by order or notice of continuance be continued or recontinued to any subsequent meeting of the state body in the same manner and to the same extent set forth in Section 11128.5 for the adjournment of meetings. A copy of the order or notice of continuance shall be conspicuously posted on or near the door of the place where the hearing was held within 24 hours after the time of the continuance; provided, that if the hearing is continued to a time less than 24 hours after the time specified in the order or notice of hearing, a copy of the order or notice of continuance of hearing shall be posted immediately following the meeting at which the order or declaration of continuance was adopted or made.

HISTORY:
Added Stats 1967 ch 1656 § 122. Amended Stats 1981 ch 968 § 19; Stats 1997 ch 949 § 12 (SB 95).

§ 11130. Action to stop or prevent violations of article; Order for recording of closed sessions; Discovery of recording

(a) The Attorney General, the district attorney, or any interested person may commence an action by mandamus, injunction, or declaratory relief for the purpose of stopping or preventing violations or threatened violations of this article or to determine the applicability of this article to past actions or threatened future action by members of the state body or to determine whether any rule or action by the state body to penalize or otherwise discourage the expression of one or more of its members is valid or invalid under the laws of this state or of the United States, or to compel the state body to audio record its closed sessions as hereinafter provided.

(b) The court in its discretion may, upon a judgment of a violation of Section 11126, order the state body to audio record its closed sessions and preserve the audio recordings for the period and under the terms of security and confidentiality the court deems appropriate.

(c)(1) Each recording so kept shall be immediately labeled with the date of the closed session recorded and the title of the clerk or other officer who shall be custodian of the recording.

(2) The audio recordings shall be subject to the following discovery procedures:

(A) In any case in which discovery or disclosure of the audio recording is sought by the Attorney General, the district attorney, or the plaintiff in a civil action pursuant to this section or Section 11130.3 alleging that a violation of this article has occurred in a closed session that has been recorded pursuant to this section, the party seeking discovery or disclosure shall file a written notice of motion with the appropriate court with notice to the governmental agency that has custody and control of the audio recording. The notice shall be given pursuant to subdivision (b) of Section 1005 of the Code of Civil Procedure.

(B) The notice shall include, in addition to the items required by Section 1010 of the Code of Civil Procedure, all of the following:

(i) Identification of the proceeding in which discovery or disclosure is sought, the party seeking discovery or disclosure, the date and time of the meeting recorded, and the governmental agency that has custody and control of the recording.

(ii) An affidavit that contains specific facts indicating that a violation of the act occurred in the closed session.

(3) If the court, following a review of the motion, finds that there is good cause to believe that a violation has occurred, the court may review, in camera, the recording of that portion of the closed session alleged to have violated the act.

(4) If, following the in camera review, the court concludes that disclosure of a portion of the recording would be likely to materially assist in the resolution of the litigation alleging violation of this article, the court shall, in its discretion, make a certified transcript of the portion of the recording a public exhibit in the proceeding.

(5) Nothing in this section shall permit discovery of communications that are protected by the attorney-client privilege.

HISTORY:

Added Stats 1967 ch 1656 § 122. Amended Stats 1969 ch 494 § 1; Stats 1981 ch 968 § 20; Stats 1997 ch 949 § 13 (SB 95); Stats 1999 ch 393 § 4 (AB 1234); Stats 2009 ch 88 § 43 (AB 176), effective January 1, 2010.

§ 11130.3. Cause of action to void action taken by state agency in violation of open meeting requirements

(a) Any interested person may commence an action by mandamus, injunction, or declaratory relief for the purpose of obtaining a judicial determination that an action taken by a state body in violation of Section 11123 or 11125 is null and void under this section. Any action seeking such a judicial determination shall be commenced within 90 days from the date the action was taken. Nothing in this section shall be construed to prevent a state body from curing or correcting an action challenged pursuant to this section.

(b) An action shall not be determined to be null and void if any of the following conditions exist:

(1) The action taken was in connection with the sale or issuance of notes, bonds, or other evidences of indebtedness or any contract, instrument, or agreement related thereto.

(2) The action taken gave rise to a contractual obligation upon which a party has, in good faith, detrimentally relied.

(3) The action taken was in substantial compliance with Sections 11123 and 11125.

(4) The action taken was in connection with the collection of any tax.

HISTORY:

Added Stats 1985 ch 936 § 1. Amended Stats 1999 ch 393 § 5 (AB 1234).

§ 11130.5. Costs and attorney fees

A court may award court costs and reasonable attorney's fees to the plaintiff in an action brought pursuant to Section 11130 or 11130.3 where it is found that a state body has violated the provisions of this article. The costs and fees shall be paid by the state body and shall not become a personal liability of any public officer or employee thereof.

A court may award court costs and reasonable attorney's fees to a defendant in any action brought pursuant to Section 11130 or 11130.3 where the defendant has prevailed in a final determination of the action and the court finds that the action was clearly frivolous and totally lacking in merit.

HISTORY:

Added Stats 1975 ch 959 § 6. Amended Stats 1981 ch 968 § 21; Stats 1985 ch 936 § 2.

§ 11130.7. Offenses

Each member of a state body who attends a meeting of that body in violation of any provision of this article, and where the member intends to deprive the public of information to which the member knows or has reason to know the public is entitled under this article, is guilty of a misdemeanor.

HISTORY:

Added Stats 1980 ch 1284 § 16. Amended Stats 1981 ch 968 § 22; Stats 1997 ch 949 § 14 (SB 95).

§ 11131. Prohibition against use of certain facilities

No state agency shall conduct any meeting, conference, or other function in any facility that prohibits the admittance of any person, or persons, on the basis of ancestry or any characteristic listed or defined in Section 11135, or that is inaccessible to disabled persons, or where members of the public may not be present without making a payment or purchase. As used in this section, "state agency" means and includes every state body, office, officer, department, division, bureau, board, council, commission, or other state agency.

HISTORY:

Added Stats 1970 ch 383 § 1. Amended Stats 1981 ch 968 § 23; Stats 1997 ch 949 § 15 (SB 95); Stats 2007 ch 568 § 32 (AB 14), effective January 1, 2008.

§ 11132. Prohibition against closed sessions except as expressly authorized

Except as expressly authorized by this article, no closed session may be held by any state body.

HISTORY:

Added Stats 1987 ch 1320 § 4.

§ 11133. Public meetings [Repealed effective July 1, 2023]

(a) Notwithstanding any other provision of this article, and subject to the notice and accessibility requirements in subdivisions (d) and (e), a state body may hold public meetings through teleconferencing and make public meetings accessible telephonically, or otherwise electronically, to all members of the public seeking to observe and to address the state body.

(b)(1) For a state body holding a public meeting through teleconferencing pursuant to this section, all requirements in this article requiring the physical presence of members, the clerk or other personnel of the state body, or the public, as a condition of participation in or quorum for a public meeting, are hereby suspended.

(2) For a state body holding a public meeting through teleconferencing pursuant to this section, all of the following requirements in this article are suspended:

(A) Each teleconference location from which a member will be participating in a public meeting or proceeding be identified in the notice and agenda of the public meeting or proceeding.

(B) Each teleconference location be accessible to the public.

(C) Members of the public may address the state body at each teleconference conference location.

(D) Post agendas at all teleconference locations.

(E) At least one member of the state body be physically present at the location specified in the notice of the meeting.

(c) A state body that holds a meeting through teleconferencing and allows members of the public to observe and address the meeting telephonically or otherwise electronically, consistent with the notice and accessibility requirements in subdivisions (d) and (e), shall have satisfied any requirement that the state body allow members of the public to attend the meeting and offer public comment. A state body need not make available any physical location from which members of the public may observe the meeting and offer public comment.

(d) If a state body holds a meeting through teleconferencing pursuant to this section and allows members of the public to observe and address the meeting telephonically or otherwise electronically, the state body shall also do both of the following:

(1) Implement a procedure for receiving and swiftly resolving requests for reasonable modification or accommodation from individuals with disabilities, consistent with the federal Americans with Disabilities Act of 1990 (42 U.S.C. Sec. 12101 et seq.), and resolving any doubt whatsoever in favor of accessibility.

(2) Advertise that procedure each time notice is given of the means by which members of the public may observe the meeting and offer public comment, pursuant to paragraph (2) of subdivision (e).

(e) Except to the extent this section provides otherwise, each state body that holds a meeting through teleconferencing pursuant to this section shall do both of the following:

(1) Give advance notice of the time of, and post the agenda for, each public meeting according to the timeframes otherwise prescribed by this article, and using the means otherwise prescribed by this article, as applicable.

(2) In each instance in which notice of the time of the meeting is otherwise given or the agenda for the meeting is otherwise posted, also give notice of the means by which members of the public may observe the meeting and offer public comment. As to any instance in which there is a change in the means of public observation and comment, or any instance prior to the effective date of this section in which the time of the meeting has been noticed or the agenda for the meeting has been posted without also including notice of the means of public observation and comment, a state body may satisfy this requirement by advertising the means of public observation and comment using the most rapid means of communication available at the time. Advertising the means of public observation and comment using the

most rapid means of communication available at the time shall include, but need not be limited to, posting such means on the state body's internet website.

(f) All state bodies utilizing the teleconferencing procedures in this section are urged to use sound discretion and to make reasonable efforts to adhere as closely as reasonably possible to the otherwise applicable provisions of this article, in order to maximize transparency and provide the public access to state body meetings.

(g) This section shall remain in effect only until July 1, 2023, and as of that date is repealed.

HISTORY:
Added Stats 2022 ch 48 § 20 (SB 189), effective June 30, 2022, repealed July 1, 2023.

PART 2.8

CIVIL RIGHTS DEPARTMENT

Chapter
6. Discrimination Prohibited.

HISTORY: Added Stats 1980 ch 992 § 4. Heading of Part 2.8, which formerly read "Department of Fair Employment and Housing," amended to read as above by Stats 2022 ch 48 § 29 (SB 189), effective June 30, 2022. Former Part 2.8, entitled "Department of General Services", consisting of §§ 12900–12986, was added Stats 1963 ch 1786 § 1, operative October 1, 1963, and repealed Stats 1965 ch 371 § 149.

CHAPTER 6

DISCRIMINATION PROHIBITED

Article
1. Unlawful Practices, Generally.

ARTICLE 1

UNLAWFUL PRACTICES, GENERALLY

Section
12944. Discrimination by licensing board.

§ 12944. Discrimination by licensing board

(a) It shall be unlawful for a licensing board to require any examination or establish any other qualification for licensing that has an adverse impact on any class by virtue of its race, creed, color, national origin or ancestry, sex, gender, gender identity, gender expression, age, medical condition, genetic information, physical disability, mental disability, reproductive health decisionmaking, or sexual orientation, unless the practice can be demonstrated to be job related.

Where the council, after hearing, determines that an examination is unlawful under this subdivision, the licensing board may continue to use and rely on the examination until such time as judicial review by the superior court of the determination is exhausted.

If an examination or other qualification for licensing is determined to be unlawful under this section, that determination shall not void, limit, repeal, or otherwise affect any right, privilege, status, or responsibility previously conferred upon any person by the examination or by a license issued in reliance on the examination or qualification.

(b) It shall be unlawful for a licensing board to fail or refuse to make reasonable accommodation to an individual's mental or physical disability or medical condition.

(c) It shall be unlawful for any licensing board, unless specifically acting in accordance with federal equal employment opportunity guidelines or regulations approved by the council, to print or circulate or cause to be printed or circulated any publication, or to make any non-job-related inquiry, either verbal or through use of an application form, which expresses, directly or indirectly, any limitation, specification, or discrimination as to race, religious creed, color, national origin, ancestry, physical disability, mental disability, medical condition, genetic information, sex, gender, gender identity, gender expression, age, reproductive health decisionmaking, or sexual orientation or any intent to make any such limitation, specification, or discrimination. Nothing in this subdivision shall prohibit any licensing board from making, in connection with prospective licensure or certification, an inquiry as to, or a request for information regarding, the physical fitness of applicants if that inquiry or request for information is directly related and pertinent to the license or the licensed position the applicant is applying for. Nothing in this subdivision shall prohibit any licensing board, in connection with prospective examinations, licensure, or certification, from inviting individuals with physical or mental disabilities to request reasonable accommodations or from making inquiries related to reasonable accommodations.

(d) It is unlawful for a licensing board to discriminate against any person because the person has filed a complaint, testified, or assisted in any proceeding under this part.

(e) It is unlawful for any licensing board to fail to keep records of applications for licensing or certification for a period of two years following the date of receipt of the applications.

(f) As used in this section, "licensing board" means any state board, agency, or authority in the Business, Consumer Services, and Housing Agency that has the authority to grant licenses or certificates which are prerequisites to employment eligibility or professional status.

HISTORY:

Added Stats 1980 ch 992 § 4. Amended Stats 1992 ch 912 § 6 (AB 1286), ch 913 § 24 (AB 1077); Stats 1999 ch 592 § 8 (AB 1001); Stats 2011 ch 261 § 15 (SB 559), effective January 1, 2012, ch 719 § 19.5 (AB 887), effective January 1, 2012; Stats 2012 ch 46 § 37 (SB 1038), effective June 27, 2012, operative January 1, 2013. See this section as modified in Governor's Reorganization Plan No. 2 § 210 of 2012; Amended Stats 2012 ch 147 § 17 (SB 1039), effective January 1, 2013, operative July 1, 2013 (ch 147 prevails); Stats 2022 ch 48 § 38 (SB 189), effective June 30, 2022; Stats 2022 ch 630 § 8 (SB 523), effective January 1, 2023.

PART 5.5
DEPARTMENT OF GENERAL SERVICES

Chapter
7. Printing.

HISTORY: Added Stats 1965 ch 371 § 179.

CHAPTER 7
PRINTING

Article
6. Distribution of State Publications.

ARTICLE 6
DISTRIBUTION OF STATE PUBLICATIONS

Section
14911. Correction of mailing lists.

§ 14911. Correction of mailing lists

If any state agency maintains a mailing list of public officials or other persons to whom publications or other printed matter is sent without charge, the state agency shall correct its mailing list and verify its accuracy at least once each year.

HISTORY:

Added Stats 1965 ch 371 § 179. Amended Stats 2020 ch 110 § 43 (SB 820), effective September 18, 2020.

TITLE 3
GOVERNMENT OF COUNTIES

Division
2. Officers.

Misc.

DIVISION 2
OFFICERS

Part
3. Other Officers.

PART 3
OTHER OFFICERS

Chapter
1. District Attorney.

CHAPTER 1
DISTRICT ATTORNEY

Article
1. Duties as Public Prosecutor.

ARTICLE 1
DUTIES AS PUBLIC PROSECUTOR

Section
26509. Consumer fraud investigations; Access by district attorney to records of other agencies.

§ 26509. Consumer fraud investigations; Access by district attorney to records of other agencies

(a) Notwithstanding any other provision of law, including any provision making records confidential, and including Title 1.8 (commencing with Section 1798) of Part 4 of Division 3 of the Civil Code, the district attorney shall be given access to, and may make copies of, any complaint against a person subject to regulation by a consumer-oriented state agency and any investigation of the person made by the agency, where that person is being investigated by the district attorney regarding possible consumer fraud.

(b) Where the district attorney does not take action with respect to the complaint or investigation, the material shall remain confidential.

(c) Where the release of the material would jeopardize an investigation or other duties of a consumer-oriented state agency, the agency shall have discretion to delay the release of the information.

(d) As used in this section, a consumer-oriented state agency is any state agency that regulates the licensure, certification, or qualification of persons to practice a profession or business within the state, where the regulation is for the protection of consumers who deal with the professionals or businesses. It includes, but is not limited to, all of the following:

(1) The Dental Board of California.
(2) The Medical Board of California.
(3) The State Board of Optometry.
(4) The California State Board of Pharmacy.
(5) The Veterinary Medical Board.
(6) The California Board of Accountancy.
(7) The California Architects Board.
(8) The State Board of Barbering and Cosmetology.
(9) The Board for Professional Engineers and Land Surveyors.

(10) The Contractors' State License Board.
(11) The Funeral Directors and Embalmers Program.
(12) The Structural Pest Control Board.
(13) The Bureau of Home Furnishings and Thermal Insulation.
(14) The Board of Registered Nursing.
(15) The State Board of Chiropractic Examiners.
(16) The Board of Behavioral Science Examiners.
(17) The State Athletic Commission.
(18) The Cemetery Program.
(19) The State Board of Guide Dogs for the Blind.
(20) The Bureau of Security and Investigative Services.
(21) The Court Reporters Board of California.
(22) The Board of Vocational Nursing and Psychiatric Technicians of the State of California.
(23) The Osteopathic Medical Board of California.
(24) The Division of Investigation.
(25) The Bureau of Automotive Repair.
(26) The State Board for Geologists and Geophysicists.
(27) The Department of Alcoholic Beverage Control.
(28) The Department of Insurance.
(29) The Public Utilities Commission.
(30) The State Department of Health Services.
(31) The New Motor Vehicle Board.

HISTORY:

Added Stats 1979 ch 559 § 1, as Gov C § 26508. Amended and renumbered by Stats 1980 ch 676 § 113; Amended Stats 1988 ch 1448 § 30; Stats 1989 ch 886 § 84. Supplemented by Governor's Reorganization Plan No. 1 of 1991 § 87, effective July 17, 1991; Amended Stats 1991 ch 359 § 35 (AB 1332); Stats 1994 ch 26 § 233 (AB 1807), effective March 30, 1994, ch 1275 § 55 (SB 2101); Stats 1995 ch 60 § 46 (SB 42), effective July 6, 1995; Stats 1998 ch 59 § 14 (AB 969); Stats 2000 ch 1055 § 35 (AB 2889), effective September 30, 2000; Amended Stats 2003 ch 325 § 8 (SB 1079).

Misc.

EXTRACTED FROM
HEALTH AND SAFETY CODE

Division
2. Licensing Provisions.
10. Uniform Controlled Substances Act.
106. Personal Health Care (Including Maternal, Child, and Adolescent).
107. Health Care Access and Information.

DIVISION 2
LICENSING PROVISIONS

Chapter
1. Clinics.
2. Health Facilities.
2.2. Health Care Service Plans.

HISTORY: Added Stats 1939 ch 60.

CHAPTER 1
CLINICS

Article
1. Definitions and General Provisions.

HISTORY: Added Stats 1978 ch 1147 § 4, effective September 26, 1978. Former Chapter 1, entitled "Clinics and Dispensaries," consisting of H & S C §§ 1200–1237, was added Stats 1953 ch 1098 § 3, effective January 1, 1954, and repealed Stats 1978 ch 1147 § 3, effective September 26, 1978. Former Chapter 1, "Clinics and Dispensaries," consisting of H & S C §§ 1200–1251, was enacted Stats 1939 ch 60 and repealed Stats 1953 ch 1098 § 1, effective January 1, 1954.

ARTICLE 1
DEFINITIONS AND GENERAL PROVISIONS

Section
1204. Clinics eligible for licensure.
1204.2. Written transfer agreement not condition of licensure; Medical records related to transfer; Primary care clinic providing services as alternative birth center.
1204.3. Alternative birth centers.

HISTORY: Added Stats 1978 ch 1147 § 4, effective September 26, 1978.

Misc.

§ 1204. Clinics eligible for licensure

Clinics eligible for licensure pursuant to this chapter are primary care clinics and specialty clinics.

(a)(1) Only the following defined classes of primary care clinics shall be eligible for licensure:

(A) A "community clinic" means a clinic operated by a tax-exempt nonprofit corporation that is supported and maintained in whole or in part by donations, bequests, gifts, grants, government funds or contributions, that may be in the form of money, goods, or services. In a community clinic, any charges to the patient shall be based on the patient's ability to pay, utilizing a sliding fee scale. No corporation other than a nonprofit corporation, exempt from federal income taxation under paragraph (3) of subsection (c) of Section 501 of the Internal Revenue Code of 1954 as amended, or a statutory successor thereof, shall operate a community clinic; provided, that the licensee of any community clinic so licensed on the effective date of this section shall not be required to obtain tax-exempt status under either federal or state law in order to be eligible for, or as a condition of, renewal of its license. No natural person or persons shall operate a community clinic.

(B) A "free clinic" means a clinic operated by a tax-exempt, nonprofit corporation supported in whole or in part by voluntary donations, bequests, gifts, grants, government funds or contributions, that may be in the form of money, goods, or services. In a free clinic there shall be no charges directly to the patient for services rendered or for drugs, medicines, appliances, or apparatuses furnished. No corporation other than a nonprofit corporation exempt from federal income taxation under paragraph (3) of subsection (c) of Section 501 of the Internal Revenue Code of 1954 as amended, or a statutory successor thereof, shall operate a free clinic; provided, that the licensee of any free clinic so licensed on the effective date of this section shall not be required to obtain tax-exempt status under either federal or state law in order to be eligible for, or as a condition of, renewal of its license. No natural person or persons shall operate a free clinic.

(2) Nothing in this subdivision shall prohibit a community clinic or a free clinic from providing services to patients whose services are reimbursed by third-party payers, or from entering into managed care contracts for services provided to private or public health plan subscribers, as long as the clinic meets the requirements identified in subparagraphs (A) and (B). For purposes of this subdivision, any payments made to a community clinic by a third-party payer, including, but not limited to, a health care service plan, shall not constitute a charge to the patient. This paragraph is a clarification of existing law.

(b) The following types of specialty clinics shall be eligible for licensure as specialty clinics pursuant to this chapter:

(1) A "surgical clinic" means a clinic that is not part of a hospital and that provides ambulatory surgical care for patients who remain less than 24 hours. A surgical clinic does not include any place or establishment owned or leased and operated as a clinic or office by one or more physicians or dentists in individual or group practice, regardless of the name used publicly to identify the place or establishment, provided, however, that physicians or dentists may, at their option, apply for licensure.

(2) A "chronic dialysis clinic" means a clinic that provides less than 24-hour care for the treatment of patients with end-stage renal disease, including renal dialysis services.

(3) A "rehabilitation clinic" means a clinic that, in addition to providing medical services directly, also provides physical rehabilitation services for patients who remain less than 24 hours. Rehabilitation clinics shall provide at least two of the following rehabilitation services: physical therapy, occupational therapy, social, speech pathology, and audiology services. A rehabilitation clinic does not include the offices of a private physician in individual or group practice.

(4) An "alternative birth center" means a clinic that is not part of a hospital and that provides comprehensive perinatal services and delivery care to pregnant women who remain less than 24 hours at the facility.

HISTORY:

Added Stats 1978 ch 1147 § 4, effective September 26, 1978. Amended Stats 1980 ch 133 § 2; Stats 1982 ch 1306 § 2, effective September 23, 1982; Stats 1985 ch 700 § 3; Stats 1992 ch 457 § 1 (SB 1593); Stats 2000 ch 27 § 1 (AB 2393).

§ 1204.2. Written transfer agreement not condition of licensure; Medical records related to transfer; Primary care clinic providing services as alternative birth center

(a) Notwithstanding any other law, and except as provided in subdivision (c), a primary care clinic described in subdivision (a) of Section 1204 that is licensed pursuant to this chapter shall not be required to enter into a written transfer agreement with a nearby hospital as a condition of licensure.

(b)(1) A primary care clinic shall send with each patient at the time of transfer, or in the case of an emergency, as promptly as possible, copies of all medical records related to the patient's transfer. To the extent practicable and applicable to the patient's transfer, the medical records shall include current medical findings, diagnoses, laboratory results, medications provided prior to transfer, a brief summary of the course of treatment provided prior to transfer, ambulation status, nursing and dietary information, name and contact information for the treating physician at the clinic, and, as appropriate, pertinent administrative and demographic information related to the patient, including name and date of birth.

(2) The requirements in paragraph (1) do not apply if the primary care clinic has entered into a written transfer agreement with a local hospital that provides for the transfer of medical records.

(c) A primary care clinic licensed pursuant to subdivision (a) of Section 1204 that provides services as an alternative birth center shall, as a condition of licensure, be required to maintain a written transfer agreement with a local hospital. The transfer agreement shall include provisions for communication and transportation to meet medical emergencies. Essential personal, health, and medical information shall either accompany the patient upon transfer or be transmitted immediately by telephone to the receiving facility. This section does not modify or supersede the requirements imposed on alternative birth centers described in Section 1204.3.

(d) This section shall become operative on January 1, 2018.

HISTORY:

Added Stats 2015 ch 704 § 2 (AB 1177), effective January 1, 2016, operative January 1, 2018. Amended Stats 2016 ch 86 § 171 (SB 1171), effective January 1, 2017, operative January 1, 2018.

§ 1204.3. Alternative birth centers

(a) An alternative birth center that is licensed as an alternative birth center specialty clinic pursuant to paragraph (4) of subdivision (b) of Section 1204 shall, as a condition of licensure, and a primary care clinic licensed pursuant to subdivision (a) of Section 1204 that provides services as an alternative birth center shall, meet all of the following requirements:

(1) Be a provider of comprehensive perinatal services as defined in Section 14134.5 of the Welfare and Institutions Code.

(2) Maintain a quality assurance program.

(3) Meet the standards for certification established by the American Association of Birth Centers, or at least equivalent standards as determined by the state department.

(4) In addition to standards of the American Association of Birth Centers regarding proximity to hospitals and presence of attendants at births, meet both of the following conditions:

(A) Be located in proximity, in time and distance, to a facility with the capacity for management of obstetrical and neonatal emergencies, including the ability to provide cesarean section delivery, within 30 minutes from time of diagnosis of the emergency.

(B) Require the presence of at least two attendants at all times during birth, one of whom shall be a physician and surgeon, a licensed midwife, or a certified nurse-midwife.

(5) Have a written policy relating to the dissemination of the following information to patients:

(A) A summary of current state laws requiring child passenger restraint systems to be used when transporting children in motor vehicles.

(B) A listing of child passenger restraint system programs located within the county, as required by Section 27362 of the Vehicle Code.

(C) Information describing the risks of death or serious injury associated with the failure to utilize a child passenger restraint system.

(b) The state department shall issue a permit to a primary care clinic licensed pursuant to subdivision (a) of Section 1204 certifying that the primary care clinic has met the requirements of this section and may provide services as an alternative birth center. Nothing in this section shall be construed to require that a licensed primary care clinic obtain an additional license in order to provide services as an alternative birth center.

(c)(1) Notwithstanding subdivision (a) of Section 1206, no place or establishment owned or leased and operated as a clinic or office by one or more licensed health care practitioners and used as an office for the practice of their profession, within the scope of their license, shall be represented or otherwise held out to be an alternative birth center licensed by the state unless it meets the requirements of this section.

(2) Nothing in this subdivision shall be construed to prohibit licensed health care practitioners from providing birth related services, within the scope of their license, in a place or establishment described in paragraph (1).

HISTORY:

Added Stats 1992 ch 457 § 2 (SB 1593). Amended Stats 1995 ch 512 § 2 (SB 503); Stats 2013 ch 665 § 8 (AB 1308), effective January 1, 2014.

CHAPTER 2
HEALTH FACILITIES

Article
1. General.
2. Administration.
3. Regulations.
9. Training Programs in Skilled Nursing and Intermediate Care Facilities.

HISTORY: Added Stats 1973 ch 1202 § 2. Former Chapter 2, entitled "Facilities," consisting of H & S C §§ 1250–1393, was added Stats 1972 ch 1148 § 3, operative July 1, 1973 and repealed Stats 1973 ch 1202 § 1. Former Chapter 2, entitled "Hospitals," consisting of H & S C §§ 1400–1433, was added Stats 1945 ch 1418 § 3 and repealed Stats 1972 ch 1148 § 2, operative July 1, 1973. Former Chapter 2, entitled "Maternity Hospitals," consisting of H & S C §§ 1400–1411, was enacted Stats 1939 ch 60 and repealed Stats 1945 ch 1418 § 2.

ARTICLE 1
GENERAL

Section
1250. Definitions.
1253.7. Observation services.
1257.7. Security and safety assessment; Security plan; Guidelines and standards on violence; Reporting.

HISTORY: Added Stats 1973 ch 1202.

§ 1250. Definitions

As used in this chapter, "health facility" means a facility, place, or building that is organized, maintained, and operated for the diagnosis, care, prevention, and treatment of human illness, physical or mental, including convalescence and rehabilitation and including care during and after pregnancy, or for any one or more of these purposes, for one or more persons, to which the persons are admitted for a 24-hour stay or longer, and includes the following types:

(a) "General acute care hospital" means a health facility having a duly constituted governing body with overall administrative and professional responsibility and an organized medical staff that provides 24-hour inpatient care, including the following basic services: medical, nursing, surgical, anesthesia, laboratory, radiology, pharmacy, and dietary services. A general acute care hospital may include more than one physical plant maintained and operated on separate premises as provided in Section 1250.8. A general acute care hospital that exclusively provides acute medical rehabilitation center services, including at least physical therapy, occupational therapy, and speech therapy, may provide for the required surgical and anesthesia services through a contract with another acute care hospital. In addition, a general acute care hospital that, on July 1, 1983, provided required surgical and anesthesia services through a contract or agreement with another acute care hospital may continue to provide these surgical and anesthesia services through a contract or agreement with an acute care hospital. The general

Misc.

acute care hospital operated by the State Department of Developmental Services at Agnews Developmental Center may, until June 30, 2007, provide surgery and anesthesia services through a contract or agreement with another acute care hospital. Notwithstanding the requirements of this subdivision, a general acute care hospital operated by the Department of Corrections and Rehabilitation or the Department of Veterans Affairs may provide surgery and anesthesia services during normal weekday working hours, and not provide these services during other hours of the weekday or on weekends or holidays, if the general acute care hospital otherwise meets the requirements of this section.

A "general acute care hospital" includes a "rural general acute care hospital." However, a "rural general acute care hospital" shall not be required by the department to provide surgery and anesthesia services. A "rural general acute care hospital" shall meet either of the following conditions:

(1) The hospital meets criteria for designation within peer group six or eight, as defined in the report entitled Hospital Peer Grouping for Efficiency Comparison, dated December 20, 1982.

(2) The hospital meets the criteria for designation within peer group five or seven, as defined in the report entitled Hospital Peer Grouping for Efficiency Comparison, dated December 20, 1982, and has no more than 76 acute care beds and is located in a census dwelling place of 15,000 or less population according to the 1980 federal census.

(b) "Acute psychiatric hospital" means a health facility having a duly constituted governing body with overall administrative and professional responsibility and an organized medical staff that provides 24-hour inpatient care for persons with mental health disorders or other patients referred to in Division 5 (commencing with Section 5000) or Division 6 (commencing with Section 6000) of the Welfare and Institutions Code, including the following basic services: medical, nursing, rehabilitative, pharmacy, and dietary services.

(c)(1) "Skilled nursing facility" means a health facility that provides skilled nursing care and supportive care to patients whose primary need is for availability of skilled nursing care on an extended basis.

(2) "Skilled nursing facility" includes a "small house skilled nursing facility (SHSNF)," as defined in Section 1323.5.

(d) "Intermediate care facility" means a health facility that provides inpatient care to ambulatory or nonambulatory patients who have recurring need for skilled nursing supervision and need supportive care, but who do not require availability of continuous skilled nursing care.

(e) "Intermediate care facility/developmentally disabled habilitative" means a facility with a capacity of 4 to 15 beds that provides 24-hour personal care, habilitation, developmental, and supportive health services to 15 or fewer persons with developmental disabilities who have intermittent recurring needs for nursing services, but have been certified by a physician and surgeon as not requiring availability of continuous skilled nursing care.

(f) "Special hospital" means a health facility having a duly constituted governing body with overall administrative and professional responsibility and an organized medical or dental staff that provides inpatient or outpatient care in dentistry or maternity.

(g) "Intermediate care facility/developmentally disabled" means a facility that provides 24-hour personal care, habilitation, developmental, and supportive health services to persons with developmental disabilities whose primary need is for developmental services and who have a recurring but intermittent need for skilled nursing services.

(h) "Intermediate care facility/developmentally disabled-nursing" means a facility with a capacity of 4 to 15 beds that provides 24-hour personal care, developmental services, and nursing supervision for persons with developmental disabilities who have intermittent recurring needs for skilled nursing care but have been certified by a physician and surgeon as not requiring continuous skilled nursing care. The facility shall serve medically fragile persons with developmental disabilities or who demonstrate significant developmental delay that may lead to a developmental disability if not treated.

(i)(1) "Congregate living health facility" means a residential home with a capacity, except as provided in paragraph (4), of no more than 18 beds, that provides inpatient care, including the following basic services: medical supervision, 24-hour skilled nursing and supportive care, pharmacy, dietary, social, recreational, and at least one type of service specified in paragraph (2). The primary need of congregate living health facility residents shall be for availability of skilled nursing care on a recurring, intermittent, extended, or continuous basis. This care is generally less intense than that provided in general acute care hospitals but more intense than that provided in skilled nursing facilities.

(2) Congregate living health facilities shall provide one or more of the following services:

(A) Services for persons who are mentally alert, persons with physical disabilities, who may be ventilator dependent.

(B) Services for persons who have a diagnosis of terminal illness, a diagnosis of a life-threatening illness, or both. Terminal illness means the individual has a life expectancy of six months or less as stated in writing by his or her attending physician and surgeon. A "life-threatening illness" means the individual has an illness that can lead to a possibility of a termination of life within five years or less as stated in writing by his or her attending physician and surgeon.

(C) Services for persons who are catastrophically and severely disabled. A person who is catastrophically and severely disabled means a person whose origin of disability was acquired through trauma or nondegenerative neurologic illness, for whom it has been determined that active rehabilitation would be beneficial and to whom these services are being provided. Services offered by a congregate living health facility to a person who is catastrophically disabled shall include, but not be limited to, speech, physical, and occupational therapy.

(3) A congregate living health facility license shall specify which of the types of persons described in paragraph (2) to whom a facility is licensed to provide services.

(4)(A) A facility operated by a city and county for the purposes of delivering services under this section may have a capacity of 59 beds.

(B) A congregate living health facility not operated by a city and county servicing persons who are terminally ill, persons who have been diagnosed with a life-threatening illness, or both, that is located in a county with a population of 500,000 or more persons, or located in a county of the 16th class pursuant to Section 28020 of the Government Code, may have not more than 25 beds for the purpose of serving persons who are terminally ill.

(5) A congregate living health facility shall have a noninstitutional, homelike environment.

(j)(1) "Correctional treatment center" means a health facility operated by the Department of Corrections and Rehabilitation, the Department of Corrections and Rehabilitation, Division of Juvenile Facilities, or a county, city, or city and county law enforcement agency that, as determined by the department, provides inpatient health services to that portion of the inmate population who do not require a general acute care level of basic services. This definition shall not apply to those areas of a law enforcement facility that houses inmates or wards who may be receiving outpatient services and are housed separately for reasons of improved access to health care, security, and protection. The health services provided by a correctional treatment center shall include, but are not limited to, all of the following basic services: physician and surgeon, psychiatrist, psychologist, nursing, pharmacy, and dietary. A correctional treatment center may provide the following services: laboratory, radiology, perinatal, and any other services approved by the department.

(2) Outpatient surgical care with anesthesia may be provided, if the correctional treatment center meets the same requirements as a surgical clinic licensed pursuant to Section 1204, with the exception of the requirement that patients remain less than 24 hours.

(3) Correctional treatment centers shall maintain written service agreements with general acute care hospitals to provide for those inmate physical health needs that cannot be met by the correctional treatment center.

(4) Physician and surgeon services shall be readily available in a correctional treatment center on a 24-hour basis.

(5) It is not the intent of the Legislature to have a correctional treatment center supplant the general acute care hospitals at the California Medical Facility, the California Men's Colony, and the California Institution for Men. This subdivision shall not be construed to prohibit the Department of Corrections and Rehabilitation from obtaining a correctional treatment center license at these sites.

(k) "Nursing facility" means a health facility licensed pursuant to this chapter that is certified to participate as a provider of care either as a skilled nursing facility in the federal Medicare Program under Title XVIII of the federal Social Security Act (42 U.S.C. Sec. 1395 et seq.) or as a nursing facility in the federal Medicaid Program under Title XIX of the federal Social Security Act (42 U.S.C. Sec. 1396 et seq.), or as both.

(*l*) Regulations defining a correctional treatment center described in subdivision (j) that is operated by a county, city, or city and county, the Department of Corrections and Rehabilitation, or the Department of Corrections and Rehabilitation, Division of Juvenile Facilities, shall not become effective prior to, or, if effective, shall be inoperative until January 1, 1996, and until that time these correctional facilities are exempt from any licensing requirements.

(m) "Intermediate care facility/developmentally disabled-continuous nursing (ICF/DD-CN)" means a homelike facility with a capacity of four to eight, inclusive, beds that provides 24-hour personal care, developmental services, and nursing supervision for persons with developmental disabilities who have continuous needs for skilled nursing care and have been certified by a physician and surgeon as warranting continuous skilled nursing care. The facility shall serve medically fragile persons who have developmental disabilities or demonstrate significant developmental delay that may lead to a developmental disability if not treated. ICF/DD-CN facilities shall be subject to licensure under this chapter upon adoption of licensing regulations in accordance with Section 1275.3. A facility providing continuous skilled nursing services to persons with developmental disabilities pursuant to Section 14132.20 or 14495.10 of the Welfare and Institutions Code shall apply for licensure under this subdivision within 90 days after the regulations become effective, and may continue to operate pursuant to those sections until its licensure application is either approved or denied.

(n) "Hospice facility" means a health facility licensed pursuant to this chapter with a capacity of no more than 24 beds that provides hospice services. Hospice services include, but are not limited to, routine care, continuous care, inpatient respite care, and inpatient hospice care as defined in subdivision (d) of Section 1339.40, and is operated by a provider of hospice services that is licensed pursuant to Section 1751 and certified as a hospice pursuant to Part 418 of Title 42 of the Code of Federal Regulations.

HISTORY:

Added Stats 1973 ch 1202 § 2. Amended Stats 1974 ch 1444 § 1; Stats 1976 ch 854 § 34, effective September 9, 1976; Stats 1978 ch 1221 § 1, effective September 27, 1978, ch 1226 § 1.5; Stats 1980 ch 569 § 1, ch 676 (ch 569 prevails); Stats 1981 ch 714 § 213, ch 743 § 3; Stats 1983 ch 695 § 1, effective September 11, 1983, ch 1003 § 1; Stats 1984 ch 497 § 2, effective July 17, 1984; Stats 1985 ch 1496 § 4; Stats 1986 ch 1111 § 1, ch 1320 § 1, ch 1459 § 1.5; Stats 1987 ch 1282 § 2; Stats 1988 ch 1478 § 3, effective September 27, ch 1608 § 1.3; Stats 1989 ch 1393 § 1, effective October 2, 1989; Stats 1990 ch 1227 § 1 (AB 3413), effective September 24, 1990, ch 1329 § 3.5 (SB 1524), effective September 25, 1990; Stats 1992 ch 697 § 11 (SB 1559), ch 1163 § 1 (SB 1570), ch 1164 § 1 (SB 1003), ch 1369 § 5 (AB 3027), effective October 27, 1992, operative January 1, 1993; Stats 1993 ch 70 § 7 (SB 86), effective June 30, 1993, ch 589 § 84 (AB 2211), ch 930 § 1 (SB 560), ch 931 § 1 (AB 972), ch 932 § 1 (SB 910), effective October 7, 1993, operative until January 1, 1994, ch 932 § 1.7 (SB 910) (ch 932 prevails), effective October 7, 1993, operative January 1, 1994; Stats 1995 ch 749 § 6 (AB 1177), effective October 10, 1995; Stats 2000 ch 451 § 2 (AB 1731); Stats 2001 ch 685 § 1 (AB 1212); Stats 2005 ch 333 § 2 (AB 1346), ch 443 § 2 (SB 666), effective January 1, 2006; Stats 2009-2010 4th Ex Sess ch 5 § 2 (ABX4 5), effective July 28, 2009; Stats 2009 ch 298 § 2 (AB 1540), effective January 1, 2010; Stats 2011 ch 331 § 1 (SB 177), effective January 1, 2012; Stats 2012 ch 671 § 1 (SB 1228), effective January 1, 2013, ch 673 § 2.5 (SB 135), effective January 1, 2013; Stats 2014 ch 144 § 25 (AB 1847), effective January 1, 2015; Stats 2015 ch 483 § 1 (AB 1211), effective October 4, 2015.

§ 1253.7. Observation services

(a) For purposes of this chapter, "observation services" means outpatient services provided by a general acute care hospital and that have been ordered by a provider, to those patients who have unstable or uncertain conditions potentially serious enough to warrant close observation, but not so serious as to warrant inpatient admission to the hospital. Observation services may include the use of a bed, monitoring by nursing and other staff, and any other services that are reasonable and necessary to safely evaluate a patient's condition or determine the need for a possible inpatient admission to the hospital.

(b) When a patient in an inpatient unit of a hospital or in an observation unit, as defined in subdivision (c), is receiving observation services, or following a change in a patient's status from inpatient to observation, the patient shall receive written notice, as soon as practicable, that he or she is on observation status. The notice shall state that while on observation status, the patient's care is being provided on an outpatient basis, which may affect his or her health care coverage reimbursement.

(c) For purposes of this chapter, "observation unit" means an area in which observation services are provided in a setting outside of any inpatient unit and that is not part of an emergency department of a general acute care hospital. A hospital may establish one or more observation units that shall be marked with signage identifying the observation unit area as an outpatient area. The signage shall use the term "outpatient" in the title of the designated area to indicate clearly to all patients and family members that the observation services provided in the center are not inpatient services. Identifying an observation unit by a name or term other than that used in this subdivision does not exempt the general acute care hospital from compliance with the requirements of this section.

(d) Notwithstanding subdivisions (d) and (e) of Section 1275, an observation unit shall comply with the same licensed nurse-to-patient ratios as supplemental emergency services. This subdivision is not intended to alter or amend the effect of any regulation adopted pursuant to Section 1276.4 as of the effective date of the act that added this subdivision.

HISTORY:

Added Stats 2016 ch 723 § 1 (SB 1076), effective January 1, 2017.

§ 1257.7. Security and safety assessment; Security plan; Guidelines and standards on violence; Reporting

(a) After July 1, 2010, all hospitals licensed pursuant to subdivisions (a), (b), and (f) of Section 1250 shall conduct, not less than annually, a security and safety assessment and, using the assessment, develop, and annually update based on the assessment, a security plan with measures to protect personnel, patients, and visitors from aggressive or violent behavior. The security and safety assessment shall examine trends of aggressive or violent behavior at the facility. These hospitals shall track incidents of aggressive or violent behavior as part of the quality assessment and improvement program and for the purposes of developing a security plan to deter and manage further aggressive or violent acts of a similar nature. The plan may include, but shall not be limited to, security considerations relating to all of the following:

(1) Physical layout.

(2) Staffing.

(3) Security personnel availability.

(4) Policy and training related to appropriate responses to violent acts.

(5) Efforts to cooperate with local law enforcement regarding violent acts in the facility.

In developing this plan, the hospital shall consider guidelines or standards on violence in health care facilities issued by the department, the Division of Occupational Safety and Health, and the federal Occupational Safety and Health Administration. As part of the security plan, a hospital shall adopt security policies including, but not limited to, personnel training policies designed to protect personnel, patients, and visitors from aggressive or violent behavior. In developing the plan and the assessment, the hospital shall consult with affected employees, including the recognized collective bargaining agent or agents, if any, and members of the hospital medical staff organized pursuant to Section 2282 of the Business and Professions Code. This consultation may occur through hospital committees.

(b) The individual or members of a hospital committee responsible for developing the security plan shall be familiar with all of the following:

(1) The role of security in hospital operations.

(2) Hospital organization.

(3) Protective measures, including alarms and access control.

(4) The handling of disturbed patients, visitors, and employees.

(5) Identification of aggressive and violent predicting factors.

(6) Hospital safety and emergency preparedness.

(7) The rudiments of documenting and reporting crimes, including, by way of example, not disturbing a crime scene.

(c) The hospital shall have sufficient personnel to provide security pursuant to the security plan developed pursuant to subdivision (a). Persons regularly assigned to provide security in a hospital setting shall be trained regarding the role of security in hospital operations, including the identification of aggressive and violent predicting factors and management of violent disturbances.

(d) Any act of assault, as defined in Section 240 of the Penal Code, or battery, as defined in Section 242 of the Penal Code, that results in injury or involves the use of a firearm or other dangerous weapon, against any on-duty hospital personnel shall be reported to the local law enforcement agency within 72 hours of the incident. Any other act of assault, as defined in Section 240 of the Penal Code, or battery, as defined in Section 242 of the Penal Code, against any on-duty hospital personnel may be reported to the local law enforcement agency within 72 hours of the incident. No health facility or employee of a health facility who reports a known or suspected instance of assault or battery pursuant to this section shall be civilly or criminally liable for any report required by this section. No health facility or employee of a health facility who reports a known or suspected instance of assault or battery that is authorized, but not required, by this section, shall be civilly or criminally liable for the report authorized by this section unless it can be proven that a false report was made and the health facility or its employee knew that the report was false or was made with reckless disregard of the truth or falsity of the report, and any health facility or employee of a health facility who makes a report known to be false or with reckless disregard of the truth or falsity of the report shall be liable for any damages caused. Any individual knowingly interfering with or obstructing the lawful reporting process shall be guilty of a misdemeanor. "Dangerous weapon," as used in this section, means any weapon the possession or concealed carrying of which is prohibited by any provision listed in Section 16590 of the Penal Code.

HISTORY:
Added Stats 1993 ch 936 § 2 (AB 508). Amended Stats 1994 ch 19X § 1 (AB 74X), effective November 30, 1994; Stats 2009 ch 506 § 1 (AB 1083), effective January 1, 2010; Stats 2010 ch 178 § 36 (SB 1115), effective January 1, 2011, operative January 1, 2012.

ARTICLE 2
ADMINISTRATION

Section
1267.61. Written notice of proposed changes to licensee or management companies of skilled nursing facilities.

HISTORY: Added Stats 1973 ch 1202.

§ 1267.61. Written notice of proposed changes to licensee or management companies of skilled nursing facilities

(a) At least 90 days prior to a finalization of the sale, transfer of operation, including management changes, assignment, lease, or other change or transfer of ownership interests, the licensee of a facility defined in subdivision (c) of Section 1250, excluding skilled nursing facilities that are operated as a distinct part of an acute care hospital, shall give a written notice of the proposed change in licensee or management company to all residents of the facility and their representatives that contains all of the following information applicable to the proposed change:

(1) The name and address of the prospective licensee, transferee, assignee, lessee, property owner, or the licensee's parent company and management company, if applicable.

(2) A list of all prospective licensee or prospective management company's owners or shareholders and their ownership percentages.

(3) A list of directors, officers, board members, and property owners of the prospective licensee and, if existing, a list of directors, officers, and board members of the prospective licensee's parent company and proposed management company.

(4) The expected date of sale, assignment, lease, or other change.

(b) The licensee shall post a copy of the notice required pursuant to this section on all entrance and exit doors of the facility.

(c) The information required by this section shall be made available to the public by the facility upon request and shall be included in the department's licensing database and consumer information website.

(d) A licensee that fails to comply with the notification requirements of this section is liable for a civil penalty in the amount of of one hundred dollars ($100) per day for each day the notice is delayed.

(e) This section applies only to license applications submitted after July 1, 2020.

HISTORY:
Added Stats 2019 ch 832 § 1 (AB 1695), effective January 1, 2020.

ARTICLE 3
REGULATIONS

Section
1276.4. Nurse to patient ratios.

HISTORY: Added Stats 1973 ch 1202 § 3.

§ 1276.4. Nurse to patient ratios

(a) By January 1, 2002, the State Department of Public Health shall adopt regulations that establish minimum, specific, and numerical licensed nurse-to-patient ratios by licensed nurse classification and by hospital unit for all health facilities licensed pursuant to subdivision (a), (b), or (f) of Section 1250. The State Department of Public Health shall adopt these regulations in accordance with the department's licensing and certification regulations as stated in Sections 70053.2, 70215, and 70217 of Title 22 of the California Code of Regulations, and the professional and vocational regulations in Section 1443.5 of Title 16 of the California Code of Regulations. The department shall review these regulations five years after adoption and shall report to the Legislature regarding any proposed changes. Flexibility shall be considered by the department for rural general acute care hospitals in response to their special needs. As used in this subdivision, "hospital unit" means a critical care unit, burn unit, labor and delivery room, postanesthesia service area, emergency department, operating room, pediatric unit, step-down/intermediate care unit, specialty care unit, telemetry unit, general medical care unit, subacute care unit, and transitional inpatient care unit. The regulation addressing the emergency department shall distinguish between regularly scheduled core staff licensed nurses and additional licensed nurses required to care for critical care patients in the emergency department.

(b) These ratios shall constitute the minimum number of registered and licensed nurses that shall be allocated. Additional staff shall be assigned in accordance with a documented patient classification system for determining nursing care requirements, including the severity of the illness, the need for specialized equipment and technology, the complexity of clinical judgment needed to design, implement, and evaluate the patient care plan and the ability for self-care, and the licensure of the personnel required for care.

(c) "Critical care unit" as used in this section means a unit that is established to safeguard and protect patients whose severity of medical conditions requires continuous monitoring, and complex intervention by licensed nurses.

(d) All health facilities licensed under subdivision (a), (b), or (f) of Section 1250 shall adopt written policies and procedures for training and orientation of nursing staff.

(e) No registered nurse shall be assigned to a nursing unit or clinical area unless that nurse has first received orientation in that clinical area sufficient to provide competent care to patients in that area, and has demonstrated current competence in providing care in that area.

(f) The written policies and procedures for orientation of nursing staff shall require that all temporary personnel shall receive orientation and be subject to competency validation consistent with Sections 70016.1and 70214 of Title 22 of the California Code of Regulations.

(g) Requests for waivers to this section that do not jeopardize the health, safety, and well-being of patients affected and that are needed for increased operational efficiency may be granted by the department to rural general acute care hospitals meeting the criteria set forth in Section 70059.1 of Title 22 of the California Code of Regulations.

(h) In case of conflict between this section and any provision or regulation defining the scope of nursing practice, the scope of practice provisions shall control.

(i) The regulations adopted by the department shall augment and not replace existing nurse-to-patient ratios that exist in regulation or law for the intensive care units, the neonatal intensive care units, or the operating room.

(j) The regulations adopted by the department shall not replace existing licensed staff-to-patient ratios for hospitals operated by the State Department of State Hospitals.

(k) The regulations adopted by the department for health facilities licensed under subdivision (b) of Section 1250 that are not operated by the State Department of State Hospitals shall take into account the special needs of the patients served in the psychiatric units.

(*l*) The department may take into consideration the unique nature of the University of California teaching hospitals as educational institutions when establishing licensed nurse-to-patient ratios. The department shall coordinate with the Board of Registered Nursing to ensure that staffing ratios are consistent with the Board of Registered Nursing approved nursing education requirements. This includes nursing clinical experience incidental to a work-study program rendered in a University of California clinical facility approved by the Board of Registered Nursing provided there will be sufficient direct care registered nurse preceptors available to ensure safe patient care.

HISTORY:

Added Stats 1999 ch 945 § 3 (AB 394). Amended Stats 2000 ch 148 § 1 (AB 1760), effective July 21, 2000; Stats 2012 ch 24 § 11 (AB 1470), effective June 27, 2012.

ARTICLE 9

TRAINING PROGRAMS IN SKILLED NURSING AND INTERMEDIATE CARE FACILITIES

Misc.

Section

1337.1. Approved training programs.
1337.15. Two year licensed vocational or registered nurse; Qualified instructor.
1337.16. Online or distance learning nurse assistant training program; Requirements.
1338.2. Work group for investigation and recommendations.
1338.4. Access to online learning tool "Building Respect for LGBT Older Adults" [Repealed].

HISTORY: Added Stats 1978 ch 351 § 1, effective July 4, 1978.

§ 1337.1. Approved training programs

A skilled nursing facility or intermediate care facility shall adopt an approved training program that meets standards established by the department. The approved training program shall consist of at least all of the following:

(a) An orientation program to be given to newly employed nurse assistants prior to providing direct patient care in skilled nursing facilities or intermediate care facilities.

(b)(1) A precertification training program consisting of at least 60 classroom hours of training on basic nursing skills, patient safety and rights, the social and psychological problems of patients, and resident abuse prevention, recognition, and reporting pursuant to subdivision (e). The 60 classroom hours of training may be conducted within a skilled nursing facility or intermediate care facility or in an educational institution or agency. A skilled nursing facility or intermediate care facility may conduct the 60 classroom hours of training in an online or distance learning course format, as approved by the department.

(2) In addition to the 60 classroom hours of training required under paragraph (1), the precertification training program shall consist of at least 100 hours of supervised and on-the-job training clinical practice. The 100 hours may consist of normal employment as a nurse assistant under the supervision of either the director of nurse training or a licensed nurse qualified to provide nurse assistant training who has no other assigned duties while providing the training.

(3) At least two hours of the 60 hours of classroom training shall address the special needs of persons with developmental and mental disorders, including intellectual disability, cerebral palsy, epilepsy, dementia, Parkinson's disease, and mental illness. At least two hours of the 60 hours of classroom training shall address the special needs of persons with Alzheimer's disease and related dementias.

(4) At least four hours of the 100 hours of supervised clinical training shall address the special needs of persons with developmental and mental disorders, including intellectual disability, cerebral palsy, epilepsy, Alzheimer's disease and related dementias, and Parkinson's disease.

(5) In a precertification training program subject to this subdivision, credit shall be given for the training received in an approved precertification training program adopted by another skilled nursing facility or intermediate care facility.

(6) This subdivision does not apply to a skilled nursing facility or intermediate care facility that demonstrates to the department that it employs only nurse assistants with a valid certification.

(c) Continuing in-service training to ensure continuing competency in existing and new nursing skills.

(d) Each facility shall consider including training regarding the characteristics and method of assessment and treatment of acquired immune deficiency syndrome (AIDS).

(e)(1) The approved training program shall include, within the 60 hours of classroom training, a minimum of six hours of instruction on preventing, recognizing, and reporting instances of resident abuse utilizing those courses developed pursuant to Section 13823.93 of the Penal Code, and a minimum of one hour of instruction on preventing, recognizing, and reporting residents' rights violations.

(2) A minimum of four hours of instruction on preventing, recognizing, and reporting instances of resident abuse, including instruction on preventing, recognizing, and reporting residents' rights violations, shall be included within the total minimum hours of continuing education or in-service training required and in effect for certified nurse assistants.

HISTORY:

Added Stats 1978 ch 351 § 1, effective July 4, 1978. Amended Stats 1987 ch 1177 § 2; Stats 1988 ch 1213 § 2; Stats 1992 ch 1169 § 1 (SB 1670); Stats 2000 ch 451 § 14 (AB 1731); Stats 2001 ch 685 § 9 (AB 1212); Stats 2004 ch 270 § 1 (AB 2791); Stats 2012 ch 448 § 27 (AB 2370), effective January 1, 2013, ch 457 § 27 (SB 1381), effective January 1, 2013 (ch 457 prevails); Stats 2017 ch 282 § 1 (SB 449), effective January 1, 2018; Stats 2018 ch 769 § 2 (AB 2850), effective January 1, 2019; Stats 2019 ch 497 § 151 (AB 991), effective January 1, 2020.

§ 1337.15. Two year licensed vocational or registered nurse; Qualified instructor

(a) A person who provides instruction or training, at a skilled nursing facility or intermediate care facility or in an educational institution, as part of a certified nurse assistant precertification training program described in Section 1337.1 or 1337.3 may be any licensed vocational nurse or registered nurse with no less than two years of nursing experience, of which no less than one year is in providing care and services to chronically ill or elderly patients in an acute care hospital, skilled nursing facility, intermediate care facility, home care, hospice care, or other long-term care setting.

(b) Notwithstanding any other law, a person described in subdivision (a) shall not be required to hold a teaching credential to provide instruction as part of a certified nurse assistant precertification training program described in Section 1337.1 or 1337.3.

HISTORY:

Added Stats 2018 ch 769 § 3 (AB 2850), effective January 1, 2019.

§ 1337.16. Online or distance learning nurse assistant training program; Requirements

(a) An online or distance learning nurse assistant training program shall comply with all of the following requirements:

(1) Provide online instruction in which the trainees and the approved instructor are online at the same or similar times and which allows them to use real-time collaborative software that combines audio, video, file sharing, or any other forms of approved interaction and communication.

(2) Require the use of a personal identification number or personal identification information that confirms the identity of the trainees and instructors, including, but not limited to, having trainees sign an affidavit attesting under penalty of perjury to their identity while completing the program.

(3) Provide safeguards to protect personal information.

(4) Include policies and procedures to ensure that instructors are accessible to trainees outside of the normal instruction times.

(5) Include policies and procedures for equipment failures, student absences, and completing assignments past original deadlines.

(6) Provide a clear explanation on its Internet Web site of all technology requirements to participate and complete the program.

(7) Provide the department with statistics about the performance of trainees in the program, including, but not limited to, exam pass rate and the rate at which trainees repeat each module of the program, and any other information requested by the department regarding trainee participation in and completion of the program.

(b) In addition to the requirements set forth in subdivision (a), an online or distance learning nurse assistant training program shall meet the same standards as a traditional, classroom-based program, and comply with any other standard established by the department for online or distance learning nurse assistant training programs. Notwithstanding any other law, the department may, without taking any regulatory actions pursuant to Chapter 3.5 (commencing with Section 11340) of Part 1 of Division 3 of Title 2 of the Government Code, implement, interpret, or make specific this section by means of an All Facilities Letter (AFL) or similar instruction.

(c) As a condition of approval by the department, an online or distance learning nurse assistant training program shall provide the department with access rights to the program for the purposes of verifying that program complies with all requirements and allowing the department to monitor online or distance learning sessions.

HISTORY:

Added Stats 2018 ch 769 § 4 (AB 2850), effective January 1, 2019.

§ 1338.2. Work group for investigation and recommendations

(a) The state department shall convene a work group to develop recommendations to the department on ways to expand the availability of training programs and certified nurse assistants available for hire in the state. The work group shall investigate, but not be limited to investigating, all of the following:

(1) Work-based learning programs for students in the regional occupational programs in the state.

(2) Utilization of apprenticeships.

(3) Promotional programs for training centers and certified nurse assistant jobs.

(4) Utilization of expanded data resources.

(b) The recommendations required by subdivision (a) shall be submitted by the work group to the state department on or before July 1, 2001.

(c) The work group shall consist of, but not be limited to, all of the following:

(1) A representative from the State Department of Education.

(2) Nurse-Assistant training center representatives.

(3) A director of staff development for a long-term health care facility.

(4) A publisher of nurse assistant training and competency curricula.

(5) An industry representative.

(6) A currently certified nurse assistant.

(7) A consumer representative.

(8) A labor union representative.

(9) A representative of the American Red Cross.

(10) The Chancellor of the California Community Colleges.

(11) A representative from the Office of Statewide Health Planning and Development.

(12) A registered nurse and a licensed vocational nurse, both of whom are currently providing long-term care nursing services.

HISTORY:
Added Stats 1999 ch 719 § 5 (AB 656).

§ 1338.4. Access to online learning tool "Building Respect for LGBT Older Adults" [Repealed]

HISTORY:
Added Stats 2017 ch 483 § 2 (SB 219), effective January 1, 2018, repealed January 1, 2019, by its own terms.

CHAPTER 2.2
HEALTH CARE SERVICE PLANS

Article
2. Administration.
5. Standards.

HISTORY: Added Stats 1975 ch 941 § 2, operative July 1, 1976.

ARTICLE 2
ADMINISTRATION

Section
1348.8. Requirements for telephone medical advice services; Forwarding of data to Department of Consumer Affairs.

HISTORY: Added Stats 1975 ch 941 § 2, operative July 1, 1976.

§ 1348.8. Requirements for telephone medical advice services; Forwarding of data to Department of Consumer Affairs

(a) A health care service plan that provides, operates, or contracts for telephone medical advice services to its enrollees and subscribers shall do all of the following:

(1) Ensure that the in-state or out-of-state telephone medical advice service complies with the requirements of Chapter 15 (commencing with Section 4999) of Division 2 of the Business and Professions Code.

(2) Ensure that the staff providing telephone medical advice services for the in-state or out-of-state telephone medical advice service are licensed as follows:

(A) For full service health care service plans, the staff hold a valid California license as a registered nurse or a valid license in the state within which they provide telephone medical advice services as a physi-

Misc.

cian and surgeon or physician assistant, and are operating in compliance with the laws governing their respective scopes of practice.

(B)(i) For specialized health care service plans providing, operating, or contracting with a telephone medical advice service in California, the staff shall be appropriately licensed, registered, or certified as a dentist pursuant to Chapter 4 (commencing with Section 1600) of Division 2 of the Business and Professions Code, as a dental hygienist pursuant to Article 7 (commencing with Section 1740) of Chapter 4 of Division 2 of the Business and Professions Code, as a physician and surgeon pursuant to Chapter 5 (commencing with Section 2000) of Division 2 of the Business and Professions Code or the Osteopathic Initiative Act, as a registered nurse pursuant to Chapter 6 (commencing with Section 2700) of Division 2 of the Business and Professions Code, as a psychologist pursuant to Chapter 6.6 (commencing with Section 2900) of Division 2 of the Business and Professions Code, as an optometrist pursuant to Chapter 7 (commencing with Section 3000) of Division 2 of the Business and Professions Code, as a marriage and family therapist pursuant to Chapter 13 (commencing with Section 4980) of Division 2 of the Business and Professions Code, as a licensed clinical social worker pursuant to Chapter 14 (commencing with Section 4991) of Division 2 of the Business and Professions Code, as a professional clinical counselor pursuant to Chapter 16 (commencing with Section 4999.10) of Division 2 of the Business and Professions Code, or as a chiropractor pursuant to the Chiropractic Initiative Act, and operating in compliance with the laws governing their respective scopes of practice.

(ii) For specialized health care service plans providing, operating, or contracting with an out-of-state telephone medical advice service, the staff shall be health care professionals, as identified in clause (i), who are licensed, registered, or certified in the state within which they are providing the telephone medical advice services and are operating in compliance with the laws governing their respective scopes of practice. All registered nurses providing telephone medical advice services to both in-state and out-of-state business entities registered pursuant to this chapter shall be licensed pursuant to Chapter 6 (commencing with Section 2700) of Division 2 of the Business and Professions Code.

(3) Ensure that every full service health care service plan provides for a physician and surgeon who is available on an on-call basis at all times the service is advertised to be available to enrollees and subscribers.

(4) Ensure that staff members handling enrollee or subscriber calls, who are not licensed, certified, or registered as required by paragraph (2), do not provide telephone medical advice. Those staff members may ask questions on behalf of a staff member who is licensed, certified, or registered as required by paragraph (2), in order to help ascertain the condition of an enrollee or subscriber so that the enrollee or subscriber can be referred to licensed staff. However, under no circumstances shall those staff members use the answers to those questions in an attempt to assess, evaluate, advise, or make any decision regarding the condition of an enrollee or subscriber or determine when an enrollee or subscriber needs to be seen by a licensed medical professional.

(5) Ensure that no staff member uses a title or designation when speaking to an enrollee or subscriber that may cause a reasonable person to believe that the staff member is a licensed, certified, or registered professional described in Section 4999.2 of the Business and Professions Code unless the staff member is a licensed, certified, or registered professional.

(6) Ensure that the in-state or out-of-state telephone medical advice service designates an agent for service of process in California and files this designation with the director.

(7) Require that the in-state or out-of-state telephone medical advice service makes and maintains records for a period of five years after the telephone medical advice services are provided, including, but not limited to, oral or written transcripts of all medical advice conversations with the health care service plan's enrollees or subscribers in California and copies of all complaints. If the records of telephone medical advice services are kept out of state, the health care service plan shall, upon the request of the director, provide the records to the director within 10 days of the request.

(8) Ensure that the telephone medical advice services are provided consistent with good professional practice.

(b) The director shall forward to the Department of Consumer Affairs, within 30 days of the end of each calendar quarter, data regarding complaints filed with the department concerning telephone medical advice services.

(c) For purposes of this section, "telephone medical advice" means a telephonic communication between a patient and a health care professional in which the health care professional's primary function is to provide to the patient a telephonic response to the patient's questions regarding his or her or a family member's medical care or treatment. "Telephone medical advice" includes assessment, evaluation, or advice provided to patients or their family members.

HISTORY:

Added Stats 1999 ch 535 § 2 (AB 285). Amended Stats 2002 ch 1013 § 83 (SB 2026); Stats 2003 ch 885 § 3 (SB 969); Stats 2008 ch 31 § 51 (SB 853), effective January 1, 2009, operative July 1, 2009 (ch 31 prevails), ch 179 § 137, effective January 1, 2008; Stats 2010 ch 328 § 113 (SB 1330), effective January 1, 2011; Stats 2011 ch 381 § 28 (SB 146), effective January 1, 2012; Stats 2016 ch 799 § 42 (SB 1039), effective January 1, 2017.

ARTICLE 5

STANDARDS

Misc.

Section

1373. Required or prohibited contract provisions.
1373.8. Contractees' right to select licensed professionals in California to perform contract services.
1374.55. Coverage for treatment of infertility; "Subsidiary".
1374.57. Exclusion of dependent child.

HISTORY: Added Stats 1975 ch 941 § 2, operative July 1, 1976.

§ 1373. Required or prohibited contract provisions

(a)(1) A plan contract may not provide an exception for other coverage if the other coverage is entitlement to Medi-Cal benefits under Chapter 7 (commencing with Section 14000) or Chapter 8 (commencing with Section 14200) of Part 3 of Division 9 of the Welfare and Institutions Code, or Medicaid benefits under Subchapter 19 (commencing with Section 1396) of Chapter 7 of Title 42 of the United States Code.

(2) Each plan contract shall be interpreted not to provide an exception for the Medi-Cal or Medicaid benefits.

(3) A plan contract shall not provide an exemption for enrollment because of an applicant's entitlement to Medi-Cal benefits under Chapter 7 (commencing with Section 14000) or Chapter 8 (commencing with Section 14200) of Part 3 of Division 9 of the Welfare and Institutions Code, or Medicaid benefits under Subchapter 19 (commencing with Section 1396) of Chapter 7 of Title 42 of the United States Code.

(4) A plan contract may not provide that the benefits payable thereunder are subject to reduction if the individual insured has entitlement to the Medi-Cal or Medicaid benefits.

(b)(1) A plan contract that provides coverage, whether by specific benefit or by the effect of general wording, for sterilization operations or procedures shall not impose any disclaimer, restriction on, or limitation of, coverage relative to the covered individual's reason for sterilization.

(2) As used in this section, "sterilization operations or procedures" shall have the same meaning as that specified in Section 10120 of the Insurance Code.

(c) Every plan contract that provides coverage to the spouse or dependents of the subscriber or spouse shall grant immediate accident and sickness coverage, from and after the moment of birth, to each newborn infant of any subscriber or spouse covered and to each minor child placed for adoption from and after the date on which the adoptive child's birth parent or other appropriate legal authority signs a written document, including, but not limited to, a health facility minor release report, a medical authorization form, or a relinquishment form, granting the subscriber or spouse the right to control health care for the adoptive child or, absent this written document, on the date there exists evidence of the subscriber's or spouse's right to control the health care of the child placed for adoption. No plan may be entered into or amended if it contains any disclaimer, waiver, or other limitation of coverage relative to the coverage or insurability of newborn infants of, or children placed for adoption with, a subscriber or spouse covered as required by this subdivision.

(d)(1) Every plan contract that provides that coverage of a dependent child of a subscriber shall terminate upon attainment of the limiting age for dependent children specified in the plan, shall also provide that attainment of the limiting age shall not operate to terminate the coverage of the child while the child is and continues to meet both of the following criteria:

(A) Incapable of self-sustaining employment by reason of a physically or mentally disabling injury, illness, or condition.

(B) Chiefly dependent upon the subscriber for support and maintenance.

(2) The plan shall notify the subscriber that the dependent child's coverage will terminate upon attainment of the limiting age unless the subscriber submits proof of the criteria described in subparagraphs (A) and (B) of paragraph (1) to the plan within 60 days of the date of receipt of the

notification. The plan shall send this notification to the subscriber at least 90 days prior to the date the child attains the limiting age. Upon receipt of a request by the subscriber for continued coverage of the child and proof of the criteria described in subparagraphs (A) and (B) of paragraph (1), the plan shall determine whether the child meets that criteria before the child attains the limiting age. If the plan fails to make the determination by that date, it shall continue coverage of the child pending its determination.

(3) The plan may subsequently request information about a dependent child whose coverage is continued beyond the limiting age under this subdivision but not more frequently than annually after the two-year period following the child's attainment of the limiting age.

(4) If the subscriber changes carriers to another plan or to a health insurer, the new plan or insurer shall continue to provide coverage for the dependent child. The new plan or insurer may request information about the dependent child initially and not more frequently than annually thereafter to determine if the child continues to satisfy the criteria in subparagraphs (A) and (B) of paragraph (1). The subscriber shall submit the information requested by the new plan or insurer within 60 days of receiving the request.

(5)(A) Except as set forth in subparagraph (B), under no circumstances shall the limiting age be less than 26 years of age with respect to plan years beginning on or after September 23, 2010.

(B) For plan years beginning before January 1, 2014, a group health care service plan contract that qualifies as a grandfathered health plan under Section 1251 of the federal Patient Protection and Affordable Care Act (Public Law 111-148) and that makes available dependent coverage of children may exclude from coverage an adult child who has not attained 26 years of age only if the adult child is eligible to enroll in an eligible employer-sponsored health plan, as defined in Section 5000A(f)(2) of the Internal Revenue Code, other than a group health plan of a parent.

(C)(i) With respect to a child (I) whose coverage under a group or individual plan contract ended, or who was denied or not eligible for coverage under a group or individual plan contract, because under the terms of the contract the availability of dependent coverage of children ended before the attainment of 26 years of age, and (II) who becomes eligible for that coverage by reason of the application of this paragraph, the health care service plan shall give the child an opportunity to enroll that shall continue for at least 30 days. This opportunity and the notice described in clause (ii) shall be provided not later than the first day of the first plan year beginning on or after September 23, 2010, consistent with the federal Patient Protection and Affordable Care Act (Public Law 111-148), as amended by the federal Health Care and Education Reconciliation Act of 2010 (Public Law 111-152), and any additional federal guidance or regulations issued by the United States Secretary of Health and Human Services.

(ii) The health care service plan shall provide written notice stating that a dependent described in clause (i) who has not attained 26 years of age is eligible to enroll in the plan for coverage. This notice may be provided to the dependent's parent on behalf of the dependent. If the notice is included with other enrollment materials for a group plan, the notice shall be prominent.

(iii) In the case of an individual who enrolls under this subparagraph, coverage shall take effect no later than the first day of the first plan year beginning on or after September 23, 2010.

(iv) A dependent enrolling in a group health plan for coverage pursuant to this subparagraph shall be treated as a special enrollee as provided under the rules of Section 146.117(d) of Title 45 of the Code of Federal Regulations. The health care service plan shall offer the recipient of the notice all of the benefit packages available to similarly situated individuals who did not lose coverage by reason of cessation of dependent status. Any difference in benefits or cost-sharing requirements shall constitute a different benefit package. A dependent enrolling in a group health plan for coverage pursuant to this subparagraph shall not be required to pay more for coverage than similarly situated individuals who did not lose coverage by reason of cessation of dependent status.

(D) Nothing in this section shall require a health care service plan to make coverage available for a child of a child receiving dependent coverage. Nothing in this section shall be construed to modify the definition of "dependent" as used in the Revenue and Taxation Code with respect to the tax treatment of the cost of coverage.

(e) A plan contract that provides coverage, whether by specific benefit or by the effect of general wording, for both an employee and one or more covered persons dependent upon the employee and provides for an extension of the coverage for any period following a termination of employment of the employee shall also provide that this extension of coverage shall apply to dependents upon the same terms and conditions precedent as applied to the covered employee, for the same period of time, subject to payment of premiums, if any, as required by the terms of the policy and subject to any applicable collective bargaining agreement.

(f) A group contract shall not discriminate against handicapped persons or against groups containing handicapped persons. Nothing in this subdivision shall preclude reasonable provisions in a plan contract against liability for services or reimbursement of the handicap condition or conditions relating thereto, as may be allowed by rules of the director.

(g) Every group contract shall set forth the terms and conditions under which subscribers and enrollees may remain in the plan in the event the group ceases to exist, the group contract is terminated, or an individual subscriber leaves the group, or the enrollees' eligibility status changes.

(h)(1) A health care service plan or specialized health care service plan may provide for coverage of, or for payment for, professional mental health services, or vision care services, or for the exclusion of these services. If the terms and conditions include coverage for services provided in a general acute care hospital or an acute psychiatric hospital as defined in Section 1250 and do not restrict or modify the choice of providers, the coverage shall extend to care provided by a psychiatric health facility as defined in Section 1250.2 operating pursuant to licensure by the State Department of Health Care Services. A health care service plan that offers outpatient mental health services but does not cover these services in all of its group contracts shall communicate to prospective group contractholders as to the availability of outpatient coverage for the treatment of mental or nervous disorders.

(2) No plan shall prohibit the member from selecting any psychologist who is licensed pursuant to the Psychology Licensing Law (Chapter 6.6 (commencing with Section 2900) of Division 2 of the Business and Professions Code), any optometrist who is the holder of a certificate issued pursuant to Chapter 7 (commencing with Section 3000) of Division 2 of the Business and Professions Code or, upon referral by a physician and surgeon licensed pursuant to the Medical Practice Act (Chapter 5 (commencing with Section 2000) of Division 2 of the Business and Professions Code), (A) any marriage and family therapist who is the holder of a license under Section 4980.50 of the Business and Professions Code, (B) any licensed clinical social worker who is the holder of a license under Section 4996 of the Business and Professions Code, (C) any registered nurse licensed pursuant to Chapter 6 (commencing with Section 2700) of Division 2 of the Business and Professions Code, who possesses a master's degree in psychiatric-mental health nursing and is listed as a psychiatric-mental health nurse by the Board of Registered Nursing, (D) any advanced practice registered nurse certified as a clinical nurse specialist pursuant to Article 9 (commencing with Section 2838) of Chapter 6 of Division 2 of the Business and Professions Code who participates in expert clinical practice in the specialty of psychiatric-mental health nursing, to perform the particular services covered under the terms of the plan, and the certificate holder is expressly authorized by law to perform these services, or (E) any professional clinical counselor who is the holder of a license under Chapter 16 (commencing with Section 4999.10) of Division 2 of the Business and Professions Code.

(3) Nothing in this section shall be construed to allow any certificate holder or licensee enumerated in this section to perform professional mental health services beyond his or her field or fields of competence as established by his or her education, training, and experience.

(4) For the purposes of this section:

(A) "Marriage and family therapist" means a licensed marriage and family therapist who has received specific instruction in assessment, diagnosis, prognosis, and counseling, and psychotherapeutic treatment of premarital, marriage, family, and child relationship dysfunctions, which is equivalent to the instruction required for licensure on January 1, 1981.

(B) "Professional clinical counselor" means a licensed professional clinical counselor who has received specific instruction in assessment, diagnosis, prognosis, counseling, and psychotherapeutic treatment of mental and emotional disorders, which is equivalent to the instruction required for licensure on January 1, 2012.

(5) Nothing in this section shall be construed to allow a member to select and obtain mental health or psychological or vision care services from a certificate holder or licenseholder who is not directly affiliated with or under contract to the health care service plan or specialized health care service plan to which the member belongs. All health care service plans and individual practice associations that offer mental health benefits shall make reasonable efforts to make available to their members the services of licensed psychologists. However, a failure of a plan or association to comply with the requirements of the preceding sentence shall not constitute a misdemeanor.

(6) As used in this subdivision, "individual practice association" means an entity as defined in subsection (5) of Section 1307 of the federal Public Health Service Act (42 U.S.C. Sec. 300e-1(5)).

(7) Health care service plan coverage for professional mental health services may include community residential treatment services that are alternatives to inpatient care and that are directly affiliated with the plan or to which enrollees are referred by providers affiliated with the plan.

(i) If the plan utilizes arbitration to settle disputes, the plan contracts shall set forth the type of disputes subject to arbitration, the process to be utilized, and how it is to be initiated.

(j) A plan contract that provides benefits that accrue after a certain time of confinement in a health care facility shall specify what constitutes a day of confinement or the number of consecutive hours of confinement that are requisite to the commencement of benefits.

(k) If a plan provides coverage for a dependent child who is over 26 years of age and enrolled as a full-time student at a secondary or postsecondary educational institution, the following shall apply:

(1) Any break in the school calendar shall not disqualify the dependent child from coverage.

(2) If the dependent child takes a medical leave of absence, and the nature of the dependent child's injury, illness, or condition would render the dependent child incapable of self-sustaining employment, the provisions of subdivision (d) shall apply if the dependent child is chiefly dependent on the subscriber for support and maintenance.

(3)(A) If the dependent child takes a medical leave of absence from school, but the nature of the dependent child's injury, illness, or condition does not meet the requirements of paragraph (2), the dependent child's coverage shall not terminate for a period not to exceed 12 months or until the date on which the coverage is scheduled to terminate pursuant to the terms and conditions of the plan, whichever comes first. The period of coverage under this paragraph shall commence on the first day of the medical leave of absence from the school or on the date the physician and surgeon determines the illness prevented the dependent child from attending school, whichever comes first. Any break in the school calendar shall not disqualify the dependent child from coverage under this paragraph.

(B) Documentation or certification of the medical necessity for a leave of absence from school shall be submitted to the plan at least 30 days prior to the medical leave of absence from the school, if the medical reason for the absence and the absence are foreseeable, or 30 days after the start date of the medical leave of absence from school and shall be considered prima facie evidence of entitlement to coverage under this paragraph.

(4) This subdivision shall not apply to a specialized health care service plan or to a Medicare supplement plan.

HISTORY:

Added Stats 1975 ch 941 § 2, operative July 1, 1976. Amended Stats 1976 ch 1185 § 94; Stats 1978 ch 648 § 1; Stats 1980 ch 11 § 1, ch 973 § 1, ch 1235 § 2, ch 1313 § 14.5; Stats 1981 ch 267 § 1, effective August 25, 1981; Stats 1982 ch 121 § 1; Stats 1983 ch 928 § 9, ch 1259 § 1.5; Stats 1984 ch 1366 § 1, ch 1367 § 1.5; Stats 1987 ch 265 § 1; Stats 1989 ch 1104 § 39; Stats 1990 ch 57 § 8 (AB 365), effective April 20, 1990; Stats 1993 ch 987 § 2 (SB 1221); Stats 1994 ch 147 § 7 (AB 2377), effective July 9, 1994; Stats 1999 ch 525 § 109 (AB 78), operative July 1, 2000; Stats 2001 ch 420 § 3 (AB 1253), effective

October 2, 2001; Stats 2002 ch 1013 § 84 (SB 2026); Stats 2007 ch 617 § 3 (AB 910), effective January 1, 2008; Stats 2008 ch 390 § 1 (SB 1168), effective January 1, 2009; Stats 2010 ch 660 § 1 (SB 1088), effective January 1, 2011; Stats 2011 ch 381 § 30 (SB 146), effective January 1, 2012; Stats 2012 ch 34 § 14 (SB 1009), effective June 27, 2012; Stats 2013 ch 23 § 14 (AB 82), effective June 27, 2013.

§ 1373.8. Contractees' right to select licensed professionals in California to perform contract services

A health care service plan contract where the plan is licensed to do business in this state and the plan provides coverage that includes California residents, but that may be written or issued for delivery outside of California, and where benefits are provided within the scope of practice of a licensed clinical social worker, a registered nurse licensed pursuant to Chapter 6 (commencing with Section 2700) of Division 2 of the Business and Professions Code who possesses a master's degree in psychiatric-mental health nursing and is listed as a psychiatric-mental health nurse by the Board of Registered Nursing, an advanced practice registered nurse who is certified as a clinical nurse specialist pursuant to Article 9 (commencing with Section 2838) of Chapter 6 of Division 2 of the Business and Professions Code who participates in expert clinical practice in the specialty of psychiatric-mental health nursing, a marriage and family therapist who is the holder of a license under Section 4980.50 of the Business and Professions Code, or a professional clinical counselor who is the holder of a license under Chapter 16 (commencing with Section 4999.10) of Division 2 of the Business and Professions Code shall not be deemed to prohibit persons covered under the contract from selecting those licensed persons in California to perform the services in California that are within the terms of the contract even though the licensees are not licensed in the state where the contract is written or issued for delivery.

It is the intent of the Legislature in amending this section in the 1984 portion of the 1983-84 Legislative Session that persons covered by the contract and those providers of health care specified in this section who are licensed in California should be entitled to the benefits provided by the plan for services of those providers rendered to those persons.

HISTORY:

Added Stats 1983 ch 673 § 1. Amended Stats 1984 ch 144 § 152 (ch 540 prevails), ch 540 § 2; Stats 2001 ch 420 § 4 (AB 1253), effective October 2, 2001; Stats 2002 ch 1013 § 85 (SB 2026); Stats 2011 ch 381 § 31 (SB 146), effective January 1, 2012.

§ 1374.55. Coverage for treatment of infertility; "Subsidiary"

(a) On and after January 1, 1990, every health care service plan contract that is issued, amended, or renewed that covers hospital, medical, or surgical expenses on a group basis, where the plan is not a health maintenance organization as defined in Section 1373.10, shall offer coverage for the treatment of infertility, except in vitro fertilization, under those terms and conditions as may be agreed upon between the group subscriber and the plan. Every plan shall communicate the availability of that coverage to all group contractholders and to all prospective group contractholders with whom they are negotiating.

(b) For purposes of this section, "infertility" means either (1) the presence of a demonstrated condition recognized by a licensed physician and surgeon as a cause of infertility, or (2) the inability to conceive a pregnancy or to carry a pregnancy to a live birth after a year or more of regular sexual relations without contraception. "Treatment for infertility" means procedures consistent with established medical practices in the treatment of infertility by licensed physicians and surgeons including, but not limited to, diagnosis, diagnostic tests, medication, surgery, and gamete intrafallopian transfer. "In vitro fertilization" means the laboratory medical procedures involving the actual in vitro fertilization process.

(c) On and after January 1, 1990, every health care service plan that is a health maintenance organization, as defined in Section 1373.10, and that issues, renews, or amends a health care service plan contract that provides group coverage for hospital, medical, or surgical expenses shall offer the coverage specified in subdivision (a), according to the terms and conditions that may be agreed upon between the group subscriber and the plan to group contractholders with at least 20 employees to whom the plan is offered. The plan shall communicate the availability of the coverage to those group contractholders and prospective group contractholders with whom the plan is negotiating.

(d) This section shall not be construed to deny or restrict in any way any existing right or benefit to coverage and treatment of infertility under an existing law, plan, or policy.

(e) This section shall not be construed to require any employer that is a religious organization to offer coverage for forms of treatment of infertility in a manner inconsistent with the religious organization's religious and ethical principles.

(f)(1) This section shall not be construed to require any plan, which is a subsidiary of an entity whose owner or corporate member is a religious organization, to offer coverage for treatment of infertility in a manner inconsistent with that religious organization's religious and ethical principles.

(2) For purposes of this subdivision, "subsidiary" of a specified corporation means a corporation more than 45 percent of the voting power of which is owned directly, or indirectly through one or more subsidiaries, by the specified corporation.

(g) Consistent with Section 1365.5, coverage for the treatment of infertility shall be offered and, if purchased, provided without discrimination on the basis of age, ancestry, color, disability, domestic partner status, gender, gender expression, gender identity, genetic information, marital status, national origin, race, religion, sex, or sexual orientation. Nothing in this subdivision shall be construed to interfere with the clinical judgment of a physician and surgeon.

HISTORY:

Added Stats 1989 ch 734 § 2. Amended Stats 1990 ch 830 § 1 (AB 2474), effective September 12, 1990; Stats 2013 ch 644 § 1 (AB 460), effective January 1, 2014.

Misc.

§ 1374.57. Exclusion of dependent child

(a) No group health care service plan that provides hospital, medical, or surgical expense benefits for employees or subscribers and their dependents shall exclude a dependent child from eligibility or benefits solely because the dependent child does not reside with the employee or subscriber.

(b) A health care service plan that provides hospital, medical, or surgical expense benefits for employees or subscribers and their dependents shall enroll, upon application by the employer or group administrator, a dependent child of the noncustodial parent when the parent is the employee or subscriber, at any time the noncustodial or custodial parent makes an application for enrollment to the employer or group administrator when a court order for medical support exists. Except as provided in Section 1374.3, the application to the employer or group administrator shall be made within 90 days of the issuance of the court order. In the case of children who are eligible for medicaid, the State Department of Health Services or the district attorney in whose jurisdiction the child resides may make that application.

(c) This section shall not be construed to require that a health care service plan enroll a dependent who resides outside the plan's geographic service area, except as provided in Section 1374.3.

(d) Notwithstanding any other provision of this section, all health care service plans shall comply with the standards set forth in Section 1374.3.

HISTORY:

Added Stats 1991 ch 1152 § 1 (AB 2118). Amended Stats 1994 ch 147 § 9 (AB 2377), effective July 9, 1994.

DIVISION 10

UNIFORM CONTROLLED SUBSTANCES ACT

Chapter
1. General Provisions and Definitions.

HISTORY: Added Stats 1972 ch 1407 § 3. Former Division 10, entitled "Narcotics," consisting of H & S C §§ 11000–11853, was enacted Stats 1939 ch 60 and repealed Stats 1972 ch 1407 § 2.

CHAPTER 1

GENERAL PROVISIONS AND DEFINITIONS

Section
11027. "Prescription"; Definitions relating to electronic transmission.

HISTORY: Added Stats 1972 ch 1407 § 3.

Misc.

§ 11027. "Prescription"; Definitions relating to electronic transmission

(a) "Prescription" means an oral order or electronic transmission prescription for a controlled substance given individually for the person(s) for whom prescribed, directly from the prescriber to the furnisher or indirectly by means of a written order of the prescriber.

(b) "Electronic transmission prescription" includes both image and data prescriptions. "Electronic image transmission prescription" is any prescription order for which a facsimile of the order is received by a pharmacy from a licensed prescriber. "Electronic data transmission prescription" is any prescription order, other than an electronic image transmission prescription, which is electronically transmitted from a licensed prescriber to a pharmacy.

HISTORY:
Added Stats 1972 ch 1407 § 3. Amended Stats 1976 ch 896 § 2; Stats 1979 ch 634 § 3; Stats 1994 ch 26 § 241 (AB 1807), effective March 30, 1994.

DIVISION 106

PERSONAL HEALTH CARE (INCLUDING MATERNAL, CHILD, AND ADOLESCENT)

Part
2. Maternal, Child, and Adolescent Health.

HISTORY: Added Stats 1995 ch 415 § 8.

PART 2

MATERNAL, CHILD, AND ADOLESCENT HEALTH

Chapter
2. Maternal Health.

HISTORY: Added Stats 1995 ch 415 § 8.

CHAPTER 2

MATERNAL HEALTH

Article
2. Abortion.

HISTORY: Added Stats 1995 ch 415 § 8.

ARTICLE 2

ABORTION

Section
123420. Misdemeanors; Employers requiring participation in abortion; Discrimination against employee for refusal.

HISTORY: Added Stats 1995 ch 415 § 8.

Misc.

§ 123420. Misdemeanors; Employers requiring participation in abortion; Discrimination against employee for refusal

(a) No employer or other person shall require a physician, a registered nurse, a licensed vocational nurse, or any other person employed or with staff privileges at a hospital, facility, or clinic to directly participate in the induction or performance of an abortion, if the employee or other person has filed a written statement with the employer or the hospital, facility, or clinic indicating a moral, ethical, or religious basis for refusal to participate in the abortion.

No such employee or person with staff privileges in a hospital, facility, or clinic shall be subject to any penalty or discipline by reason of his or her refusal to participate in an abortion. No such employee of a hospital, facility, or clinic that does not permit the performance of abortions, or person with staff privileges therein, shall be subject to any penalty or discipline on account of the person's participation in the performance of an abortion in other than the hospital, facility, or clinic.

No employer shall refuse to employ any person because of the person's refusal for moral, ethical, or religious reasons to participate in an abortion, unless the person would be assigned in the normal course of business of any hospital, facility, or clinic to work in those parts of the hospital, facility, or clinic where abortion patients are cared for. No provision of this article prohibits any hospital, facility, or clinic that permits the performance of abortions from inquiring whether an employee or prospective employee would advance a moral, ethical, or religious basis for refusal to participate in an abortion before hiring or assigning that person to that part of a hospital, facility, or clinic where abortion patients are cared for.

The refusal of a physician, nurse, or any other person to participate or aid in the induction or performance of an abortion pursuant to this subdivision shall not form the basis of any claim for damages.

(b) No medical school or other facility for the education or training of physicians, nurses, or other medical personnel shall refuse admission to a person or penalize the person in any way because of the person's unwillingness to participate in the performance of an abortion for moral, ethical, or religious reasons. No hospital, facility, or clinic shall refuse staff privileges to a physician because of the physician's refusal to participate in the performance of abortion for moral, ethical, or religious reasons.

(c) Nothing in this article shall require a nonprofit hospital or other facility or clinic that is organized or operated by a religious corporation or other religious organization and licensed pursuant to Chapter 1 (commencing with Section 1200) or Chapter 2 (commencing with Section 1250) of Division 2, or any administrative officer, employee, agent, or member of the governing board thereof, to perform or to permit the performance of an abortion in the facility or clinic or to provide abortion services. No such nonprofit facility or clinic organized or operated by a religious corporation or other religious organization, nor its administrative officers, employees, agents, or members of its governing board shall be liable, individually or collectively, for failure or refusal to participate in any such act. The failure or refusal of any such corporation, unincorporated association or individual person to perform or to permit the performance of such medical procedures shall not be the basis for any disciplinary or other recriminatory action against such corporations, unincorporated associations, or individuals. Any such facility or clinic that does not permit the performance of abortions on its premises shall post notice of that proscription in an area of the facility or clinic that is open to patients and prospective admittees.

(d) This section shall not apply to medical emergency situations and spontaneous abortions.

Any violation of this section is a misdemeanor.

HISTORY:
Added Stats 1995 ch 415 § 8 (SB 1360).

DIVISION 107

HEALTH CARE ACCESS AND INFORMATION

Part
3. Health Professions Development.

HISTORY: Added Stats 1995 ch 415 § 9. The heading of Division 107, which formerly read "Statewide Health Planning and Development," amended to read as above by Stats 2021 ch 143 § 28 (AB 133), effective July 27, 2021.

PART 3

HEALTH PROFESSIONS DEVELOPMENT

Chapter
1. Health Professions Planning.
4. Health Care Workforce Training Programs.
5. Health Professions Education Programs.

HISTORY: Added Stats 1995 ch 415 § 9.

CHAPTER 1

HEALTH PROFESSIONS PLANNING

Article
1. Health Personnel Planning [Repealed].

HISTORY: Added Stats 1995 ch 415 § 9.

ARTICLE 1

HEALTH PERSONNEL PLANNING [REPEALED]

Section
127760. Legislative findings and declarations [Repealed].
127765. Collection of data from licentiates [Repealed].
127770. Contents of data [Repealed].
127775. Confidentiality of data in transmission [Repealed].
127780. Confidentiality of information received [Repealed].
127785. Collection of data on health care trainees [Repealed].
127790. Contents of data on health care trainees [Repealed].
127795. Implementation of data collection process [Repealed].

Section
127800. Provision of information as condition of relicensure [Repealed].

HISTORY: Added Stats 1995 ch 415 § 9. Repealed Stats 2021 ch 143 § 115 (AB 133), effective July 27, 2021.

§ 127760. Legislative findings and declarations [Repealed]

HISTORY:
Added Stats 1995 ch 415 § 9 (SB 1360). Amended Stats 1996 ch 1023 § 357 (SB 1497), effective September 19, 1996; Stats 2004 ch 183 § 233 (AB 3082). Repealed Stats 2021 ch 143 § 115 (AB 133), effective July 27, 2021.

§ 127765. Collection of data from licentiates [Repealed]

HISTORY:
Added Stats 1995 ch 415 § 9 (SB 1360). Repealed Stats 2021 ch 143 § 115 (AB 133), effective July 27, 2021.

§ 127770. Contents of data [Repealed]

HISTORY:
Added Stats 1995 ch 415 § 9 (SB 1360). Repealed Stats 2021 ch 143 § 115 (AB 133), effective July 27, 2021.

§ 127775. Confidentiality of data in transmission [Repealed]

HISTORY:
Added Stats 1995 ch 415 § 9 (SB 1360). Repealed Stats 2021 ch 143 § 115 (AB 133), effective July 27, 2021.

§ 127780. Confidentiality of information received [Repealed]

HISTORY:
Added Stats 1995 ch 415 § 9 (SB 1360). Amended Stats 1996 ch 1023 § 358 (SB 1497), effective September 29, 1996. Repealed Stats 2021 ch 143 § 115 (AB 133), effective July 27, 2021.

§ 127785. Collection of data on health care trainees [Repealed]

HISTORY:
Added Stats 1995 ch 415 § 9 (SB 1360). Repealed Stats 2021 ch 143 § 115 (AB 133), effective July 27, 2021.

§ 127790. Contents of data on health care trainees [Repealed]

HISTORY:
Added Stats 1995 ch 415 § 9 (SB 1360). Repealed Stats 2021 ch 143 § 115 (AB 133), effective July 27, 2021.

§ 127795. Implementation of data collection process [Repealed]

HISTORY:
Added Stats 1995 ch 415 § 9 (SB 1360). Repealed Stats 2021 ch 143 § 115 (AB 133), effective July 27, 2021.

§ 127800. Provision of information as condition of relicensure [Repealed]

HISTORY:
Added Stats 1995 ch 415 § 9 (SB 1360). Repealed Stats 2021 ch 143 § 115 (AB 133), effective July 27, 2021.

CHAPTER 4

HEALTH CARE WORKFORCE TRAINING PROGRAMS

Article
4. Midwifery Workforce Training Act.

HISTORY: Added Stats 1996 ch 1023 § 360 (SB 1497), effective September 29, 1996. The heading of Chapter 4, which formerly read "Family Physician Training Programs," amended to read as above by Stats 2006 ch 259 § 5 (SB 1850), effective January 1, 2007. Former Chapter 4, entitled "Family Practice Physician Programs (Reserved)," consisting of Article 1, entitled "Family Physician Training Program (Reserved)," and Article 2, entitled "Additional Duties of the Health Manpower Policy Commission (HMPC) (Reserved)," was added Stats 1995 ch 415 § 9, effective January 1, 1996, and repealed Stats 2015 ch 303 § 360, effective January 1, 2016.

ARTICLE 4

MIDWIFERY WORKFORCE TRAINING ACT

Section
128297. Definitions.
128298. Program to contract with certified nurse-midwives and licensed midwives training programs.

HISTORY: Added Stats 2021 ch 449 § 5 (SB 65), effective January 1, 2022, operative January 1, 2022.

§ 128297. Definitions

For purposes of this article, the following definitions apply:

(a) "Certified nurse-midwife" means an advanced practice nurse with training in midwifery, as specified in, and a certificate issued pursuant to, Article 2.5 (commencing with Section 2746) of Chapter 6 of Division 2 of the Business and Professions Code.

(b) "Licensed midwife" means an individual who has been issued a license to practice midwifery pursuant to Article 24 (commencing with Section 2505) of Chapter 5 of Division 2 of the Business and Professions Code.

(c) "Office" means the Office of Statewide Health Planning and Development (OSHPD).

(d) "Programs that train certified nurse-midwives" means a nurse-midwifery education program that is operated by a California school of nursing and approved by the Accreditation Commission for Midwifery Education, or that is authorized by the Regents of the University of California or by the

Trustees of the California State University, or that is approved by the Board of Registered Nursing.

(e) "Programs that train licensed midwives" means a midwifery education program operated by a California school of midwifery, and accredited by the Midwifery Education Accreditation Council (MEAC), or approved by the Bureau for Private and Postsecondary Education, or approved by the state licensing and regulatory board for licensed midwives.

HISTORY:

Added Stats 2021 ch 449 § 5 (SB 65), effective January 1, 2022, operative January 1, 2022.

§ 128298. Program to contract with certified nurse-midwives and licensed midwives training programs

(a) It is the intent of the Legislature to provide for a program designed primarily to increase the number of students receiving quality education and training as a certified nurse-midwife or a licensed midwife in accordance with the global standards for midwifery education and the international definition of "midwife" as established by the International Confederation of Midwives, in order to maximize the delivery of reproductive services to specific areas of California where there is a recognized unmet priority need.

(b)(1) The office shall establish a program to contract with programs that train certified nurse-midwives and programs that train licensed midwives in accordance with the global standards for midwifery education and the international definition of "midwife" as established by the International Confederation of Midwives in order to increase the number of students receiving quality education and training as a certified nurse-midwife or as a licensed midwife.

(2) The office shall only contract with programs that train certified nurse-midwives and programs that train licensed midwives that, at minimum, include, or that intend to create, a component of training designed for medically underserved multicultural communities, lower socioeconomic neighborhoods, or rural communities, and that are organized to prepare program graduates for service in those neighborhoods and communities, or that seek to recruit and retain racially and ethnically diverse students, underrepresented groups, or people from underserved or historically marginalized communities.

(3) The office may adopt standards and regulations necessary to carry out this article. In adopting eligibility standards for programs that train certified nurse-midwives and that train licensed midwives in accordance with the standards set forth in subdivisions (a) and (b), the office may accept those educational standards and competencies established by the respective state licensing and regulatory bodies for certified nurse-midwives and for licensed midwives. The office shall take care not to implement education or competency standards beyond what is required for the training programs by their respective state licensing and regulatory bodies that could inadvertently create an unnecessary barrier for training programs to obtain funding for the training of midwives in California.

(4) The office shall develop alternative strategies to provide long-term stability for, or expansion of, this act, such as through funding provided by

private foundations and administered by the office for the purposes of carrying out this article.

(5) Nothing in this article prevents the office from developing a protocol to contract with potential programs that train nurse-midwives or that train licensed midwives, in order to support the initial startup of new training programs, as long as the eligibility requirements of this article are met or can be met through the award of funds.

(6) The office may pay contracted programs that train certified nurse-midwives and programs that train licensed midwives in an amount calculated based on a single per-student capitation formula, or through another method, in order to cover the costs of innovative special projects or programs.

(7) Funds appropriated to the office for purposes of this article and awarded by the office to eligible programs that train certified nurse-midwives or programs that train licensed midwives may be used by the training program to develop new initiatives, projects, or curriculum, or to expand existing initiatives, projects, or curriculum. Awarded funds may also be used for general support and sustainability of the overall training program, or to sustain specific components of the training program, including, but not limited to, tuition assistance for students, or support for preceptor recruitment, or to sustain preceptor training sites for students.

(c) This section shall be implemented only upon an appropriation by the Legislature for these purposes in the annual Budget Act or another act.

HISTORY:
Added Stats 2021 ch 449 § 5 (SB 65), effective January 1, 2022, operative January 1, 2022.

CHAPTER 5
HEALTH PROFESSIONS EDUCATION PROGRAMS

Article
1. Health Professions Education Programs.
2. California Registered Nurse Education Program.
3. Geriatric Nurse Practitioner and Clinical Nurse Specialist Scholarship Program [Repealed].

HISTORY: Added Stats 1995 ch 415 § 9. The heading of former Chapter 5 which read "Minority Health Professions Education Foundation Programs," amended to read as above by Stats 1999 ch 149 § 4 (SB 308), effective July 22, 1999; The heading of Chapter 5, which formerly read "Health Professions Education Foundation Programs," amended to read as above by Stats 2021 ch 143 § 159 (AB 133), effective July 27, 2021.

ARTICLE 1
HEALTH PROFESSIONS EDUCATION PROGRAMS

Section
128330. Definitions.
128335. Health Professions Education Foundation [Repealed].
128337. Dissolution of Health Professions Education Foundation.
128338. Post-dissolution reference to Health Professions Education Foundation as reference to department.

Section
128340. Board members [Repealed].
128345. Duties and powers of department.
128350. Duties of Department of Health Care Access and Information.
128355. Health Professions Education Fund.
128360. Exemption from certain regulations and rulemaking requirements; Notice to public of Health Professions Education Programs information; Repeal of prior regulations.
128365. Financial assistance applications and other private documentation exempt from disclosure provisions.
128370. Exemption of donation-related documents from public disclosure.
128371. Legislative findings and declarations; Denial of admission to certain programs on the basis on immigration or citizenship status.

HISTORY: Added Stats 1996 ch 1023 § 362, effective September 29, 1996. The heading of former Article 1 which formerly read "Minority Health Professions Education Foundation," amended to read as above by Stats 1999 ch 149 § 5, effective July 22, 1999. Former Article 1, entitled "Minority Health Professions Education Foundation" (Reserved), was repealed Stats 1996 ch 1023 § 356, effective September 29, 1996. The heading of Article 1, which formerly read "Health Professions Education Foundation," amended to read as above by Stats 2021 ch 143 § 160 (AB 133), effective July 27, 2021.

§ 128330. Definitions

As used in this article:

(a) "Board" means the Board of Trustees of the Health Professions Education Foundation.

(b) "Council" means the California Health Workforce Education and Training Council.

(c) "Director" means the Director of the of Department of Health Care Access and Information.

(d) "Foundation" means the Health Professions Education Foundation.

(e) "Health professions" or "health professionals" means physicians and surgeons licensed pursuant to Chapter 5 (commencing with Section 2000) of Division 2 of the Business and Professions Code or pursuant to the Osteopathic Act, dentists, registered nurses, and other health professionals determined by the department to be needed in medically underserved areas.

(f) "Department" means the Department of Health Care Access and Information.

(g) "Underrepresented groups" means populations that are underrepresented in medicine, dentistry, nursing, or other health professions as determined by the department. The department, upon a finding that the action is necessary to meet the health care needs of medically underserved areas, may add a group comprising the economically disadvantaged to those groups authorized to receive assistance under this article. The department shall recognize that it is especially important that medical and dental care be provided in a way that is sensitive to the sociocultural variables that affect a person's health.

HISTORY:

Added Stats 1996 ch 1023 § 362 (SB 1497), effective September 29, 1996. Amended Stats 1999 ch 149 § 6 (SB 308), effective July 22, 1999; Stats 2003 ch 582 § 18 (AB 1627); Stats 2009 ch 600 § 4 (SB 606), effective January 1, 2010; Stats 2021 ch 143 § 161 (AB 133), effective July 27, 2021.

§ 128335. Health Professions Education Foundation [Repealed]

HISTORY:

Added Stats 2005 ch 317 § 3.5 (AB 920), effective January 1, 2006. Amended Stats 2010 ch 451 §

4 (AB 1767), effective January 1, 2011, operative January 1, 2016; Stats 2017 ch 775 § 113 (SB 798), effective January 1, 2018; Stats 2021 ch 143 § 162 (AB 133), effective July 27, 2021, repealed January 1, 2022.

§ 128337. Dissolution of Health Professions Education Foundation

Notwithstanding any other law, on or before October 1, 2021, the nonprofit public benefit corporation known as the Health Professions Education Foundation shall be dissolved. All assets, including records, and any liabilities shall be transferred to the department.

HISTORY:

Added Stats 2021 ch 143 § 163 (AB 133), effective July 27, 2021.

§ 128338. Post-dissolution reference to Health Professions Education Foundation as reference to department

Effective with the dissolution of the Health Professions Education Foundation, any reference to the Health Professions Education Foundation, or the Foundation, in this chapter shall be deemed a reference to the department.

HISTORY:

Added Stats 2021 ch 143 § 164 (AB 133), effective July 27, 2021.

§ 128340. Board members [Repealed]

HISTORY:

Added Stats 1996 ch 1023 § 362 (SB 1497), effective September 29, 1996. Repealed Stats 2021 ch 143 § 165 (AB 133), effective July 27, 2021.

§ 128345. Duties and powers of department

The department may do any of the following:

(a) Solicit and receive funds from business, industry, foundations, and other private or public sources for the purpose of providing financial assistance in the form of scholarships or loans to students from underrepresented groups. These funds shall be expended by the department after transfer to the Health Professions Education Fund, created pursuant to Section 128355.

(b) Disburse private sector moneys deposited in the Health Professions Education Fund to students from underrepresented groups enrolled in or graduated from schools of medicine, dentistry, nursing, or other health professions in the form of loans or scholarships.

(c) Encourage private sector institutions, including hospitals, community clinics, and other health agencies to identify and provide educational experiences to students from underrepresented groups who are potential applicants to schools of medicine, dentistry, nursing, or other health professions.

(d) Implement the Steven M. Thompson Physician Corps Loan Repayment Program and the Volunteer Physician Program, as provided under Article 5 (commencing with Section 128550).

HISTORY:

Added Stats 1996 ch 1023 § 362 (SB 1497), effective September 29, 1996. Amended Stats 1999 ch 149 § 8 (SB 308), effective July 22, 1999; Stats 2005 ch 317 § 4 (AB 920), effective January 1, 2006; Stats 2021 ch 143 § 166 (AB 133), effective July 27, 2021.

§ 128350. Duties of Department of Health Care Access and Information

The department shall do all of the following:

(a) Provide technical and staff support to the programs in meeting all of its responsibilities.

(b) Provide financial management for the Health Professions Education Fund.

(c) Enter into contractual agreements with students from underrepresented groups for the disbursement of scholarships or loans in return for the commitment of these students to practice their profession in an area in California designated as deficient in primary care services.

(d) Disseminate information regarding the areas in the state that are deficient in primary care services to potential applicants for the scholarships or loans.

(e) Monitor the practice locations of the recipients of the scholarships or loans.

(f) Recover funds, in accordance with the terms of the contractual agreements, from recipients of scholarships or loans who fail to begin or complete their obligated service. Funds so recovered shall be redeposited in the Health Professions Education Fund.

(g) Contract with the institutions that train family practice residents, in order to increase the participation of students from underrepresented groups in entering the specialty of family practice. The director may seek the recommendations of the council as to what programs best demonstrate the ability to meet this objective.

(h) Contract with training institutions that are involved in osteopathic postgraduate training in general or family practice medicine, in order to increase the participation of students from underrepresented groups participating in the practice of osteopathic medicine. The director may seek the recommendations of the council as to what programs have demonstrated the ability to meet this objective.

(i) Enter into contractual agreements with graduated health professionals to repay some or all of the debts they incurred in health professional schools in return for practicing their professions in an area in California designated as deficient in primary care services.

(j) Contract with institutions that award baccalaureate of science degrees in nursing in order to increase the participation of students from underrepresented groups in the nursing profession. The director may seek the recommendations of the council as to what programs have demonstrated the ability to meet this objective.

HISTORY:

Added Stats 1996 ch 1023 § 362 (SB 1497), effective September 29, 1996. Amended Stats 1999 ch 149 § 9 (SB 308), effective July 22, 1999; Stats 2021 ch 143 § 167 (AB 133), effective July 27, 2021.

§ 128355. Health Professions Education Fund

There is hereby created within the department a Health Professions Education Fund. The primary purpose of this fund is to provide scholarships and loans to students from underrepresented groups who are accepted to or enrolled in schools of medicine, dentistry, nursing, or other health professions.

The fund shall also be used to pay for the cost of administering the program and for any other purpose authorized by this article. The level of expenditure by the department for the administrative support of the program created pursuant to this article shall be subject to review and approval annually through the State Budget process. The department may receive private donations to be deposited into this fund. All money in the fund is continuously appropriated to the department for the purposes of this article. The department shall manage this fund prudently in accordance with other provisions of law.

HISTORY:
Added Stats 1996 ch 1023 § 362 (SB 1497), effective September 29, 1996. Amended Stats 1999 ch 149 § 10 (SB 308), effective July 22, 1999; Stats 2021 ch 143 § 168 (AB 133), effective July 27, 2021.

§ 128360. Exemption from certain regulations and rulemaking requirements; Notice to public of Health Professions Education Programs information; Repeal of prior regulations

(a) In administering this chapter, the department shall be exempt from the requirements of Chapter 3.5 (commencing with Section 11340) of Part 1 of Division 3 of Title 2 of the Government Code. The department shall provide opportunities for public participation as it administers the Health Professions Education Programs. Information about each type of scholarship or loan repayment opportunity shall be publicly available at least 60 days prior to any application deadline. This information shall include eligibility criteria and the application process, materials, and deadlines, and shall be posted on the department's internet website and be available directly from the department. All the information shall remain posted and available during the entire application period for a funding cycle.

(b) Regulations that have been adopted to administer this chapter prior to the effective date of this section are repealed as of the effective date of this section.

HISTORY:
Added Stats 2021 ch 143 § 170 (AB 133), effective July 27, 2021.

§ 128365. Financial assistance applications and other private documentation exempt from disclosure provisions

Notwithstanding any other provision, applications for financial assistance under this article, or other documents that the department reasonably determines should not be discussed in public due to privacy considerations shall be exempt from the disclosure provisions of the Public Records Act (Division 10 (commencing with Section 7920.000) of Title 1 of the Government Code).

HISTORY:
Added Stats 1996 ch 1023 § 362 (SB 1497), effective September 29, 1996. Amended Stats 2021 ch 143 § 171 (AB 133), effective July 27, 2021; Stats 2022 ch 28 § 107 (SB 1380), effective January 1, 2023.

§ 128370. Exemption of donation-related documents from public disclosure

Notwithstanding any other law, the department may exempt from public disclosure any document in the possession of the department that pertains to a donation made pursuant to this article if the donor has requested anonymity.

HISTORY:

Added Stats 1996 ch 1023 § 362 (SB 1497), effective September 29, 1996. Amended Stats 2021 ch 143 § 172 (AB 133), effective July 27, 2021.

§ 128371. Legislative findings and declarations; Denial of admission to certain programs on the basis on immigration or citizenship status

(a) The Legislature finds and declares that it is in the best interest of the State of California to provide persons who are not lawfully present in the United States with the state benefits provided by those programs listed in subdivision (d), and therefore, enacts this section pursuant to Section 1621(d) of Title 8 of the United States Code.

(b) A program listed in subdivision (d) shall not deny an application based on the citizenship status or immigration status of the applicant.

(c) For any program listed in subdivision (d), when mandatory disclosure of a social security number is required, an applicant shall provide their social security number, if one has been issued, or an individual tax identification number that has been or will be submitted.

(d) This section applies to all of the following:

(1) Programs supported through the Health Professions Education Fund pursuant to Section 128355.

(2) The Registered Nurse Education Fund created pursuant to Section 128400.

(3) The Mental Health Practitioner Education Fund created pursuant to Section 128458.

(4) The Vocational Nurse Education Fund created pursuant to Section 128500.

(5) The Medically Underserved Account for Physicians created pursuant to Section 128555.

(6) Loan forgiveness and scholarship programs created pursuant to Part 3.1 (commencing with Section 5820) of Division 5 of the Welfare and Institutions Code.

(7) The Song-Brown Health Care Workforce Training Act created pursuant to Article 1 (commencing with Section 128200) of Chapter 4.

(8) To the extent permitted under federal law, the program administered by the department pursuant to the federal National Health Service Corps State Loan Repayment Program (42 U.S.C. Sec. 254q-1), commonly known as the California State Loan Repayment Program.

(9) The programs administered by the department pursuant to the Health Professions Career Opportunity Program (Section 127885), commonly known as the Mini Grants Program, and California's Student/Resident Experiences and Rotations in Community Health, commonly known as the CalSEARCH program.

HISTORY:

Added Stats 2016 ch 786 § 3 (SB 1139), effective January 1, 2017. Amended Stats 2017 ch 561 § 136 (AB 1516), effective January 1, 2018; Stats 2021 ch 143 § 173 (AB 133), effective July 27, 2021.

ARTICLE 2

CALIFORNIA REGISTERED NURSE EDUCATION PROGRAM

Section
128375. Legislative findings and declarations.
128380. Legislative intent.
128385. Registered Nurse Education Program.
128390. Use of funds.
128395. Solicitation of advice [Repealed].
128400. Registered Nurse Education Fund.

HISTORY: Added Stats 1995 ch 415 § 9.

§ 128375. Legislative findings and declarations

(a) The Legislature hereby finds and declares that an adequate supply of professional nurses is critical to assuring the health and well-being of the citizens of California, particularly those who live in medically underserved areas.

(b) The Legislature further finds that changes in the health care system of this state have increased the need for more highly skilled nurses. These changes include advances in medical technology and pharmacology, that necessitate the use of more highly skilled nurses in acute care facilities. Further, the containment of health care costs has led to increased reliance on home health care and outpatient services and to a higher proportion of more acutely ill patients in acute care facilities. Long-term care facilities also need more highly educated nursing personnel. Both shifts require a larger number of skilled nursing personnel.

(c) The Legislature further finds and declares that in nursing, as in other professions, certain populations are underrepresented. The Legislature also finds and declares that it is especially important that nursing care be provided in a way that is sensitive to the sociocultural variables that affect a person's health. The Legislature recognizes that the financial burden of obtaining a baccalaureate degree is considerable and that persons from families lacking adequate financial resources may need financial assistance to complete a baccalaureate degree.

HISTORY:

Added Stats 1995 ch 415 § 9 (SB 1360). Amended Stats 1999 ch 149 § 11 (SB 308), effective July 22, 1999; Stats 2000 ch 135 § 106 (AB 2539); Stats 2021 ch 143 § 174 (AB 133), effective July 27, 2021.

§ 128380. Legislative intent

It is the intent of the Legislature to accomplish the following:

(a) Assure an adequate supply of appropriately trained professional nurses.

(b) Encourage persons from populations that are currently underrepresented in the nursing profession to enter that profession.

(c) Encourage professional nurses to work in medically underserved areas.

HISTORY:

Added Stats 1995 ch 415 § 9 (SB 1360).

§ 128385. Registered Nurse Education Program

(a) There is hereby created the Registered Nurse Education Program within the department. Persons participating in this program shall be persons who agree in writing prior to graduation to serve in an eligible county health facility, an eligible state-operated health facility, a health workforce shortage area, or a California nursing school, as designated by the director of the department. Persons agreeing to serve in eligible county health facilities, eligible state-operated health facilities, or health workforce shortage areas, and master's or doctoral students agreeing to serve in a California nursing school may apply for scholarship or loan repayment. The Registered Nurse Education Program shall be administered in accordance with Article 1 (commencing with Section 128330), except that all funds in the Registered Nurse Education Fund shall be used only for the purpose of promoting the education of registered nurses and related administrative costs. The department shall adopt both of the following:

(1) A standard contractual agreement to be signed by the director and any student who has received an award to work in an eligible county health facility, an eligible state-operated health facility, or in a health workforce shortage area that would require a period of obligated professional service in the areas of California designated by the department as deficient in primary care services. The obligated professional service shall be in direct patient care. The agreement shall include a clause entitling the state to recover the funds awarded plus the maximum allowable interest for failure to begin or complete the service obligation.

(2) Maximum allowable amounts for scholarships, educational loans, and loan repayment programs in order to assure the most effective use of these funds.

(b) Applicants may be persons licensed as registered nurses, graduates of associate degree nursing programs prior to entering a program granting a baccalaureate of science degree in nursing, or students entering an entry-level master's degree program in registered nursing or other registered nurse master's or doctoral degree program approved by the Board of Registered Nursing. Priority shall be given to applicants who hold associate degrees in nursing.

(c) Registered nurses and students shall commit to teaching nursing in a California nursing school for five years in order to receive a scholarship or loan repayment for a doctoral degree program.

(d) As used in this section, "eligible county health facility" means a county health facility that has been determined by the department to have a nursing vacancy rate greater than noncounty health facilities located in the same health facility planning area.

(e) As used in this section, "eligible state-operated health facility" means a state-operated health facility that has been determined by the department to have a nursing vacancy rate greater than noncounty health facilities located in the same health facility planning area.

Misc.

HISTORY:

Added Stats 1995 ch 415 § 9 (SB 1360). Amended Stats 1999 ch 149 § 12 (SB 308), effective July

22, 1999; Stats 2000 ch 360 § 1 (AB 2516); Stats 2003 ch 582 § 19 (AB 1627); Stats 2005 ch 611 § 2 (AB 702), effective January 1, 2006; Stats 2006 ch 259 § 9 (SB 1850), effective January 1, 2007; Stats 2021 ch 143 § 175 (AB 133), effective July 27, 2021.

§ 128390. Use of funds

The funds made available pursuant to this article shall be used as specified in Article 14 (commencing with Section 69795) of Chapter 2 of Part 42 of the Education Code, except that the funds shall be used only for the purpose of assisting students in completing nursing programs meeting the standards specified in subdivision (j) of Section 69799 of the Education Code.

HISTORY:
Added Stats 1995 ch 415 § 9 (SB 1360).

§ 128395. Solicitation of advice [Repealed]

HISTORY:
Added Stats 1995 ch 415 § 9 (SB 1360). Amended Stats 1999 ch 149 § 13 (SB 308), effective July 22, 1999. Repealed Stats 2021 ch 143 § 176 (AB 133), effective July 27, 2021.

§ 128400. Registered Nurse Education Fund

There is hereby established in the State Treasury the Registered Nurse Education Fund. All money in the fund shall be used for the purposes specified in the California Registered Nurse Education Program established pursuant to this article. This fund shall receive money collected pursuant to subdivision (d) of Section 2815 and Section 2815.1 of the Business and Professions Code.

HISTORY:
Added Stats 1995 ch 415 § 9 (SB 1360). Amended Stats 1999 ch 149 § 14 (SB 308), effective July 22, 1999; Stats 2013 ch 384 § 1 (SB 271), effective January 1, 2014.

ARTICLE 3

GERIATRIC NURSE PRACTITIONER AND CLINICAL NURSE SPECIALIST SCHOLARSHIP PROGRAM [REPEALED]

Section
128425. Legislative findings and declarations [Repealed].
128430. Definitions [Repealed].
128435. Creation of program [Repealed].
128440. Coordination of awards with other financial assistance [Repealed].
128445. Solicitation of advice from other professional and educational groups [Repealed].
128450. Funding of program [Repealed].

HISTORY: Added Stats 1995 ch 415 § 9. Repealed Stats 2021 ch 143 § 178 (AB 133), effective July 27, 2021.

§ 128425. Legislative findings and declarations [Repealed]

HISTORY:
Added Stats 1995 ch 415 § 9 (SB 1360). Repealed Stats 2021 ch 143 § 178 (AB 133), effective July 27, 2021.

§ 128430. Definitions [Repealed]

HISTORY:
Added Stats 1995 ch 415 § 9 (SB 1360). Repealed Stats 2021 ch 143 § 178 (AB 133), effective July 27, 2021.

§ 128435. Creation of program [Repealed]

HISTORY:
Added Stats 1995 ch 415 § 9 (SB 1360). Amended Stats 1999 ch 149 § 16 (SB 308), effective July 22, 1999. Repealed Stats 2021 ch 143 § 178 (AB 133), effective July 27, 2021.

§ 128440. Coordination of awards with other financial assistance [Repealed]

HISTORY:
Added Stats 1996 ch 1023 § 363 (SB 1497), effective September 29, 1996. Repealed Stats 2021 ch 143 § 178 (AB 133), effective July 27, 2021.

§ 128445. Solicitation of advice from other professional and educational groups [Repealed]

HISTORY:
Added Stats 1996 ch 1023 § 364 (SB 1497), effective September 29, 1996. Amended Stats 1999 ch 149 § 17 (SB 308), effective July 22, 1999. Repealed Stats 2021 ch 143 § 178 (AB 133), effective July 27, 2021.

§ 128450. Funding of program [Repealed]

HISTORY:
Added Stats 1996 ch 1023 § 365 (SB 1497), effective September 29, 1996. Amended Stats 1999 ch 149 § 18 (SB 308), effective July 22, 1999. Repealed Stats 2021 ch 143 § 178 (AB 133), effective July 27, 2021.

EXTRACTED FROM
INSURANCE CODE

Division
2. Classes of Insurance.

DIVISION 2
CLASSES OF INSURANCE

Part
2. Life and Disability Insurance.

HISTORY: Enacted Stats 1935 ch 145.

PART 2
LIFE AND DISABILITY INSURANCE

Chapter
1. The Contract.
4. Standard Provisions in Disability Policies.

HISTORY: Enacted Stats 1935 ch 145.

CHAPTER 1
THE CONTRACT

Article
4. Payment and Proceeds.

HISTORY: Enacted 1935 ch 145.

ARTICLE 4
PAYMENT AND PROCEEDS

Section
10176. Freedom to choose specified health care professionals.
10176.7. Mental health or respiratory care licensure requirements for out of state disability policies.
10177. Professional mental health expenses under self–insured plan.
10177.8. Mental health care licensure requirements for out of state self–insured plans.

HISTORY: Enacted Stats 1935 ch 145.

§ 10176. Freedom to choose specified health care professionals

(a) In disability insurance, the policy may provide for payment of medical, surgical, chiropractic, physical therapy, speech pathology, audiology, acupuncture, professional mental health, dental, hospital, or optometric expenses upon a reimbursement basis, or for the exclusion of any of those services, and provision may be made therein for payment of all or a portion of the amount of charge for these services without requiring that the insured first pay the expenses. The policy shall not prohibit the insured from selecting any psychologist or other person who is the holder of a certificate or license under Section 1000, 1634, 2050, 2472, 2553, 2630, 2948, 3055, or 4938 of the Business and Professions Code, to perform the particular services covered under the terms of the policy, the certificate holder or licensee being expressly authorized by law to perform those services.

(b) If the insured selects any person who is a holder of a certificate under Section 4938 of the Business and Professions Code, a disability insurer or nonprofit hospital service plan shall pay the bona fide claim of an acupuncturist holding a certificate pursuant to Section 4938 of the Business and Professions Code for the treatment of an insured person only if the insured's policy or contract expressly includes acupuncture as a benefit and includes coverage for the injury or illness treated. Unless the policy or contract expressly includes acupuncture as a benefit, no person who is the holder of any license or certificate set forth in this section shall be paid or reimbursed under the policy for acupuncture.

(c) The policy shall not prohibit the insured, upon referral by a physician and surgeon licensed under Section 2050 of the Business and Professions Code, from selecting any licensed clinical social worker who is the holder of a license issued under Section 4996 of the Business and Professions Code, any occupational therapist as specified in Section 2570.2 of the Business and Professions Code, any marriage and family therapist who is the holder of a license under Section 4980.50 of the Business and Professions Code, or any professional clinical counselor who is the holder of a license under Chapter 16 (commencing with Section 4999.10) of Division 2 of the Business and Professions Code, to perform the particular services covered under the terms of the policy, or from selecting any speech-language pathologist or audiologist licensed under Section 2532 of the Business and Professions Code or any registered nurse licensed pursuant to Chapter 6 (commencing with Section 2700) of Division 2 of the Business and Professions Code who possesses a master's degree in psychiatric-mental health nursing and is listed as a psychiatric-mental health nurse by the Board of Registered Nursing, or any advanced practice registered nurse certified as a clinical nurse specialist pursuant to Article 9 (commencing with Section 2838) of Chapter 6 of Division 2 of the Business and Professions Code who participates in expert clinical practice in the specialty of psychiatric-mental health nursing, or any respiratory care practitioner certified pursuant to Chapter 8.3 (commencing with Section 3700) of Division 2 of the Business and Professions Code to perform services deemed necessary by the referring physician and surgeon, that certificate holder, licensee or otherwise regulated person, being expressly authorized by law to perform the services.

(d) Nothing in this section shall be construed to allow any certificate holder or licensee enumerated in this section to perform professional mental health services beyond his or her field or fields of competence as established by his or her education, training, and experience.

(e) For the purposes of this section:

(1) "Marriage and family therapist" means a licensed marriage and family therapist who has received specific instruction in assessment, diagnosis, prognosis, and counseling, and psychotherapeutic treatment of premarital, marriage, family, and child relationship dysfunctions, which is equivalent to the instruction required for licensure on January 1, 1981.

(2) "Professional clinical counselor" means a licensed professional clinical counselor who has received specific instruction in assessment, diagnosis, prognosis, counseling, and psychotherapeutic treatment of mental and emotional disorders, which is equivalent to the instruction required for licensure on January 1, 2012.

(f) An individual disability insurance policy, which is issued, renewed, or amended on or after January 1, 1988, which includes mental health services coverage may not include a lifetime waiver for that coverage with respect to any applicant. The lifetime waiver of coverage provision shall be deemed unenforceable.

HISTORY:

Added Stats 1943 ch 909 § 1. Amended Stats 1959 ch 138 § 1; Stats 1961 ch 2000 § 1; Stats 1963 ch 606 § 9; Stats 1965 ch 663 § 1; Stats 1968 ch 1286 § 1; Stats 1969 ch 296 § 1; Stats 1971 ch 1490 § 1; Stats 1974 ch 958 § 2; Stats 1976 ch 432 § 2; Stats 1978 ch 439 § 1, ch 1130 § 2.5; Stats 1980 ch 973 § 2; Stats 1982 ch 121 § 2; Stats 1983 ch 928 § 10; Stats 1984 ch 1067 § 3; Stats 1987 ch 1163 § 2; Stats 1989 ch 786 § 1; Stats 1990 ch 1569 § 1 (AB 2459); Stats 2001 ch 420 § 5 (AB 1253), effective October 2, 2001; Stats 2002 ch 1013 § 90 (SB 2026); Stats 2011 ch 381 § 37 (SB 146), effective January 1, 2012.

§ 10176.7. Mental health or respiratory care licensure requirements for out of state disability policies

(a) Disability insurance where the insurer is licensed to do business in this state and which provides coverage under a contract of insurance which includes California residents but which may be written or issued for delivery outside of California where benefits are provided within the scope of practice of a licensed clinical social worker, a registered nurse licensed pursuant to Chapter 6 (commencing with Section 2700) of Division 2 of the Business and Professions Code who possesses a master's degree in psychiatric-mental health nursing and two years of supervised experience in psychiatric-mental health nursing, a marriage and family therapist who is the holder of a license under Chapter 13 (commencing with Section 4980) of Division 2 of the Business and Professions Code, a professional clinical counselor who is the holder of a license under Chapter 16 (commencing with Section 4999.10) of Division 2 of the Business and Professions Code, or a respiratory care practitioner certified pursuant to Chapter 8.3 (commencing with Section 3700) of Division 2 of the Business and Professions Code shall not be deemed to prohibit persons covered under the contract from selecting those licensees in California to perform the services in California that are within the terms of the contract even though the licensees are not licensed in the state where the contract is written or issued for delivery.

(b) It is the intent of the Legislature in amending this section in the 1984 portion of the 1983–84 Legislative Session that persons covered by the insurance and those providers of health care specified in this section who are licensed in California should be entitled to the benefits provided by the insurance for services of those providers rendered to those persons.

HISTORY:

Added Stats 1983 ch 673 § 2. Amended Stats 1984 ch 540 § 3; Stats 1989 ch 786 § 2; Stats 2002 ch 1013 § 91 (SB 2026); Stats 2011 ch 381 § 38 (SB 146), effective January 1, 2012.

§ 10177. Professional mental health expenses under self-insured plan

(a) A self-insured employee welfare benefit plan may provide for payment of professional mental health expenses upon a reimbursement basis, or for the exclusion of those services, and provision may be made therein for payment of all or a portion of the amount of charge for those services without requiring that the employee first pay those expenses. The plan shall not prohibit the employee from selecting any psychologist who is the holder of a certificate issued under Section 2948 of the Business and Professions Code or, upon referral by a physician and surgeon licensed under Section 2135 of the Business and Professions Code, any licensed clinical social worker who is the holder of a license issued under Section 4996 of the Business and Professions Code or any marriage and family therapist who is the holder of a certificate or license under Section 4980.50 of the Business and Professions Code, any professional clinical counselor who is the holder of a license under Chapter 16 (commencing with Section 4999.10) of Division 2 of the Business and Professions Code, or any registered nurse licensed pursuant to Chapter 6 (commencing with Section 2700) of Division 2 of the Business and Professions Code, who possesses a master's degree in psychiatric-mental health nursing and is listed as a psychiatric-mental health nurse by the Board of Registered Nursing or any advanced practice registered nurse certified as a clinical nurse specialist pursuant to Article 9 (commencing with Section 2838) of Chapter 6 of Division 2 of the Business and Professions Code who participates in expert clinical practice in the specialty of psychiatric-mental health nursing, to perform the particular services covered under the terms of the plan, the certificate or license holder being expressly authorized by law to perform these services.

(b) Nothing in this section shall be construed to allow any certificate holder or licensee enumerated in this section to perform professional services beyond his or her field or fields of competence as established by his or her education, training, and experience.

(c) For the purposes of this section:

(1) "Marriage and family therapist" shall mean a licensed marriage and family therapist who has received specific instruction in assessment, diagnosis, prognosis, and counseling, and psychotherapeutic treatment of premarital, marriage, family, and child relationship dysfunctions, which is equivalent to the instruction required for licensure on January 1, 1981.

(2) "Professional clinical counselor" means a licensed professional clinical counselor who has received specific instruction in assessment, diagnosis, prognosis, counseling, and psychotherapeutic treatment of mental and emotional disorders, which is equivalent to the instruction required for licensure on January 1, 2012.

(d) A self-insured employee welfare benefit plan, which is issued, renewed, or amended on or after January 1, 1988, that includes mental health services coverage in nongroup contracts may not include a lifetime waiver for that coverage with respect to any employee. The lifetime waiver of coverage provision shall be deemed unenforceable.

HISTORY:
Added Stats 1974 ch 958 § 3. Amended Stats 1976 ch 432 § 3; Stats 1980 ch 973 § 3; Stats 1982 ch 121 § 3; Stats 1983 ch 928 § 11; Stats 1987 ch 1163 § 3; Stats 1989 ch 1104 § 40; Stats 2001 ch 420 § 6 (AB 1253), effective October 2, 2001; Stats 2002 ch 1013 § 92 (SB 2026); Stats 2011 ch 381 § 39 (SB 146), effective January 1, 2012.

§ 10177.8. Mental health care licensure requirements for out of state self-insured plans

(a) A self-insured employee welfare benefit plan doing business in this state and providing coverage that includes California residents but that may be written or issued for delivery outside of California where benefits are provided within the scope of practice of a licensed clinical social worker, a registered nurse licensed pursuant to Chapter 6 (commencing with Section 2700) of Division 2 of the Business and Professions Code who possesses a master's degree in psychiatric-mental health nursing and two years of supervised experience in psychiatric-mental health nursing, a marriage and family therapist who is the holder of a license under Chapter 13 (commencing with Section 4980) of Division 2 of the Business and Professions Code, or a professional clinical counselor who is the holder of a license under Chapter 16 (commencing with Section 4999.10) of Division 2 of the Business and Professions Code, shall not be deemed to prohibit persons covered under the plan from selecting those licensees in California to perform the services in California that are within the terms of the contract even though the licensees are not licensed in the state where the contract is written or issued.

(b) It is the intent of the Legislature in amending this section in the 1984 portion of the 1983–84 Legislative Session that persons covered by the plan and those providers of health care specified in this section who are licensed in California should be entitled to the benefits provided by the plan for services of those providers rendered to those persons.

HISTORY:
Added Stats 1983 ch 673 § 3. Amended Stats 1984 ch 540 § 4; Stats 2002 ch 1013 § 93 (SB 2026). Stats 2011 ch 381 § 40 (SB 146), effective January 1, 2012.

CHAPTER 4

STANDARD PROVISIONS IN DISABILITY POLICIES

Article
1. Scope of Chapter and Definitions.

HISTORY: Enacted 1935 ch 145.

Misc.

ARTICLE 1

SCOPE OF CHAPTER AND DEFINITIONS

Section
10279. Requirements for telephone medical advice services.

HISTORY: Enacted 1935 ch 145.

§ 10279. Requirements for telephone medical advice services

(a) Every disability insurer that provides group or individual policies of disability, or both, that provides, operates, or contracts for, telephone medical advice services to its insureds shall do all of the following:

(1) Ensure that the in-state or out-of-state telephone medical advice service complies with the requirements of Chapter 15 (commencing with Section 4999) of Division 2 of the Business and Professions Code.

(2) Ensure that the staff providing telephone medical advice services for the in-state or out-of-state telephone medical advice service hold a valid California license as a registered nurse or a valid license in the state within which they provide telephone medical advice services as a physician and surgeon or physician assistant and are operating consistent with the laws governing their respective scopes of practice.

(3) Ensure that a physician and surgeon is available on an on-call basis at all times the service is advertised to be available to enrollees and subscribers.

(4) Ensure that the in-state or out-of-state telephone medical advice service designates an agent for service of process in California and files this designation with the commissioner.

(5) Require that the in-state or out-of-state telephone medical advice service makes and maintains records for a period of five years after the telephone medical advice services are provided, including, but not limited to, oral or written transcripts of all medical advice conversations with the disability insurer's insureds in California and copies of all complaints. If the records of telephone medical advice services are kept out of state, the insurer shall, upon the request of the director, provide the records to the director within 10 days of the request.

(6) Ensure that the telephone medical advice services are provided consistent with good professional practice.

(b) The commissioner shall forward to the Department of Consumer Affairs, within 30 days of the end of each calendar quarter, data regarding complaints filed with the department concerning telephone medical advice services.

HISTORY:

Added Stats 1999 ch 535 § 3 (AB 285). Amended Stats 2016 ch 799 § 43 (SB 1039), effective January 1, 2017.

Misc.

EXTRACTED FROM
PENAL CODE

Part
1. Of Crimes and Punishments.
4. Prevention of Crimes and Apprehension of Criminals.

PART 1

OF CRIMES AND PUNISHMENTS

Title
13. Of Crimes Against Property.

TITLE 13

OF CRIMES AGAINST PROPERTY

Chapter
4. Forgery and Counterfeiting.

CHAPTER 4

FORGERY AND COUNTERFEITING

Section
471.5. Falsification of medical records.

§ 471.5. Falsification of medical records

Any person who alters or modifies the medical record of any person, with fraudulent intent, or who, with fraudulent intent, creates any false medical record, is guilty of a misdemeanor.

HISTORY:
Added Stats 1974 ch 888 § 10. Amended Stats 1979 ch 644 § 2.

PART 4

PREVENTION OF CRIMES AND APPREHENSION OF CRIMINALS

Title
1. Investigation and Control of Crimes and Criminals.

HISTORY: Added Stats 1953 ch 1385 § 1 p 2964.

TITLE 1
INVESTIGATION AND CONTROL OF CRIMES AND CRIMINALS

Chapter
2. Control of Crimes and Criminals.

CHAPTER 2
CONTROL OF CRIMES AND CRIMINALS

Article
2. Reports of Injuries.
2.5. Child Abuse and Neglect Reporting Act.

HISTORY: Added Stats 1953 ch 70 § 1.

ARTICLE 2
REPORTS OF INJURIES

Section
11160. Injuries required to be reported; Method of reporting; Team reports; Internal procedures.
11161. Report by physician or surgeon; Medical records; Referrals.
11161.5. Legislative intent regarding development of protocols for interagency investigations of a physician's prescription of medication to patients.
11161.9. Immunity from liability.
11162. Violation of article; Punishment.
11162.5. Definitions.
11162.7. Application of article when reports required under other provisions.
11163. Claim for attorney's fees incurred in action based on reporting.
11163.2. Application of privileges; Confidentiality of reports.

HISTORY: Added Stats 1953 ch 34 § 1. Heading of Article 2, consisting of §§ 11160–11163.6, was amended Stats 1993 ch 992 § 1.

Misc.

§ 11160. Injuries required to be reported; Method of reporting; Team reports; Internal procedures

(a) A health practitioner, as defined in subdivision (a) of Section 11162.5, employed by a health facility, clinic, physician's office, local or state public health department, local government agency, or a clinic or other type of facility operated by a local or state public health department who, in the health practitioner's professional capacity or within the scope of the health practitioner's employment, provides medical services for a physical condition to a patient whom the health practitioner knows or reasonably suspects is a person described as follows, shall immediately make a report in accordance with subdivision (b):

(1) A person suffering from a wound or other physical injury inflicted by the person's own act or inflicted by another where the injury is by means of a firearm.

(2) A person suffering from a wound or other physical injury inflicted upon the person where the injury is the result of assaultive or abusive conduct.

(b) A health practitioner, as defined in subdivision (a) of Section 11162.5, employed by a health facility, clinic, physician's office, local or state public health department, local government agency, or a clinic or other type of facility operated by a local or state public health department shall make a report regarding persons described in subdivision (a) to a local law enforcement agency as follows:

(1) A report by telephone shall be made immediately or as soon as practically possible.

(2) A written report shall be prepared on the standard form developed in compliance with paragraph (4), and adopted by the Office of Emergency Services, or on a form developed and adopted by another state agency that otherwise fulfills the requirements of the standard form. The completed form shall be sent to a local law enforcement agency within two working days of receiving the information regarding the person.

(3) A local law enforcement agency shall be notified and a written report shall be prepared and sent pursuant to paragraphs (1) and (2) even if the person who suffered the wound, other injury, or assaultive or abusive conduct has expired, regardless of whether or not the wound, other injury, or assaultive or abusive conduct was a factor contributing to the death, and even if the evidence of the conduct of the perpetrator of the wound, other injury, or assaultive or abusive conduct was discovered during an autopsy.

(4) The report shall include, but shall not be limited to, the following:

(A) The name of the injured person, if known.

(B) The injured person's whereabouts.

(C) The character and extent of the person's injuries.

(D) The identity of any person the injured person alleges inflicted the wound, other injury, or assaultive or abusive conduct upon the injured person.

(c) For the purposes of this section, "injury" does not include any psychological or physical condition brought about solely through the voluntary administration of a narcotic or restricted dangerous drug.

(d) For the purposes of this section, "assaultive or abusive conduct" includes any of the following offenses:

(1) Murder, in violation of Section 187.

(2) Manslaughter, in violation of Section 192 or 192.5.

(3) Mayhem, in violation of Section 203.

(4) Aggravated mayhem, in violation of Section 205.

(5) Torture, in violation of Section 206.

(6) Assault with intent to commit mayhem, rape, sodomy, or oral copulation, in violation of Section 220.

(7) Administering controlled substances or anesthetic to aid in commission of a felony, in violation of Section 222.

(8) Battery, in violation of Section 242.

(9) Sexual battery, in violation of Section 243.4.

(10) Incest, in violation of Section 285.

(11) Throwing any vitriol, corrosive acid, or caustic chemical with intent to injure or disfigure, in violation of Section 244.

(12) Assault with a stun gun or taser, in violation of Section 244.5.

(13) Assault with a deadly weapon, firearm, assault weapon, or machinegun, or by means likely to produce great bodily injury, in violation of Section 245.

(14) Rape, in violation of Section 261 or former Section 262.

(15) Procuring a person to have sex with another person, in violation of Section 266, 266a, 266b, or 266c.

(16) Child abuse or endangerment, in violation of Section 273a or 273d.

(17) Abuse of spouse or cohabitant, in violation of Section 273.5.

(18) Sodomy, in violation of Section 286.

(19) Lewd and lascivious acts with a child, in violation of Section 288.

(20) Oral copulation, in violation of Section 287 or former Section 288a.

(21) Sexual penetration, in violation of Section 289.

(22) Elder abuse, in violation of Section 368.

(23) An attempt to commit any crime specified in paragraphs (1) to (22), inclusive.

(e) When two or more persons who are required to report are present and jointly have knowledge of a known or suspected instance of violence that is required to be reported pursuant to this section, and when there is an agreement among these persons to report as a team, the team may select by mutual agreement a member of the team to make a report by telephone and a single written report, as required by subdivision (b). The written report shall be signed by the selected member of the reporting team. Any member who has knowledge that the member designated to report has failed to do so shall thereafter make the report.

(f) The reporting duties under this section are individual, except as provided in subdivision (e).

(g) A supervisor or administrator shall not impede or inhibit the reporting duties required under this section and a person making a report pursuant to this section shall not be subject to any sanction for making the report. However, internal procedures to facilitate reporting and apprise supervisors and administrators of reports may be established, except that these procedures shall not be inconsistent with this article. The internal procedures shall not require an employee required to make a report under this article to disclose the employee's identity to the employer.

(h) For the purposes of this section, it is the Legislature's intent to avoid duplication of information.

(i) For purposes of this section only, "employed by a local government agency" includes an employee of an entity under contract with a local government agency to provide medical services.

HISTORY:

Added Stats 1993 ch 992 § 3 (AB 1652). Amended Stats 1st Ex Sess 1993–94 ch 19 § 2 (AB 74X), effective November 30, 1994; Stats 2000 ch 287 § 20 (SB 1955); Stats 2002 ch 249 § 2 (SB 580); Stats 2003 ch 229 § 15 (AB 1757); Stats 2010 ch 618 § 206 (AB 2791), effective January 1, 2011; Stats 2013 ch 352 § 418 (AB 1317), effective September 26, 2013, operative July 1, 2013; Stats 2018 ch 164 § 1 (AB 1973), effective January 1, 2019; Stats 2018 ch 423 § 111 (SB 1494), effective January 1, 2019 (ch

164 prevails); Stats 2019 ch 497 § 207 (AB 991), effective January 1, 2020; Stats 2021 ch 626 § 63 (AB 1171), effective January 1, 2022.

§ 11161. Report by physician or surgeon; Medical records; Referrals

Notwithstanding Section 11160, the following shall apply to every physician or surgeon who has under his or her charge or care any person described in subdivision (a) of Section 11160:

(a) The physician or surgeon shall make a report in accordance with subdivision (b) of Section 11160 to a local law enforcement agency.

(b) It is recommended that any medical records of a person about whom the physician or surgeon is required to report pursuant to subdivision (a) include the following:

(1) Any comments by the injured person regarding past domestic violence, as defined in Section 13700, or regarding the name of any person suspected of inflicting the wound, other physical injury, or assaultive or abusive conduct upon the person.

(2) A map of the injured person's body showing and identifying injuries and bruises at the time of the health care.

(3) A copy of the law enforcement reporting form.

(c) It is recommended that the physician or surgeon refer the person to local domestic violence services if the person is suffering or suspected of suffering from domestic violence, as defined in Section 13700.

HISTORY:

Added Stats 1993 ch 992 § 5 (AB 1652).

§ 11161.5. Legislative intent regarding development of protocols for interagency investigations of a physician's prescription of medication to patients

(a) It is the intent of the Legislature that on or before January 1, 2006, the California District Attorneys Association, in conjunction with interested parties, including, but not limited to, the Department of Justice, the California Narcotic Officers' Association, the California Police Chiefs' Association, the California State Sheriffs' Association, the California Medical Association, the American Pain Society, the American Academy of Pain Medicine, the California Society of Anesthesiologists, the California Chapter of the American College of Emergency Physicians, the California Medical Board, the California Orthopedic Association, and other medical and patient advocacy entities specializing in pain control therapies, shall develop protocols for the development and implementation of interagency investigations in connection with a physician's prescription of medication to patients. The protocols are intended to assure the competent review of, and that relevant investigation procedures are followed for, the suspected undertreatment, undermedication, overtreatment, and overmedication of pain cases. Consideration shall be made for the special circumstances of urban and rural communities. The investigation protocol shall be designed to facilitate communication between the medical and law enforcement communities and the timely return of medical records pertaining to the identity, diagnosis, prognosis, or treatment of any patient that are seized by law enforcement from a physician who is suspected of engaging in or having engaged in criminal activity related to the documents.

(b) The costs incurred by the California District Attorneys Association in implementing this section shall be solicited and funded from nongovernmental entities.

HISTORY:
Added Stats 2004 ch 864 § 2 (SB 1782).

§ 11161.9. Immunity from liability

(a) A health practitioner who makes a report in accordance with this article shall not incur civil or criminal liability as a result of any report required or authorized by this article.

(b)(1) No person required or authorized to report pursuant to this article, or designated by a person required or authorized to report pursuant to this article, who takes photographs of a person suspected of being a person described in this article about whom a report is required or authorized shall incur any civil or criminal liability for taking the photographs, causing the photographs to be taken, or disseminating the photographs to local law enforcement with the reports required by this article in accordance with this article. However, this subdivision shall not be deemed to grant immunity from civil or criminal liability with respect to any other use of the photographs.

(2) A court may award attorney's fees to a commercial film and photographic print processor when a suit is brought against the processor because of a disclosure mandated by this article and the court finds that the suit is frivolous.

(c) A health practitioner who, pursuant to a request from an adult protective services agency or a local law enforcement agency, provides the requesting agency with access to the victim of a known or suspected instance of abuse shall not incur civil or criminal liability as a result of providing that access.

(d) No employee shall be discharged, suspended, disciplined, or harassed for making a report pursuant to this section.

(e) This section does not apply to mandated reporting of child abuse, as provided for in Article 2.5 (commencing with Section 11164).

HISTORY:
Added Stats 1993 ch 992 § 6 (AB 1652).

§ 11162. Violation of article; Punishment

A violation of this article is a misdemeanor, punishable by imprisonment in a county jail not exceeding six months, or by a fine not exceeding one thousand dollars ($1,000), or by both that fine and imprisonment.

HISTORY:
Added Stats 1953 ch 34 § 1. Amended Stats 1993 ch 992 § 7 (AB 1652).

§ 11162.5. Definitions

As used in this article, the following definitions shall apply:

(a) "Health practitioner" has the same meaning as provided in paragraphs (21) to (28), inclusive, of subdivision (a) of Section 11165.7.

(b) "Clinic" is limited to include any clinic specified in Sections 1204 and 1204.3 of the Health and Safety Code.

(c) "Health facility" has the same meaning as provided in Section 1250 of the Health and Safety Code.

(d) "Reasonably suspects" means that it is objectively reasonable for a person to entertain a suspicion, based upon facts that could cause a reasonable person in a like position, drawing, when appropriate, on his or her training and experience, to suspect.

HISTORY:

Added Stats 1993 ch 992 § 8 (AB 1652). Amended Stats 2006 ch 701 § 1 (AB 525), effective January 1, 2007.

§ 11162.7. Application of article when reports required under other provisions

This article shall not apply when a report is required to be made pursuant to the Child Abuse and Neglect Reporting Act (Article 2.5 (commencing with Section 11164)), and Chapter 11 (commencing with Section 15600) of Part 3 of Division 9 of the Welfare and Institutions Code.

HISTORY:

Added Stats 1993 ch 992 § 9 (AB 1652).

§ 11163. Claim for attorney's fees incurred in action based on reporting

(a) The Legislature finds and declares that even though the Legislature has provided for immunity from liability, pursuant to Section 11161.9, for persons required or authorized to report pursuant to this article, that immunity does not eliminate the possibility that actions may be brought against those persons based upon required reports of abuse pursuant to other laws.

In order to further limit the financial hardship that those persons may incur as a result of fulfilling their legal responsibility, it is necessary that they not be unfairly burdened by legal fees incurred in defending those actions.

(b)(1) Therefore, a health practitioner may present a claim to the Department of General Services for reasonable attorney's fees incurred in any action against that person on the basis of that person reporting in accordance with this article if the court dismisses the action upon a demurrer or motion for summary judgment made by that person or if that person prevails in the action.

(2) The Department of General Services shall allow the claim pursuant to paragraph (1) if the requirements of paragraph (1) are met, and the claim shall be paid from an appropriation to be made for that purpose. Attorney's fees awarded pursuant to this section shall not exceed an hourly rate greater than the rate charged by the Attorney General at the time the award is made and shall not exceed an aggregate amount of fifty thousand dollars ($50,000).

(3) This subdivision shall not apply if a public entity has provided for the defense of the action pursuant to Section 995 of the Government Code.

HISTORY:

Added Stats 1993 ch 992 § 10 (AB 1652). Amended Stats 2006 ch 538 § 524 (SB 1852), effective January 1, 2007; Stats 2016 ch 31 § 256 (SB 836), effective June 27, 2017.

§ 11163.2. Application of privileges; Confidentiality of reports

(a) In any court proceeding or administrative hearing, neither the physician–patient privilege nor the psychotherapist privilege applies to the information required to be reported pursuant to this article.

(b) The reports required by this article shall be kept confidential by the health facility, clinic, or physician's office that submitted the report, and by local law enforcement agencies, and shall only be disclosed by local law enforcement agencies to those involved in the investigation of the report or the enforcement of a criminal law implicated by a report. In no case shall the person suspected or accused of inflicting the wound, other injury, or assaultive or abusive conduct upon the injured person or his or her attorney be allowed access to the injured person's whereabouts.

(c) For the purposes of this article, reports of suspected child abuse and information contained therein may be disclosed only to persons or agencies with whom investigations of child abuse are coordinated under the regulations promulgated under Section 11174.

(d) The Board of Prison Terms may subpoena reports that are not unfounded and reports that concern only the current incidents upon which parole revocation proceedings are pending against a parolee.

HISTORY:
Added Stats 1993 ch 992 § 11 (AB 1652).

ARTICLE 2.5

CHILD ABUSE AND NEGLECT REPORTING ACT

Section
11165.2. "Neglect"; "Severe neglect"; "General neglect".
11165.7. "Mandated reporter"; Training.
11166.5. Statement acknowledging awareness of reporting duties and promising compliance; Exemptions; Distribution in connection with licensure or certification.
11167.5. Confidentiality and disclosure of reports.

HISTORY: Added Stats 1980 ch 1071 § 4, effective January 1, 1981. Heading of Article 2.5, which formerly read "Child Abuse Reporting," amended to read as above by Stats 1987 ch 1444 § 1, effective January 1, 1988.

§ 11165.2. "Neglect"; "Severe neglect"; "General neglect"

Misc.

As used in this article, "neglect" means the negligent treatment or the maltreatment of a child by a person responsible for the child's welfare under circumstances indicating harm or threatened harm to the child's health or welfare. The term includes both acts and omissions on the part of the responsible person.

(a) "Severe neglect" means the negligent failure of a person having the care or custody of a child to protect the child from severe malnutrition or medically diagnosed nonorganic failure to thrive. "Severe neglect" also means those situations of neglect where any person having the care or custody of a child willfully causes or permits the person or health of the child to be placed in a situation such that their person or health is endangered as proscribed by Section 11165.3, including the intentional failure to provide adequate food, clothing, shelter, or medical care.

(b) "General neglect" means the negligent failure of a person having the care or custody of a child to provide adequate food, clothing, shelter, medical care, or supervision where no physical injury to the child has occurred but the child is at substantial risk of suffering serious physical harm or illness. "General neglect" does not include a parent's economic disadvantage.

For the purposes of this chapter, a child receiving treatment by spiritual means as provided in Section 16509.1 of the Welfare and Institutions Code or not receiving specified medical treatment for religious reasons, shall not for that reason alone be considered a neglected child. An informed and appropriate medical decision made by parent or guardian after consultation with a physician or physicians who have examined the minor does not constitute neglect.

HISTORY:

Added Stats 1987 ch 1459 § 7. Amended Stats 2022 ch 770 § 1 (AB 2085), effective January 1, 2023.

§ 11165.7. "Mandated reporter"; Training

(a) As used in this article, "mandated reporter" is defined as any of the following:

(1) A teacher.

(2) An instructional aide.

(3) A teacher's aide or teacher's assistant employed by a public or private school.

(4) A classified employee of a public school.

(5) An administrative officer or supervisor of child welfare and attendance, or a certificated pupil personnel employee of a public or private school.

(6) An administrator of a public or private day camp.

(7) An administrator or employee of a public or private youth center, youth recreation program, or youth organization.

(8) An administrator, board member, or employee of a public or private organization whose duties require direct contact and supervision of children, including a foster family agency.

(9) An employee of a county office of education or the State Department of Education whose duties bring the employee into contact with children on a regular basis.

(10) A licensee, an administrator, or an employee of a licensed community care or child daycare facility.

(11) A Head Start program teacher.

(12) A licensing worker or licensing evaluator employed by a licensing agency, as defined in Section 11165.11.

(13) A public assistance worker.

(14) An employee of a childcare institution, including, but not limited to, foster parents, group home personnel, and personnel of residential care facilities.

(15) A social worker, probation officer, or parole officer.

(16) An employee of a school district police or security department.

(17) A person who is an administrator or presenter of, or a counselor in, a child abuse prevention program in a public or private school.

(18) A district attorney investigator, inspector, or local child support agency caseworker, unless the investigator, inspector, or caseworker is working with an attorney appointed pursuant to Section 317 of the Welfare and Institutions Code to represent a minor.

(19) A peace officer, as defined in Chapter 4.5 (commencing with Section 830) of Title 3 of Part 2, who is not otherwise described in this section.

(20) A firefighter, except for volunteer firefighters.

(21) A physician and surgeon, psychiatrist, psychologist, dentist, resident, intern, podiatrist, chiropractor, licensed nurse, dental hygienist, optometrist, marriage and family therapist, clinical social worker, professional clinical counselor, or any other person who is currently licensed under Division 2 (commencing with Section 500) of the Business and Professions Code.

(22) An emergency medical technician I or II, paramedic, or other person certified pursuant to Division 2.5 (commencing with Section 1797) of the Health and Safety Code.

(23) A psychological assistant registered pursuant to Section 2913 of the Business and Professions Code.

(24) A marriage and family therapist trainee, as defined in subdivision (c) of Section 4980.03 of the Business and Professions Code.

(25) An unlicensed associate marriage and family therapist registered under Section 4980.44 of the Business and Professions Code.

(26) A state or county public health employee who treats a minor for venereal disease or any other condition.

(27) A coroner.

(28) A medical examiner or other person who performs autopsies.

(29) A commercial film and photographic print or image processor as specified in subdivision (e) of Section 11166. As used in this article, "commercial film and photographic print or image processor" means a person who develops exposed photographic film into negatives, slides, or prints, or who makes prints from negatives or slides, or who prepares, publishes, produces, develops, duplicates, or prints any representation of information, data, or an image, including, but not limited to, any film, filmstrip, photograph, negative, slide, photocopy, videotape, video laser disc, computer hardware, computer software, computer floppy disk, data storage medium, CD-ROM, computer-generated equipment, or computer-generated image, for compensation. The term includes any employee of that person; it does not include a person who develops film or makes prints or images for a public agency.

(30) A child visitation monitor. As used in this article, "child visitation monitor" means a person who, for financial compensation, acts as a monitor of a visit between a child and another person when the monitoring of that visit has been ordered by a court of law.

(31) An animal control officer or humane society officer. For the purposes of this article, the following terms have the following meanings:

(A) "Animal control officer" means a person employed by a city, county, or city and county for the purpose of enforcing animal control laws or regulations.

(B) "Humane society officer" means a person appointed or employed by a public or private entity as a humane officer who is qualified pursuant to Section 14502 or 14503 of the Corporations Code.

(32) A clergy member, as specified in subdivision (d) of Section 11166. As used in this article, "clergy member" means a priest, minister, rabbi, religious practitioner, or similar functionary of a church, temple, or recognized denomination or organization.

(33) Any custodian of records of a clergy member, as specified in this section and subdivision (d) of Section 11166.

(34) An employee of any police department, county sheriff's department, county probation department, or county welfare department.

(35) An employee or volunteer of a Court Appointed Special Advocate program, as defined in Rule 5.655 of the California Rules of Court.

(36) A custodial officer, as defined in Section 831.5.

(37) A person providing services to a minor child under Section 12300 or 12300.1 of the Welfare and Institutions Code.

(38) An alcohol and drug counselor. As used in this article, an "alcohol and drug counselor" is a person providing counseling, therapy, or other clinical services for a state licensed or certified drug, alcohol, or drug and alcohol treatment program. However, alcohol or drug abuse, or both alcohol and drug abuse, is not, in and of itself, a sufficient basis for reporting child abuse or neglect.

(39) A clinical counselor trainee, as defined in subdivision (g) of Section 4999.12 of the Business and Professions Code.

(40) An associate professional clinical counselor registered under Section 4999.42 of the Business and Professions Code.

(41) An employee or administrator of a public or private postsecondary educational institution, whose duties bring the administrator or employee into contact with children on a regular basis, or who supervises those whose duties bring the administrator or employee into contact with children on a regular basis, as to child abuse or neglect occurring on that institution's premises or at an official activity of, or program conducted by, the institution. Nothing in this paragraph shall be construed as altering the lawyer-client privilege as set forth in Article 3 (commencing with Section 950) of Chapter 4 of Division 8 of the Evidence Code.

(42) An athletic coach, athletic administrator, or athletic director employed by any public or private school that provides any combination of instruction for kindergarten, or grades 1 to 12, inclusive.

(43)(A) A commercial computer technician as specified in subdivision (e) of Section 11166. As used in this article, "commercial computer technician" means a person who works for a company that is in the business of repairing, installing, or otherwise servicing a computer or computer component, including, but not limited to, a computer part, device, memory storage or recording mechanism, auxiliary storage recording or memory capacity, or any other material relating to the operation and maintenance of a computer or computer network system, for a fee. An employer who provides an electronic communications service or a remote computing service to the public shall be deemed to comply with this article if that employer complies with Section 2258A of Title 18 of the United States Code.

(B) An employer of a commercial computer technician may implement internal procedures for facilitating reporting consistent with this article. These procedures may direct employees who are mandated reporters under this paragraph to report materials described in subdivision (e) of Section 11166 to an employee who is designated by the employer to receive the reports. An employee who is designated to receive reports under this subparagraph shall be a commercial computer technician for purposes of this article. A commercial computer technician who makes a report to the designated employee pursuant to this subparagraph shall be deemed to have complied with the requirements of this article and shall be subject to the protections afforded to mandated reporters, including, but not limited to, those protections afforded by Section 11172.

(44) Any athletic coach, including, but not limited to, an assistant coach or a graduate assistant involved in coaching, at public or private postsecondary educational institutions.

(45) An individual certified by a licensed foster family agency as a certified family home, as defined in Section 1506 of the Health and Safety Code.

(46) An individual approved as a resource family, as defined in Section 1517 of the Health and Safety Code and Section 16519.5 of the Welfare and Institutions Code.

(47) A qualified autism service provider, a qualified autism service professional, or a qualified autism service paraprofessional, as defined in Section 1374.73 of the Health and Safety Code and Section 10144.51 of the Insurance Code.

(48) A human resource employee of a business subject to Part 2.8 (commencing with Section 12900) of Division 3 of Title 2 of the Government Code that employs minors. For purposes of this section, a "human resource employee" is the employee or employees designated by the employer to accept any complaints of misconduct as required by Chapter 6 (commencing with Section 12940) of Part 2.8 of Division 3 of Title 2 of the Government Code.

(49) An adult person whose duties require direct contact with and supervision of minors in the performance of the minors' duties in the workplace of a business subject to Part 2.8 (commencing with Section 12900) of Division 3 of Title 2 of the Government Code is a mandated reporter of sexual abuse, as defined in Section 11165.1. Nothing in this paragraph shall be construed to modify or limit the person's duty to report known or suspected child abuse or neglect when the person is acting in some other capacity that would otherwise make the person a mandated reporter.

(b) Except as provided in paragraph (35) of subdivision (a), volunteers of public or private organizations whose duties require direct contact with and supervision of children are not mandated reporters but are encouraged to obtain training in the identification and reporting of child abuse and neglect and are further encouraged to report known or suspected instances of child abuse or neglect to an agency specified in Section 11165.9.

(c)(1) Except as provided in subdivision (d) and paragraph (2), employers are strongly encouraged to provide their employees who are mandated reporters with training in the duties imposed by this article. This training shall include training in child abuse and neglect identification and training in child abuse and neglect reporting. Whether or not employers provide their employees with training in child abuse and neglect identification and reporting, the employers shall provide their employees who are mandated reporters with the statement required pursuant to subdivision (a) of Section 11166.5.

(2) Employers subject to paragraphs (48) and (49) of subdivision (a) shall provide their employees who are mandated reporters with training in the duties imposed by this article. This training shall include training in child abuse and neglect identification and training in child abuse and neglect reporting. The training requirement may be met by completing the general online training for mandated reporters offered by the Office of Child Abuse Prevention in the State Department of Social Services.

(d) Pursuant to Section 44691 of the Education Code, school districts, county offices of education, state special schools and diagnostic centers operated by the State Department of Education, and charter schools shall annually train their employees and persons working on their behalf specified in subdivision (a) in the duties of mandated reporters under the child abuse reporting laws. The training shall include, but not necessarily be limited to, training in child abuse and neglect identification and child abuse and neglect reporting.

(e)(1) On and after January 1, 2018, pursuant to Section 1596.8662 of the Health and Safety Code, a childcare licensee applicant shall take training in the duties of mandated reporters under the child abuse reporting laws as a condition of licensure, and a childcare administrator or an employee of a licensed child daycare facility shall take training in the duties of mandated reporters during the first 90 days when that administrator or employee is employed by the facility.

(2) A person specified in paragraph (1) who becomes a licensee, administrator, or employee of a licensed child daycare facility shall take renewal mandated reporter training every two years following the date on which that person completed the initial mandated reporter training. The training shall include, but not necessarily be limited to, training in child abuse and neglect identification and child abuse and neglect reporting.

(f) Unless otherwise specifically provided, the absence of training shall not excuse a mandated reporter from the duties imposed by this article.

(g) Public and private organizations are encouraged to provide their volunteers whose duties require direct contact with and supervision of children with training in the identification and reporting of child abuse and neglect.

HISTORY:

Added Stats 1987 ch 1459 § 14. Amended Stats 1991 ch 132 § 1 (AB 1133); Stats 1992 ch 459 § 1 (SB 1695); Stats 2000 ch 916 § 5 (AB 1241); Stats 2001 ch 133 § 3 (AB 102), effective July 31, 2001, ch 754 § 4 (AB 1697); Stats 2002 ch 927 § 10.7 (AB 3032), ch 936 § 1 (AB 299), effective September 27, 2002; Stats 2003 ch 122 § 1 (SB 316); Stats 2004 ch 762 § 1 (AB 2531), ch 842 § 5.5 (SB 1313); Stats 2006 ch 901 § 9.5 (SB 1422), effective January 1, 2007; Stats 2008 ch 456 § 1 (AB 2337), effective January 1, 2009; Stats 2011 ch 381 § 41 (SB 146), effective January 1, 2012; Stats 2012 ch 162 § 136 (SB 1171), effective January 1, 2013, ch 517 § 1 (AB 1713), effective January 1, 2013, ch 518 § 1 (SB 1264), effective January 1, 2013, ch 519 § 1 (AB 1434), effective January 1, 2013, ch 520 § 1 (AB 1435), effective January 1, 2013, ch 521 § 1.15 (AB 1817), effective January 1, 2013 (ch 521 prevails); Stats 2013 ch 76 § 164 (AB 383), effective January 1, 2014; Stats 2014 ch 797 § 4 (AB 1432), effective January 1, 2015; Stats 2015 ch 414 § 3 (AB 1207), effective January 1, 2016; Stats 2016 ch 612 § 57 (AB 1997), effective January 1, 2017; Stats 2016 ch 850 § 4.5 (AB 1001), effective January 1, 2017;

Stats 2017 ch 573 § 77 (SB 800), effective January 1, 2018; Stats 2019 ch 674 § 1 (AB 189), effective January 1, 2020; Stats 2020 ch 243 § 1 (AB 1963), effective January 1, 2021.

§ 11166.5. Statement acknowledging awareness of reporting duties and promising compliance; Exemptions; Distribution in connection with licensure or certification

(a)(1) On and after January 1, 1985, any mandated reporter as specified in Section 11165.7, with the exception of child visitation monitors, prior to commencing his or her employment, and as a prerequisite to that employment, shall sign a statement on a form provided to him or her by his or her employer to the effect that he or she has knowledge of the provisions of Section 11166 and will comply with those provisions. The statement shall inform the employee that he or she is a mandated reporter and inform the employee of his or her reporting obligations under Section 11166 and of his or her confidentiality rights under subdivision (d) of Section 11167. The employer shall provide a copy of Sections 11165.7, 11166, and 11167 to the employee.

On and after January 1, 1993, any person who acts as a child visitation monitor, as defined in paragraph (31) of subdivision (a) of Section 11165.7, prior to engaging in monitoring the first visit in a case, shall sign a statement on a form provided to him or her by the court which ordered the presence of that third person during the visit, to the effect that he or she has knowledge of the provisions of Section 11166 and will comply with those provisions.

(2) The signed statements shall be retained by the employer or the court, as the case may be. The cost of printing, distribution, and filing of these statements shall be borne by the employer or the court.

(3) This subdivision is not applicable to persons employed by public or private youth centers, youth recreation programs, and youth organizations as members of the support staff or maintenance staff and who do not work with, observe, or have knowledge of children as part of their official duties.

(b) On and after January 1, 1986, when a person is issued a state license or certificate to engage in a profession or occupation, the members of which are required to make a report pursuant to Section 11166, the state agency issuing the license or certificate shall send a statement substantially similar to the one contained in subdivision (a) to the person at the same time as it transmits the document indicating licensure or certification to the person. In addition to the requirements contained in subdivision (a), the statement also shall indicate that failure to comply with the requirements of Section 11166 is a misdemeanor, punishable by up to six months in a county jail, by a fine of one thousand dollars ($1,000), or by both that imprisonment and fine.

(c) As an alternative to the procedure required by subdivision (b), a state agency may cause the required statement to be printed on all application forms for a license or certificate printed on or after January 1, 1986.

(d) On and after January 1, 1993, any child visitation monitor, as defined in paragraph (31) of subdivision (a) of Section 11165.7, who desires to act in that capacity shall have received training in the duties imposed by this article, including training in child abuse identification and child abuse reporting. The person, prior to engaging in monitoring the first visit in a case, shall sign a statement on a form provided to him or her by the court which ordered the presence of that third person during the visit, to the effect that he or she has received this training. This statement may be included in the statement required by subdivision (a) or it may be a separate statement. This statement shall be filed, along with the statement required by subdivision (a), in the court file of the case for which the visitation monitoring is being provided.

(e) Any person providing services to a minor child, as described in paragraph (38) of subdivision (a) of Section 11165.7, shall not be required to make a report pursuant to Section 11166 unless that person has received training, or instructional materials in the appropriate language, on the duties imposed by this article, including identifying and reporting child abuse and neglect.

HISTORY:

Added Stats 1984 ch 1718 § 1. Amended Stats 1985 ch 464 § 1; Stats 1985 ch 1598 § 5.1; Stats 1986 ch 248 § 168; Stats 1987 ch 1459 § 21; Stats 1990 ch 931 § 1 (AB 3521); Stats 1991 ch 132 § 2 (AB 1133); Stats 1992 ch 459 § 4 (SB 1695); Stats 1993 ch 510 § 2 (SB 665); Stats 1996 ch 1081 § 4 (AB 3354); Stats 2000 ch 916 § 20 (AB 1241); Stats 2001 ch 133 § 9 (AB 102), effective July 31, 2001; Stats 2004 ch 762 § 2 (AB 2531), ch 842 § 10.5 (SB 1313); Stats 2012 ch 518 § 2 (SB 1264), effective January 1, 2013.

§ 11167.5. Confidentiality and disclosure of reports

(a) The reports required by Sections 11166 and 11166.2, or authorized by Section 11166.05, and child abuse or neglect investigative reports that result in a summary report being filed with the Department of Justice pursuant to subdivision (a) of Section 11169 shall be confidential and may be disclosed only as provided in subdivision (b). Any violation of the confidentiality provided by this article is a misdemeanor punishable by imprisonment in a county jail not to exceed six months, by a fine of five hundred dollars ($500), or by both that imprisonment and fine.

(b) Reports of suspected child abuse or neglect and information contained therein may be disclosed only to the following:

(1) Persons or agencies to whom disclosure of the identity of the reporting party is permitted under Section 11167.

(2) Persons or agencies to whom disclosure of information is permitted under subdivision (b) of Section 11170 or subdivision (a) of Section 11170.5.

(3) Persons or agencies with whom investigations of child abuse or neglect are coordinated under the regulations promulgated under Section 11174.

(4) Multidisciplinary personnel teams as defined in subdivision (d) of Section 18951 of the Welfare and Institutions Code.

(5) Persons or agencies responsible for the licensing of facilities which care for children, as specified in Section 11165.7.

(6) The State Department of Social Services or any county, as specified in paragraph (4) of subdivision (b) of Section 11170, when an individual has applied for a license to operate a community care facility or child daycare facility, or for a certificate of approval to operate a certified family home or resource family home, or for employment or presence in a licensed facility, certified family home, or resource family home, or when a complaint alleges child abuse or neglect by a licensee or employee of, or individual approved to be present in, a licensed facility, certified family home, or resource family home.

(7) Hospital scan teams. As used in this paragraph, "hospital scan team" means a team of three or more persons established by a hospital, or two or

more hospitals in the same county, consisting of health care professionals and representatives of law enforcement and child protective services, the members of which are engaged in the identification of child abuse or neglect. The disclosure authorized by this section includes disclosure among all hospital scan teams.

(8) Coroners and medical examiners when conducting a post mortem examination of a child.

(9) The Board of Parole Hearings, which may subpoena an employee of a county welfare department who can provide relevant evidence and reports that both (A) are not unfounded, pursuant to Section 11165.12, and (B) concern only the current incidents upon which parole revocation proceedings are pending against a parolee charged with child abuse or neglect. The reports and information shall be confidential pursuant to subdivision (d) of Section 11167.

(10) Personnel from an agency responsible for making a placement of a child pursuant to Section 361.3 of, and Article 7 (commencing with Section 305) of Chapter 2 of Part 1 of Division 2 of, the Welfare and Institutions Code.

(11) Persons who have been identified by the Department of Justice as listed in the Child Abuse Central Index pursuant to paragraph (7) of subdivision (b) of Section 11170 or subdivision (c) of Section 11170, or persons who have verified with the Department of Justice that they are listed in the Child Abuse Central Index as provided in subdivision (f) of Section 11170. Disclosure under this paragraph is required notwithstanding the California Public Records Act, (Division 10 (commencing with Section 7920.000) of Title 1 of the Government Code). Nothing in this paragraph shall preclude a submitting agency prior to disclosure from redacting any information necessary to maintain confidentiality as required by law.

(12) Out-of-state law enforcement agencies conducting an investigation of child abuse or neglect only when an agency makes the request for reports of suspected child abuse or neglect in writing and on official letterhead, or as designated by the Department of Justice, identifying the suspected abuser or victim by name and date of birth or approximate age. The request shall be signed by the department supervisor of the requesting law enforcement agency. The written request shall cite the out-of-state statute or interstate compact provision that requires that the information contained within these reports is to be disclosed only to law enforcement, prosecutorial entities, or multidisciplinary investigative teams, and shall cite the safeguards in place to prevent unlawful disclosure provided by the requesting state or the applicable interstate compact provision.

(13) Out-of-state agencies responsible for approving prospective foster or adoptive parents for placement of a child only when the agency makes the request in compliance with the Adam Walsh Child Protection and Safety Act of 2006 (Public Law 109-248). The request shall also cite the safeguards in place to prevent unlawful disclosure provided by the requesting state or the applicable interstate compact provision and indicate that the requesting state shall maintain continual compliance with the requirement in paragraph (20) of subdivision (a) of Section 671 of Title 42 of the United States Code that requires the state have in place safeguards to prevent the

unauthorized disclosure of information in any child abuse and neglect registry maintained by the state and prevent the information from being used for a purpose other than the conducting of background checks in foster or adoptive placement cases.

(14) Each chairperson of a county child death review team, or the chairperson's designee, to whom disclosure of information is permitted under this article, relating to the death of one or more children and any prior child abuse or neglect investigation reports maintained involving the same victim, siblings, or suspects. Local child death review teams may share any relevant information regarding case reviews involving child death with other child death review teams.

(c) Authorized persons within county health departments shall be permitted to receive copies of any reports made by health practitioners, as defined in paragraphs (21) to (28), inclusive, of subdivision (a) of Section 11165.7, and pursuant to Section 11165.13, and copies of assessments completed pursuant to Sections 123600 and 123605 of the Health and Safety Code, to the extent permitted by federal law. Any information received pursuant to this subdivision is protected by subdivision (e).

(d) Nothing in this section requires the Department of Justice to disclose information contained in records maintained under Section 11170 or under the regulations promulgated pursuant to Section 11174, except as otherwise provided in this article.

(e) This section shall not be interpreted to allow disclosure of any reports or records relevant to the reports of child abuse or neglect if the disclosure would be prohibited by any other provisions of state or federal law applicable to the reports or records relevant to the reports of child abuse or neglect.

HISTORY:

Added Stats 1983 ch 1082 § 1. Amended Stats 1985 ch 1593 § 4, effective October 2, 1985, ch 1598 § 7.5; Stats 1987 ch 167 § 1, ch 1459 § 22; Stats 1988 ch 1580 § 5; Stats 1989 ch 153 § 1, ch 1169 § 2; Stats 1995 ch 391 § 1 (AB 1440); Stats 1997 ch 24 § 1 (AB 1536), ch 842 § 4 (SB 644), ch 844 § 1.5 (AB 1065); Stats 1998 ch 485 § 135 (AB 2803); Stats 2000 ch 916 § 25 (AB 1241); Stats 2002 ch 187 § 2 (SB 1745); Stats 2004 ch 842 § 16 (SB 1313); Stats 2006 ch 701 § 5 (AB 525), effective January 1, 2007; Stats 2007 ch 583 § 18 (SB 703), effective January 1, 2008; Stats 2008 ch 699 § 17 (SB 1241), effective January 1, 2009, ch 701 § 9 (AB 2651) (ch 701 prevails), effective September 30, 2008; Stats 2017 ch 732 § 41 (AB 404), effective January 1, 2018; Stats 2021 ch 615 § 346 (AB 474), effective January 1, 2022.

EXTRACTED FROM
UNEMPLOYMENT INSURANCE CODE

Division
1. Unemployment and Disability Compensation.

DIVISION 1
UNEMPLOYMENT AND DISABILITY COMPENSATION

Part
2. Disability Compensation.

PART 2
DISABILITY COMPENSATION

Chapter
2. Disability Benefits.

CHAPTER 2
DISABILITY BENEFITS

Article
4. Filing, Determination and Payment of Disability Benefit Claims.

ARTICLE 4
FILING, DETERMINATION AND PAYMENT OF DISABILITY BENEFIT CLAIMS

Section
2708. Medical practitioner's certificate; "Physician"; "Practitioner".

Misc.

§ 2708. Medical practitioner's certificate; "Physician"; "Practitioner"

(a)(1) In accordance with the director's authorized regulations, and except as provided in subdivision (c) and Sections 2708.1 and 2709, a claimant shall establish medical eligibility for each uninterrupted period of disability by filing a first claim for disability benefits supported by the certificate of a treating physician or practitioner that establishes the sickness, injury, or pregnancy of the employee, or the condition of the family member that warrants the care of the employee. For subsequent periods of uninterrupted disability after the period covered by the initial certificate or any preceding continued claim, a claimant shall file a continued claim for those benefits supported by the certificate of a treating physician or practitioner. A certificate filed to establish medical eligibility for the employee's own sickness, injury, or pregnancy shall contain a diagnosis and diagnostic code prescribed in the International Classification of Diseases, or, if no diagnosis has yet been obtained, a detailed statement of symptoms.

(2) A certificate filed to establish medical eligibility of the employee's own sickness, injury, or pregnancy shall also contain a statement of medical facts, including secondary diagnoses when applicable, within the physician's or practitioner's knowledge, based on a physical examination and a documented medical history of the claimant by the physician or practitioner, indicating the physician's or practitioner's conclusion as to the claimant's disability, and a statement of the physician's or practitioner's opinion as to the expected duration of the disability.

(b) An employee shall be required to file a certificate to establish eligibility when taking leave to care for a family member with a serious health condition. The certificate shall be developed by the department. In order to establish medical eligibility of the serious health condition of the family member that warrants the care of the employee, the information shall be within the physician's or practitioner's knowledge and shall be based on a physical examination and documented medical history of the family member and shall contain all of the following:

(1) A diagnosis and diagnostic code prescribed in the International Classification of Diseases, or, if no diagnosis has yet been obtained, a detailed statement of symptoms.

(2) The date, if known, on which the condition commenced.

(3) The probable duration of the condition.

(4) An estimate of the amount of time that the physician or practitioner believes the employee needs to care for the child, parent, grandparent, grandchild, sibling, spouse, or domestic partner.

(5)(A) A statement that the serious health condition warrants the participation of the employee to provide care for his or her child, parent, grandparent, grandchild, sibling, spouse, or domestic partner.

(B) "Warrants the participation of the employee" includes, but is not limited to, providing psychological comfort, and arranging "third party" care for the child, parent, grandparent, grandchild, sibling, spouse, or domestic partner, as well as directly providing, or participating in, the medical care.

(c) The department shall develop a certification form for bonding that is separate and distinct from the certificate required in subdivision (a) for an employee taking leave to bond with a minor child within the first year of the child's birth or placement in connection with foster care or adoption.

(d) The first and any continuing claim of an individual who obtains care and treatment outside this state shall be supported by a certificate of a treating physician or practitioner duly licensed or certified by the state or foreign country in which the claimant is receiving the care and treatment. If a physician or practitioner licensed by and practicing in a foreign country is under investigation by the department for filing false claims and the department does not have legal remedies to conduct a criminal investigation or prosecution in that country, the department may suspend the processing of all further certifications until the physician or practitioner fully cooperates, and continues to cooperate, with the investigation. A physician or practitioner licensed by, and practicing in, a foreign country who has been convicted of filing false claims with the department may not file a certificate in support of a claim for disability benefits for a period of five years.

(e) For purposes of this part:

(1) "Physician" has the same meaning as defined in Section 3209.3 of the Labor Code.

(2)(A) "Practitioner" means a person duly licensed or certified in California acting within the scope of his or her license or certification who is a dentist, podiatrist, or a nurse practitioner, and in the case of a nurse practitioner, after performance of a physical examination by a nurse practitioner and collaboration with a physician and surgeon, or as to normal pregnancy or childbirth, a midwife or nurse midwife, or nurse practitioner.

(B) "Practitioner" also means a physician assistant who has performed a physical examination under the supervision of a physician and surgeon. Funds appropriated to cover the costs required to implement this subparagraph shall come from the Unemployment Compensation Disability Fund. This subparagraph shall be implemented on or before January 1, 2017.

(f) For a claimant who is hospitalized in or under the authority of a county hospital in this state, a certificate of initial and continuing medical disability, if any, shall satisfy the requirements of this section if the disability is shown by the claimant's hospital chart, and the certificate is signed by the hospital's registrar. For a claimant hospitalized in or under the care of a medical facility of the United States government, a certificate of initial and continuing medical disability, if any, shall satisfy the requirements of this section if the disability is shown by the claimant's hospital chart, and the certificate is signed by a medical officer of the facility duly authorized to do so.

(g) Nothing in this section shall be construed to preclude the department from requesting additional medical evidence to supplement the first or any continued claim if the additional evidence can be procured without additional cost to the claimant. The department may require that the additional evidence include any or all of the following:

(1) Identification of diagnoses.

(2) Identification of symptoms.

(3) A statement setting forth the facts of the claimant's disability. The statement shall be completed by any of the following individuals:

(A) The physician or practitioner treating the claimant.

(B) The registrar, authorized medical officer, or other duly authorized official of the hospital or health facility treating the claimant.

(C) An examining physician or other representative of the department.

(h) This section shall become operative on July 1, 2014.

HISTORY:

Added Stats 2013 ch 350 § 2 (SB 770), effective January 1, 2014, operative July 1, 2014. Amended Stats 2014 ch 438 § 2 (SB 1083), effective January 1, 2015.

EXTRACTED FROM
WELFARE AND INSTITUTIONS CODE

Division
9. Public Social Services.

DIVISION 9
PUBLIC SOCIAL SERVICES

Part
3. Aid and Medical Assistance.

HISTORY: Added Stats 1965 ch 1784 § 5.

PART 3
AID AND MEDICAL ASSISTANCE

Chapter
7. Basic Health Care.
11. Elder Abuse and Dependent Adult Civil Protection Act.

HISTORY: Added Stats 1965 ch 1784 § 5.

CHAPTER 7
BASIC HEALTH CARE

Article
3. Administration.
4. The Medi-Cal Benefits Program.

HISTORY: Added Stats 1965 2d Ex Sess ch 4 § 2, effective November 15, 1965, operative March 1, 1966. Former Chapter 7, entitled "Medical Care for Public Assistance Recipients," consisting of §§ 14000–14108, was added Stats 1965 ch 1784 § 5 and repealed Stats 1965 2d Ex Sess ch 4 § 1, effective November 15, 1965, operative March 1, 1966.

ARTICLE 3
ADMINISTRATION

Section
14111. Delegation of duties to nurse practitioner in long-term health care facility.
14111.5. Tasks of nurse practitioner in long-term health care facility.

HISTORY: Added Stats 1965 2d Ex Sess ch 4 § 2, effective November 15, 1965, operative March 1, 1966. Former Article 3, entitled "Fiscal Provisions," consisting of §§ 14100–14108, was added Stats 1965 ch 1784 § 5 and repealed Stats 1965 2d Ex Sess ch 4 § 1, effective November 15, 1965, operative March 1, 1966.

§ 14111. Delegation of duties to nurse practitioner in long-term health care facility

(a) As permitted by federal law or regulations, for health care services provided in a long-term health care facility that are reimbursed by Medicare, a physician and surgeon may delegate any of the following to a nurse practitioner:

(1) Alternating visits required by federal law and regulations with a physician and surgeon.

(2) Any duties consistent with federal law and regulations within the scope of practice of nurse practitioners, so long as all of the following conditions are met:

(A) A physician and surgeon approves, in writing, the admission of the individual to the facility.

(B) The medical care of each resident is supervised by a physician and surgeon.

(C) A physician and surgeon performs the initial visit and alternate required visits.

(b) This section does not authorize benefits not otherwise authorized by federal law or regulation.

(c) All responsibilities delegated to a nurse practitioner pursuant to this section shall be performed under the supervision of the physician and surgeon and pursuant to a standardized procedure among the physician and surgeon, nurse practitioner, and facility.

(d) No task that is required by federal law or regulation to be performed personally by a physician may be delegated to a nurse practitioner.

(e) Nothing in this section shall be construed as limiting the authority of a long-term health care facility to hire and employ nurse practitioners so long as that employment is consistent with federal law and within the scope of practice of a nurse practitioner.

HISTORY:

Added Stats 1992 ch 1048 § 2 (AB 2849). Amended Stats 1994 ch 646 § 1 (AB 2879).

§ 14111.5. Tasks of nurse practitioner in long-term health care facility

(a) As permitted by federal law or regulations, for health care services provided in a long-term health care facility that are reimbursed under this chapter, a nurse practitioner may, to the extent consistent with his or her scope of practice, perform any of the following tasks otherwise required of a physician and surgeon:

(1) With respect to visits required by federal law or regulations, making alternating visits, or more frequent visits if the physician and surgeon is not available.

(2) Any duty or task that is consistent with federal and state law or regulation within the scope of practice of nurse practitioners, so long as all of the following conditions are met:

(A) A physician and surgeon approves, in writing, the admission of the individual to the facility.

(B) The medical care of each resident is supervised by a physician and surgeon.

(C) A physician and surgeon performs the initial visit and alternate required visits.

(b) This section does not authorize benefits not otherwise authorized by federal or state law or regulation.

(c) All responsibilities undertaken by a nurse practitioner pursuant to this section shall be performed in collaboration with the physician and surgeon and pursuant to a standardized procedure among the physician and surgeon, nurse practitioner, and facility.

(d) Except as provided in subdivisions (a) to (c), inclusive, any task that is required by federal law or regulation to be performed personally by a physician may be delegated to a nurse practitioner who is not an employee of the long-term health care facility.

(e) Nothing in this section shall be construed as limiting the authority of a long-term health care facility to hire and employ nurse practitioners so long as that employment is consistent with federal law and with the scope of practice of a nurse practitioner.

HISTORY:
Added Stats 1992 ch 1048 § 3 (AB 2849). Amended Stats 1994 ch 646 § 2 (AB 2879); Stats 1995 ch 91 § 186 (SB 975).

ARTICLE 4
THE MEDI-CAL BENEFITS PROGRAM

Section
14132.06. Medi-Cal benefits provided by local educational agency.

HISTORY: Added Stats 1971 ch 577 § 38, effective August 13, 1971, operative October 1, 1971, as Article 4.2. Renumbered by Stats 1977 ch 1252 § 847, operative July 1, 1978. Former Article 4, entitled "Health Care Commission," consisting of §§ 14125–14126, was added Stats 1971 ch 577 § 37.7, effective August 13, 1971, operative October 1, 1971, and repealed Stats 1976 ch 737 § 1. Former Article 4, entitled "Health Review and Program Council," consisting of §§ 14125–14130, was added Stats 1965 2d Ex Sess ch 4 § 2, effective November 15, 1965, operative March 1, 1966, and repealed Stats 1971 ch 577 § 37.6, effective August 13, 1971, operative October 1, 1971.

§ 14132.06. Medi-Cal benefits provided by local educational agency

(a) Services specified in this section that are provided by a local educational agency are covered Medi-Cal benefits, to the extent federal financial participation is available, and subject to utilization controls and standards adopted by the department, and consistent with Medi-Cal requirements for physician prescription, order, and supervision.

(b) Any provider enrolled on or after January 1, 1993, to provide services pursuant to this section may bill for those services provided on or after January 1, 1993.

(c) This section shall not be interpreted to expand the current category of professional health care practitioners permitted to directly bill the Medi-Cal program.

(d) This section is not intended to increase the scope of practice of any health professional providing services under this section or Medi-Cal requirements for physician prescription, order, and supervision.

(e)(1) For the purposes of this section, the local educational agency, as a condition of enrollment to provide services under this section, shall be considered the provider of services. A local educational agency provider, as a condition of enrollment to provide services under this section, shall enter into, and maintain, a contract with the department in accordance with guidelines contained in regulations adopted by the director and published in Title 22 of the California Code of Regulations.

(2) Notwithstanding paragraph (1), a local educational agency providing services pursuant to this section shall utilize current safety net and traditional health care providers, when those providers are accessible to specific schoolsites identified by the local educational agency to participate in this program, rather than adding duplicate capacity.

(f) For the purposes of this section, covered services may include all of the following local educational agency services:

(1) Health and mental health evaluations and health and mental health education.

(2) Medical transportation.

(A) The following provisions shall not apply to medical transportation eligible to be billed under this section:

(i) Section 51323(a)(2)(A) of Title 22 of the California Code of Regulations.

(ii) Section 51323(a)(3)(B) of Title 22 of the California Code of Regulations.

(iii) For students whose medical or physical condition does not require the use of a gurney, Section 51231.1(f) of Title 22 of the California Code of Regulations.

(B)(i) Subparagraph (A) shall become inoperative on January 1, 2018, or on the date the director executes a declaration stating that the regulations implementing subparagraph (A) and Section 14115.8 have been updated, whichever is later.

(ii) The department shall post the declaration executed under clause (i) on its Internet Web site and transmit a copy of the declaration to the Assembly Committee on Budget and the Senate Committee on Budget and Fiscal Review and the LEA Ad Hoc Workgroup.

(iii) If subparagraph (A) becomes inoperative on January 1, 2018, subparagraph (A) and this subparagraph shall be inoperative on January 1, 2018, unless a later enacted statute enacted before that date, deletes or extends that date.

(iv) If subparagraph (A) becomes inoperative on the date the director executes a declaration as described in clause (i), subparagraph (A) and this subparagraph shall be inoperative on the January 1 immediately following the date subparagraph (A) becomes inoperative, unless a later enacted statute enacted before that date, deletes or extends that date.

(3) Nursing services.

(4) Occupational therapy.

(5) Physical therapy.

(6) Physician services.

(7) Mental health and counseling services.

(8) School health aide services.

(9) Speech pathology services. These services may be provided by either of the following:

(A) A licensed speech pathologist.

(B) A credentialed speech-language pathologist, to the extent authorized by Chapter 5.3 (commencing with Section 2530) of Division 2 of the Business and Professions Code.

(10) Audiology services.

(11) Targeted case management services for children regardless of whether the child has an individualized education plan (IEP) or an individualized family service plan (IFSP).

(g) Local educational agencies may, but need not, provide any or all of the services specified in subdivision (f).

(h) For the purposes of this section, "local educational agency" means the governing body of any school district or community college district, the county office of education, a charter school, a state special school, a California State University campus, or a University of California campus.

(i) Notwithstanding any other law, a community college district, a California State University campus, or a University of California campus, consistent with the requirements of this section, may bill for services provided to any student, regardless of age, who is a Medi-Cal recipient.

(j) No later than July 1, 2013, and every year thereafter, the department shall make publicly accessible an annual accounting of all funds collected by the department from federal Medicaid payments allocable to local educational agencies, including, but not limited to, the funds withheld pursuant to subdivision (g) of Section 14115.8. The accounting shall detail amounts withheld from federal Medicaid payments to each participating local educational agency for that year. One-time costs for the development of this accounting shall not exceed two hundred fifty thousand dollars ($250,000).

(k)(1) If the requirements in paragraphs (2) and (4) are satisfied, the department shall seek federal financial participation for covered services that are provided by a local educational agency pursuant to subdivision (a) to a child who is an eligible Medi-Cal beneficiary, regardless of either of the following:

(A) Whether the child has an IEP or an IFSP.

(B) Whether those same services are provided at no charge to the beneficiary or to the community at large.

(2) The local educational agency shall take all reasonable measures to ascertain and pursue claims for payment of covered services specified in this section against legally liable third parties pursuant to Section 1902(a)(25) of the federal Social Security Act (42 U.S.C. Sec. 1396a(a)(25)).

(3) If a legally liable third party receives a claim submitted by a local educational agency pursuant to paragraph (2), the legally liable third party shall either reimburse the claim or issue a notice of denial of noncoverage of services or benefits. If there is no response to a claim submitted to a legally liable third party by a local educational agency within 45 days, the local educational agency may bill the Medi-Cal program pursuant to subdivision

(b). The local educational agency shall retain a copy of the claim submitted to the legally liable third party for a period of three years.

(4) This subdivision shall not be implemented until the department obtains any necessary federal approvals.

HISTORY:

Added Stats 1993 ch 654 § 5 (SB 256). Amended Stats 1995 ch 305 § 15 (AB 911), effective August 3, 1995; Stats 1997 ch 211 § 1 (AB 1294), effective August 4, 1997, ch 883 § 2 (AB 549); Stats 2006 ch 581 § 2 (AB 2837), effective September 28, 2006; Stats 2012 ch 755 § 2 (AB 2608), effective January 1, 2013; Stats 2015 ch 653 § 2 (SB 276), effective January 1, 2016; Stats 2016 ch 86 § 320 (SB 1171), effective January 1, 2017.

CHAPTER 11

ELDER ABUSE AND DEPENDENT ADULT CIVIL PROTECTION ACT

Article

2. Definitions.
3. Mandatory and Nonmandatory Reports of Abuse.
4. Confidentiality.
8. Prosecution of Elder and Dependent Adult Abuse Cases.
10. Employee Statement.

HISTORY: Added Stats 1982 ch 1184 § 3. The heading of Chapter 11, which formerly read "Abuse of the Elderly and Other Dependent Adults," amended to read "Abuse of the Elderly and Dependent Adults," by Stats 1986 ch 769 § 2, effective September 15, 1986, and amended to read as above by Stats 1991 ch 774 § 1.

ARTICLE 2

DEFINITIONS

Section

15610. Construction of chapter.
15610.02. Legislative findings, declarations, and intent.
15610.05. "Abandonment".
15610.07. "Abuse of an elder or a dependent adult".
15610.10. "Adult protective services".
15610.13. "Adult protective services agency".
15610.15. Division.
15610.17. "Care custodian".
15610.20. "Clients' rights advocate".
15610.23. "Dependent adult".
15610.25. "Developmentally disabled person".
15610.27. "Elder".
15610.30. "Financial abuse" of elder or dependent adult.
15610.35. "Goods and services necessary to avoid physical harm or mental suffering".
15610.37. "Health practitioner".
15610.40. "Investigation".
15610.43. "Isolation".
15610.47. "Long-term care facility".
15610.50. "Long-term care ombudsman".
15610.53. "Mental suffering".
15610.57. "Neglect".

Misc.

Section
15610.60. "Patients' rights advocate".
15610.63. "Physical abuse".
15610.65. "Reasonable suspicion".
15610.67. "Serious bodily injury".
15610.70. Undue influence.

HISTORY: Added Stats 1994 ch 594 § 3. Former Article 2, also entitled "Definitions," consisting of §§ 15610, 15610.1, was added Stats 1982 ch 1184 § 3 and repealed Stats 1994 ch 594 § 2.

§ 15610. Construction of chapter

The definitions contained in this article shall govern the construction of this chapter, unless the context requires otherwise.

HISTORY:
Added Stats 1994 ch 594 § 3 (SB 1681).

§ 15610.02. Legislative findings, declarations, and intent

(a) The Legislature finds and declares all of the following:

(1) The adult protective services program (program), established by the Legislature as a statewide program in 1998, is a critical component of the state's safety net for vulnerable adults.

(2) The population served by the county-run, state-overseen program has grown and changed significantly since the program's inception and will continue to do so at a rapid pace, given the increasing number of older adults in California. California's over-65 years of age population is expected to be 87 percent higher in 2030 than in 2012, an increase of more than 4,000,000 people. The population over 85 years of age will increase at an even faster rate, with 489 percent growth between 2010 and 2060.

(3) The increasing population of older adults often has more complex needs, including persons with cognitive impairments and a growing number of those experiencing homelessness. Research indicates that approximately 50 percent of homeless individuals are over 50 years of age, and one-half of those individuals became homeless after 50 years of age.

(b) In order to address the safety and well-being of the growing number of diverse older adults who will need adult protective services, it is the intent of the Legislature to enhance the program in a number of ways, including enabling the program to provide longer term case management for those with more complex cases, expanding and making more flexible the Home Safe Program to aid clients facing homelessness, and encouraging the use of collaborative, multidisciplinary best practices across the state, including financial abuse specialist teams and forensic centers. It is further the intent of the Legislature to expand the age of clients served under the program in order to intervene earlier with aging adults before their situations reach a crisis point.

HISTORY:
Added Stats 2021 ch 85 § 62 (AB 135), effective July 16, 2021.

§ 15610.05. "Abandonment"

"Abandonment" means the desertion or willful forsaking of an elder or a dependent adult by anyone having care or custody of that person under circumstances in which a reasonable person would continue to provide care and custody.

HISTORY:
Added Stats 1994 ch 594 § 3 (SB 1681).

§ 15610.07. "Abuse of an elder or a dependent adult"

(a) "Abuse of an elder or a dependent adult" means any of the following:

(1) Physical abuse, neglect, abandonment, isolation, abduction, or other treatment with resulting physical harm or pain or mental suffering.

(2) The deprivation by a care custodian of goods or services that are necessary to avoid physical harm or mental suffering.

(3) Financial abuse, as defined in Section 15610.30.

(b) This section shall become operative on July 1, 2016.

HISTORY:
Added Stats 2015 ch 285 § 2 (SB 196), effective January 1, 2016, operative July 1, 2016.

§ 15610.10. "Adult protective services"

"Adult protective services" means those activities performed on behalf of elders and dependent adults who have come to the attention of the adult protective services agency due to potential abuse or neglect.

HISTORY:
Added Stats 1994 ch 594 § 3 (SB 1681). Amended Stats 1998 ch 946 § 3 (SB 2199); Stats 2021 ch 85 § 63 (AB 135), effective July 16, 2021.

§ 15610.13. "Adult protective services agency"

"Adult protective services agency" means a county welfare department, except persons who do not work directly with elders or dependent adults as part of their official duties, including members of support staff and maintenance staff.

HISTORY:
Added Stats 1994 ch 594 § 3 (SB 1681).

§ 15610.15. Division

"Division" means the Division of Medi-Cal Fraud and Elder Abuse within the office of the Attorney General.

HISTORY:
Added Stats 1994 ch 594 § 3 (SB 1681). Amended Stats 2021 ch 554 § 13 (SB 823), effective January 1, 2022.

§ 15610.17. "Care custodian"

"Care custodian" means an administrator or an employee of any of the following public or private facilities or agencies, or persons providing care or services for elders or dependent adults, including members of the support staff and maintenance staff:

(a) Twenty-four-hour health facilities, as defined in Sections 1250, 1250.2, and 1250.3 of the Health and Safety Code.

(b) Clinics.

(c) Home health agencies.

(d) Agencies providing publicly funded in-home supportive services, nutrition services, or other home and community-based support services.

(e) Adult day health care centers and adult day care.

(f) Secondary schools that serve 18- to 22-year-old dependent adults and postsecondary educational institutions that serve dependent adults or elders.

(g) Independent living centers.

(h) Camps.

(i) Alzheimer's Disease day care resource centers.

(j) Community care facilities, as defined in Section 1502 of the Health and Safety Code, and residential care facilities for the elderly, as defined in Section 1569.2 of the Health and Safety Code.

(k) Respite care facilities.

(*l*) Foster homes.

(m) Vocational rehabilitation facilities and work activity centers.

(n) Designated area agencies on aging.

(o) Regional centers for persons with developmental disabilities.

(p) State Department of Social Services and State Department of Health Services licensing divisions.

(q) County welfare departments.

(r) Offices of patients' rights advocates and clients' rights advocates, including attorneys.

(s) The office of the long-term care ombudsman.

(t) Offices of public conservators, public guardians, and court investigators.

(u) Any protection or advocacy agency or entity that is designated by the Governor to fulfill the requirements and assurances of the following:

(1) The federal Developmental Disabilities Assistance and Bill of Rights Act of 2000, contained in Chapter 144 (commencing with Section 15001) of Title 42 of the United States Code, for protection and advocacy of the rights of persons with developmental disabilities.

(2) The Protection and Advocacy for the Mentally Ill Individuals Act of 1986, as amended, contained in Chapter 114 (commencing with Section 10801) of Title 42 of the United States Code, for the protection and advocacy of the rights of persons with mental illness.

(v) Humane societies and animal control agencies.

(w) Fire departments.

(x) Offices of environmental health and building code enforcement.

(y) Any other protective, public, sectarian, mental health, or private assistance or advocacy agency or person providing health services or social services to elders or dependent adults.

Misc.

HISTORY:

Added Stats 1994 ch 594 § 3 (SB 1681). Amended Stats 1998 ch 946 § 4 (SB 2199); Stats 2002 ch 54 § 2 (AB 255).

§ 15610.20. "Clients' rights advocate"

"Clients' rights advocate" means the individual or individuals assigned by a regional center or state hospital developmental center to be responsible for clients' rights assurance for persons with developmental disabilities.

HISTORY:

Added Stats 1994 ch 594 § 3 (SB 1681).

§ 15610.23. "Dependent adult"

(a) "Dependent adult" means a person, regardless of whether the person lives independently, between the ages of 18 and 64 years who resides in this state and who has physical or mental limitations that restrict his or her ability to carry out normal activities or to protect his or her rights, including, but not limited to, persons who have physical or developmental disabilities, or whose physical or mental abilities have diminished because of age.

(b) "Dependent adult" includes any person between the ages of 18 and 64 years who is admitted as an inpatient to a 24-hour health facility, as defined in Sections 1250, 1250.2, and 1250.3 of the Health and Safety Code.

HISTORY:

Added Stats 1994 ch 594 § 3 (SB 1681). Amended Stats 2002 ch 54 § 4 (AB 255); Stats 2018 ch 70 § 5 (AB 1934), effective January 1, 2019.

§ 15610.25. "Developmentally disabled person"

"Developmentally disabled person" means a person with a developmental disability specified by or as described in subdivision (a) of Section 4512.

HISTORY:

Added Stats 1994 ch 594 § 3 (SB 1681).

§ 15610.27. "Elder"

"Elder" means any person residing in this state, 65 years of age or older.

HISTORY:

Added Stats 1994 ch 594 § 3 (SB 1681).

§ 15610.30. "Financial abuse" of elder or dependent adult

(a) "Financial abuse" of an elder or dependent adult occurs when a person or entity does any of the following:

(1) Takes, secretes, appropriates, obtains, or retains real or personal property of an elder or dependent adult for a wrongful use or with intent to defraud, or both.

(2) Assists in taking, secreting, appropriating, obtaining, or retaining real or personal property of an elder or dependent adult for a wrongful use or with intent to defraud, or both.

(3) Takes, secretes, appropriates, obtains, or retains, or assists in taking, secreting, appropriating, obtaining, or retaining, real or personal property of an elder or dependent adult by undue influence, as defined in Section 15610.70.

(b) A person or entity shall be deemed to have taken, secreted, appropriated, obtained, or retained property for a wrongful use if, among other things, the person or entity takes, secretes, appropriates, obtains, or retains the property and the person or entity knew or should have known that this conduct is likely to be harmful to the elder or dependent adult.

(c) For purposes of this section, a person or entity takes, secretes, appropriates, obtains, or retains real or personal property when an elder or dependent adult is deprived of any property right, including by means of an agreement, donative transfer, or testamentary bequest, regardless of whether the property is held directly or by a representative of an elder or dependent adult.

(d) For purposes of this section, "representative" means a person or entity that is either of the following:

(1) A conservator, trustee, or other representative of the estate of an elder or dependent adult.

(2) An attorney-in-fact of an elder or dependent adult who acts within the authority of the power of attorney.

HISTORY:

Added Stats 1994 ch 594 § 3 (SB 1681). Amended Stats 1997 ch 724 § 37 (AB 1172); Stats 1998 ch 946 § 5 (SB 2199); Stats 2000 ch 442 § 5 (AB 2107) (ch 442 prevails), ch 813 § 2 (SB 1742); Stats 2008 ch 475 § 1 (SB 1140), effective January 1, 2009; Stats 2013 ch 668 § 2 (AB 140), effective January 1, 2014.

§ 15610.35. "Goods and services necessary to avoid physical harm or mental suffering"

"Goods and services necessary to avoid physical harm or mental suffering" include, but are not limited to, all of the following:

(a) The provision of medical care for physical and mental health needs.

(b) Assistance in personal hygiene.

(c) Adequate clothing.

(d) Adequately heated and ventilated shelter.

(e) Protection from health and safety hazards.

(f) Protection from malnutrition, under those circumstances where the results include, but are not limited to, malnutrition and deprivation of necessities or physical punishment.

(g) Transportation and assistance necessary to secure any of the needs set forth in subdivisions (a) to (f), inclusive.

HISTORY:

Added Stats 1994 ch 594 § 3 (SB 1681).

§ 15610.37. "Health practitioner"

"Health practitioner" means a physician and surgeon, psychiatrist, psychologist, dentist, resident, intern, podiatrist, chiropractor, registered nurse, dental hygienist, licensed clinical social worker or associate clinical social worker, marriage and family therapist, licensed professional clinical counselor, or any other person who is currently licensed under Division 2 (commencing with Section 500) of the Business and Professions Code, any emergency medical technician I or II, paramedic, or person certified pursuant to Division 2.5 (commencing with Section 1797) of the Health and Safety Code, a psychological assistant registered pursuant to Section 2913 of the Business and Professions Code, a marriage and family therapist trainee, as defined in subdivision (c) of Section 4980.03 of the Business and Professions Code, an unlicensed marriage and family therapist intern registered under Section 4980.44 of the Business and Professions Code, a clinical counselor trainee, as defined in subdivision (g) of Section 4999.12 of the Business and Professions Code, a clinical counselor intern registered under Section 4999.42 of the Business and Professions Code, a state or county public health or social service employee who treats an elder or a dependent adult for any condition, a coroner, or a substance use disorder counselor. As used in this section, a "substance use disorder counselor" is a person providing counseling services in an alcoholism or drug abuse recovery and treatment program licensed, certified, or funded under Part 2 (commencing with Section 11760) of Division 10.5 of the Health and Safety Code.

HISTORY:
Added Stats 1994 ch 594 § 3 (SB 1681). Amended Stats 2002 ch 54 § 5 (AB 255); Stats 2003 ch 62 § 334 (SB 600); Stats 2011 ch 381 § 49 (SB 146), effective January 1, 2012; Stats 2017 ch 407 § 1 (AB 575), effective January 1, 2018.

§ 15610.40. "Investigation"

"Investigation" means that activity undertaken to determine the validity of a report of elder or dependent adult abuse.

HISTORY:
Added Stats 1994 ch 594 § 3 (SB 1681).

§ 15610.43. "Isolation"

(a) "Isolation" means any of the following:

(1) Acts intentionally committed for the purpose of preventing, and that do serve to prevent, an elder or dependent adult from receiving his or her mail or telephone calls.

(2) Telling a caller or prospective visitor that an elder or dependent adult is not present, or does not wish to talk with the caller, or does not wish to meet with the visitor where the statement is false, is contrary to the express wishes of the elder or the dependent adult, whether he or she is competent or not, and is made for the purpose of preventing the elder or dependent adult from having contact with family, friends, or concerned persons.

(3) False imprisonment, as defined in Section 236 of the Penal Code.

(4) Physical restraint of an elder or dependent adult, for the purpose of preventing the elder or dependent adult from meeting with visitors.

(b) The acts set forth in subdivision (a) shall be subject to a rebuttable presumption that they do not constitute isolation if they are performed pursuant to the instructions of a physician and surgeon licensed to practice medicine in the state, who is caring for the elder or dependent adult at the time the instructions are given, and who gives the instructions as part of his or her medical care.

(c) The acts set forth in subdivision (a) shall not constitute isolation if they are performed in response to a reasonably perceived threat of danger to property or physical safety.

HISTORY:
Added Stats 1994 ch 594 § 3 (SB 1681).

§ 15610.47. "Long-term care facility"

"Long-term care facility" means any of the following:

(a) Any long-term health care facility, as defined in subdivision (a) of Section 1418 of the Health and Safety Code.

(b) Any community care facility, as defined in paragraphs (1) and (2) of subdivision (a) of Section 1502 of the Health and Safety Code, whether licensed or unlicensed.

(c) Any swing bed in an acute care facility, or any extended care facility.

(d) Any adult day health care facility as defined in subdivision (b) of Section 1570.7 of the Health and Safety Code.

(e) Any residential care facility for the elderly as defined in Section 1569.2 of the Health and Safety Code.

HISTORY:

Added Stats 1994 ch 594 § 3 (SB 1681).

§ 15610.50. "Long-term care ombudsman"

"Long-term care ombudsman" means the State Long-Term Care Ombudsman, local ombudsman coordinators, and other persons currently certified as ombudsmen by the Department of Aging as described in Chapter 11 (commencing with Section 9700) of Division 8.5.

HISTORY:

Added Stats 1994 ch 594 § 3 (SB 1681). Amended Stats 2002 ch 54 § 7 (AB 255).

§ 15610.53. "Mental suffering"

"Mental suffering" means fear, agitation, confusion, severe depression, or other forms of serious emotional distress that is brought about by forms of intimidating behavior, threats, harassment, or by deceptive acts performed or false or misleading statements made with malicious intent to agitate, confuse, frighten, or cause severe depression or serious emotional distress of the elder or dependent adult.

HISTORY:

Added Stats 1994 ch 594 § 3 (SB 1681). Amended Stats 2000 ch 559 § 3 (AB 1819).

§ 15610.57. "Neglect"

(a) "Neglect" means either of the following:

(1) The negligent failure of any person having the care or custody of an elder or a dependent adult to exercise that degree of care that a reasonable person in a like position would exercise.

(2) The negligent failure of an elder or dependent adult to exercise that degree of self care that a reasonable person in a like position would exercise.

(b) Neglect includes, but is not limited to, all of the following:

(1) Failure to assist in personal hygiene, or in the provision of food, clothing, or shelter.

(2) Failure to provide medical care for physical and mental health needs. A person shall not be deemed neglected or abused for the sole reason that the person voluntarily relies on treatment by spiritual means through prayer alone in lieu of medical treatment.

(3) Failure to protect from health and safety hazards.

(4) Failure to prevent malnutrition or dehydration.

(5) Substantial inability or failure of an elder or dependent adult to manage their own finances.

(6) Failure of an elder or dependent adult to satisfy any of the needs specified in paragraphs (1) to (5), inclusive, for themselves as a result of poor

cognitive functioning, mental limitation, substance abuse, or chronic poor health.

(c) Neglect includes being homeless if the elder or dependent adult is also unable to meet any of the needs specified in paragraphs (1) to (5), inclusive, of subdivision (b).

HISTORY:

Added Stats 1994 ch 594 § 3 (SB 1681). Amended Stats 1998 ch 946 § 7 (SB 2199); Stats 2002 ch 54 § 8 (AB 255); Stats 2021 ch 85 § 65 (AB 135), effective July 16, 2021.

§ 15610.60. "Patients' rights advocate"

"Patients' rights advocate" means a person who has no direct or indirect clinical or administrative responsibility for the patient, and who is responsible for ensuring that laws, regulations, and policies on the rights of the patient are observed.

HISTORY:

Added Stats 1994 ch 594 § 3 (SB 1681).

§ 15610.63. "Physical abuse"

"Physical abuse" means any of the following:

(a) Assault, as defined in Section 240 of the Penal Code.

(b) Battery, as defined in Section 242 of the Penal Code.

(c) Assault with a deadly weapon or force likely to produce great bodily injury, as defined in Section 245 of the Penal Code.

(d) Unreasonable physical constraint, or prolonged or continual deprivation of food or water.

(e) Sexual assault, that means any of the following:

(1) Sexual battery, as defined in Section 243.4 of the Penal Code.

(2) Rape, as defined in Section 261 of the Penal Code, or former Section 262 of the Penal Code.

(3) Rape in concert, as described in Section 264.1 of the Penal Code.

(4) Incest, as defined in Section 285 of the Penal Code.

(5) Sodomy, as defined in Section 286 of the Penal Code.

(6) Oral copulation, as defined in Section 287 or former Section 288a of the Penal Code.

(7) Sexual penetration, as defined in Section 289 of the Penal Code.

(8) Lewd or lascivious acts, as defined in paragraph (2) of subdivision (b) of Section 288 of the Penal Code.

(f) Use of a physical or chemical restraint or psychotropic medication under any of the following conditions:

(1) For punishment.

(2) For a period beyond that for which the medication was ordered pursuant to the instructions of a physician and surgeon licensed in the State of California, who is providing medical care to the elder or dependent adult at the time the instructions are given.

(3) For any purpose not authorized by the physician and surgeon.

HISTORY:

Added Stats 1994 ch 594 § 3 (SB 1681). Amended Stats 1996 ch 1075 § 22 (SB 1444); Stats 2000 ch 287 § 29 (SB 1955); Stats 2004 ch 823 § 18 (AB 20); Stats 2018 ch 423 § 129 (SB 1494), effective

January 1, 2019; Stats 2021 ch 626 § 75 (AB 1171), effective January 1, 2022; Stats 2022 ch 197 § 39 (SB 1493), effective January 1, 2023.

§ 15610.65. "Reasonable suspicion"

"Reasonable suspicion" means an objectively reasonable suspicion that a person would entertain, based upon facts that could cause a reasonable person in a like position, drawing when appropriate upon his or her training and experience, to suspect abuse.

HISTORY:

Added Stats 1994 ch 594 § 3 (SB 1681).

§ 15610.67. "Serious bodily injury"

"Serious bodily injury" means an injury involving extreme physical pain, substantial risk of death, or protracted loss or impairment of function of a bodily member, organ, or of mental faculty, or requiring medical intervention, including, but not limited to, hospitalization, surgery, or physical rehabilitation.

HISTORY:

Added Stats 2012 ch 659 § 1 (AB 40), effective January 1, 2013.

§ 15610.70. Undue influence

(a) "Undue influence" means excessive persuasion that causes another person to act or refrain from acting by overcoming that person's free will and results in inequity. In determining whether a result was produced by undue influence, all of the following shall be considered:

(1) The vulnerability of the victim. Evidence of vulnerability may include, but is not limited to, incapacity, illness, disability, injury, age, education, impaired cognitive function, emotional distress, isolation, or dependency, and whether the influencer knew or should have known of the alleged victim's vulnerability.

(2) The influencer's apparent authority. Evidence of apparent authority may include, but is not limited to, status as a fiduciary, family member, care provider, health care professional, legal professional, spiritual adviser, expert, or other qualification.

(3) The actions or tactics used by the influencer. Evidence of actions or tactics used may include, but is not limited to, all of the following:

(A) Controlling necessaries of life, medication, the victim's interactions with others, access to information, or sleep.

(B) Use of affection, intimidation, or coercion.

(C) Initiation of changes in personal or property rights, use of haste or secrecy in effecting those changes, effecting changes at inappropriate times and places, and claims of expertise in effecting changes.

(4) The equity of the result. Evidence of the equity of the result may include, but is not limited to, the economic consequences to the victim, any divergence from the victim's prior intent or course of conduct or dealing, the relationship of the value conveyed to the value of any services or consideration received, or the appropriateness of the change in light of the length and nature of the relationship.

(b) Evidence of an inequitable result, without more, is not sufficient to prove undue influence.

HISTORY:

Added Stats 2013 ch 668 § 3 (AB 140), effective January 1, 2014.

ARTICLE 3

MANDATORY AND NONMANDATORY REPORTS OF ABUSE

Section

15630. Duties of mandated reporter; Punishment for failure to report.
15630.1. Civil penalty for failure to report financial abuse.
15630.2. Report suspected financial abuse by mandated reporter; Elder or dependent adult; Liability; Definitions.
15631. Other persons who may report abuse.
15632. Application of physician-patient or psychotherapist-patient privilege.

HISTORY: Added Stats 1982 ch 1184 § 3, as Article 4. The heading of Article 4, which formerly read "Reports of Abuse," amended and renumbered to read as above by Stats 1994 ch 594 § 5.
Former Article 3, entitled "Data Base Method of Reporting Requirements," consisting of §§ 15620–15621, was added Stats 1982 ch 1184 § 3 and repealed Stats 1994 ch 594 § 4.

§ 15630. Duties of mandated reporter; Punishment for failure to report

(a) A person who has assumed full or intermittent responsibility for the care or custody of an elder or dependent adult, whether or not they receive compensation, including administrators, supervisors, and any licensed staff of a public or private facility that provides care or services for elder or dependent adults, or any elder or dependent adult care custodian, health practitioner, clergy member, or employee of a county adult protective services agency or a local law enforcement agency, is a mandated reporter.

(b)(1) A mandated reporter who, in their professional capacity, or within the scope of their employment, has observed or has knowledge of an incident that reasonably appears to be physical abuse, as defined in Section 15610.63, abandonment, abduction, isolation, financial abuse, or neglect, or is told by an elder or dependent adult that they have experienced behavior, including an act or omission, constituting physical abuse, as defined in Section 15610.63, abandonment, abduction, isolation, financial abuse, or neglect, or reasonably suspects that abuse, shall report the known or suspected instance of abuse by telephone or through a confidential internet reporting tool, as authorized by Section 15658, immediately or as soon as practicably possible. If reported by telephone, a written report shall be sent, or an internet report shall be made through the confidential internet reporting tool established in Section 15658, within two working days.

(A) If the suspected or alleged abuse is physical abuse, as defined in Section 15610.63, and the abuse occurred in a long-term care facility, except a state mental health hospital or a state developmental center, the following shall occur:

Misc.

(i) If the suspected abuse results in serious bodily injury, a telephone report shall be made to the local law enforcement agency immediately, but also no later than within two hours of the mandated reporter observing, obtaining knowledge of, or suspecting the physical abuse, and a written report shall be made to the local ombudsman, the corresponding licensing agency, and the local law enforcement agency within two hours of the mandated reporter observing, obtaining knowledge of, or suspecting the physical abuse.

(ii) If the suspected abuse does not result in serious bodily injury, a telephone report shall be made to the local law enforcement agency within 24 hours of the mandated reporter observing, obtaining knowledge of, or suspecting the physical abuse, and a written report shall be made to the local ombudsman, the corresponding licensing agency, and the local law enforcement agency within 24 hours of the mandated reporter observing, obtaining knowledge of, or suspecting the physical abuse.

(iii) When the suspected abuse is allegedly caused by a resident with a physician's diagnosis of dementia, and there is no serious bodily injury, as reasonably determined by the mandated reporter, drawing upon their training or experience, the reporter shall report to the local ombudsman or law enforcement agency by telephone, immediately or as soon as practicably possible, and by written report, within 24 hours.

(iv) When applicable, reports made pursuant to clauses (i) and (ii) shall be deemed to satisfy the reporting requirements of the federal Elder Justice Act of 2009, as set out in Subtitle H of the federal Patient Protection and Affordable Care Act (Public Law 111-148), Section 1418.91ofthe Health and Safety Code, and Section 72541 of Title 22 of the California Code of Regulations. When a local law enforcement agency receives an initial report of suspected abuse in a long-term care facility pursuant to this subparagraph, the local law enforcement agency may coordinate efforts with the local ombudsman to provide the most immediate and appropriate response warranted to investigate the mandated report. The local ombudsman and local law enforcement agencies may collaborate to develop protocols to implement this subparagraph.

(B) Notwithstanding the rulemaking provisions of Chapter 3.5 (commencing with Section 11340) of Part 1 of Division 3 of Title 2 of the Government Code, or any other law, the department may implement subparagraph (A), in whole or in part, by means of all-county letters, provider bulletins, or other similar instructions without taking regulatory action.

(C) If the suspected or alleged abuse is abuse other than physical abuse, and the abuse occurred in a long-term care facility, except a state mental health hospital or a state developmental center, a telephone report and a written report shall be made to the local ombudsman or the local law enforcement agency.

(D) With regard to abuse reported pursuant to subparagraph (C), the local ombudsman and the local law enforcement agency shall, as soon as practicable, except in the case of an emergency or pursuant to a report

Misc.

required to be made pursuant to clause (v), in which case these actions shall be taken immediately, do all of the following:

(i) Report to the State Department of Public Health any case of known or suspected abuse occurring in a long-term health care facility, as defined in subdivision (a) of Section 1418 of the Health and Safety Code.

(ii) Report to the State Department of Social Services any case of known or suspected abuse occurring in a residential care facility for the elderly, as defined in Section 1569.2 of the Health and Safety Code, or in an adult day program, as defined in paragraph (2) of subdivision (a) of Section 1502 of the Health and Safety Code.

(iii) Report to the State Department of Public Health and the California Department of Aging any case of known or suspected abuse occurring in an adult day health care center, as defined in subdivision (b) of Section 1570.7 of the Health and Safety Code.

(iv) Report to the Division of Medi-Cal Fraud and Elder Abuse any case of known or suspected criminal activity.

(v) Report all cases of known or suspected physical abuse and financial abuse to the local district attorney's office in the county where the abuse occurred.

(E)(i) If the suspected or alleged abuse or neglect occurred in a state mental hospital or a state developmental center, and the suspected or alleged abuse or neglect resulted in any of the following incidents, a report shall be made immediately, but no later than within two hours of the mandated reporter observing, obtaining knowledge of, or suspecting abuse, to designated investigators of the State Department of State Hospitals or the State Department of Developmental Services, and to the local law enforcement agency:

(I) A death.

(II) A sexual assault, as defined in Section 15610.63.

(III) An assault with a deadly weapon, as described in Section 245 of the Penal Code, by a nonresident of the state mental hospital or state developmental center.

(IV) An assault with force likely to produce great bodily injury, as described in Section 245 of the Penal Code.

(V) An injury to the genitals when the cause of the injury is undetermined.

(VI) A broken bone when the cause of the break is undetermined.

(ii) All other reports of suspected or alleged abuse or neglect that occurred in a state mental hospital or a state developmental center shall be made immediately, but no later than within two hours of the mandated reporter observing, obtaining knowledge of, or suspecting abuse, to designated investigators of the State Department of State Hospitals or the State Department of Developmental Services, or to the local law enforcement agency.

(iii) When a local law enforcement agency receives an initial report of suspected or alleged abuse or neglect in a state mental hospital or a state developmental center pursuant to clause (i), the local law enforcement agency shall coordinate efforts with the designated investigators of the State Department of State Hospitals or the State Department of Developmental Services to provide the most immediate and appropriate response warranted to investigate the mandated report. The designated investigators of the State Department of State Hospitals or the State Department of Developmental Services and local law enforcement agencies may collaborate to develop protocols to implement this clause.

(iv) Except in an emergency, the local law enforcement agency shall, as soon as practicable, report any case of known or suspected criminal activity to the Division of Medi-Cal Fraud and Elder Abuse.

(v) Notwithstanding any other law, a mandated reporter who is required to report pursuant to Section 4427.5 shall not be required to report under clause (i).

(F) If the abuse has occurred in any place other than a long-term care facility, a state mental hospital, or a state developmental center, the report shall be made to the adult protective services agency or the local law enforcement agency.

(2)(A) A mandated reporter who is a clergy member who acquires knowledge or reasonable suspicion of elder or dependent adult abuse during a penitential communication is not subject to paragraph (1). For purposes of this subdivision, "penitential communication" means a communication that is intended to be in confidence, including, but not limited to, a sacramental confession made to a clergy member who, in the course of the discipline or practice of their church, denomination, or organization is authorized or accustomed to hear those communications and under the discipline tenets, customs, or practices of their church, denomination, or organization, has a duty to keep those communications secret.

(B) This subdivision shall not modify or limit a clergy member's duty to report known or suspected elder and dependent adult abuse if they are acting in the capacity of a care custodian, health practitioner, or employee of an adult protective services agency.

(C) Notwithstanding this section, a clergy member who is not regularly employed on either a full-time or part-time basis in a long-term care facility or does not have care or custody of an elder or dependent adult shall not be responsible for reporting abuse or neglect that is not reasonably observable or discernible to a reasonably prudent person having no specialized training or experience in elder or dependent care.

(3)(A) A mandated reporter who is a physician and surgeon, a registered nurse, or a psychotherapist, as defined in Section 1010 of the Evidence Code, shall not be required to report, pursuant to paragraph (1), an incident if all of the following conditions exist:

(i) The mandated reporter has been told by an elder or dependent adult that they have experienced behavior constituting physical abuse, as defined in Section 15610.63, abandonment, abduction, isolation, financial abuse, or neglect.

(ii) The mandated reporter is unaware of any independent evidence that corroborates the statement that the abuse has occurred.

(iii) The elder or dependent adult has been diagnosed with a mental illness or dementia, or is the subject of a court-ordered conservatorship because of a mental illness or dementia.

(iv) In the exercise of clinical judgment, the physician and surgeon, the registered nurse, or the psychotherapist, as defined in Section 1010 of the Evidence Code, reasonably believes that the abuse did not occur.

(B) This paragraph shall not impose upon mandated reporters a duty to investigate a known or suspected incident of abuse and shall not lessen or restrict any existing duty of mandated reporters.

(4)(A) In a long-term care facility, a mandated reporter shall not be required to report as a suspected incident of abuse, as defined in Section 15610.07, an incident if all of the following conditions exist:

(i) The mandated reporter is aware that there is a proper plan of care.

(ii) The mandated reporter is aware that the plan of care was properly provided or executed.

(iii) A physical, mental, or medical injury occurred as a result of care provided pursuant to clause (i) or (ii).

(iv) The mandated reporter reasonably believes that the injury was not the result of abuse.

(B) This paragraph shall neither require a mandated reporter to seek, nor preclude a mandated reporter from seeking, information regarding a known or suspected incident of abuse before reporting. This paragraph shall apply only to those categories of mandated reporters that the State Department of Public Health determines, upon approval by the Division of Medi-Cal Fraud and Elder Abuse and the state long-term care ombudsman, have access to plans of care and have the training and experience necessary to determine whether the conditions specified in this section have been met.

(c)(1) Any mandated reporter who has knowledge, or reasonably suspects, that types of elder or dependent adult abuse for which reports are not mandated have been inflicted upon an elder or dependent adult, or that their emotional well-being is endangered in any other way, may report the known or suspected instance of abuse.

(2) If the suspected or alleged abuse occurred in a long-term care facility other than a state mental health hospital or a state developmental center, the report may be made to the long-term care ombudsman program. Except in an emergency, the local ombudsman shall report any case of known or suspected abuse to the State Department of Public Health and any case of known or suspected criminal activity to the Division of Medi-Cal Fraud and Elder Abuse, as soon as is practicable.

(3) If the suspected or alleged abuse occurred in a state mental health hospital or a state developmental center, the report may be made to the designated investigator of the State Department of State Hospitals or the State Department of Developmental Services or to a local law enforcement agency. Except in an emergency, the local law enforcement agency shall report any case of known or suspected criminal activity to the Division of Medi-Cal Fraud and Elder Abuse, as soon as is practicable.

(4) If the suspected or alleged abuse occurred in a place other than a place described in paragraph (2) or (3), the report may be made to the county adult protective services agency.

(5) If the conduct involves criminal activity not covered in subdivision (b), it may be immediately reported to the appropriate law enforcement agency.

(d) If two or more mandated reporters are present and jointly have knowledge or reasonably suspect that types of abuse of an elder or a dependent adult for which a report is or is not mandated have occurred, and there is agreement among them, the telephone report or internet report, as authorized by Section 15658, may be made by a member of the team selected by mutual agreement, and a single report may be made and signed by the selected member of the reporting team. Any member who has knowledge that the member designated to report has failed to do so shall thereafter make the report.

(e) A telephone report or internet report, as authorized by Section 15658, of a known or suspected instance of elder or dependent adult abuse shall include, if known, the name of the person making the report, the name and age of the elder or dependent adult, the present location of the elder or dependent adult, the names and addresses of family members or any other adult responsible for the elder's or dependent adult's care, the nature and extent of the elder's or dependent adult's condition, the date of the incident, and any other information, including information that led that person to suspect elder or dependent adult abuse, as requested by the agency receiving the report.

(f) The reporting duties under this section are individual, and no supervisor or administrator shall impede or inhibit the reporting duties, and no person making the report shall be subject to any sanction for making the report. However, internal procedures to facilitate reporting, ensure confidentiality, and apprise supervisors and administrators of reports may be established, provided they are not inconsistent with this chapter.

(g)(1) Whenever this section requires a county adult protective services agency to report to a law enforcement agency, the law enforcement agency shall, immediately upon request, provide a copy of its investigative report concerning the reported matter to that county adult protective services agency.

(2) Whenever this section requires a law enforcement agency to report to a county adult protective services agency, the county adult protective services agency shall, immediately upon request, provide to that law enforcement agency a copy of its investigative report concerning the reported matter.

(3) The requirement to disclose investigative reports pursuant to this subdivision shall not include the disclosure of social services records or case files that are confidential, nor shall this subdivision allow disclosure of any reports or records if the disclosure would be prohibited by any other state or federal law.

(h) Failure to report, or impeding or inhibiting a report of, physical abuse, as defined in Section 15610.63, abandonment, abduction, isolation, financial abuse, or neglect of an elder or dependent adult, in violation of this section, is a misdemeanor, punishable by not more than six months in the county jail, by a fine of not more than one thousand dollars ($1,000), or by both that fine and imprisonment. A mandated reporter who willfully fails to report, or impedes or inhibits a report of, physical abuse, as defined in Section 15610.63, abandonment, abduction, isolation, financial abuse, or neglect of an elder or dependent adult, in violation of this section, if that abuse results in death or great bodily injury, shall be punished by not more than one year in a county jail, by a fine of not more than five thousand dollars ($5,000), or by both that fine and imprisonment. If a mandated reporter intentionally conceals their failure to report an incident known by the mandated reporter to be abuse or severe neglect under this section, the failure to report is a continuing offense until a law enforcement agency specified in paragraph (1) of subdivision (b) of Section 15630 discovers the offense.

(i) For purposes of this section, "dependent adult" has the same meaning as that term is defined in Section 15610.23.

HISTORY:

Added Stats 1994 ch 594 § 7 (SB 1681). Amended Stats 1995 ch 813 § 1 (AB 1836); Stats 1998 ch 946 § 8 (SB 2199), ch 980 § 1 (AB 1780); Stats 1999 ch 236 § 1 (AB 739); Stats 2002 ch 54 § 9 (AB 255); Stats 2004 ch 823 § 19 (AB 20); Stats 2005 ch 163 § 2 (AB 1188), effective January 1, 2006; Stats 2008 ch 481 § 1 (AB 2100), effective January 1, 2009; Stats 2011 ch 373 § 1 (SB 718), effective January 1, 2012; Stats 2012 ch 24 § 202 (AB 1470), effective June 27, 2012, ch 660 § 4 (SB 1051), effective September 27, 2012, operative until January 1, 2013, ch 660 § 4.5 (SB 1051), effective September 27, 2012, operative January 1, 2013; Stats 2013 ch 76 § 223 (AB 383), effective January 1, 2014, ch 673 § 3 (AB 602), effective January 1, 2014 (ch 673 prevails); Stats 2021 ch 85 § 66 (AB 135), effective July 16, 2021; Stats 2021 ch 554 § 14 (SB 823), effective January 1, 2022.

§ 15630.1. Civil penalty for failure to report financial abuse

(a) As used in this section, "mandated reporter of suspected financial abuse of an elder or dependent adult" means all officers and employees of financial institutions.

(b) As used in this section, the term "financial institution" means any of the following:

(1) A depository institution, as defined in Section 3(c) of the Federal Deposit Insurance Act (12 U.S.C. Sec. 1813(c)).

(2) An institution-affiliated party, as defined in Section 3(u) of the Federal Deposit Insurance Act (12 U.S.C. Sec. 1813(u)).

(3) A federal credit union or state credit union, as defined in Section 101 of the Federal Credit Union Act (12 U.S.C. Sec. 1752), including, but not limited to, an institution-affiliated party of a credit union, as defined in Section 206(r) of the Federal Credit Union Act (12 U.S.C. Sec. 1786(r)).

(c) As used in this section, "financial abuse" has the same meaning as in Section 15610.30.

(d)(1) Any mandated reporter of suspected financial abuse of an elder or dependent adult who has direct contact with the elder or dependent adult or who reviews or approves the elder or dependent adult's financial documents, records, or transactions, in connection with providing financial services with respect to an elder or dependent adult, and who, within the scope of his or her employment or professional practice, has observed or has knowledge of an incident, that is directly related to the transaction or matter that is within that scope of employment or professional practice, that reasonably appears to be financial abuse, or who reasonably suspects that abuse, based solely on the information before him or her at the time of reviewing or approving the document, record, or transaction in the case of mandated reporters who do not have direct contact with the elder or dependent adult, shall report the known or suspected instance of financial abuse by telephone or through a confidential Internet reporting tool, as authorized pursuant to Section 15658, immediately, or as soon as practicably possible. If reported by telephone, a written report shall be sent, or an Internet report shall be made through the confidential Internet reporting tool established in Section 15658, within two working days to the local adult protective services agency or the local law enforcement agency.

(2) When two or more mandated reporters jointly have knowledge or reasonably suspect that financial abuse of an elder or a dependent adult for which the report is mandated has occurred, and when there is an agreement among them, the telephone report or Internet report, as authorized by Section 15658, may be made by a member of the reporting team who is selected by mutual agreement. A single report may be made and signed by the selected member of the reporting team. Any member of the team who has knowledge that the member designated to report has failed to do so shall thereafter make that report.

(3) If the mandated reporter knows that the elder or dependent adult resides in a long-term care facility, as defined in Section 15610.47, the report shall be made to the local ombudsman or local law enforcement agency.

(e) An allegation by the elder or dependent adult, or any other person, that financial abuse has occurred is not sufficient to trigger the reporting requirement under this section if both of the following conditions are met:

(1) The mandated reporter of suspected financial abuse of an elder or dependent adult is aware of no other corroborating or independent evidence of the alleged financial abuse of an elder or dependent adult. The mandated reporter of suspected financial abuse of an elder or dependent adult is not required to investigate any accusations.

(2) In the exercise of his or her professional judgment, the mandated reporter of suspected financial abuse of an elder or dependent adult reasonably believes that financial abuse of an elder or dependent adult did not occur.

(f) Failure to report financial abuse under this section shall be subject to a civil penalty not exceeding one thousand dollars ($1,000) or if the failure to report is willful, a civil penalty not exceeding five thousand dollars ($5,000), which shall be paid by the financial institution that is the employer of the mandated reporter to the party bringing the action. Subdivision (h) of Section 15630 shall not apply to violations of this section.

(g)(1) The civil penalty provided for in subdivision (f) shall be recovered only in a civil action brought against the financial institution by the Attorney General, district attorney, or county counsel. No action shall be brought under this section by any person other than the Attorney General, district attorney, or county counsel. Multiple actions for the civil penalty may not be brought for the same violation.

(2) Nothing in the Financial Elder Abuse Reporting Act of 2005 shall be construed to limit, expand, or otherwise modify any civil liability or remedy that may exist under this or any other law.

(h) As used in this section, "suspected financial abuse of an elder or dependent adult" occurs when a person who is required to report under subdivision (a) observes or has knowledge of behavior or unusual circumstances or transactions, or a pattern of behavior or unusual circumstances or transactions, that would lead an individual with like training or experience, based on the same facts, to form a reasonable belief that an elder or dependent adult is the victim of financial abuse as defined in Section 15610.30.

(i) Reports of suspected financial abuse of an elder or dependent adult made by an employee or officer of a financial institution pursuant to this section are covered under subdivision (b) of Section 47 of the Civil Code.

(j)(1) A mandated reporter of suspected financial abuse of an elder or dependent adult is authorized to not honor a power of attorney described in Division 4.5 (commencing with Section 4000) of the Probate Code as to an attorney-in-fact, if the mandated reporter of suspected financial abuse of an elder or dependent adult makes a report to an adult protective services agency or a local law enforcement agency of any state that the principal may be subject to financial abuse, as described in this chapter or as defined in similar laws of another state, by that attorney-in-fact or person acting for or with that attorney-in-fact.

(2) If a mandated reporter of suspected financial abuse of an elder or dependent adult does not honor a power of attorney as to an attorney-in-fact pursuant to paragraph (1), the power of attorney shall remain enforceable as to every other attorney-in-fact also designated in the power of attorney about whom a report has not been made.

(3) For purposes of this subdivision, the terms "principal" and "attorney-in-fact" shall have the same meanings as those terms are used in Division 4.5 (commencing with Section 4000) of the Probate Code.

HISTORY:

Added Stats 2005 ch 140 § 4 (SB 1018), effective January 1, 2006, operative January 1, 2007, repealed January 1, 2013. Amended Stats 2011 ch 372 § 1 (SB 33), effective January 1, 2012, ch 373 § 2.5 (SB 718), effective January 1, 2012; Stats 2017 ch 408 § 1 (AB 611), effective January 1, 2018.

§ 15630.2. Report suspected financial abuse by mandated reporter; Elder or dependent adult; Liability; Definitions

(a) For purposes of this section, the following terms have the following definitions:

(1) "Financial abuse" has the same meaning as in Section 15610.30.

(2) "Broker-dealer" has the same meaning as in Section 25004 of the Corporations Code.

(3) "Investment adviser" has the same meaning as in Section 25009 of the Corporations Code.

(4) "Mandated reporter of suspected financial abuse of an elder or dependent adult" means a broker-dealer or an investment adviser.

(b)(1) Any mandated reporter of suspected financial abuse of an elder or dependent adult who has direct contact with the elder or dependent adult or who reviews or approves the elder or dependent adult's financial documents, records, or transactions, in connection with providing financial services with respect to an elder or dependent adult, and who, within the scope of their employment or professional practice, has observed or has knowledge of an incident that is directly related to the transaction or matter that is within that scope of employment or professional practice, that reasonably appears to be financial abuse, or who reasonably suspects that abuse, based solely on the information before them at the time of reviewing or approving the document, record, or transaction in the case of mandated reporters who do not have direct contact with the elder or dependent adult, shall report the known or suspected instance of financial abuse by telephone or through a confidential internet reporting tool, as authorized pursuant to Section 15658, immediately, or as soon as practicably possible. If reported by telephone, a written report shall be sent, or an internet report shall be made through the confidential internet reporting tool established in Section 15658, within two working days to the local adult protective services agency, the local law enforcement agency, and the Department of Financial Protection and Innovation.

(2) When two or more mandated reporters jointly have knowledge or reasonably suspect that financial abuse of an elder or a dependent adult for which the report is mandated has occurred, and when there is an agreement among them, the telephone report or internet report, as authorized by Section 15658, may be made by a member of the reporting team who is selected by mutual agreement. A single report may be made and signed by the selected member of the reporting team. Any member of the team who has knowledge that the member designated to report has failed to do so shall thereafter make that report.

(3) If the mandated reporter knows that the elder or dependent adult resides in a long-term care facility, as defined in Section 15610.47, the report shall be made to the local ombudsman, local law enforcement agency, and the Department of Financial Protection and Innovation.

(c) An allegation by the elder or dependent adult, or any other person, that financial abuse has occurred is not sufficient to trigger the reporting requirement under this section if both of the following conditions are met:

(1) The mandated reporter of suspected financial abuse of an elder or dependent adult is aware of no other corroborating or independent evidence of the alleged financial abuse of an elder or dependent adult. The mandated reporter of suspected financial abuse of an elder or dependent adult is not required to investigate any accusations.

(2) In the exercise of their professional judgment, the mandated reporter of suspected financial abuse of an elder or dependent adult reasonably believes that financial abuse of an elder or dependent adult did not occur.

(d) Failure to report financial abuse under this section shall be subject to a civil penalty not exceeding one thousand dollars ($1,000) or if the failure to report is willful, a civil penalty not exceeding five thousand dollars ($5,000), which shall be paid by the employer of the mandated reporter of suspected financial abuse of an elder or dependent adult to the party bringing the action. Subdivision (h) of Section 15630 shall not apply to violations of this section.

(e) The civil penalty provided for in subdivision (d) shall be recovered only in a civil action brought against the broker-dealer or investment adviser by the Attorney General, district attorney, or county counsel. An action shall not be brought under this section by any person other than the Attorney General, district attorney, or county counsel. Multiple actions for the civil penalty may not be brought for the same violation.

(f) As used in this section, "suspected financial abuse of an elder or dependent adult" occurs when a person who is required to report under subdivision (b) observes or has knowledge of behavior or unusual circumstances or transactions, or a pattern of behavior or unusual circumstances or transactions, that would lead an individual with like training or experience, based on the same facts, to form a reasonable belief that an elder or dependent adult is the victim of financial abuse as defined in Section 15610.30.

(g) Reports of suspected financial abuse of an elder or dependent adult made pursuant to this section are covered under subdivision (b) of Section 47 of the Civil Code.

(h)(1) A mandated reporter of suspected financial abuse of an elder or dependent adult who makes a report pursuant to this section may notify any trusted contact person who had previously been designated by the elder or dependent adult to receive notification of any known or suspected financial abuse, unless the trusted contact person is suspected of the financial abuse. This authority does not affect the ability of the mandated reporter to make any other notifications otherwise permitted by law.

(2) A mandated reporter of suspected financial abuse of an elder or dependent adult shall not be civilly liable for any notification made in good faith and with reasonable care pursuant to this subdivision.

(i)(1) A mandated reporter of suspected financial abuse of an elder or dependent adult is authorized to not honor a power of attorney described in Division 4.5 (commencing with Section 4000) of the Probate Code as to an attorney-in-fact, if the mandated reporter of suspected financial abuse of an elder or dependent adult makes a report to an adult protective services agency or a local law enforcement agency of any state that the principal may be subject to financial abuse, as described in this chapter or as defined in similar laws of another state, by that attorney-in-fact or person acting for or with that attorney-in-fact.

(2) If a mandated reporter of suspected financial abuse of an elder or dependent adult does not honor a power of attorney as to an attorney-in-fact pursuant to paragraph (1), the power of attorney shall remain enforceable as to every other attorney-in-fact also designated in the power of attorney about whom a report has not been made.

(3) For purposes of this subdivision, the terms "principal" and "attorney-in-fact" have the same meanings as those terms are used in Division 4.5 (commencing with Section 4000) of the Probate Code.

(j)(1) A mandated reporter of suspected financial abuse of an elder or dependent adult may temporarily delay a requested disbursement from, or a requested transaction involving, an account of an elder or dependent adult or an account to which an elder or dependent adult is a beneficiary if the mandated reporter meets all of following conditions:

(A) They have a reasonable belief, after initiating an internal review of the requested disbursement or transaction and the suspected financial abuse, that the requested disbursement or transaction may result in the financial abuse of an elder or dependent adult.

(B) Immediately, but no later than two business days after the requested disbursement or transaction is delayed, they provide written notification of the delay and the reason for the delay to all parties authorized to transact business on the account, unless a party is reasonably believed to have engaged in suspected financial abuse of the elder or dependent.

(C) Immediately, but no later than two business days after the requested disbursement or transaction is delayed, they notify the local county adult protective services agency, local law enforcement agency, and the Department of Financial Protection and Innovation about the delay.

Misc.

(D) They provide any updates relevant to the report to the local adult protective services agency, the local law enforcement agency, and the Department of Financial Protection and Innovation.

(2) Any delay of a requested disbursement or transaction authorized by this subdivision shall expire upon either of the following, whichever is sooner:

(A) A determination by the mandated reporter that the requested disbursement or transaction will not result in financial abuse of the elder or dependent adult provided that the mandated reporter first consults with the local county adult protective services agency, local law enforcement agency, and the Department of Financial Protection and Innovation, and receives no objection from those entities.

(B) Fifteen business days after the date on which the mandated reporter first delayed the requested disbursement or transaction, unless the adult protective services agency, local law enforcement agency, or the Department of Financial Protection and Innovation requests that the mandated reporter extend the delay, in which case the delay shall expire no more than 25 business days after the date on which the mandated reporter first delayed the requested disbursement or transaction, unless sooner terminated by the adult protective services agency, local law enforcement agency, the Department of Financial Protection and Innovation, or an order of a court of competent jurisdiction.

(3) A court of competent jurisdiction may enter an order extending the delay of the requested disbursement or transaction or may order other protective relief based on the petition of the adult protective services agency, the mandated reporter who initiated the delay, or any other interested party.

(4) A mandated reporter of suspected financial abuse of an elder or dependent adult shall not be civilly liable for any temporary disbursement delay or transaction made in good faith and with reasonable care on an account pursuant to this subdivision.

(k) Notwithstanding any provision of law, a local adult protective services agency, a local law enforcement agency, and the Department of Financial Protection and Innovation may disclose to a mandated reporter of suspected financial abuse of an elder or dependent adult or their employer, upon request, the general status or final disposition of any investigation that arose from a report made by that mandated reporter of suspected financial abuse of an elder or dependent adult pursuant to this section.

HISTORY:

Added Stats 2019 ch 272 § 1 (SB 496), effective January 1, 2020. Amended Stats 2022 ch 452 § 210 (SB 1498), effective January 1, 2023.

§ 15631. Other persons who may report abuse

(a) Any person who is not a mandated reporter under Section 15630, who knows, or reasonably suspects, that an elder or a dependent adult has been the victim of abuse may report that abuse to a long-term care ombudsman program or local law enforcement agency, or both the long-term care ombudsman program and local law enforcement agency when the abuse is alleged to have occurred in a long-term care facility.

(b) Any person who is not a mandated reporter under Section 15630, who knows, or reasonably suspects, that an elder or a dependent adult has been the victim of abuse in any place other than a long-term care facility may report the abuse to the county adult protective services agency or local law enforcement agency.

HISTORY:
Added Stats 1994 ch 594 § 9 (SB 1681). Amended Stats 2012 ch 659 § 3 (AB 40), effective January 1, 2013.

§ 15632. Application of physician-patient or psychotherapist-patient privilege

(a) In any court proceeding or administrative hearing, neither the physician-patient privilege nor the psychotherapist-patient privilege applies to the specific information reported pursuant to this chapter.

(b) Nothing in this chapter shall be interpreted as requiring an attorney to violate his or her oath and duties pursuant to Section 6067 or subdivision (e) of Section 6068 of the Business and Professions Code, and Article 3 (commencing with Section 950) of Chapter 4 of Division 8 of the Evidence Code.

HISTORY:
Added Stats 1994 ch 594 § 11 (SB 1681).

ARTICLE 4

CONFIDENTIALITY

Section
15633. Disclosure; Penalties.
15633.5. Other persons to whom disclosure may be made.
15634. Immunity from liability of persons authorized to report abuse; Attorney fees.

HISTORY: Heading added Stats 1994 ch 594 § 13. Former Article 4, entitled "Reports of Abuse," consisting of §§ 15630–15632, was added Stats 1982 ch 1184 § 3 and amended and renumbered Article 3 by Stats 1994 ch 594 § 5.

§ 15633. Disclosure; Penalties

(a) The reports made pursuant to Sections 15630, 15630.1, 15630.2, and 15631 shall be confidential and may be disclosed only as provided in subdivision (b). Any violation of the confidentiality required by this chapter is a misdemeanor punishable by not more than six months in the county jail, by a fine of five hundred dollars ($500), or by both that fine and imprisonment.

(b) Reports of suspected abuse of an elder or dependent adult and information contained in the report may be disclosed only to the following:

(1) Persons or agencies to whom disclosure of information or the identity of the reporting party is permitted under Section 15633.5.

(2)(A) Persons who are trained and qualified to serve on multidisciplinary personnel teams may disclose to one another information and records that are relevant to the prevention, identification, or treatment of abuse of elderly or dependent persons.

(B) Except as provided in subparagraph (A), any personnel of the multidisciplinary team or agency who receives information pursuant to this chapter shall be under the same obligations and subject to the same confidentiality penalties as the person disclosing or providing that information. The information obtained shall be maintained in a manner that ensures the maximum protection of privacy and confidentiality rights.

(3) A trusted contact person, as specified in subdivision (h) of Section 15630.2.

(c) This section does not allow disclosure of any reports or records relevant to the reports of abuse of an elder or dependent adult if the disclosure would be prohibited by any other provisions of state or federal law applicable to the reports or records relevant to the reports of the abuse, nor does it prohibit the disclosure by a financial institution, broker-dealer, or investment adviser of any reports or records relevant to the reports of abuse of an elder or dependent adult if the disclosure would be required of a financial institution, broker-dealer, or investment adviser by otherwise applicable state or federal law or court order.

(d) This section does not prohibit employees of a county's adult protective services agency or a county's child welfare agency from disclosing information with each other for the purpose of multidisciplinary teamwork in the prevention, intervention, management, or treatment of the abuse or neglect of a child or abuse or neglect of an elder or dependent adult.

HISTORY:

Added Stats 1994 ch 594 § 14 (SB 1681). Amended Stats 1998 ch 946 § 9 (SB 2199), ch 980 § 2 (AB 1780); Stats 2005 ch 140 § 5 (SB 1018), effective January 1, 2006, operative January 1, 2007, repealed January 1, 2013; Stats 2011 ch 372 § 2 (SB 33), effective January 1, 2012; Stats 2019 ch 272 § 2 (SB 496), effective January 1, 2020; Stats 2022 ch 506 § 2 (SB 1054), effective January 1, 2023.

§ 15633.5. Other persons to whom disclosure may be made

(a)(1) Information relevant to the incident of elder or dependent adult abuse shall be given to an investigator from an adult protective services agency, a local law enforcement agency, the office of the district attorney, the office of the public guardian, the probate court, the division, the Department of Financial Protection and Innovation, or an investigator of the Department of Consumer Affairs, Division of Investigation, who is investigating a known or suspected case of elder or dependent adult abuse.

(2)(A) If the incident of elder or dependent adult financial abuse may be within the jurisdiction of a federal law enforcement agency, information relevant to the incident may be given to the federal law enforcement agency for the sole purpose of investigating a financial crime committed against the elder or dependent adult.

(B) Information relevant to the incident of elder or dependent adult abuse may be provided to a local code enforcement agency for the sole purpose of investigating an unlicensed care facility where the health and safety of an elder or dependent adult resident is at risk.

(b) The identity of a person who reports under this chapter shall be confidential and disclosed only among the following agencies or persons representing an agency:

(1) An adult protective services agency.

(2) A long-term care ombudsperson program.
(3) A licensing agency.
(4) A local law enforcement agency.
(5) The office of the district attorney.
(6) The office of the public guardian.
(7) The probate court.
(8) The division.
(9) The Department of Financial Protection and Innovation.
(10) The Department of Consumer Affairs, Division of Investigation.
(11) Counsel representing an adult protective services agency.

(c) The identity of a person who reports pursuant to this chapter may also be disclosed under the following circumstances:

(1) To the district attorney in a criminal prosecution.
(2) When a person reporting waives confidentiality.
(3) By court order.

(d) Notwithstanding subdivisions (a) to (c), inclusive, a person reporting pursuant to Section 15631 shall not be required to include their name in the report.

HISTORY:

Added Stats 1994 ch 594 § 15 (SB 1681). Amended Stats 1998 ch 970 § 211 (AB 2802); Stats 2002 ch 54 § 10 (AB 255), ch 552 § 2 (AB 2735); Stats 2019 ch 272 § 3 (SB 496), effective January 1, 2020; Stats 2021 ch 554 § 15 (SB 823), effective January 1, 2022; Stats 2021 ch 621 § 1.5 (AB 636), effective January 1, 2022 (ch 621 prevails).

§ 15634. Immunity from liability of persons authorized to report abuse; Attorney fees

(a) No care custodian, clergy member, health practitioner, mandated reporter of suspected financial abuse of an elder or dependent adult, or employee of an adult protective services agency or a local law enforcement agency who reports a known or suspected instance of abuse of an elder or dependent adult shall be civilly or criminally liable for any report required or authorized by this article. Any other person reporting a known or suspected instance of abuse of an elder or dependent adult shall not incur civil or criminal liability as a result of any report authorized by this article, unless it can be proven that a false report was made and the person knew that the report was false. No person required to make a report pursuant to this article, or any person taking photographs at his or her discretion, shall incur any civil or criminal liability for taking photographs of a suspected victim of abuse of an elder or dependent adult or causing photographs to be taken of such a suspected victim or for disseminating the photographs with the reports required by this article. However, this section shall not be construed to grant immunity from this liability with respect to any other use of the photographs.

(b) No care custodian, clergy member, health practitioner, mandated reporter of suspected financial abuse of an elder or dependent adult, or employee of an adult protective services agency or a local law enforcement agency who, pursuant to a request from an adult protective services agency or a local law enforcement agency investigating a report of known or suspected abuse of an elder or dependent adult, provides the requesting agency with access to the victim of a known or suspected instance of abuse of an elder or dependent adult, shall incur civil or criminal liability as a result of providing that access.

(c) The Legislature finds that, even though it has provided immunity from liability to persons required to report abuse of an elder or dependent adult, immunity does not eliminate the possibility that actions may be brought against those persons based upon required reports of abuse. In order to further limit the financial hardship that those persons may incur as a result of fulfilling their legal responsibilities, it is necessary that they not be unfairly burdened by legal fees incurred in defending those actions. Therefore, a care custodian, clergy member, health practitioner, or an employee of an adult protective services agency or a local law enforcement agency may present to the Department of General Services a claim for reasonable attorneys' fees incurred in any action against that person on the basis of making a report required or authorized by this article if the court has dismissed the action upon a demurrer or motion for summary judgment made by that person, or if he or she prevails in the action. The Department of General Services shall allow that claim if the requirements of this subdivision are met, and the claim shall be paid from an appropriation to be made for that purpose. Attorneys' fees awarded pursuant to this section shall not exceed an hourly rate greater than the rate charged by the Attorney General at the time the award is made and shall not exceed an aggregate amount of fifty thousand dollars ($50,000). This subdivision shall not apply if a public entity has provided for the defense of the action pursuant to Section 995 of the Government Code.

HISTORY:
Added Stats 1985 ch 1164 § 11, effective September 28, 1985. Amended Stats 1986 ch 769 § 14, effective September 15, 1986; Stats 1990 ch 241 § 2 (SB 1911); Stats 2002 ch 54 § 11 (AB 255); Stats 2005 ch 140 § 7 (SB 1018), effective January 1, 2006, repealed January 1, 2013; Stats 2011 ch 372 § 4 (SB 33), effective January 1, 2012; Stats 2016 ch 31 § 285 (SB 836), effective June 27, 2016.

ARTICLE 8

PROSECUTION OF ELDER AND DEPENDENT ADULT ABUSE CASES

Section
15656. Penalties for abuse of elder or dependent adult.

HISTORY: Added Stats 1994 ch 594 § 23.

§ 15656. Penalties for abuse of elder or dependent adult

(a) Any person who knows or reasonably should know that a person is an elder or dependent adult and who, under circumstances or conditions likely to produce great bodily harm or death, willfully causes or permits any elder or dependent adult to suffer, or inflicts unjustifiable physical pain or mental suffering upon him or her, or having the care or custody of any elder or dependent adult, willfully causes or permits the person or health of the elder or dependent adult to be injured, or willfully causes or permits the elder or dependent adult to be placed in a situation such that his or her person or health is endangered, is punishable by imprisonment in the county jail not exceeding one year, or in the state prison for two, three, or four years.

(b) Any person who knows or reasonably should know that a person is an elder or dependent adult and who, under circumstances or conditions other than those likely to produce great bodily harm or death, willfully causes or permits any elder or dependent adult to suffer, or inflicts unjustifiable physical pain or mental suffering on him or her, or having the care or custody of any elder or dependent adult, willfully causes or permits the person or health of the elder or dependent adult to be injured or willfully causes or permits the elder or dependent adult to be placed in a situation such that his or her person or health may be endangered, is guilty of a misdemeanor.

(c) Any caretaker of an elder or a dependent adult who violates any provision of law prescribing theft or embezzlement, with respect to the property of that elder or dependent adult, is punishable by imprisonment in the county jail not exceeding one year, or in the state prison for two, three, or four years when the money, labor, or real or personal property taken is of a value exceeding nine hundred fifty dollars ($950), and by a fine not exceeding one thousand dollars ($1,000), or by imprisonment in the county jail not exceeding one year, or by both that imprisonment and fine, when the money, labor, or real or personal property taken is of a value not exceeding nine hundred fifty dollars ($950).

(d) As used in this section, "caretaker" means any person who has the care, custody, or control of or who stands in a position of trust with, an elder or a dependent adult.

(e) Conduct covered in subdivision (b) of Section 15610.57 shall not be subject to this section.

HISTORY:

Added Stats 1994 ch 594 § 23 (SB 1681). Amended Stats 2004 ch 886 § 2 (AB 2611); Stats 2009–2010 3d Ex Sess ch 28 § 57 (SBX3 18), effective January 25, 2010.

ARTICLE 10

EMPLOYEE STATEMENT

Section

15659. Statement as to knowledge of compliance with reporting requirements.

HISTORY: Added Stats 1994 ch 594 § 25.

Misc.

§ 15659. Statement as to knowledge of compliance with reporting requirements

(a) Any person who enters into employment on or after January 1, 1995, as a care custodian, clergy member, health practitioner, or with an adult protective services agency or a local law enforcement agency, prior to commencing his or her employment and as a prerequisite to that employment, shall sign a statement on a form that shall be provided by the prospective employer, to the effect that he or she has knowledge of Section 15630 and will comply with its provisions. The employer shall provide a copy of Section 15630 to the employee. The statement shall inform the employee that he or she is a mandated reporter and inform the employee of his or her reporting obligations under Section 15630. The signed statement shall be retained by the employer.

(b) Agencies or facilities that employ persons who were employed prior to January 1, 1995, and who are required to make reports pursuant to Section 15630, shall inform those persons of their responsibility to make reports by delivering to them a copy of the statement specified in subdivision (a).

(c) The cost of printing, distribution, and filing of these statements shall be borne by the employer.

(d) On and after January 1, 1995, when a person is issued a state license or certificate to engage in a profession or occupation the members of which are required to make a report pursuant to Section 15630, the state agency issuing the license or certificate shall send to the person a statement substantially similar to the one contained in subdivision (a) at the same time that it transmits to the person the document indicating licensure or certification.

(e) As an alternative to the procedure required by subdivision (d), a state agency may cause the required statement to be printed on all application forms for a license or certificate printed on or after January 1, 1995.

(f) The retention of statements required by subdivision (a), and the delivery of statements required by subdivision (b), shall be the full extent of the employer's duty pursuant to this section. The failure of any employee or other person associated with the employer to report abuse of elders or dependent adults pursuant to Section 15630 or otherwise meet the requirements of this chapter shall be the sole responsibility of that person. The employer or facility shall incur no civil or other liability for the failure of these persons to comply with the requirements of this chapter.

HISTORY:

Added Stats 1994 ch 594 § 25 (SB 1681). Amended Stats 1998 ch 946 § 12 (SB 2199); Stats 2002 ch 54 § 12.7 (AB 255).

ADMINISTRATIVE PROCEDURE ACT AND ADMINISTRATIVE ADJUDICATIONS

EXTRACTED FROM

CODE OF CIVIL PROCEDURE

Part
4. Miscellaneous Provisions.

PART 4

MISCELLANEOUS PROVISIONS

Title
3. Of the Production of Evidence.

HISTORY: The heading of Part 4, which formerly read "Evidence," amended to read as above by Stats 1965 ch 299 § 23, operative January 1, 1967.

TITLE 3

OF THE PRODUCTION OF EVIDENCE

Chapter
2. Means of Production.

HISTORY: Enacted 1872.

CHAPTER 2

MEANS OF PRODUCTION

Section
1985. "Subpoena"; Issuance; Affidavit.
1985.1. Agreement to appear at time not specified in subpoena.
1985.2. Subpoena requiring attendance of witness; Notice.
1985.3. Subpoena duces tecum for production of personal records; Definitions; Application of section.
1985.4. Production of consumer records maintained by state or local agency.
1985.6. Subpoena duces tecum for production of employment records; Definitions, Procedures and requirements; Application of section and exceptions.
1987. Service of subpoena, or of written notice.

HISTORY: Enacted 1872.

§ 1985. "Subpoena"; Issuance; Affidavit

(a) The process by which the attendance of a witness is required is the subpoena. It is a writ or order directed to a person and requiring the person's attendance at a particular time and place to testify as a witness. It may also require a witness to bring any books, documents, electronically stored information, or other things under the witness's control which the witness is bound by law to produce in evidence. When a county recorder is using the microfilm system for recording, and a witness is subpoenaed to present a record, the witness shall be deemed to have complied with the subpoena if the witness produces a certified copy thereof.

(b) A copy of an affidavit shall be served with a subpoena duces tecum issued before trial, showing good cause for the production of the matters and things described in the subpoena, specifying the exact matters or things desired to be produced, setting forth in full detail the materiality thereof to the issues involved in the case, and stating that the witness has the desired matters or things in his or her possession or under his or her control.

(c) The clerk, or a judge, shall issue a subpoena or subpoena duces tecum signed and sealed but otherwise in blank to a party requesting it, who shall fill it in before service. An attorney at law who is the attorney of record in an action or proceeding, may sign and issue a subpoena to require attendance before the court in which the action or proceeding is pending or at the trial of an issue therein, or upon the taking of a deposition in an action or proceeding pending therein; the subpoena in such a case need not be sealed. An attorney at law who is the attorney of record in an action or proceeding, may sign and issue a subpoena duces tecum to require production of the matters or things described in the subpoena.

HISTORY:

Enacted 1872. Amended Stats 1933 ch 567 § 1; Stats 1961 ch 496 § 1; Stats 1967 ch 431 § 1; Stats 1968 ch 95 § 1; Stats 1979 ch 458 § 1; Stats 1982 ch 452 § 1; Stats 1986 ch 603 § 3; Stats 1990 ch 511 § 1 (SB 163); Stats 2012 ch 72 § 1 (SB 1574), effective January 1, 2013.

§ 1985.1. Agreement to appear at time not specified in subpoena

Any person who is subpoenaed to appear at a session of court, or at the trial of an issue therein, may, in lieu of appearance at the time specified in the subpoena, agree with the party at whose request the subpoena was issued to appear at another time or upon such notice as may be agreed upon. Any failure to appear pursuant to such agreement may be punished as a contempt by the court issuing the subpoena. The facts establishing or disproving such agreement and the failure to appear may be proved by an affidavit of any person having personal knowledge of the facts.

HISTORY:

Added Stats 1969 ch 140 § 1.

§ 1985.2. Subpoena requiring attendance of witness; Notice

Any subpoena which requires the attendance of a witness at any civil trial shall contain the following notice in a type face designed to call attention to the notice:

Contact the attorney requesting this subpoena, listed above, before the date on which you are required to be in court, if you have any question about the time or date for you to appear, or if you want to be certain that your presence in court is required.

HISTORY:
Added Stats 1978 ch 431 § 1, operative July 1, 1979.

§ 1985.3. Subpoena duces tecum for production of personal records; Definitions; Application of section

(a) For purposes of this section, the following definitions apply:

(1) "Personal records" means the original, any copy of books, documents, other writings, or electronically stored information pertaining to a consumer and which are maintained by any "witness" which is a physician, dentist, ophthalmologist, optometrist, chiropractor, physical therapist, acupuncturist, podiatrist, veterinarian, veterinary hospital, veterinary clinic, pharmacist, pharmacy, hospital, medical center, clinic, radiology or MRI center, clinical or diagnostic laboratory, state or national bank, state or federal association (as defined in Section 5102 of the Financial Code), state or federal credit union, trust company, anyone authorized by this state to make or arrange loans that are secured by real property, security brokerage firm, insurance company, title insurance company, underwritten title company, escrow agent licensed pursuant to Division 6 (commencing with Section 17000) of the Financial Code or exempt from licensure pursuant to Section 17006 of the Financial Code, attorney, accountant, institution of the Farm Credit System, as specified in Section 2002 of Title 12 of the United States Code, or telephone corporation which is a public utility, as defined in Section 216 of the Public Utilities Code, or psychotherapist, as defined in Section 1010 of the Evidence Code, or a private or public preschool, elementary school, secondary school, or postsecondary school as described in Section 76244 of the Education Code.

(2) "Consumer" means any individual, partnership of five or fewer persons, association, or trust which has transacted business with, or has used the services of, the witness or for whom the witness has acted as agent or fiduciary.

(3) "Subpoenaing party" means the person or persons causing a subpoena duces tecum to be issued or served in connection with any civil action or proceeding pursuant to this code, but shall not include the state or local agencies described in Section 7465 of the Government Code, or any entity provided for under Article VI of the California Constitution in any proceeding maintained before an adjudicative body of that entity pursuant to Chapter 4 (commencing with Section 6000) of Division 3 of the Business and Professions Code.

(4) "Deposition officer" means a person who meets the qualifications specified in Section 2020.420.

(b) Prior to the date called for in the subpoena duces tecum for the production of personal records, the subpoenaing party shall serve or cause to be served on the consumer whose records are being sought a copy of the subpoena duces tecum, of the affidavit supporting the issuance of the subpoena, if any, and of the notice described in subdivision (e), and proof of service as indicated in paragraph (1) of subdivision (c). This service shall be made as follows:

(1) To the consumer personally, or at his or her last known address, or in accordance with Chapter 5 (commencing with Section 1010) of Title 14 of

Part 3, or, if he or she is a party, to his or her attorney of record. If the consumer is a minor, service shall be made on the minor's parent, guardian, conservator, or similar fiduciary, or if one of them cannot be located with reasonable diligence, then service shall be made on any person having the care or control of the minor or with whom the minor resides or by whom the minor is employed, and on the minor if the minor is at least 12 years of age.

(2) Not less than 10 days prior to the date for production specified in the subpoena duces tecum, plus the additional time provided by Section 1013 if service is by mail.

(3) At least five days prior to service upon the custodian of the records, plus the additional time provided by Section 1013 if service is by mail.

(c) Prior to the production of the records, the subpoenaing party shall do either of the following:

(1) Serve or cause to be served upon the witness a proof of personal service or of service by mail attesting to compliance with subdivision (b).

(2) Furnish the witness a written authorization to release the records signed by the consumer or by his or her attorney of record. The witness may presume that any attorney purporting to sign the authorization on behalf of the consumer acted with the consent of the consumer, and that any objection to release of records is waived.

(d) A subpoena duces tecum for the production of personal records shall be served in sufficient time to allow the witness a reasonable time, as provided in Section 2020.410, to locate and produce the records or copies thereof.

(e) Every copy of the subpoena duces tecum and affidavit, if any, served on a consumer or his or her attorney in accordance with subdivision (b) shall be accompanied by a notice, in a typeface designed to call attention to the notice, indicating that (1) records about the consumer are being sought from the witness named on the subpoena; (2) if the consumer objects to the witness furnishing the records to the party seeking the records, the consumer must file papers with the court or serve a written objection as provided in subdivision (g) prior to the date specified for production on the subpoena; and (3) if the party who is seeking the records will not agree in writing to cancel or limit the subpoena, an attorney should be consulted about the consumer's interest in protecting his or her rights of privacy. If a notice of taking of deposition is also served, that other notice may be set forth in a single document with the notice required by this subdivision.

(f) A subpoena duces tecum for personal records maintained by a telephone corporation which is a public utility, as defined in Section 216 of the Public Utilities Code, shall not be valid or effective unless it includes a consent to release, signed by the consumer whose records are requested, as required by Section 2891 of the Public Utilities Code.

(g) Any consumer whose personal records are sought by a subpoena duces tecum and who is a party to the civil action in which this subpoena duces tecum is served may, prior to the date for production, bring a motion under Section 1987.1 to quash or modify the subpoena duces tecum. Notice of the bringing of that motion shall be given to the witness and deposition officer at least five days prior to production. The failure to provide notice to the deposition officer shall not invalidate the motion to quash or modify the subpoena duces tecum but may be raised by the deposition officer as an affirmative defense in any action for liability for improper release of records.

Any other consumer or nonparty whose personal records are sought by a subpoena duces tecum may, prior to the date of production, serve on the subpoenaing party, the witness, and the deposition officer, a written objection that cites the specific grounds on which production of the personal records should be prohibited.

No witness or deposition officer shall be required to produce personal records after receipt of notice that the motion has been brought by a consumer, or after receipt of a written objection from a nonparty consumer, except upon order of the court in which the action is pending or by agreement of the parties, witnesses, and consumers affected.

The party requesting a consumer's personal records may bring a motion under Section 1987.1 to enforce the subpoena within 20 days of service of the written objection. The motion shall be accompanied by a declaration showing a reasonable and good faith attempt at informal resolution of the dispute between the party requesting the personal records and the consumer or the consumer's attorney.

(h) Upon good cause shown and provided that the rights of witnesses and consumers are preserved, a subpoenaing party shall be entitled to obtain an order shortening the time for service of a subpoena duces tecum or waiving the requirements of subdivision (b) where due diligence by the subpoenaing party has been shown.

(i) Nothing contained in this section shall be construed to apply to any subpoena duces tecum which does not request the records of any particular consumer or consumers and which requires a custodian of records to delete all information which would in any way identify any consumer whose records are to be produced.

(j) This section shall not apply to proceedings conducted under Division 1 (commencing with Section 50), Division 4 (commencing with Section 3200), Division 4.5 (commencing with Section 6100), or Division 4.7 (commencing with Section 6200), of the Labor Code.

(k) Failure to comply with this section shall be sufficient basis for the witness to refuse to produce the personal records sought by a subpoena duces tecum.

(*l*) If the subpoenaing party is the consumer, and the consumer is the only subject of the subpoenaed records, notice to the consumer, and delivery of the other documents specified in subdivision (b) to the consumer, is not required under this section.

HISTORY:

Added Stats 1980 ch 976 § 1, operative July 1, 1981. Amended Stats 1981 ch 227 § 1, effective July 20, 1981, operative July 1, 1981, ch 1014 § 1; Stats 1982 ch 666 § 1; Stats 1984 ch 603 § 1; Stats 1985 ch 983 § 1, effective September 26, 1985; Stats 1986 ch 248 § 21, ch 605 § 1, ch 1209 § 2; Stats 1987 ch 20 § 1, ch 149 § 1, effective July 10, 1987, ch 1080 § 10, ch 1492 § 2; Stats 1988 ch 184 § 1; Stats 1990 ch 1220 § 1 (AB 2980); Stats 1996 ch 679 § 1 (SB 1821); Stats 1997 ch 442 § 10 (AB 758); Stats 1998 ch 932 § 19 (AB 1094); Stats 1999 ch 444 § 1 (AB 794); Stats 2004 ch 182 § 18 (AB 3081), operative July 1, 2005; Stats 2005 ch 300 § 6 (AB 496), effective January 1, 2006; Stats 2012 ch 72 § 2 (SB 1574), effective January 1, 2013.

§ 1985.4. Production of consumer records maintained by state or local agency

The procedures set forth in Section 1985.3 are applicable to a subpoena duces tecum for records containing "personal information," as defined in

Section 1798.3 of the Civil Code that are otherwise exempt from public disclosure under a provision listed in Section 7920.505 of the Government Code that are maintained by a state or local agency as defined in Section 7920.510 or 7920.540 of the Government Code. For the purposes of this section, "witness" means a state or local agency as defined in Section 7920.510 or 7920.540 of the Government Code and "consumer" means any employee of any state or local agency as defined in Section 7920.510 or 7920.540 of the Government Code, or any other natural person. Nothing in this section shall pertain to personnel records as defined in Section 832.8 of the Penal Code.

HISTORY:

Added Stats 1984 ch 437 § 1. Amended Stats 1988 ch 441 § 1; Stats 2021 ch 615 § 57 (AB 474), effective January 1, 2022.

§ 1985.6. Subpoena duces tecum for production of employment records; Definitions, Procedures and requirements; Application of section and exceptions

(a) For purposes of this section, the following terms have the following meanings:

(1) "Deposition officer" means a person who meets the qualifications specified in Section 2020.420.

(2) "Employee" means any individual who is or has been employed by a witness subject to a subpoena duces tecum. "Employee" also means any individual who is or has been represented by a labor organization that is a witness subject to a subpoena duces tecum.

(3) "Employment records" means the original or any copy of books, documents, other writings, or electronically stored information pertaining to the employment of any employee maintained by the current or former employer of the employee, or by any labor organization that has represented or currently represents the employee.

(4) "Labor organization" has the meaning set forth in Section 1117 of the Labor Code.

(5) "Subpoenaing party" means the person or persons causing a subpoena duces tecum to be issued or served in connection with any civil action or proceeding, but does not include the state or local agencies described in Section 7465 of the Government Code, or any entity provided for under Article VI of the California Constitution in any proceeding maintained before an adjudicative body of that entity pursuant to Chapter 4 (commencing with Section 6000) of Division 3 of the Business and Professions Code.

(b) Prior to the date called for in the subpoena duces tecum of the production of employment records, the subpoenaing party shall serve or cause to be served on the employee whose records are being sought a copy of: the subpoena duces tecum; the affidavit supporting the issuance of the subpoena, if any; the notice described in subdivision (e); and proof of service as provided in paragraph (1) of subdivision (c). This service shall be made as follows:

(1) To the employee personally, or at his or her last known address, or in accordance with Chapter 5 (commencing with Section 1010) of Title 14 of Part 2, or, if he or she is a party, to his or her attorney of record. If the employee is a minor, service shall be made on the minor's parent, guardian, conservator, or similar fiduciary, or if one of them cannot be located with

reasonable diligence, then service shall be made on any person having the care or control of the minor, or with whom the minor resides, and on the minor if the minor is at least 12 years of age.

(2) Not less than 10 days prior to the date for production specified in the subpoena duces tecum, plus the additional time provided by Section 1013 if service is by mail.

(3) At least five days prior to service upon the custodian of the employment records, plus the additional time provided by Section 1013 if service is by mail.

(c) Prior to the production of the records, the subpoenaing party shall either:

(1) Serve or cause to be served upon the witness a proof of personal service or of service by mail attesting to compliance with subdivision (b).

(2) Furnish the witness a written authorization to release the records signed by the employee or by his or her attorney of record. The witness may presume that the attorney purporting to sign the authorization on behalf of the employee acted with the consent of the employee, and that any objection to the release of records is waived.

(d) A subpoena duces tecum for the production of employment records shall be served in sufficient time to allow the witness a reasonable time, as provided in Section 2020.410, to locate and produce the records or copies thereof.

(e) Every copy of the subpoena duces tecum and affidavit served on an employee or his or her attorney in accordance with subdivision (b) shall be accompanied by a notice, in a typeface designed to call attention to the notice, indicating that (1) employment records about the employee are being sought from the witness named on the subpoena; (2) the employment records may be protected by a right of privacy; (3) if the employee objects to the witness furnishing the records to the party seeking the records, the employee shall file papers with the court prior to the date specified for production on the subpoena; and (4) if the subpoenaing party does not agree in writing to cancel or limit the subpoena, an attorney should be consulted about the employee's interest in protecting his or her rights of privacy. If a notice of taking of deposition is also served, that other notice may be set forth in a single document with the notice required by this subdivision.

(f)(1) Any employee whose employment records are sought by a subpoena duces tecum may, prior to the date for production, bring a motion under Section 1987.1 to quash or modify the subpoena duces tecum. Notice of the bringing of that motion shall be given to the witness and the deposition officer at least five days prior to production. The failure to provide notice to the deposition officer does not invalidate the motion to quash or modify the subpoena duces tecum but may be raised by the deposition officer as an affirmative defense in any action for liability for improper release of records.

(2) Any nonparty employee whose employment records are sought by a subpoena duces tecum may, prior to the date of production, serve on the subpoenaing party, the deposition officer, and the witness a written objection that cites the specific grounds on which production of the employment records should be prohibited.

(3) No witness or deposition officer shall be required to produce employment records after receipt of notice that the motion has been brought by an employee, or after receipt of a written objection from a nonparty employee,

except upon order of the court in which the action is pending or by agreement of the parties, witnesses, and employees affected.

(4) The party requesting an employee's employment records may bring a motion under subdivision (c) of Section 1987 to enforce the subpoena within 20 days of service of the written objection. The motion shall be accompanied by a declaration showing a reasonable and good faith attempt at informal resolution of the dispute between the party requesting the employment records and the employee or the employee's attorney.

(g) Upon good cause shown and provided that the rights of witnesses and employees are preserved, a subpoenaing party shall be entitled to obtain an order shortening the time for service of a subpoena duces tecum or waiving the requirements of subdivision (b) if due diligence by the subpoenaing party has been shown.

(h) This section may not be construed to apply to any subpoena duces tecum that does not request the records of any particular employee or employees and that requires a custodian of records to delete all information that would in any way identify any employee whose records are to be produced.

(i) This section does not apply to proceedings conducted under Division 1 (commencing with Section 50), Division 4 (commencing with Section 3200), Division 4.5 (commencing with Section 6100), or Division 4.7 (commencing with Section 6200), of the Labor Code.

(j) Failure to comply with this section shall be sufficient basis for the witness to refuse to produce the employment records sought by subpoena duces tecum.

(k) If the subpoenaing party is the employee, and the employee is the only subject of the subpoenaed records, notice to the employee, and delivery of the other documents specified in subdivision (b) to the employee, are not required under this section.

HISTORY:

Added Stats 1995 ch 299 § 1 (AB 617). Amended Stats 1996 ch 679 § 1 (SB 1821); Stats 1997 ch 442 § 11 (AB 758); Stats 1998 ch 932 § 20 (AB 1094); Stats 1999 ch 444 § 2 (AB 794); Stats 2004 ch 101 § 1 (SB 1465) (ch 101 prevails), ch 182 § 19 (AB 3081), operative July 1, 2005; Stats 2005 ch 22 § 20 (SB 1108), ch 294 § 5 (AB 333), ch 300 § 7.5 (AB 496), effective January 1, 2006; Stats 2006 ch 538 § 76 (SB 1852), effective January 1, 2007; Stats 2012 ch 72 § 3 (SB 1574), effective January 1, 2013.

§ 1987. Service of subpoena, or of written notice

(a) Except as provided in Sections 68097.1 to 68097.8, inclusive, of the Government Code, the service of a subpoena is made by delivering a copy, or a ticket containing its substance, to the witness personally, giving or offering to the witness at the same time, if demanded by him or her, the fees to which he or she is entitled for travel to and from the place designated, and one day's attendance there. The service shall be made so as to allow the witness a reasonable time for preparation and travel to the place of attendance. The service may be made by any person. If service is to be made on a minor, service shall be made on the minor's parent, guardian, conservator, or similar fiduciary, or if one of those persons cannot be located with reasonable diligence, service shall be made on any person having the care or control of the minor or with whom the minor resides or by whom the minor is employed, and on the minor if the minor is 12 years of age or older. If the minor is alleged to come within the description of Section 300, 601, or 602 of the Welfare and Institutions Code and the minor is not in the custody of a parent or guardian, regardless of the age of the minor, service also shall be made upon the designated agent for service of process at the county child welfare department or the probation department under whose jurisdiction the minor has been placed.

(b) In the case of the production of a party to the record of any civil action or proceeding or of a person for whose immediate benefit an action or proceeding is prosecuted or defended or of anyone who is an officer, director, or managing agent of any such party or person, the service of a subpoena upon any such witness is not required if written notice requesting the witness to attend before a court, or at a trial of an issue therein, with the time and place thereof, is served upon the attorney of that party or person. The notice shall be served at least 10 days before the time required for attendance unless the court prescribes a shorter time. If entitled thereto, the witness, upon demand, shall be paid witness fees and mileage before being required to testify. The giving of the notice shall have the same effect as service of a subpoena on the witness, and the parties shall have those rights and the court may make those orders, including the imposition of sanctions, as in the case of a subpoena for attendance before the court.

(c) If the notice specified in subdivision (b) is served at least 20 days before the time required for attendance, or within any shorter period of time as the court may order, it may include a request that the party or person bring with him or her books, documents, electronically stored information, or other things. The notice shall state the exact materials or things desired and that the party or person has them in his or her possession or under his or her control. Within five days thereafter, or any other time period as the court may allow, the party or person of whom the request is made may serve written objections to the request or any part thereof, with a statement of grounds. Thereafter, upon noticed motion of the requesting party, accompanied by a showing of good cause and of materiality of the items to the issues, the court may order production of items to which objection was made, unless the objecting party or person establishes good cause for nonproduction or production under limitations or conditions. The procedure of this subdivision is alternative to the procedure provided by Sections 1985 and 1987.5 in the cases herein provided for, and no subpoena duces tecum shall be required.

Subject to this subdivision, the notice provided in this subdivision shall have the same effect as is provided in subdivision (b) as to a notice for attendance of that party or person.

HISTORY:

Enacted 1872. Amended Stats 1963 ch 1485 § 3; Stats 1968 ch 933 § 1; Stats 1969 ch 311 § 1, ch 1034 § 1.5; Stats 1981 ch 184 § 2; Stats 1986 ch 605 § 2; Stats 1989 ch 1416 § 28; Stats 2002 ch 1008 § 6 (AB 3028); Stats 2012 ch 72 § 5 (SB 1574), effective January 1, 2013.

EXTRACTED FROM
GOVERNMENT CODE

Title
2. Government of the State of California.

TITLE 2

GOVERNMENT OF THE STATE OF CALIFORNIA

Division
3. Executive Department.

DIVISION 3

EXECUTIVE DEPARTMENT

Part
1. State Departments and Agencies.

HISTORY: Added Stats 1945 ch 111 § 3.

PART 1

STATE DEPARTMENTS AND AGENCIES

Chapter
3.5. Administrative Regulations and Rulemaking.
4. Office of Administrative Hearings.
4.5. Administrative Adjudication: General Provisions.
5. Administrative Adjudication: Formal Hearing.

CHAPTER 3.5

ADMINISTRATIVE REGULATIONS AND RULEMAKING

Article
1. General.
2. Definitions.
3. Filing and Publication.
4. The California Code of Regulations, the California Code of Regulations Supplement, and the California Regulatory Notice Register.
5. Public Participation: Procedure for Adoption of Regulations.
6. Review of Proposed Regulations.
7. Review of Existing Regulations.
8. Judicial Review.
9. Special Procedures.
10. California Taxpayers' Right to Self-Governance and Participation [Repealed].

HISTORY: Added Stats 1979 ch 567 § 1. Heading amended Stats 1994 ch 1039 § 2.

ARTICLE 1
GENERAL

Section
11340. Legislative findings and declarations.
11340.1. Declarations and intent regarding establishment of Office of Administrative Law.
11340.2. Office of Administrative Law; Director and deputy director.
11340.3. Employment and compensation of assistants and other employees.
11340.4. Recommendations on administrative rulemaking.
11340.5. Adoption of guidelines, bulletins and manuals as regulations.
11340.6. Petition requesting adoption, amendment, or repeal of regulation; Contents.
11340.7. Procedure upon petition requesting adoption, amendment or repeal of regulation.
11340.85. Electronic communications.
11340.9. Inapplicable provisions.
11341. Identification numbers.
11342.1. Authority not conferred on state agencies.
11342.2. Consistency with statute; Effectuation of purpose of statute.
11342.4. Regulations.

§ 11340. Legislative findings and declarations

The Legislature finds and declares as follows:

(a) There has been an unprecedented growth in the number of administrative regulations in recent years.

(b) The language of many regulations is frequently unclear and unnecessarily complex, even when the complicated and technical nature of the subject matter is taken into account. The language is often confusing to the persons who must comply with the regulations.

(c) Substantial time and public funds have been spent in adopting regulations, the necessity for which has not been established.

(d) The imposition of prescriptive standards upon private persons and entities through regulations where the establishment of performance standards could reasonably be expected to produce the same result has placed an unnecessary burden on California citizens and discouraged innovation, research, and development of improved means of achieving desirable social goals.

(e) There exists no central office in state government with the power and duty to review regulations to ensure that they are written in a comprehensible manner, are authorized by statute, and are consistent with other law.

(f) Correcting the problems that have been caused by the unprecedented growth of regulations in California requires the direct involvement of the Legislature as well as that of the executive branch of state government.

(g) The complexity and lack of clarity in many regulations put small businesses, which do not have the resources to hire experts to assist them, at a distinct disadvantage.

HISTORY:

Added Stats 1979 ch 567 § 1, operative July 1, 1980. Amended Stats 1981 ch 865 § 2; Stats 1983 ch 874 § 1; Stats 1993 ch 870 § 1 (SB 726).

§ 11340.1. Declarations and intent regarding establishment of Office of Administrative Law

(a) The Legislature therefore declares that it is in the public interest to establish an Office of Administrative Law which shall be charged with the orderly review of adopted regulations. It is the intent of the Legislature that the purpose of such review shall be to reduce the number of administrative regulations and to improve the quality of those regulations which are adopted. It is the intent of the Legislature that agencies shall actively seek to reduce the unnecessary regulatory burden on private individuals and entities by substituting performance standards for prescriptive standards wherever performance standards can be reasonably expected to be as effective and less burdensome, and that this substitution shall be considered during the course of the agency rulemaking process. It is the intent of the Legislature that neither the Office of Administrative Law nor the court should substitute its judgment for that of the rulemaking agency as expressed in the substantive content of adopted regulations. It is the intent of the Legislature that while the Office of Administrative Law will be part of the executive branch of state government, that the office work closely with, and upon request report directly to, the Legislature in order to accomplish regulatory reform in California.

(b) It is the intent of the Legislature that the California Code of Regulations made available on the Internet by the office pursuant to Section 11344 include complete authority and reference citations and history notes.

HISTORY:

Added Stats 1979 ch 567 § 1, operative July 1, 1980. Amended Stats 1981 ch 865 § 3; Stats 1983 ch 874 § 2; Stats 1996 ch 501 § 1 (SB 1910).

§ 11340.2. Office of Administrative Law; Director and deputy director

(a) The Office of Administrative Law is hereby established in state government in the Government Operations Agency. The office shall be under the direction and control of an executive officer who shall be known as the director. There shall also be a deputy director. The director's term and the deputy director's term of office shall be coterminous with that of the appointing power, except that they shall be subject to reappointment.

(b) The director and deputy director shall have the same qualifications as a hearing officer and shall be appointed by the Governor subject to the confirmation of the Senate.

HISTORY:

Added Stats 1979 ch 567 § 1, operative July 1, 1980. Amended Stats 1980 ch 992 § 1.5. See this section as modified in Governor's Reorganization Plan No. 2 § 175 of 2012; Amended Stats 2013 ch 352 § 235 (AB 1317), effective September 26, 2013, operative July 1, 2013.

§ 11340.3. Employment and compensation of assistants and other employees

The director may employ and fix the compensation, in accordance with law, of such professional assistants and clerical and other employees as is deemed necessary for the effective conduct of the work of the office.

HISTORY:

Added Stats 1979 ch 567 § 1, operative July 1, 1980.

§ 11340.4. Recommendations on administrative rulemaking

(a) The office is authorized and directed to do the following:

(1) Study the subject of administrative rulemaking in all its aspects.

(2) In the interest of fairness, uniformity, and the expedition of business, submit its suggestions to the various agencies.

(3) Report its recommendations to the Governor and Legislature at the commencement of each general session.

(b) All agencies of the state shall give the office ready access to their records and full information and reasonable assistance in any matter of research requiring recourse to them or to data within their knowledge or control. Nothing in this subdivision authorizes an agency to provide access to records required by statute to be kept confidential.

HISTORY:

Added Stats 1995 ch 938 § 14 (SB 523), operative July 1, 1997.

§ 11340.5. Adoption of guidelines, bulletins and manuals as regulations

(a) No state agency shall issue, utilize, enforce, or attempt to enforce any guideline, criterion, bulletin, manual, instruction, order, standard of general application, or other rule, which is a regulation as defined in Section 11342.600, unless the guideline, criterion, bulletin, manual, instruction, order, standard of general application, or other rule has been adopted as a regulation and filed with the Secretary of State pursuant to this chapter.

(b) If the office is notified of, or on its own, learns of the issuance, enforcement of, or use of, an agency guideline, criterion, bulletin, manual, instruction, order, standard of general application, or other rule that has not been adopted as a regulation and filed with the Secretary of State pursuant to this chapter, the office may issue a determination as to whether the guideline, criterion, bulletin, manual, instruction, order, standard of general application, or other rule, is a regulation as defined in Section 11342.600.

(c) The office shall do all of the following:

(1) File its determination upon issuance with the Secretary of State.

(2) Make its determination known to the agency, the Governor, and the Legislature.

(3) Publish its determination in the California Regulatory Notice Register within 15 days of the date of issuance.

(4) Make its determination available to the public and the courts.

(d) Any interested person may obtain judicial review of a given determination by filing a written petition requesting that the determination of the office be modified or set aside. A petition shall be filed with the court within 30 days of the date the determination is published.

(e) A determination issued by the office pursuant to this section shall not be considered by a court, or by an administrative agency in an adjudicatory proceeding if all of the following occurs:

(1) The court or administrative agency proceeding involves the party that sought the determination from the office.

(2) The proceeding began prior to the party's request for the office's determination.

(3) At issue in the proceeding is the question of whether the guideline, criterion, bulletin, manual, instruction, order, standard of general application, or other rule that is the legal basis for the adjudicatory action is a regulation as defined in Section 11342.600.

HISTORY:

Added Stats 1994 ch 1039 § 4 (AB 2531). Amended Stats 1995 ch 938 § 15 (SB 523), operative January 1, 1996; Stats 2000 ch 1060 § 3 (AB 1822).

§ 11340.6. Petition requesting adoption, amendment, or repeal of regulation; Contents

Except where the right to petition for adoption of a regulation is restricted by statute to a designated group or where the form of procedure for such a petition is otherwise prescribed by statute, any interested person may petition a state agency requesting the adoption, amendment, or repeal of a regulation as provided in Article 5 (commencing with Section 11346). This petition shall state the following clearly and concisely:

(a) The substance or nature of the regulation, amendment, or repeal requested.

(b) The reason for the request.

(c) Reference to the authority of the state agency to take the action requested.

HISTORY:

Added Stats 1994 ch 1039 § 5 (AB 2531).

§ 11340.7. Procedure upon petition requesting adoption, amendment or repeal of regulation

(a) Upon receipt of a petition requesting the adoption, amendment, or repeal of a regulation pursuant to Article 5 (commencing with Section 11346), a state agency shall notify the petitioner in writing of the receipt and shall within 30 days deny the petition indicating why the agency has reached its decision on the merits of the petition in writing or schedule the matter for public hearing in accordance with the notice and hearing requirements of that article.

(b) A state agency may grant or deny the petition in part, and may grant any other relief or take any other action as it may determine to be warranted by the petition and shall notify the petitioner in writing of this action.

(c) Any interested person may request a reconsideration of any part or all of a decision of any agency on any petition submitted. The request shall be submitted in accordance with Section 11340.6 and include the reason or reasons why an agency should reconsider its previous decision no later than 60 days after the date of the decision involved. The agency's reconsideration of any matter relating to a petition shall be subject to subdivision (a).

(d) Any decision of a state agency denying in whole or in part or granting in whole or in part a petition requesting the adoption, amendment, or repeal of a regulation pursuant to Article 5 (commencing with Section 11346) shall be in writing and shall be transmitted to the Office of Administrative Law for publication in the California Regulatory Notice Register at the earliest practicable date. The decision shall identify the agency, the party submitting the petition, the provisions of the California Code of Regulations requested to be affected, reference to authority to take the action requested, the reasons supporting the agency determination, an agency contact person, and the right of interested persons to obtain a copy of the petition from the agency.

HISTORY:

Added Stats 1994 ch 1994 ch 1039 § 6 (AB 2531).

§ 11340.85. Electronic communications

(a) As used in this section, "electronic communication" includes electronic transmission of written or graphical material by electronic mail, facsimile, or other means, but does not include voice communication.

(b) Notwithstanding any other provision of this chapter that refers to mailing or sending, or to oral or written communication:

(1) An agency may permit and encourage use of electronic communication, but may not require use of electronic communication.

(2) An agency may publish or distribute a document required by this chapter or by a regulation implementing this chapter by means of electronic communication, but shall not make that the exclusive means by which the document is published or distributed.

(3) A notice required or authorized by this chapter or by a regulation implementing this chapter may be delivered to a person by means of electronic communication if the person has expressly indicated a willingness to receive the notice by means of electronic communication.

(4) A comment regarding a regulation may be delivered to an agency by means of electronic communication.

(5) A petition regarding a regulation may be delivered to an agency by means of electronic communication if the agency has expressly indicated a willingness to receive a petition by means of electronic communication.

(c) An agency that maintains an Internet Web site or other similar forum for the electronic publication or distribution of written material shall publish on that Web site or other forum information regarding a proposed regulation or regulatory repeal or amendment, that includes, but is not limited to, the following:

(1) Any public notice required by this chapter or by a regulation implementing this chapter.

(2) The initial statement of reasons prepared pursuant to subdivision (b) of Section 11346.2.

(3) The final statement of reasons prepared pursuant to subdivision (a) of Section 11346.9.

(4) Notice of a decision not to proceed prepared pursuant to Section 11347.

(5) The text of a proposed action or instructions on how to obtain a copy of the text.

(6) A statement of any decision made by the office regarding a proposed action.

(7) The date a rulemaking action is filed with the Secretary of State.

(8) The effective date of a rulemaking action.

(9) A statement to the effect that a business or person submitting a comment regarding a proposed action has the right to request a copy of the final statement of reasons.

(10) The text of a proposed emergency adoption, amendment, or repeal of a regulation pursuant to Section 11346.1 and the date it was submitted to the office for review and filing.

(d) A document that is required to be posted pursuant to subdivision (c) shall be posted within a reasonable time after issuance of the document, and shall remain posted until at least 15 days after (1) the rulemaking action is filed with the Secretary of State, or (2) notice of a decision not to proceed is published pursuant to Section 11347. Publication under subdivision (c) supplements any other required form of publication or distribution. Failure to comply with this section is not grounds for disapproval of a proposed regulation. Subdivision (c) does not require an agency to establish or maintain a Web site or other forum for the electronic publication or distribution of written material.

(e) Nothing in this section precludes the office from requiring that the material submitted to the office for publication in the California Code of Regulations or the California Regulatory Notice Register be submitted in electronic form.

(f) This section is intended to make the regulatory process more user-friendly and to improve communication between interested parties and the regulatory agencies.

HISTORY:

Added Stats 2000 ch 1060 § 4 (AB 1822). Amended Stats 2001 ch 59 § 2 (SB 561); Stats 2002 ch 389 § 2 (AB 1857); Stats 2006 ch 713 § 1 (AB 1302), effective January 1, 2007.

§ 11340.9. Inapplicable provisions

This chapter does not apply to any of the following:

(a) An agency in the judicial or legislative branch of the state government.

(b) A legal ruling of counsel issued by the Franchise Tax Board or State Board of Equalization.

(c) A form prescribed by a state agency or any instructions relating to the use of the form, but this provision is not a limitation on any requirement that a regulation be adopted pursuant to this chapter when one is needed to implement the law under which the form is issued.

(d) A regulation that relates only to the internal management of the state agency.

(e) A regulation that establishes criteria or guidelines to be used by the staff of an agency in performing an audit, investigation, examination, or inspection, settling a commercial dispute, negotiating a commercial arrangement, or in the defense, prosecution, or settlement of a case, if disclosure of the criteria or guidelines would do any of the following:

(1) Enable a law violator to avoid detection.

(2) Facilitate disregard of requirements imposed by law.

(3) Give clearly improper advantage to a person who is in an adverse position to the state.

(f) A regulation that embodies the only legally tenable interpretation of a provision of law.

(g) A regulation that establishes or fixes rates, prices, or tariffs.

(h) A regulation that relates to the use of public works, including streets and highways, when the effect of the regulation is indicated to the public by means of signs or signals or when the regulation determines uniform standards and specifications for official traffic control devices pursuant to Section 21400 of the Vehicle Code.

(i) A regulation that is directed to a specifically named person or to a group of persons and does not apply generally throughout the state.

HISTORY:

Added Stats 2000 ch 1060 § 5 (AB 1822).

§ 11341. Identification numbers

(a) The office shall establish a system to give a unique identification number to each regulatory action.

(b) The office and the state agency taking the regulatory action shall use the identification number given by the office pursuant to subdivision (a) to refer to the regulatory action for which a notice has already been published in the California Regulatory Notice Register.

(c) The identification number shall be sufficient information for a member of the public to identify and track a regulatory action both with the office and the state agency taking the regulatory action. No other information pertaining to the regulatory action shall be required of a member of the public if the identification number of the regulatory action has been provided.

HISTORY:

Added Stats 2000 ch 1059 § 5 (AB 505).

§ 11342.1. Authority not conferred on state agencies

Except as provided in Section 11342.4, nothing in this chapter confers authority upon or augments the authority of any state agency to adopt, administer, or enforce any regulation. Each regulation adopted, to be effective, shall be within the scope of authority conferred and in accordance with standards prescribed by other provisions of law.

HISTORY:

Added Stats 1979 ch 567 § 1, operative July 1, 1980. Amended Stats 1987 ch 1375 § 2.

§ 11342.2. Consistency with statute; Effectuation of purpose of statute

Whenever by the express or implied terms of any statute a state agency has authority to adopt regulations to implement, interpret, make specific or otherwise carry out the provisions of the statute, no regulation adopted is valid or effective unless consistent and not in conflict with the statute and reasonably necessary to effectuate the purpose of the statute.

HISTORY:

Added Stats 1979 ch 567 § 1, operative July 1, 1980.

§ 11342.4. Regulations

The office shall adopt, amend, or repeal regulations for the purpose of carrying out the provisions of this chapter.

HISTORY:

Added Stats 1981 ch 865 § 19, as Gov C § 11344.6. Amended Stats 1982 ch 1573 § 1. Renumbered by Stats 1983 ch 797 § 12.

ARTICLE 2
DEFINITIONS

Section
11342.510. Governing definitions.
11342.520. "Agency".
11342.530. "Building standard".
11342.535. "Cost impact".
11342.540. "Director".
11342.545. "Emergency".
11342.548. "Major regulation".
11342.550. "Office".
11342.560. "Order of repeal".
11342.570. "Performance standard".
11342.580. "Plain English".
11342.590. "Prescriptive standard".
11342.595. "Proposed action".
11342.600. "Regulation".
11342.610. "Small Business".

HISTORY: Added Stats 2000 ch 1060 § 8. Heading of former heading of Article 2, entitled "Rules and Regulations", consisting of §§ 11342–11342.5, was repealed Stats 2000 ch 1060 § 6.

§ 11342.510. Governing definitions

Unless the provision or context otherwise requires, the definitions in this article govern the construction of this chapter.

HISTORY:
Added Stats 2000 ch 1060 § 8 (AB 1822).

§ 11342.520. "Agency"

"Agency" means state agency.

HISTORY:
Added Stats 2000 ch 1060 § 8 (AB 1822).

§ 11342.530. "Building standard"

"Building standard" has the same meaning provided in Section 18909 of the Health and Safety Code.

HISTORY:
Added Stats 2000 ch 1060 § 8 (AB 1822).

§ 11342.535. "Cost impact"

"Cost impact" means the amount of reasonable range of direct costs, or a description of the type and extent of direct costs, that a representative private person or business necessarily incurs in reasonable compliance with the proposed action.

HISTORY:
Added Stats 2000 ch 1059 § 6.5 (AB 505).

§ 11342.540. "Director"

"Director" means the director of the office.

HISTORY:

Added Stats 2000 ch 1060 § 8 (AB 1822).

§ 11342.545. "Emergency"

"Emergency" means a situation that calls for immediate action to avoid serious harm to the public peace, health, safety, or general welfare.

HISTORY:

Added Stats 2006 ch 713 § 2 (AB 1302), effective January 1, 2007.

§ 11342.548. "Major regulation"

"Major regulation" means any proposed adoption, amendment, or repeal of a regulation subject to review by the Office of Administrative Law pursuant to Article 6 (commencing with Section 11349) that will have an economic impact on California business enterprises and individuals in an amount exceeding fifty million dollars ($50,000,000), as estimated by the agency.

HISTORY:

Added Stats 2011 ch 496 § 1 (SB 617), effective January 1, 2012.

§ 11342.550. "Office"

"Office" means the Office of Administrative Law.

HISTORY:

Added Stats 2000 ch 1060 § 8 (AB 1822).

§ 11342.560. "Order of repeal"

"Order of repeal" means any resolution, order, or other official act of a state agency that expressly repeals a regulation in whole or in part.

HISTORY:

Added Stats 2000 ch 1060 § 8 (AB 1822).

§ 11342.570. "Performance standard"

"Performance standard" means a regulation that describes an objective with the criteria stated for achieving the objective.

HISTORY:

Added Stats 2000 ch 1060 § 8 (AB 1822).

§ 11342.580. "Plain English"

"Plain English" means language that satisfies the standard of clarity provided in Section 11349.

HISTORY:

Added Stats 2000 ch 1060 § 8 (AB 1822).

§ 11342.590. "Prescriptive standard"

"Prescriptive standard" means a regulation that specifies the sole means of compliance with a performance standard by specific actions, measurements, or other quantifiable means.

HISTORY:
Added Stats 2000 ch 1060 § 8 (AB 1822).

§ 11342.595. "Proposed action"

"Proposed action" means the regulatory action, notice of which is submitted to the office for publication in the California Regulatory Notice Register.

HISTORY:
Added Stats 2000 ch 1059 § 6.7 (AB 505). Amended Stats 2001 ch 59 § 3 (SB 561).

§ 11342.600. "Regulation"

"Regulation" means every rule, regulation, order, or standard of general application or the amendment, supplement, or revision of any rule, regulation, order, or standard adopted by any state agency to implement, interpret, or make specific the law enforced or administered by it, or to govern its procedure.

HISTORY:
Added Stats 2000 ch 1060 § 8 (AB 1822).

§ 11342.610. "Small Business"

(a) "Small business" means a business activity in agriculture, general construction, special trade construction, retail trade, wholesale trade, services, transportation and warehousing, manufacturing, generation and transmission of electric power, or a health care facility, unless excluded in subdivision (b), that is both of the following:

(1) Independently owned and operated.

(2) Not dominant in its field of operation.

(b) "Small business" does not include the following professional and business activities:

(1) A financial institution including a bank, a trust, a savings and loan association, a thrift institution, a consumer finance company, a commercial finance company, an industrial finance company, a credit union, a mortgage and investment banker, a securities broker-dealer, or an investment adviser.

(2) An insurance company, either stock or mutual.

(3) A mineral, oil, or gas broker.

(4) A subdivider or developer.

(5) A landscape architect, an architect, or a building designer.

(6) An entity organized as a nonprofit institution.

(7) An entertainment activity or production, including a motion picture, a stage performance, a television or radio station, or a production company.

(8) A utility, a water company, or a power transmission company generating and transmitting more than 4.5 million kilowatt hours annually.

(9) A petroleum producer, a natural gas producer, a refiner, or a pipeline.

(10) A manufacturing enterprise exceeding 250 employees.

(11) A health care facility exceeding 150 beds or one million five hundred thousand dollars ($1,500,000) in annual gross receipts.

(c) "Small business" does not include the following business activities:

(1) Agriculture, where the annual gross receipts exceed one million dollars ($1,000,000).

(2) General construction, where the annual gross receipts exceed nine million five hundred thousand dollars ($9,500,000).

(3) Special trade construction, where the annual gross receipts exceed five million dollars ($5,000,000).

(4) Retail trade, where the annual gross receipts exceed two million dollars ($2,000,000).

(5) Wholesale trade, where the annual gross receipts exceed nine million five hundred thousand dollars ($9,500,000).

(6) Services, where the annual gross receipts exceed two million dollars ($2,000,000).

(7) Transportation and warehousing, where the annual gross receipts exceed one million five hundred thousand dollars ($1,500,000).

HISTORY:

Added Stats 2000 ch 1060 § 8 (AB 1822).

ARTICLE 3

FILING AND PUBLICATION

Section

11343. Procedure.
11343.1. Style of regulations; Endorsement.
11343.2. Endorsement of time and date of filing and maintenance of file for public inspection.
11343.3. Vehicle weight impacts and ability of vehicle manufacturers or operators to comply with laws limiting weight of vehicles to be taken into account when promulgating administrative regulations.
11343.4. Effective date of regulation or order of repeal; Applicability.
11343.5. Filing copies of Code of Regulations or Regulatory Code Supplement.
11343.6. Rebuttable presumptions raised by filing of certified copy.
11343.8. Filing and publication of regulation or order of repeal not required to be filed.

§ 11343. Procedure

Every state agency shall:

(a) Transmit to the office for filing with the Secretary of State a certified copy of every regulation adopted or amended by it except one that is a building standard.

(b) Transmit to the office for filing with the Secretary of State a certified copy of every order of repeal of a regulation required to be filed under subdivision (a).

(c)(1) Within 15 days of the office filing a state agency's regulation with the Secretary of State, post the regulation on its internet website in an easily marked and identifiable location. The state agency shall keep the regulation on its internet website for at least six months from the date the regulation is filed with the Secretary of State.

(2) Within five days of posting, the state agency shall send to the office the internet website link of each regulation that the agency posts on its internet website pursuant to paragraph (1).

(3) This subdivision shall not apply to a state agency that does not maintain an internet website.

(d) Deliver to the office, at the time of transmittal for filing a regulation or order of repeal, a citation of the authority pursuant to which it or any part thereof was adopted.

(e) Deliver to the office a copy of the notice of proposed action required by Section 11346.4.

(f) Transmit to the California Building Standards Commission for approval a certified copy of every regulation, or order of repeal of a regulation, that is a building standard, together with a citation of authority pursuant to which it or any part thereof was adopted, a copy of the notice of proposed action required by Section 11346.4, and any other records prescribed by the California Building Standards Law (Part 2.5 (commencing with Section 18901) of Division 13 of the Health and Safety Code).

(g) Whenever a certification is required by this section, it shall be made by the head of the state agency that is adopting, amending, or repealing the regulation, or by a designee of the agency head, and the certification and delegation shall be in writing.

HISTORY:

Added Stats 1979 ch 567 § 1. Amended Stats 1979 ch 1152 § 12.2, operative July 1, 1980; Stats 1980 ch 204 § 1, effective June 20, 1980; Stats 1981 ch 865 § 5; Stats 1982 ch 749 § 1, effective September 8, 1982; Stats 1983 ch 291 § 1; Stats 1987 ch 1375 § 3; Stats 1988 ch 1194 sec 1.2, operative January 1, 1989; Stats 2000 ch 1060 § 9 (AB 1822); Stats 2002 ch 389 § 3 (AB 1857); Stats 2012 ch 295 § 1 (SB 1099), effective January 1, 2013; Stats 2022 ch 48 § 22 (SB 189), effective June 30, 2022.

§ 11343.1. Style of regulations; Endorsement

(a) All regulations transmitted to the Office of Administrative Law for filing with the Secretary of State shall conform to the style prescribed by the office.

(b) Regulations approved by the office shall bear an endorsement by the office affixed to the certified copy which is filed with the Secretary of State.

HISTORY:

Added Stats 1983 ch 797 § 2. Amended Stats 1994 ch 1039 § 12 (AB 2531).

§ 11343.2. Endorsement of time and date of filing and maintenance of file for public inspection

The Secretary of State shall endorse on the certified copy of each regulation or order of repeal filed with or delivered to him or her, the time and date of filing and shall maintain a permanent file of the certified copies of regulations and orders of repeal for public inspection.

No fee shall be charged by any state officer or public official for the performance of any official act in connection with the certification or filing of regulations pursuant to this article.

HISTORY:

Added Stats 1994 ch 1039 § 14 (AB 2531).

§ 11343.3. Vehicle weight impacts and ability of vehicle manufacturers or operators to comply with laws limiting weight of vehicles to be taken into account when promulgating administrative regulations

Notwithstanding any other law, a state agency that is required to promulgate administrative regulations, including, but not limited to, the State Air Resources Board, the California Environmental Protection Agency, the State Energy Resources Conservation and Development Commission, and the Department of Motor Vehicles, shall take into account vehicle weight impacts and the ability of vehicle manufacturers or vehicle operators to comply with laws limiting the weight of vehicles.

HISTORY:

Added Stats 2012 ch 771 § 2 (AB 1706), effective January 1, 2013.

§ 11343.4. Effective date of regulation or order of repeal; Applicability

(a) Except as otherwise provided in subdivision (b), a regulation or an order of repeal required to be filed with the Secretary of State shall become effective on a quarterly basis as follows:

(1) January 1 if the regulation or order of repeal is filed on September 1 to November 30, inclusive.

(2) April 1 if the regulation or order of repeal is filed on December 1 to February 29, inclusive.

(3) July 1 if the regulation or order of repeal is filed on March 1 to May 31, inclusive.

(4) October 1 if the regulation or order of repeal is filed on June 1 to August 31, inclusive.

(b) The effective dates in subdivision (a) shall not apply in all of the following:

(1) The effective date is specifically provided by the statute pursuant to which the regulation or order of repeal was adopted, in which event it becomes effective on the day prescribed by the statute.

(2) A later date is prescribed by the state agency in a written instrument filed with, or as part of, the regulation or order of repeal.

(3) The agency makes a written request to the office demonstrating good cause for an earlier effective date, in which case the office may prescribe an earlier date.

(4)(A) A regulation adopted by the Fish and Game Commission that is governed by Article 2 (commencing with Section250) of Chapter 2 of Division 1 of the Fish and Game Code.

(B) A regulation adopted by the Fish and Game Commission that requires a different effective date in order to conform to a federal regulation.

HISTORY:

Added Stats 1994 ch 1039 § 16 (AB 2531). Amended Stats 2000 ch 1060 § 10 (AB 1822); Stats 2012 ch 295 § 2 (SB 1099), effective January 1, 2013; Stats 2016 ch 546 § 26 (SB 1473), effective January 1, 2017.

§ 11343.5. Filing copies of Code of Regulations or Regulatory Code Supplement

Within 10 days from the receipt of printed copies of the California Code of Regulations or of the California Code of Regulations Supplement from the State Printing Office, the office shall file one copy of the particular issue of the code or supplement in the office of the county clerk of each county in this state, or if the authority to accept filings on his or her behalf has been delegated by the county clerk of any county pursuant to Section 26803.5, in the office of the person to whom that authority has been delegated.

HISTORY:

Added Stats 1979 ch 567 § 1, operative July 1, 1980, as Gov C § 11343.6. Amended and renumbered by Stats 1981 ch 865 § 9; Amended Stats 1987 ch 1375 § 3.2; Stats 2000 ch 1060 § 11 (AB 1822).

§ 11343.6. Rebuttable presumptions raised by filing of certified copy

The filing of a certified copy of a regulation or an order of repeal with the Secretary of State raises the rebuttable presumptions that:

(a) It was duly adopted.

(b) It was duly filed and made available for public inspection at the day and hour endorsed on it.

(c) All requirements of this chapter and the regulations of the office relative to such regulation have been complied with.

(d) The text of the certified copy of a regulation or order of repeal is the text of the regulation or order of repeal as adopted.

The courts shall take judicial notice of the contents of the certified copy of each regulation and of each order of repeal duly filed.

HISTORY:

Added Stats 1979 ch 567 § 1, operative July 1, 1980, as Gov C § 11343.7. Renumbered by Stats 1981 ch 865 § 10.

§ 11343.8. Filing and publication of regulation or order of repeal not required to be filed

Upon the request of a state agency, the office may file with the Secretary of State and the office may publish in such manner as it believes proper, any regulation or order of repeal of a regulation not required by this article to be filed with the Secretary of State.

HISTORY:

Added Stats 1979 ch 567 § 1, operative July 1, 1980, as § 11343.9. Amended and renumbered by Stats 1981 ch 865 § 12.

ARTICLE 4

THE CALIFORNIA CODE OF REGULATIONS, THE CALIFORNIA CODE OF REGULATIONS SUPPLEMENT, AND THE CALIFORNIA REGULATORY NOTICE REGISTER

Section

11344. Publication of Code of Regulations and Code of Regulations Supplement; Availability of regulations on internet.
11344.1. Publication of Regulatory Notice Register.
11344.2. Furnishing Code and Supplement to county clerks or delegatees.
11344.3. Time of publication of documents.
11344.4. Sale of Code, Supplement and Regulatory Notice Register.

Section
11344.6. Rebuttable presumption raised by publication of regulations.
11344.7. Authority of state agencies to purchase copies of Code, Supplement, or Register or to print and distribute special editions.
11344.9. "California Administrative Code"; "California Administrative Notice Register"; "California Administrative Code Supplement".
11345. Identification number not required.

HISTORY: Heading of Article 4, consisting of §§ 11344–11345, amended Stats 2000 ch 1060 § 12.

§ 11344. Publication of Code of Regulations and Code of Regulations Supplement; Availability of regulations on internet

The office shall do all of the following:

(a) Provide for the official compilation, printing, and publication of adoption, amendment, or repeal of regulations, which shall be known as the California Code of Regulations. On and after July 1, 1998, the office shall make available on the Internet, free of charge, the full text of the California Code of Regulations, and may contract with another state agency or a private entity in order to provide this service.

(b) Make available on its Internet Web site a list of, and a link to the full text of, each regulation filed with the Secretary of State that is pending effectiveness pursuant to Section 11343.4.

(c) Provide for the compilation, printing, and publication of weekly updates of the California Code of Regulations. This publication shall be known as the California Code of Regulations Supplement and shall contain amendments to the code.

(d) Provide for the publication dates and manner and form in which regulations shall be printed and distributed and ensure that regulations are available in printed form at the earliest practicable date after filing with the Secretary of State.

(e) Ensure that each regulation is printed together with a reference to the statutory authority pursuant to which it was enacted and the specific statute or other provision of law which the regulation is implementing, interpreting, or making specific.

HISTORY:

Added Stats 1983 ch 797 § 7. Amended Stats 1987 ch 1375 § 3.5; Stats 1994 ch 1039 § 17 (AB 2531); Stats 1996 ch 501 § 2 (SB 1910); Stats 2000 ch 1060 § 13 (AB 1822); Stats 2012 ch 295 § 3 (SB 1099), effective January 1, 2013.

§ 11344.1. Publication of Regulatory Notice Register

The office shall do all of the following:

(a) Provide for the publication of the California Regulatory Notice Register, which shall be an official publication of the State of California and which shall contain the following:

(1) Notices of proposed action prepared by regulatory agencies, subject to the notice requirements of this chapter, and which have been approved by the office.

(2) A summary of all regulations filed with the Secretary of State in the previous week.

(3) Summaries of all regulation decisions issued in the previous week detailing the reasons for disapproval of a regulation, the reasons for not filing an emergency regulation, and the reasons for repealing an emergency regulation. The California Regulatory Notice Register shall also include a quarterly index of regulation decisions.

(4) Material that is required to be published under Sections 11349.5, 11349.7, and 11349.9.

(5) Determinations issued pursuant to Section 11340.5.

(b) Establish the publication dates and manner and form in which the California Regulatory Notice Register shall be prepared and published and ensure that it is published and distributed in a timely manner to the presiding officer and rules committee of each house of the Legislature and to all subscribers.

(c) Post on its website, on a weekly basis:

(1) The California Regulatory Notice Register. Each issue of the California Regulatory Notice Register on the office's website shall remain posted for a minimum of 18 months.

(2) One or more Internet links to assist the public to gain access to the text of regulations proposed by state agencies.

HISTORY:

Added Stats 1983 ch 797 § 9. Amended Stats 1987 ch 1375 § 4; Stats 1994 ch 1039 § 18 (AB 2531); Stats 2000 ch 1059 § 7 (AB 505), ch 1060 § 14.5 (AB 1822).

§ 11344.2. Furnishing Code and Supplement to county clerks or delegatees

The office shall supply a complete set of the California Code of Regulations, and of the California Code of Regulations Supplement to the county clerk of any county or to the delegatee of the county clerk pursuant to Section 26803.5, provided the director makes the following two determinations:

(a) The county clerk or the delegatee of the county clerk pursuant to Section 26803.5 is maintaining the code and supplement in complete and current condition in a place and at times convenient to the public.

(b) The California Code of Regulations and California Code of Regulations Supplement are not otherwise reasonably available to the public in the community where the county clerk or the delegatee of the county clerk pursuant to Section 26803.5 would normally maintain the code and supplements by distribution to libraries pursuant to Article 6 (commencing with Section 14900) of Chapter 7 of Part 5.5.

HISTORY:

Added Stats 1979 ch 567 § 1, operative July 1, 1980. Amended Stats 1979 ch 1203 § 2; Stats 1981 ch 865 § 14; Stats 1987 ch 1375 § 4.5; Stats 2000 ch 1060 § 15 (AB 1822).

§ 11344.3. Time of publication of documents

Every document, other than a notice of proposed rulemaking action, required to be published in the California Regulatory Notice Register by this chapter, shall be published in the first edition of the California Regulatory Notice Register following the date of the document.

HISTORY:

Added Stats 1985 ch 1044 § 9 as § 11349.9. Amended and renumbered by Stats 1987 ch 1375 § 23.

§ 11344.4. Sale of Code, Supplement and Regulatory Notice Register

(a) The California Code of Regulations, the California Code of Regulations Supplement, and the California Regulatory Notice Register shall be sold at prices which will reimburse the state for all costs incurred for printing, publication, and distribution.

(b) All money received by the state from the sale of the publications listed in subdivision (a) shall be deposited in the treasury and credited to the General Fund, except that, where applicable, an amount necessary to cover the printing, publication, and distribution costs shall be credited to the fund from which the costs have been paid.

HISTORY:

Added Stats 1979 ch 567 § 1, operative July 1, 1980. Amended Stats 1979 ch 1203 § 4; Stats 1981 ch 865 § 16; Stats 1987 ch 1375 § 5; Stats 1988 ch 1194 § 1.3, operative January 1, 1989; Stats 2000 ch 1060 § 16 (AB 1822).

§ 11344.6. Rebuttable presumption raised by publication of regulations

The publication of a regulation in the California Code of Regulations or California Code of Regulations Supplement raises a rebuttable presumption that the text of the regulation as so published is the text of the regulation adopted.

The courts shall take judicial notice of the contents of each regulation which is printed or which is incorporated by appropriate reference into the California Code of Regulations as compiled by the office.

The courts shall also take judicial notice of the repeal of a regulation as published in the California Code of Regulations Supplement compiled by the office.

HISTORY:

Added Stats 1979 ch 567 § 1, operative July 1, 1980, as Gov C § 11343.8. Amended and renumbered Gov C § 11343.7 by Stats 1981 ch 865 § 11; Amended and renumbered by Stats 1983 ch 797 § 5; Amended Stats 1987 ch 1375 § 6; Stats 2000 ch 1060 § 17 (AB 1822).

§ 11344.7. Authority of state agencies to purchase copies of Code, Supplement, or Register or to print and distribute special editions

Nothing in this chapter precludes any person or state agency from purchasing copies of the California Code of Regulations, the California Code of Regulations Supplement, or the California Regulatory Notice Register or of any unit of either, nor from printing special editions of any such units and distributing the same. However, where the purchase and printing is by a state agency, the state agency shall do so at the cost or at less than the cost to the agency if it is authorized to do so by other provisions of law.

HISTORY:

Added Stats 1979 ch 567 § 1, operative July 1, 1980. Amended Stats 1981 ch 865 § 20; Stats 1987 ch 1375 § 6.5; Stats 2000 ch 1060 § 18 (AB 1822).

§ 11344.9. "California Administrative Code"; "California Administrative Notice Register"; "California Administrative Code Supplement"

(a) Whenever the term "California Administrative Code" appears in law, official legal paper, or legal publication, it means the "California Code of Regulations."

(b) Whenever the term "California Administrative Notice Register" appears in any law, official legal paper, or legal publication, it means the "California Regulatory Notice Register."

(c) Whenever the term "California Administrative Code Supplement" or "California Regulatory Code Supplement" appears in any law, official legal paper, or legal publication, it means the "California Code of Regulations Supplement."

HISTORY:

Added Stats 1988 ch 1194 § 1, operative January 1, 1989, as Gov C § 11342.02. Renumbered by Stats 1994 ch 1039 § 9 (AB 2531). Amended Stats 2000 ch 1060 § 19 (AB 1822).

§ 11345. Identification number not required

The office is not required to develop a unique identification number system for each regulatory action pursuant to Section 11341 or to make the California Regulatory Notice Register available on its website pursuant to subdivision (c) of Section 11344.1 until January 1, 2002.

HISTORY:

Added Stats 2000 ch 1059 § 8 (AB 505).

ARTICLE 5

PUBLIC PARTICIPATION: PROCEDURE FOR ADOPTION OF REGULATIONS

Section

11346. Purpose and applicability of article; Subsequent legislation.
11346.1. Emergency regulations and orders of repeal.
11346.2. Availability to public of copy of proposed regulation; Initial statement of reasons for proposed action.
11346.3. Assessment of potential for adverse economic impact on businesses and individuals.
11346.36. Adoption of regulations for conducting standardized regulatory impact analyses; Submission; Publication.
11346.4. Notice of proposed action.
11346.45. Increased public participation.
11346.5. Contents of notice of proposed adoption, amendment, or repeal of regulation.
11346.6. Duty of agency, upon request from person with certain disability, to provide narrative description of proposed regulation.
11346.7. Link on website.
11346.8. Hearing.
11346.9. Final statements of reasons for proposing adoption or amendment of regulation; Informative digest.
11347. Decision not to proceed with proposed action.
11347.1. Addition to rulemaking file.
11347.3. File of rulemaking; Contents and availability of file.
11348. Rulemaking records.

HISTORY: Heading amended Stats 1994 ch 1039 § 19.

§ 11346. Purpose and applicability of article; Subsequent legislation

(a) It is the purpose of this chapter to establish basic minimum procedural requirements for the adoption, amendment, or repeal of administrative regulations. Except as provided in Section 11346.1, the provisions of this chapter are applicable to the exercise of any quasi-legislative power conferred by any statute heretofore or hereafter enacted, but nothing in this chapter repeals or diminishes additional requirements imposed by any statute. This chapter shall not be superseded or modified by any subsequent legislation except to the extent that the legislation shall do so expressly.

(b) An agency that is considering adopting, amending, or repealing a regulation may consult with interested persons before initiating regulatory action pursuant to this article.

HISTORY:

Added Stats 1979 ch 567 § 1, operative July 1, 1980. Amended Stats 1994 ch 1039 § 20 (AB 2531); Stats 2000 ch 1060 § 20 (AB 1822).

§ 11346.1. Emergency regulations and orders of repeal

(a)(1) The adoption, amendment, or repeal of an emergency regulation is not subject to any provision of this article or Article 6 (commencing with Section 11349), except this section and Sections 11349.5 and 11349.6.

(2) At least five working days before submitting an emergency regulation to the office, the adopting agency shall, except as provided in paragraph (3), send a notice of the proposed emergency action to every person who has filed a request for notice of regulatory action with the agency. The notice shall include both of the following:

(A) The specific language proposed to be adopted.

(B) The finding of emergency required by subdivision (b).

(3) An agency is not required to provide notice pursuant to paragraph (2) if the emergency situation clearly poses such an immediate, serious harm that delaying action to allow public comment would be inconsistent with the public interest.

(b)(1) Except as provided in subdivision (c), if a state agency makes a finding that the adoption of a regulation or order of repeal is necessary to address an emergency, the regulation or order of repeal may be adopted as an emergency regulation or order of repeal.

(2) Any finding of an emergency shall include a written statement that contains the information required by paragraphs (2) to (6), inclusive, of subdivision (a) of Section 11346.5 and a description of the specific facts demonstrating the existence of an emergency and the need for immediate action, and demonstrating, by substantial evidence, the need for the proposed regulation to effectuate the statute being implemented, interpreted, or made specific and to address only the demonstrated emergency. The finding of emergency shall also identify each technical, theoretical, and empirical study, report, or similar document, if any, upon which the agency relies. The enactment of an urgency statute shall not, in and of itself, constitute a need for immediate action.

A finding of emergency based only upon expediency, convenience, best interest, general public need, or speculation, shall not be adequate to demonstrate the existence of an emergency. If the situation identified in the finding of emergency existed and was known by the agency adopting the emergency regulation in sufficient time to have been addressed through nonemergency regulations adopted in accordance with the provisions of Article 5 (commencing with Section 11346), the finding of emergency shall include facts explaining the failure to address the situation through nonemergency regulations.

(3) The statement and the regulation or order of repeal shall be filed immediately with the office.

(c) Notwithstanding any other provision of law, no emergency regulation that is a building standard shall be filed, nor shall the building standard be effective, unless the building standard is submitted to the California Building Standards Commission, and is approved and filed pursuant to Sections 18937 and 18938 of the Health and Safety Code.

(d) The emergency regulation or order of repeal shall become effective upon filing or upon any later date specified by the state agency in a written instrument filed with, or as a part of, the regulation or order of repeal.

(e) No regulation, amendment, or order of repeal initially adopted as an emergency regulatory action shall remain in effect more than 180 days unless the adopting agency has complied with Sections 11346.2 to 11347.3, inclusive, either before adopting an emergency regulation or within the 180-day period. The adopting agency, prior to the expiration of the 180-day period, shall transmit to the office for filing with the Secretary of State the adopted regulation, amendment, or order of repeal, the rulemaking file, and a certification that Sections 11346.2 to 11347.3, inclusive, were complied with either before the emergency regulation was adopted or within the 180-day period.

(f) If an emergency amendment or order of repeal is filed and the adopting agency fails to comply with subdivision (e), the regulation as it existed prior to the emergency amendment or order of repeal shall thereupon become effective and after notice to the adopting agency by the office shall be reprinted in the California Code of Regulations.

(g) If a regulation is originally adopted and filed as an emergency and the adopting agency fails to comply with subdivision (e), this failure shall constitute a repeal of the regulation and after notice to the adopting agency by the office, shall be deleted.

(h) The office may approve not more than two readoptions, each for a period not to exceed 90 days, of an emergency regulation that is the same as or substantially equivalent to an emergency regulation previously adopted by that agency. Readoption shall be permitted only if the agency has made substantial progress and proceeded with diligence to comply with subdivision (e).

HISTORY:

Added Stats 1979 ch 567 § 1, operative July 1, 1980. Amended Stats 1979 ch 1152 § 12.4, operative July 1, 1980; Stats 1980 ch 204 § 2, effective June 20, 1980, ch 1238 § 1, effective September 29, 1980; Stats 1981 ch 274 § 7, effective August 27, 1981, ch 865 § 22; Stats 1982 ch 86 § 3, effective March 1, 1982; Stats 1982 ch 86 § 3, effective March 1, 1982, ch 1573 § 2; Stats 1983 ch 797 § 13; Stats 1984 ch 287 § 45, effective July 6, 1984; Stats 1985 ch 956 § 10, effective September 26, 1985; Stats 1987 ch 1375 § 7; Stats 1994 ch 1039 § 21 (AB 2531); Stats 2000 ch 1060 § 21 (AB 1822); Stats 2006 ch 713 § 3 (AB 1302), effective January 1, 2007.

§ 11346.2. Availability to public of copy of proposed regulation; Initial statement of reasons for proposed action

Every agency subject to this chapter shall prepare, submit to the office with the notice of the proposed action as described in Section 11346.5, and make available to the public upon request, all of the following:

(a) A copy of the express terms of the proposed regulation.

(1) The agency shall draft the regulation in plain, straightforward language, avoiding technical terms as much as possible, and using a coherent and easily readable style. The agency shall draft the regulation in plain English.

(2) The agency shall include a notation following the express terms of each California Code of Regulations section, listing the specific statutes or other provisions of law authorizing the adoption of the regulation and listing the specific statutes or other provisions of law being implemented, interpreted, or made specific by that section in the California Code of Regulations.

(3) The agency shall use underline or italics to indicate additions to, and strikeout to indicate deletions from, the California Code of Regulations.

(b) An initial statement of reasons for proposing the adoption, amendment, or repeal of a regulation. This statement of reasons shall include, but not be limited to, all of the following:

(1) A statement of the specific purpose of each adoption, amendment, or repeal, the problem the agency intends to address, and the rationale for the determination by the agency that each adoption, amendment, or repeal is reasonably necessary to carry out the purpose and address the problem for which it is proposed. The statement shall enumerate the benefits anticipated from the regulatory action, including the benefits or goals provided in the authorizing statute. These benefits may include, to the extent applicable, nonmonetary benefits such as the protection of public health and safety, worker safety, or the environment, the prevention of discrimination, the promotion of fairness or social equity, and the increase in openness and transparency in business and government, among other things. Where the adoption or amendment of a regulation would mandate the use of specific technologies or equipment, a statement of the reasons why the agency believes these mandates or prescriptive standards are required.

(2)(A) For a regulation that is not a major regulation, the economic impact assessment required by subdivision (b) of Section 11346.3.

(B) For a major regulation proposed on or after November 1, 2013, the standardized regulatory impact analysis required by subdivision (c) of Section 11346.3.

(3) An identification of each technical, theoretical, and empirical study, report, or similar document, if any, upon which the agency relies in proposing the adoption, amendment, or repeal of a regulation.

(4)(A) A description of reasonable alternatives to the regulation and the agency's reasons for rejecting those alternatives. Reasonable alternatives to be considered include, but are not limited to, alternatives that are proposed as less burdensome and equally effective in achieving the purposes of the regulation in a manner that ensures full compliance with the authorizing statute or other law being implemented or made specific by the proposed regulation. In the case of a regulation that would mandate the use of specific technologies or equipment or prescribe specific actions or procedures, the imposition of performance standards shall be considered as an alternative.

(B) A description of reasonable alternatives to the regulation that would lessen any adverse impact on small business and the agency's reasons for rejecting those alternatives.

(C) Notwithstanding subparagraph (A) or (B), an agency is not required to artificially construct alternatives or describe unreasonable alternatives.

(5)(A) Facts, evidence, documents, testimony, or other evidence on which the agency relies to support an initial determination that the action will not have a significant adverse economic impact on business.

(B)(i) If a proposed regulation is a building standard, the initial statement of reasons shall include the estimated cost of compliance, the estimated potential benefits, and the related assumptions used to determine the estimates.

(ii) The model codes adopted pursuant to Section 18928 of the Health and Safety Code shall be exempt from the requirements of this subparagraph. However, if an interested party has made a request in writing to the agency, at least 30 days before the submittal of the initial statement of reasons, to examine a specific section for purposes of estimating the cost of compliance and the potential benefits for that section, and including the related assumptions used to determine the estimates, then the agency shall comply with the requirements of this subparagraph with regard to that requested section.

(6) A department, board, or commission within the Environmental Protection Agency, the Natural Resources Agency, or the Office of the State Fire Marshal shall describe its efforts, in connection with a proposed rulemaking action, to avoid unnecessary duplication or conflicts with federal regulations contained in the Code of Federal Regulations addressing the same issues. These agencies may adopt regulations different from federal regulations contained in the Code of Federal Regulations addressing the same issues upon a finding of one or more of the following justifications:

(A) The differing state regulations are authorized by law.

(B) The cost of differing state regulations is justified by the benefit to human health, public safety, public welfare, or the environment.

(c) A state agency that adopts or amends a regulation mandated by federal law or regulations, the provisions of which are identical to a previously adopted or amended federal regulation, shall be deemed to have complied with subdivision (b) if a statement to the effect that a federally mandated regulation or amendment to a regulation is being proposed, together with a citation to where an explanation of the regulation can be found, is included in the notice of proposed adoption or amendment prepared pursuant to Section 11346.5. However, the agency shall comply fully with this chapter with respect to any provisions in the regulation that the agency proposes to adopt or amend that are different from the corresponding provisions of the federal regulation.

(d) This section shall be inoperative from January 1, 2012, until January 1, 2014.

HISTORY:

Added Stats 1994 ch 1039 § 23 (AB 2531). Amended Stats 1995 ch 938 § 15.3 (SB 523), operative January 1, 1996; Stats 2000 ch 1059 § 9 (AB 505), ch 1060 § 22.5 (AB 1822); Stats 2002 ch 389 § 4

(AB 1857); Stats 2010 ch 398 § 1 (AB 2738), effective September 27, 2010, inoperative January 1, 2012 until January 1, 2014; Stats 2011 ch 496 § 3 (SB 617), effective January 1, 2012; Stats 2012 ch 471 § 2 (AB 1612), effective January 1, 2013, inoperative January 1, 2012, until January 1, 2014; Stats 2013 ch 212 § 2 (SB 401), effective January 1, 2014, inoperative January 1, 2014; Stats 2014 ch 779 § 1 (AB 1711), effective January 1, 2015.

§ 11346.3. Assessment of potential for adverse economic impact on businesses and individuals

(a) A state agency proposing to adopt, amend, or repeal any administrative regulation shall assess the potential for adverse economic impact on California business enterprises and individuals, avoiding the imposition of unnecessary or unreasonable regulations or reporting, recordkeeping, or compliance requirements. For purposes of this subdivision, assessing the potential for adverse economic impact shall require agencies, when proposing to adopt, amend, or repeal a regulation, to adhere to the following requirements, to the extent that these requirements do not conflict with other state or federal laws:

(1) The proposed adoption, amendment, or repeal of a regulation shall be based on adequate information concerning the need for, and consequences of, proposed governmental action.

(2) The state agency, before submitting a proposal to adopt, amend, or repeal a regulation to the office, shall consider the proposal's impact on business, with consideration of industries affected including the ability of California businesses to compete with businesses in other states. For purposes of evaluating the impact on the ability of California businesses to compete with businesses in other states, an agency shall consider, but not be limited to, information supplied by interested parties.

(3) An economic impact assessment prepared pursuant to this subdivision for a proposed regulation that is not a major regulation or that is a major regulation proposed before November 1, 2013, shall be prepared in accordance with subdivision (b), and shall be included in the initial statement of reasons as required by Section 11346.2. An economic assessment prepared pursuant to this subdivision for a major regulation proposed on or after November 1, 2013, shall be prepared in accordance with subdivision (c), and shall be included in the initial statement of reasons as required by Section 11346.2.

(b)(1) A state agency proposing to adopt, amend, or repeal a regulation that is not a major regulation or that is a major regulation proposed before November 1, 2013, shall prepare an economic impact assessment that assesses whether and to what extent it will affect the following:

(A) The creation or elimination of jobs within the state.

(B) The creation of new businesses or the elimination of existing businesses within the state.

(C) The expansion of businesses currently doing business within the state.

(D) The benefits of the regulation to the health and welfare of California residents, worker safety, and the state's environment.

(2) This subdivision does not apply to the University of California, the college named in Section 92200 of the Education Code, or the Fair Political Practices Commission.

(3) Information required from a state agency for the purpose of completing the assessment may come from existing state publications.

(4)(A) For purposes of conducting the economic impact assessment pursuant to this subdivision, a state agency may use the consolidated definition of small business in subparagraph (B) in order to determine the number of small businesses within the economy, a specific industry sector, or geographic region. The state agency shall clearly identify the use of the consolidated small business definition in its rulemaking package.

(B) For the exclusive purpose of undertaking the economic impact assessment, a "small business" means a business that is all of the following:

(i) Independently owned and operated.

(ii) Not dominant in its field of operation.

(iii) Has fewer than 100 employees.

(C) Subparagraph (A) shall not apply to a regulation adopted by the Department of Insurance that applies to an insurance company.

(c)(1) Each state agency proposing to adopt, amend, or repeal a major regulation on or after November 1, 2013, shall prepare a standardized regulatory impact analysis in the manner prescribed by the Department of Finance pursuant to Section 11346.36. The standardized regulatory impact analysis shall address all of the following:

(A) The creation or elimination of jobs within the state.

(B) The creation of new businesses or the elimination of existing businesses within the state.

(C) The competitive advantages or disadvantages for businesses currently doing business within the state.

(D) The increase or decrease of investment in the state.

(E) The incentives for innovation in products, materials, or processes.

(F) The benefits of the regulations, including, but not limited to, benefits to the health, safety, and welfare of California residents, worker safety, and the state's environment and quality of life, among any other benefits identified by the agency.

(2) This subdivision shall not apply to the University of California, the college named in Section 92200 of the Education Code, or the Fair Political Practices Commission.

(3) Information required from state agencies for the purpose of completing the analysis may be derived from existing state, federal, or academic publications.

(d) Any administrative regulation adopted on or after January 1, 1993, that requires a report shall not apply to businesses, unless the state agency adopting the regulation makes a finding that it is necessary for the health, safety, or welfare of the people of the state that the regulation apply to businesses.

(e) Analyses conducted pursuant to this section are intended to provide agencies and the public with tools to determine whether the regulatory proposal is an efficient and effective means of implementing the policy decisions enacted in statute or by other provisions of law in the least burdensome manner. Regulatory impact analyses shall inform the agencies and the public of the economic consequences of regulatory choices, not reassess statutory policy. The baseline for the regulatory analysis shall be the most cost-effective set of regulatory measures that are equally effective in achieving the purpose of the regulation in a manner that ensures full compliance with the authorizing statute or other law being implemented or made specific by the proposed regulation.

(f) Each state agency proposing to adopt, amend, or repeal a major regulation on or after November 1, 2013, and that has prepared a standardized regulatory impact analysis pursuant to subdivision (c), shall submit that analysis to the Department of Finance upon completion. The department shall comment, within 30 days of receiving that analysis, on the extent to which the analysis adheres to the regulations adopted pursuant to Section 11346.36. Upon receiving the comments from the department, the agency may update its analysis to reflect any comments received from the department and shall summarize the comments and the response of the agency along with a statement of the results of the updated analysis for the statement required by paragraph (10) of subdivision (a) of Section 11346.5.

HISTORY:

Added Stats 1994 ch 1039 § 24 (AB 2531). Amended Stats 2000 ch 1059 § 10 (AB 505), ch 1060 § 23 (AB 1822); Stats 2011 ch 496 § 4 (SB 617), effective January 1, 2012; Stats 2012 ch 766 § 2 (SB 1520), effective September 29, 2012; Stats 2014 ch 779 § 2 (AB 1711), effective January 1, 2015; Stats 2016 ch 346 § 1 (AB 1033), effective January 1, 2017; Stats 2022 ch 478 § 59 (AB 1936), effective January 1, 2023.

§ 11346.36. Adoption of regulations for conducting standardized regulatory impact analyses; Submission; Publication

(a) Prior to November 1, 2013, the Department of Finance, in consultation with the office and other state agencies, shall adopt regulations for conducting the standardized regulatory impact analyses required by subdivision (c) of Section 11346.3.

(b) The regulations, at a minimum, shall assist the agencies in specifying the methodologies for:

(1) Assessing and determining the benefits and costs of the proposed regulation, expressed in monetary terms to the extent feasible and appropriate. Assessing the value of nonmonetary benefits such as the protection of public health and safety, worker safety, or the environment, the prevention of discrimination, the promotion of fairness or social equity, the increase in the openness and transparency of business and government and other nonmonetary benefits consistent with the statutory policy or other provisions of law.

(2) Comparing proposed regulatory alternatives with an established baseline so agencies can make analytical decisions for the adoption, amendment, or repeal of regulations necessary to determine that the proposed action is the most effective, or equally effective and less burdensome, alternative in carrying out the purpose for which the action is proposed, or the most cost-effective alternative to the economy and to affected private persons that would be equally effective in implementing the statutory policy or other provision of law.

(3) Determining the impact of a regulatory proposal on the state economy, businesses, and the public welfare, as described in subdivision (c) of Section 11346.3.

(4) Assessing the effects of a regulatory proposal on the General Fund and special funds of the state and affected local government agencies attributable to the proposed regulation.

(5) Determining the cost of enforcement and compliance to the agency and to affected business enterprises and individuals.

(6) Making the estimation described in Section 11342.548.

(c) To the extent required by this chapter, the department shall convene a public hearing or hearings and take public comment on any draft regulation. Representatives from state agencies and the public at large shall be afforded the opportunity to review and comment on the draft regulation before the regulation is adopted in final form.

(d) State agencies shall provide the Director of Finance and the office ready access to their records and full information and reasonable assistance in any matter requested for purposes of developing the regulations required by this section. This subdivision shall not be construed to authorize an agency to provide access to records required by statute to be kept confidential.

(e) The standardized regulatory impact analysis prepared by the proposing agency shall be included in the initial statement of reasons for the regulation as provided in subdivision (b) of Section 11346.2.

(f) On or before November 1, 2013, the department shall submit the adopted regulations to the Senate and Assembly Committees on Governmental Organization and shall publish the adopted regulations in the State Administrative Manual.

HISTORY:

Added Stats 2011 ch 496 § 5 (SB 617), effective January 1, 2012.

§ 11346.4. Notice of proposed action

(a) At least 45 days prior to the hearing and close of the public comment period on the adoption, amendment, or repeal of a regulation, notice of the proposed action shall be:

(1) Mailed to every person who has filed a request for notice of regulatory actions with the state agency. Each state agency shall give a person filing a request for notice of regulatory actions the option of being notified of all proposed regulatory actions or being notified of regulatory actions concerning one or more particular programs of the state agency.

(2) In cases in which the state agency is within a state department, mailed or delivered to the director of the department.

(3) Mailed to a representative number of small business enterprises or their representatives that are likely to be affected by the proposed action. "Representative" for the purposes of this paragraph includes, but is not limited to, a trade association, industry association, professional association, or any other business group or association of any kind that represents a business enterprise or employees of a business enterprise.

(4) When appropriate in the judgment of the state agency, mailed to any person or group of persons whom the agency believes to be interested in the proposed action and published in the form and manner as the state agency shall prescribe.

(5) Published in the California Regulatory Notice Register as prepared by the office for each state agency's notice of regulatory action.

(6) Posted on the state agency's website if the agency has a website.

(b) The effective period of a notice issued pursuant to this section shall not exceed one year from the date thereof. If the adoption, amendment, or repeal of a regulation proposed in the notice is not completed and transmitted to the office within the period of one year, a notice of the proposed action shall again be issued pursuant to this article.

(c) Once the adoption, amendment, or repeal is completed and approved by the office, no further adoption, amendment, or repeal to the noticed regulation shall be made without subsequent notice being given.

(d) The office may refuse to publish a notice submitted to it if the agency has failed to comply with this article.

(e) The office shall make the California Regulatory Notice Register available to the public and state agencies at a nominal cost that is consistent with a policy of encouraging the widest possible notice distribution to interested persons.

(f) Where the form or manner of notice is prescribed by statute in any particular case, in addition to filing and mailing notice as required by this section, the notice shall be published, posted, mailed, filed, or otherwise publicized as prescribed by that statute. The failure to mail notice to any person as provided in this section shall not invalidate any action taken by a state agency pursuant to this article.

HISTORY:

Added Stats 1979 ch 567 § 1, operative July 1, 1980. Amended Stats 1979 ch 1203 § 5; Stats 1981 ch 865 § 24; Stats 1982 ch 1083 § 3; Stats 1985 ch 1044 § 1; Stats 1987 ch 1375 § 9; Stats 1994 ch 1039 § 25 (AB 2531); Stats 2000 ch 1059 § 11 (AB 505).

§ 11346.45. Increased public participation

(a) In order to increase public participation and improve the quality of regulations, state agencies proposing to adopt regulations shall, prior to publication of the notice required by Section 11346.5, involve parties who would be subject to the proposed regulations in public discussions regarding those proposed regulations, when the proposed regulations involve complex proposals or a large number of proposals that cannot easily be reviewed during the comment period.

(b) This section does not apply to a state agency in any instance where that state agency is required to implement federal law and regulations for which there is little or no discretion on the part of the state to vary.

(c) If the agency does not or cannot comply with the provisions of subdivision (a), it shall state the reasons for noncompliance with reasonable specificity in the rulemaking record.

(d) The provisions of this section shall not be subject to judicial review or to the provisions of Section 11349.1.

HISTORY:

Added Stats 2000 ch 1059 § 12 (AB 505).

§ 11346.5. Contents of notice of proposed adoption, amendment, or repeal of regulation

(a) The notice of proposed adoption, amendment, or repeal of a regulation shall include the following:

(1) A statement of the time, place, and nature of proceedings for adoption, amendment, or repeal of the regulation.

(2) Reference to the authority under which the regulation is proposed and a reference to the particular code sections or other provisions of law that are being implemented, interpreted, or made specific.

(3) An informative digest drafted in plain English in a format similar to the Legislative Counsel's digest on legislative bills. The informative digest shall include the following:

(A) A concise and clear summary of existing laws and regulations, if any, related directly to the proposed action and of the effect of the proposed action.

(B) If the proposed action differs substantially from an existing comparable federal regulation or statute, a brief description of the significant differences and the full citation of the federal regulations or statutes.

(C) A policy statement overview explaining the broad objectives of the regulation and the specific benefits anticipated by the proposed adoption, amendment, or repeal of a regulation, including, to the extent applicable, nonmonetary benefits such as the protection of public health and safety, worker safety, or the environment, the prevention of discrimination, the promotion of fairness or social equity, and the increase in openness and transparency in business and government, among other things.

(D) An evaluation of whether the proposed regulation is inconsistent or incompatible with existing state regulations.

(4) Any other matters as are prescribed by statute applicable to the specific state agency or to any specific regulation or class of regulations.

(5) A determination as to whether the regulation imposes a mandate on local agencies or school districts and, if so, whether the mandate requires state reimbursement pursuant to Part 7 (commencing with Section 17500) of Division 4.

(6) An estimate, prepared in accordance with instructions adopted by the Department of Finance, of the cost or savings to any state agency, the cost to any local agency or school district that is required to be reimbursed under Part 7 (commencing with Section 17500) of Division 4, other nondiscretionary cost or savings imposed on local agencies, and the cost or savings in federal funding to the state.

For purposes of this paragraph, "cost or savings" means additional costs or savings, both direct and indirect, that a public agency necessarily incurs in reasonable compliance with regulations.

(7) If a state agency, in proposing to adopt, amend, or repeal any administrative regulation, makes an initial determination that the action may have a significant, statewide adverse economic impact directly affecting business, including the ability of California businesses to compete with businesses in other states, it shall include the following information in the notice of proposed action:

(A) Identification of the types of businesses that would be affected.

(B) A description of the projected reporting, recordkeeping, and other compliance requirements that would result from the proposed action.

(C) The following statement: "The (name of agency) has made an initial determination that the (adoption/amendment/repeal) of this regulation may have a significant, statewide adverse economic impact directly affecting business, including the ability of California businesses to compete with businesses in other states. The (name of agency) (has/has not) considered proposed alternatives that would lessen any adverse economic impact on business and invites you to submit proposals. Submissions may include the following considerations:

(i) The establishment of differing compliance or reporting requirements or timetables that take into account the resources available to businesses.

(ii) Consolidation or simplification of compliance and reporting requirements for businesses.

(iii) The use of performance standards rather than prescriptive standards.

(iv) Exemption or partial exemption from the regulatory requirements for businesses."

(8) If a state agency, in adopting, amending, or repealing any administrative regulation, makes an initial determination that the action will not have a significant, statewide adverse economic impact directly affecting business, including the ability of California businesses to compete with businesses in other states, it shall make a declaration to that effect in the notice of proposed action. In making this declaration, the agency shall provide in the record facts, evidence, documents, testimony, or other evidence upon which the agency relies to support its initial determination.

An agency's initial determination and declaration that a proposed adoption, amendment, or repeal of a regulation may have or will not have a significant, adverse impact on businesses, including the ability of California businesses to compete with businesses in other states, shall not be grounds for the office to refuse to publish the notice of proposed action.

(9) A description of all cost impacts, known to the agency at the time the notice of proposed action is submitted to the office, that a representative private person or business would necessarily incur in reasonable compliance with the proposed action.

If no cost impacts are known to the agency, it shall state the following: "The agency is not aware of any cost impacts that a representative private person or business would necessarily incur in reasonable compliance with the proposed action."

(10) A statement of the results of the economic impact assessment required by subdivision (b) of Section 11346.3 or the standardized regulatory impact analysis if required by subdivision (c) of Section 11346.3, a summary of any comments submitted to the agency pursuant to subdivision (f) of Section 11346.3 and the agency's response to those comments.

(11) The finding prescribed by subdivision (d) of Section 11346.3, if required.

(12)(A) A statement that the action would have a significant effect on housing costs, if a state agency, in adopting, amending, or repealing any administrative regulation, makes an initial determination that the action would have that effect.

(B) The agency officer designated in paragraph (14) shall make available to the public, upon request, the agency's evaluation, if any, of the effect of the proposed regulatory action on housing costs.

(C) The statement described in subparagraph (A) shall also include the estimated costs of compliance and potential benefits of a building standard, if any, that were included in the initial statement of reasons.

(D) For purposes of model codes adopted pursuant to Section 18928 of the Health and Safety Code, the agency shall comply with the requirements of this paragraph only if an interested party has made a request to the agency to examine a specific section for purposes of estimating the costs of compliance and potential benefits for that section, as described in Section 11346.2.

(13) A statement that the adopting agency must determine that no reasonable alternative considered by the agency or that has otherwise been identified and brought to the attention of the agency would be more effective in carrying out the purpose for which the action is proposed, would be as effective and less burdensome to affected private persons than the proposed action, or would be more cost effective to affected private persons and equally effective in implementing the statutory policy or other provision of law. For a major regulation, as defined by Section 11342.548, proposed on or after November 1, 2013, the statement shall be based, in part, upon the standardized regulatory impact analysis of the proposed regulation, as required by Section 11346.3, as well as upon the benefits of the proposed regulation identified pursuant to subparagraph (C) of paragraph (3).

(14) The name and telephone number of the agency representative and designated backup contact person to whom inquiries concerning the proposed administrative action may be directed.

(15) The date by which comments submitted in writing must be received to present statements, arguments, or contentions in writing relating to the proposed action in order for them to be considered by the state agency before it adopts, amends, or repeals a regulation.

(16) Reference to the fact that the agency proposing the action has prepared a statement of the reasons for the proposed action, has available all the information upon which its proposal is based, and has available the express terms of the proposed action, pursuant to subdivision (b).

(17) A statement that if a public hearing is not scheduled, any interested person or his or her duly authorized representative may request, no later than 15 days prior to the close of the written comment period, a public hearing pursuant to Section 11346.8.

(18) A statement indicating that the full text of a regulation changed pursuant to Section 11346.8 will be available for at least 15 days prior to the date on which the agency adopts, amends, or repeals the resulting regulation.

(19) A statement explaining how to obtain a copy of the final statement of reasons once it has been prepared pursuant to subdivision (a) of Section 11346.9.

(20) If the agency maintains an Internet Web site or other similar forum for the electronic publication or distribution of written material, a statement explaining how materials published or distributed through that forum can be accessed.

(21) If the proposed regulation is subject to Section 11346.6, a statement that the agency shall provide, upon request, a description of the proposed changes included in the proposed action, in the manner provided by Section

11346.6, to accommodate a person with a visual or other disability for which effective communication is required under state or federal law and that providing the description of proposed changes may require extending the period of public comment for the proposed action.

(b) The agency representative designated in paragraph (14) of subdivision (a) shall make available to the public upon request the express terms of the proposed action. The representative shall also make available to the public upon request the location of public records, including reports, documentation, and other materials, related to the proposed action. If the representative receives an inquiry regarding the proposed action that the representative cannot answer, the representative shall refer the inquiry to another person in the agency for a prompt response.

(c) This section shall not be construed in any manner that results in the invalidation of a regulation because of the alleged inadequacy of the notice content or the summary or cost estimates, or the alleged inadequacy or inaccuracy of the housing cost estimates, if there has been substantial compliance with those requirements.

HISTORY:

Added Stats 1979 ch 567 § 1, operative July 1, 1980. Amended Stats 1979 ch 1203 § 6; Stats 1981 ch 865 § 25; Stats 1982 ch 327 § 30, effective June 30, 1982; Stats 1983 ch 797 § 15; Stats 1986 ch 879 § 1; Stats 1987 ch 1375 § 10; Stats 1993 ch 1046 § 1 (AB 1144); Stats 1994 ch 1039 § 26 (AB 2531); Stats 2000 ch 1059 § 13 (AB 505), ch 1060 § 24.5 (AB 1822); Stats 2002 ch 389 § 5 (AB 1857); Stats 2011 ch 495 § 2 (AB 410), ch 496 § 6 (SB 617), effective January 1, 2012; Stats 2012 ch 471 § 3 (AB 1612), effective January 1, 2013, ch 723 § 1.5 (AB 2041), effective January 1, 2013.

§ 11346.6. Duty of agency, upon request from person with certain disability, to provide narrative description of proposed regulation

(a) This section shall only apply to the following proposed regulations:

(1) Regulations proposed by the Department of Rehabilitation.

(2) Regulations that must be submitted to the California Building Standards Commission that pertain to disability access compliance, including, but not limited to, regulations proposed by the State Fire Marshal, the Department of Housing and Community Development, the Division of the State Architect, and the California Commission on Disability Access.

(3) Regulations proposed by the State Department of Education that pertain to special education.

(4) Regulations proposed by the State Department of Health Care Services that pertain to the Medi-Cal program.

(b) Upon request from a person with a visual disability or other disability for which effective communication is required under state or federal law, the agency shall provide that person a narrative description of the additions to, and deletions from, the California Code of Regulations or other publication. The description shall identify each addition to or deletion from the California Code of Regulations by reference to the subdivision, paragraph, subparagraph, clause, or subclause within the proposed regulation containing the addition or deletion. The description shall provide the express language proposed to be added to or deleted from the California Code of Regulations or other publication and any portion of the surrounding language necessary to understand the change in a manner that allows for accurate translation by reading software used by the visually impaired.

(c) The agency shall provide the information described in subdivision (b) within 10 business days, unless the agency determines that compliance with this requirement would be impractical and notifies the requester of the date on which the information will be provided.

(d) Notwithstanding any other law, if information is provided to a requester pursuant to this section, the agency shall provide that requester at least 45 days from the date upon which the information was provided to the requester to submit a public comment regarding the proposed regulation. The agency shall not take final action to adopt the regulation until the requester has submitted a public comment or the extended 45-day comment period expires, whichever occurs first.

(e) The requirements imposed pursuant to subdivisions (b) to (d), inclusive, for a proposed regulation described in subdivision (a) shall apply to an agency only for purposes of that proposed regulation until the proposed regulation is filed with the Secretary of State or until the agency otherwise concludes the regulatory adoption process.

(f)(1) Not later than February 1, 2014, an agency that adopted a proposed regulation subject to the requirements of this section shall submit a report, for both the 2012 and 2013 calendar years, to the Governor, the fiscal committee in each house of the Legislature, and the appropriate policy committee in each house of the Legislature, that specifies the number of requests submitted for a narrative description of a proposed regulation, and the number of narrative descriptions actually provided pursuant to this section.

(2) The report shall be submitted to the Legislature in the manner required pursuant to Section 9795.

(3) The reporting requirement imposed by this subdivision shall become inoperative on February 1, 2018, as required pursuant to Section 10231.5.

(4) It is the intent of the Legislature to evaluate the reports submitted pursuant to this subdivision to determine whether the requirements of this section should be applied to all regulations adopted by all agencies.

HISTORY:

Added Stats 2011 ch 495 § 3 (AB 410), effective January 1, 2012.

§ 11346.7. Link on website

The office shall maintain a link on its website to the website maintained by the Small Business Advocate that also includes the telephone number of the Small Business Advocate.

HISTORY:

Added Stats 2000 ch 1059 § 17 (AB 505).

§ 11346.8. Hearing

(a) If a public hearing is held, both oral and written statements, arguments, or contentions, shall be permitted. The agency may impose reasonable limitations on oral presentations. If a public hearing is not scheduled, the state agency shall, consistent with Section 11346.4, afford any interested person or his or her duly authorized representative, the opportunity to present statements, arguments or contentions in writing. In addition, a public hearing shall be held if, no later than 15 days prior to the close of the written comment period, an interested person or his or her duly authorized representative submits in writing to the state agency, a request to hold a public hearing. The state agency shall, to the extent practicable, provide notice of the time, date, and place of the hearing by mailing the notice to every person who has filed a request for notice thereby with the state agency. The state agency shall consider all relevant matter presented to it before adopting, amending, or repealing any regulation.

(b) In any hearing under this section, the state agency or its duly authorized representative shall have authority to administer oaths or affirmations. An agency may continue or postpone a hearing from time to time to the time and at the place as it determines. If a hearing is continued or postponed, the state agency shall provide notice to the public as to when it will be resumed or rescheduled.

(c) No state agency may adopt, amend, or repeal a regulation which has been changed from that which was originally made available to the public pursuant to Section 11346.5, unless the change is (1) nonsubstantial or solely grammatical in nature, or (2) sufficiently related to the original text that the public was adequately placed on notice that the change could result from the originally proposed regulatory action. If a sufficiently related change is made, the full text of the resulting adoption, amendment, or repeal, with the change clearly indicated, shall be made available to the public for at least 15 days before the agency adopts, amends, or repeals the resulting regulation. Any written comments received regarding the change must be responded to in the final statement of reasons required by Section 11346.9.

(d) No state agency shall add any material to the record of the rulemaking proceeding after the close of the public hearing or comment period, unless the agency complies with Section 11347.1. This subdivision does not apply to material prepared pursuant to Section 11346.9.

(e) If a comment made at a public hearing raises a new issue concerning a proposed regulation and a member of the public requests additional time to respond to the new issue before the state agency takes final action, it is the intent of the Legislature that rulemaking agencies consider granting the request for additional time if, under the circumstances, granting the request is practical and does not unduly delay action on the regulation.

HISTORY:

Added Stats 1981 ch 865 § 29. Amended Stats 1981 ch 1091 § 2; Stats 1982 ch 86 § 4, effective March 1, 1982; Stats 1983 ch 797 § 19; Stats 1987 ch 1375 § 15; Stats 1994 ch 1039 § 32 (AB 2531); Stats 2000 ch 1059 § 16 (AB 505), ch 1060 § 26.5 (AB 1822).

§ 11346.9. Final statements of reasons for proposing adoption or amendment of regulation; Informative digest

Every agency subject to this chapter shall do the following:

(a) Prepare and submit to the office with the adopted regulation a final statement of reasons that shall include all of the following:

(1) An update of the information contained in the initial statement of reasons. If the update identifies any data or any technical, theoretical or empirical study, report, or similar document on which the agency is relying in proposing the adoption, amendment, or repeal of a regulation that was

not identified in the initial statement of reasons, or which was otherwise not identified or made available for public review prior to the close of the public comment period, the agency shall comply with Section 11347.1.

(2) A determination as to whether adoption, amendment, or repeal of the regulation imposes a mandate on local agencies or school districts. If the determination is that adoption, amendment, or repeal of the regulation would impose a local mandate, the agency shall state whether the mandate is reimbursable pursuant to Part 7 (commencing with Section 17500) of Division 4. If the agency finds that the mandate is not reimbursable, it shall state the reasons for that finding.

(3) A summary of each objection or recommendation made regarding the specific adoption, amendment, or repeal proposed, together with an explanation of how the proposed action has been changed to accommodate each objection or recommendation, or the reasons for making no change. This requirement applies only to objections or recommendations specifically directed at the agency's proposed action or to the procedures followed by the agency in proposing or adopting the action. The agency may aggregate and summarize repetitive or irrelevant comments as a group, and may respond to repetitive comments or summarily dismiss irrelevant comments as a group. For the purposes of this paragraph, a comment is "irrelevant" if it is not specifically directed at the agency's proposed action or to the procedures followed by the agency in proposing or adopting the action.

(4) A determination with supporting information that no alternative considered by the agency would be more effective in carrying out the purpose for which the regulation is proposed, would be as effective and less burdensome to affected private persons than the adopted regulation, or would be more cost effective to affected private persons and equally effective in implementing the statutory policy or other provision of law. For a major regulation, as defined by Section 11342.548 proposed on or after November 1, 2013, the determination shall be based, in part, upon the standardized regulatory impact analysis of the proposed regulation and, in part, upon the statement of benefits identified in subparagraph (C) of paragraph (3) of subdivision (a) of Section 11346.5.

(5) An explanation setting forth the reasons for rejecting any proposed alternatives that would lessen the adverse economic impact on small businesses. The agency shall include, as supporting information, the standardized regulatory impact analysis for a major regulation, if required by subdivision (c) of Section 11346.3, as well as the benefits of the proposed regulation identified pursuant to paragraph (3) of subdivision (a) of Section 11346.5.

(b) Prepare and submit to the office with the adopted regulation an updated informative digest containing a clear and concise summary of the immediately preceding laws and regulations, if any, relating directly to the adopted, amended, or repealed regulation and the effect of the adopted, amended, or repealed regulation. The informative digest shall be drafted in a format similar to the Legislative Counsel's Digest on legislative bills.

(c) A state agency that adopts or amends a regulation mandated by federal law or regulations, the provisions of which are identical to a previously adopted or amended federal regulation, shall be deemed to have complied with this section if a statement to the effect that a federally mandated regulation or amendment to a regulation is being proposed, together with a citation to where an explanation of the provisions of the regulation can be found, is included in the notice of proposed adoption or amendment prepared pursuant to Section 11346.5. However, the agency shall comply fully with this chapter with respect to any provisions in the regulation which the agency proposes to adopt or amend that are different from the corresponding provisions of the federal regulation.

(d) If an agency determines that a requirement of this section can be satisfied by reference to an agency statement made pursuant to Sections 11346.2 to 11346.5, inclusive, the agency may satisfy the requirement by incorporating the relevant statement by reference.

HISTORY:

Added Stats 1994 ch 1039 § 33 (AB 2531). Amended Stats 2000 ch 1060 § 27 (AB 1822); Stats 2011 ch 496 § 7 (SB 617), effective January 1, 2012.

§ 11347. Decision not to proceed with proposed action

(a) If, after publication of a notice of proposed action pursuant to Section 11346.4, but before the notice of proposed action becomes ineffective pursuant to subdivision (b) of that section, an agency decides not to proceed with the proposed action, it shall deliver notice of its decision to the office for publication in the California Regulatory Notice Register.

(b) Publication of a notice under this section terminates the effect of the notice of proposed action referred to in the notice. Nothing in this section precludes an agency from proposing a new regulatory action that is similar or identical to a regulatory action that was previously the subject of a notice published under this section.

HISTORY:

Added Stats 2000 ch 1059 § 17 (AB 505), ch 1060 § 28 (AB 1822).

§ 11347.1. Addition to rulemaking file

(a) An agency that adds any technical, theoretical, or empirical study, report, or similar document to the rulemaking file after publication of the notice of proposed action and relies on the document in proposing the action shall make the document available as required by this section.

(b) At least 15 calendar days before the proposed action is adopted by the agency, the agency shall mail to all of the following persons a notice identifying the added document and stating the place and business hours that the document is available for public inspection:

(1) Persons who testified at the public hearing.

(2) Persons who submitted written comments at the public hearing.

(3) Persons whose comments were received by the agency during the public comment period.

(4) Persons who requested notification from the agency of the availability of changes to the text of the proposed regulation.

(c) The document shall be available for public inspection at the location described in the notice for at least 15 calendar days before the proposed action is adopted by the agency.

(d) Written comments on the document or information received by the agency during the availability period shall be summarized and responded to in the final statement of reasons as provided in Section 11346.9.

(e) The rulemaking file shall contain a statement confirming that the agency complied with the requirements of this section and stating the date on which the notice was mailed.

(f) If there are no persons in categories listed in subdivision (b), then the rulemaking file shall contain a confirming statement to that effect.

HISTORY:

Added Stats 2000 ch 1060 § 29 (AB 1822).

§ 11347.3. File of rulemaking; Contents and availability of file

(a) Every agency shall maintain a file of each rulemaking that shall be deemed to be the record for that rulemaking proceeding. Commencing no later than the date that the notice of the proposed action is published in the California Regulatory Notice Register, and during all subsequent periods of time that the file is in the agency's possession, the agency shall make the file available to the public for inspection and copying during regular business hours.

(b) The rulemaking file shall include:

(1) Copies of any petitions received from interested persons proposing the adoption, amendment, or repeal of the regulation, and a copy of any decision provided for by subdivision (d) of Section 11340.7, which grants a petition in whole or in part.

(2) All published notices of proposed adoption, amendment, or repeal of the regulation, and an updated informative digest, the initial statement of reasons, and the final statement of reasons.

(3) The determination, together with the supporting data required by paragraph (5) of subdivision (a) of Section 11346.5.

(4) The determination, together with the supporting data required by paragraph (8) of subdivision (a) of Section 11346.5.

(5) The estimate, together with the supporting data and calculations, required by paragraph (6) of subdivision (a) of Section 11346.5.

(6) All data and other factual information, any studies or reports, and written comments submitted to the agency in connection with the adoption, amendment, or repeal of the regulation.

(7) All data and other factual information, technical, theoretical, and empirical studies or reports, if any, on which the agency is relying in the adoption, amendment, or repeal of a regulation, including any economic impact assessment or standardized regulatory impact analysis as required by Section 11346.3.

(8) A transcript, recording, or minutes of any public hearing connected with the adoption, amendment, or repeal of the regulation.

(9) The date on which the agency made the full text of the proposed regulation available to the public for 15 days prior to the adoption, amendment, or repeal of the regulation, if required to do so by subdivision (c) of Section 11346.8.

(10) The text of regulations as originally proposed and the modified text of regulations, if any, that were made available to the public prior to adoption.

(11) Any other information, statement, report, or data that the agency is required by law to consider or prepare in connection with the adoption, amendment, or repeal of a regulation.

(12) An index or table of contents that identifies each item contained in the rulemaking file. The index or table of contents shall include an affidavit or a declaration under penalty of perjury in the form specified by Section 2015.5 of the Code of Civil Procedure by the agency official who has compiled the rulemaking file, specifying the date upon which the record was closed, and that the file or the copy, if submitted, is complete.

(c) Every agency shall submit to the office with the adopted regulation, the rulemaking file or a complete copy of the rulemaking file.

(d) The rulemaking file shall be made available by the agency to the public, and to the courts in connection with the review of the regulation.

(e) Upon filing a regulation with the Secretary of State pursuant to Section 11349.3, the office shall return the related rulemaking file to the agency, after which no item contained in the file shall be removed, altered, or destroyed or otherwise disposed of. The agency shall maintain the file unless it elects to transmit the file to the State Archives pursuant to subdivision (f).

(f) The agency may transmit the rulemaking file to the State Archives. The file shall include instructions that the Secretary of State shall not remove, alter, or destroy or otherwise dispose of any item contained in the file. Pursuant to Section 12223.5, the Secretary of State may designate a time for the delivery of the rulemaking file to the State Archives in consideration of document processing or storage limitations.

HISTORY:

Added Stats 1979 ch 567 § 1, operative July 1, 1980. Amended Stats 1979 ch 1203 § 8; Stats 1981 ch 865 § 31; Stats 1982 ch 327 § 35, effective June 30, 1982; Stats 1983 ch 797 § 21; Stats 1984 ch 1444 § 5, effective September 26, 1984; Stats 1987 ch 1375 § 16; Stats 1991 ch 899 § 3 (SB 327), effective October 12, 1991; Stats 1994 ch 1039 § 36 (AB 2531); Stats 1996 ch 928 § 3 (SB 1507); Stats 2000 ch 1060 § 30 (AB 1822); 2011 ch 496 § 8 (SB 617), effective January 1, 2012.

§ 11348. Rulemaking records

Each agency subject to this chapter shall keep its rulemaking records on all of that agency's pending rulemaking actions, in which the notice has been published in the California Regulatory Notice Register, current and in one central location.

HISTORY:

Added Stats 2000 ch 1059 § 19 (AB 505).

ARTICLE 6

REVIEW OF PROPOSED REGULATIONS

Section

11349. Definitions.
11349.1. Review of regulations; Regulations to govern review process; Return to adopting agency.
11349.1.5. Review of standardized regulatory impact analyses; Report; Notice of noncompliance.
11349.2. Adding material to file.
11349.3. Time for review of regulations; Procedure on disapproval; Return of regulations.
11349.4. Rewriting and resubmission of regulation; Review.

Section
11349.5. Governor's review of decisions.
11349.6. Review by office of emergency regulation.

HISTORY: Heading amended Stats 1994 ch 1039 § 38.

§ 11349. Definitions

The following definitions govern the interpretation of this chapter:

(a) "Necessity" means the record of the rulemaking proceeding demonstrates by substantial evidence the need for a regulation to effectuate the purpose of the statute, court decision, or other provision of law that the regulation implements, interprets, or makes specific, taking into account the totality of the record. For purposes of this standard, evidence includes, but is not limited to, facts, studies, and expert opinion.

(b) "Authority" means the provision of law which permits or obligates the agency to adopt, amend, or repeal a regulation.

(c) "Clarity" means written or displayed so that the meaning of regulations will be easily understood by those persons directly affected by them.

(d) "Consistency" means being in harmony with, and not in conflict with or contradictory to, existing statutes, court decisions, or other provisions of law.

(e) "Reference" means the statute, court decision, or other provision of law which the agency implements, interprets, or makes specific by adopting, amending, or repealing a regulation.

(f) "Nonduplication" means that a regulation does not serve the same purpose as a state or federal statute or another regulation. This standard requires that an agency proposing to amend or adopt a regulation must identify any state or federal statute or regulation which is overlapped or duplicated by the proposed regulation and justify any overlap or duplication. This standard is not intended to prohibit state agencies from printing relevant portions of enabling legislation in regulations when the duplication is necessary to satisfy the clarity standard in paragraph (3) of subdivision (a) of Section 11349.1. This standard is intended to prevent the indiscriminate incorporation of statutory language in a regulation.

HISTORY:
Added Stats 1979 ch 567 § 1, operative July 1, 1980. Amended Stats 1981 ch 983 § 4; Stats 1982 ch 1573 § 4; Stats 1983 ch 797 § 22; Stats 1985 ch 1044 § 3; Stats 1994 ch 1039 § 39 (AB 2531); Stats 2000 ch 1060 § 31 (AB 1822).

§ 11349.1. Review of regulations; Regulations to govern review process; Return to adopting agency

(a) The office shall review all regulations adopted, amended, or repealed pursuant to the procedure specified in Article 5 (commencing with Section 11346) and submitted to it for publication in the California Code of Regulations Supplement and for transmittal to the Secretary of State and make determinations using all of the following standards:

(1) Necessity.
(2) Authority.
(3) Clarity.
(4) Consistency.

(5) Reference.
(6) Nonduplication.

In reviewing regulations pursuant to this section, the office shall restrict its review to the regulation and the record of the rulemaking proceeding. The office shall approve the regulation or order of repeal if it complies with the standards set forth in this section and with this chapter.

(b) In reviewing proposed regulations for the criteria in subdivision (a), the office may consider the clarity of the proposed regulation in the context of related regulations already in existence.

(c) The office shall adopt regulations governing the procedures it uses in reviewing regulations submitted to it. The regulations shall provide for an orderly review and shall specify the methods, standards, presumptions, and principles the office uses, and the limitations it observes, in reviewing regulations to establish compliance with the standards specified in subdivision (a). The regulations adopted by the office shall ensure that it does not substitute its judgment for that of the rulemaking agency as expressed in the substantive content of adopted regulations.

(d) The office shall return any regulation subject to this chapter to the adopting agency if any of the following occur:

(1) The adopting agency has not prepared the estimate required by paragraph (6) of subdivision (a) of Section 11346.5 and has not included the data used and calculations made and the summary report of the estimate in the file of the rulemaking.

(2) The agency has not complied with Section 11346.3. "Noncompliance" means that the agency failed to complete the economic impact assessment or standardized regulatory impact analysis required by Section 11346.3 or failed to include the assessment or analysis in the file of the rulemaking proceeding as required by Section 11347.3.

(3) The adopting agency has prepared the estimate required by paragraph (6) of subdivision (a) of Section 11346.5, the estimate indicates that the regulation will result in a cost to local agencies or school districts that is required to be reimbursed under Part 7 (commencing with Section 17500) of Division 4, and the adopting agency fails to do any of the following:

(A) Cite an item in the Budget Act for the fiscal year in which the regulation will go into effect as the source from which the Controller may pay the claims of local agencies or school districts.

(B) Cite an accompanying bill appropriating funds as the source from which the Controller may pay the claims of local agencies or school districts.

(C) Attach a letter or other documentation from the Department of Finance which states that the Department of Finance has approved a request by the agency that funds be included in the Budget Bill for the next following fiscal year to reimburse local agencies or school districts for the costs mandated by the regulation.

(D) Attach a letter or other documentation from the Department of Finance which states that the Department of Finance has authorized the augmentation of the amount available for expenditure under the agency's appropriation in the Budget Act which is for reimbursement pursuant to Part 7 (commencing with Section 17500) of Division 4 to local agencies or school districts from the unencumbered balances of other appropriations in the Budget Act and that this augmentation is sufficient to reimburse local agencies or school districts for their costs mandated by the regulation.

(4) The proposed regulation conflicts with an existing state regulation and the agency has not identified the manner in which the conflict may be resolved.

(5) The agency did not make the alternatives determination as required by paragraph (4) of subdivision (a) of Section 11346.9.

(e) The office shall notify the Department of Finance of all regulations returned pursuant to subdivision (d).

(f) The office shall return a rulemaking file to the submitting agency if the file does not comply with subdivisions (a) and (b) of Section 11347.3. Within three state working days of the receipt of a rulemaking file, the office shall notify the submitting agency of any deficiency identified. If no notice of deficiency is mailed to the adopting agency within that time, a rulemaking file shall be deemed submitted as of the date of its original receipt by the office. A rulemaking file shall not be deemed submitted until each deficiency identified under this subdivision has been corrected.

(g) Notwithstanding any other law, return of the regulation to the adopting agency by the office pursuant to this section is the exclusive remedy for a failure to comply with subdivision (c) of Section 11346.3 or paragraph (10) of subdivision (a) of Section 11346.5.

HISTORY:

Added Stats 1979 ch 567 § 1, operative July 1, 1980. Amended Stats 1979 ch 1152 § 12.8, operative July 1, 1980; Stats 1981 ch 865 § 32; Stats 1982 ch 86 § 5, effective March 1, 1982, ch 327 § 36, effective June 30, 1982, ch 1544 § 1, ch 1573 § 5; Stats 1985 ch 1044 § 4; Stats 1987 ch 1375 § 17.5; Stats 1991 ch 794 § 4 (AB 2061); Stats 1994 ch 1039 § 40 (AB 2531); Stats 2000 ch 1060 § 32 (AB 1822); Stats 2011 ch 496 § 9 (SB 617), effective January 1, 2012.

§ 11349.1.5. Review of standardized regulatory impact analyses; Report; Notice of noncompliance

(a) The Department of Finance and the office shall, from time to time, review the standardized regulatory impact analyses required by subdivision (c) of Section 11346.3 and submitted to the office pursuant to Section 11347.3, for adherence to the regulations adopted by the department pursuant to Section 11346.36.

(b) On or before November 1, 2015, the office shall submit to the Senate and Assembly Committees on Governmental Organization a report describing the extent to which submitted standardized regulatory impact analyses for proposed major regulations adhere to the regulations adopted pursuant to Section 11346.36. The report shall include a discussion of agency adherence to the regulations as well as a comparison between various state agencies on the question of adherence. The report may also include any recommendations from the office for actions the Legislature might consider for improving state agency performance.

(c) In addition to the report required by subdivision (b), the office may notify the Legislature of noncompliance by a state agency with the regulations adopted pursuant to Section 11346.36, in any manner or form determined by the office.

HISTORY:

Added Stats 2011 ch 496 § 10 (SB 617), effective January 1, 2012.

§ 11349.2. Adding material to file

An agency may add material to a rulemaking file that has been submitted to the office for review pursuant to this article if addition of the material does not violate other requirements of this chapter.

HISTORY:

Added Stats 2000 ch 1060 § 33 (AB 1822).

§ 11349.3. Time for review of regulations; Procedure on disapproval; Return of regulations

(a) The office shall either approve a regulation submitted to it for review and transmit it to the Secretary of State for filing or disapprove it within 30 working days after the regulation has been submitted to the office for review. If the office fails to act within 30 days, the regulation shall be deemed to have been approved and the office shall transmit it to the Secretary of State for filing.

(b) If the office disapproves a regulation, it shall return it to the adopting agency within the 30-day period specified in subdivision (a) accompanied by a notice specifying the reasons for disapproval. Within seven calendar days of the issuance of the notice, the office shall provide the adopting agency with a written decision detailing the reasons for disapproval. No regulation shall be disapproved except for failure to comply with the standards set forth in Section 11349.1 or for failure to comply with this chapter.

(c) If an agency determines, on its own initiative, that a regulation submitted pursuant to subdivision (a) should be returned by the office prior to completion of the office's review, it may request the return of the regulation. All requests for the return of a regulation shall be memorialized in writing by the submitting agency no later than one week following the request. Any regulation returned pursuant to this subdivision shall be resubmitted to the office for review within the one-year period specified in subdivision (b) of Section 11346.4 or shall comply with Article 5 (commencing with Section 11346) prior to resubmission.

(d) The office shall not initiate the return of a regulation pursuant to subdivision (c) as an alternative to disapproval pursuant to subdivision (b).

HISTORY:

Added Stats 1979 ch 567 § 1, operative July 1, 1980. Amended Stats 1981 ch 865 § 33; Stats 1982 ch 1236 § 1; Stats 1985 ch 1044 § 5; Stats 1987 ch 1375 § 19; Stats 1991 ch 794 § 5 (AB 2061); Stats 1992 ch 1306 § 2 (AB 3511).

§ 11349.4. Rewriting and resubmission of regulation; Review

(a) A regulation returned to an agency because of failure to meet the standards of Section 11349.1, because of an agency's failure to comply with this chapter may be rewritten and resubmitted within 120 days of the agency's receipt of the written opinion required by subdivision (b) of Section 11349.3 without complying with the notice and public hearing requirements of Sections 11346.4, 11346.5, and 11346.8 unless the substantive provisions of the regulation have been significantly changed. If the regulation has been significantly changed or was not submitted within 120 days of receipt of the written opinion, the agency shall comply with Article 5 (commencing with Section 11346) and readopt the regulation. The director of the office may, upon a showing of good cause, grant an extension to the 120-day time period specified in this subdivision.

(b) Upon resubmission of a disapproved regulation to the office pursuant to subdivision (a), the office shall only review the resubmitted regulation for those reasons expressly identified in the written opinion required by subdivision (b) of Section 11349.3, or for those issues arising as a result of a substantial change to a provision of the resubmitted regulation or as a result of intervening statutory changes or intervening court orders or decisions.

(c) When an agency resubmits a withdrawn or disapproved regulation to the office it shall identify the prior withdrawn or disapproved regulation by date of submission to the office, shall specify the portion of the prior rulemaking record that should be included in the resubmission, and shall submit to the office a copy of the prior rulemaking record if that record has been returned to the agency by the office.

(d) The office shall expedite the review of a regulation submitted without significant substantive change.

HISTORY:

Added Stats 1979 ch 567 § 1, operative July 1, 1980. Amended Stats 1981 ch 865 § 34; Stats 1982 ch 1573 § 7; Stats 1983 ch 142 § 37; Stats 1985 ch 1044 § 6; Stats 1987 ch 1375 § 20.

§ 11349.5. Governor's review of decisions

(a) To initiate a review of a decision by the office, the agency shall file a written Request for Review with the Governor's Legal Affairs Secretary within 10 days of receipt of the written opinion provided by the office pursuant to subdivision (b) of Section 11349.3. The Request for Review shall include a complete statement as to why the agency believes the decision is incorrect and should be overruled. Along with the Request for Review, the agency shall submit all of the following:

(1) The office's written decision detailing the reasons for disapproval required by subdivision (b) of Section 11349.3.

(2) Copies of all regulations, notices, statements, and other documents which were submitted to the office.

(b) A copy of the agency's Request for Review shall be delivered to the office on the same day it is delivered to the Governor's office. The office shall file its written response to the agency's request with the Governor's Legal Affairs Secretary within 10 days and deliver a copy of its response to the agency on the same day it is delivered to the Governor's office.

(c) The Governor's office shall provide the requesting agency and the office with a written decision within 15 days of receipt of the response by the office to the agency's Request for Review. Upon receipt of the decision, the office shall publish in the California Regulatory Notice Register the agency' s Request for Review, the office's response thereto, and the decision of the Governor's office.

(d) The time requirements set by subdivisions (a) and (b) may be shortened by the Governor's office for good cause.

(e) The Governor may overrule the decision of the office disapproving a proposed regulation, an order repealing an emergency regulation adopted pursuant to subdivision (b) of Section 11346.1, or a decision refusing to allow the readoption of an emergency regulation pursuant to Section 11346.1. In that event, the office shall immediately transmit the regulation to the Secretary of State for filing.

(f) Upon overruling the decision of the office, the Governor shall immediately transmit to the Committees on Rules of both houses of the Legislature a statement of his or her reasons for overruling the decision of the office, along with copies of the adopting agency's initial statement of reasons issued pursuant to Section 11346.2 and the office's statement regarding the disapproval of a regulation issued pursuant to subdivision (b) of Section 11349.3. The Governor's action and the reasons therefor shall be published in the California Regulatory Notice Register.

HISTORY:

Added Stats 1979 ch 567 § 1, operative July 1, 1980. Amended Stats 1980 ch 1238 § 5, effective September 29, 1980; Stats 1981 ch 865 § 34.5; Stats 1982 ch 86 § 6, effective March 1, 1982, ch 1236 § 2; Stats 1983 ch 724 § 1; Stats 1985 ch 1044 § 7; Stats 1987 ch 1375 § 20.2; Stats 1994 ch 1039 § 41 (AB 2531); Stats 1995 ch 938 § 15.6 (SB 523), operative January 1, 1996.

§ 11349.6. Review by office of emergency regulation

(a) If the adopting agency has complied with Sections 11346.2 to 11347.3, inclusive, prior to the adoption of the regulation as an emergency, the office shall approve or disapprove the regulation in accordance with this article.

(b) Emergency regulations adopted pursuant to subdivision (b) of Section 11346.1 shall be reviewed by the office within 10 calendar days after their submittal to the office. After posting a notice of the filing of a proposed emergency regulation on its Internet Web site, the office shall allow interested persons five calendar days to submit comments on the proposed emergency regulations unless the emergency situation clearly poses such an immediate serious harm that delaying action to allow public comment would be inconsistent with the public interest. The office shall disapprove the emergency regulations if it determines that the situation addressed by the regulations is not an emergency, or if it determines that the regulation fails to meet the standards set forth in Section 11349.1, or if it determines the agency failed to comply with Section 11346.1.

(c) If the office considers any information not submitted to it by the rulemaking agency when determining whether to file emergency regulations, the office shall provide the rulemaking agency with an opportunity to rebut or comment upon that information.

(d) Within 30 working days of the filing of a certificate of compliance, the office shall review the regulation and hearing record and approve or order the repeal of an emergency regulation if it determines that the regulation fails to meet the standards set forth in Section 11349.1, or if it determines that the agency failed to comply with this chapter.

HISTORY:

Added Stats 1979 ch 567 § 1, operative July 1, 1980. Amended Stats 1979 ch 1203 § 9; Stats 1980 ch 1238 § 6, effective September 29, 1980; Stats 1981 ch 865 § 35; Stats 1982 ch 1236 § 3, ch 1573 § 8; Stats 1983 ch 797 § 23; Stats 1985 ch 1044 § 8; Stats 1987 ch 1375 § 20.5; Stats 1994 ch 1039 § 42 (AB 2531); Stats 2000 ch 1060 § 34 (AB 1822); Stats 2006 ch 713 § 4 (AB 1302), effective January 1, 2007.

ARTICLE 7
REVIEW OF EXISTING REGULATIONS

Section

11349.7. Priority review of regulations.
11349.8. Repeal of regulation for which statutory authority is repealed, ineffective or inoperative.
11349.9. Review of notice of repeal.

HISTORY: Added Stats 1994 ch 1039 § 43. Former Article 7, consisting of § 11350, added Stats 1979 ch 567 § 1, operative July 1, 1980. Renumbered Article 8 by Stats 1994 ch 1039 § 46.

§ 11349.7. Priority review of regulations

The office, at the request of any standing, select, or joint committee of the Legislature, shall initiate a priority review of any regulation, group of regulations, or series of regulations that the committee believes does not meet the standards set forth in Section 11349.1.

The office shall notify interested persons and shall publish notice in the California Regulatory Notice Register that a priority review has been requested, shall consider the written comments submitted by interested persons, the information contained in the rulemaking record, if any, and shall complete each priority review made pursuant to this section within 90 calendar days of the receipt of the committee's written request. During the period of any priority review made pursuant to this section, all information available to the office relating to the priority review shall be made available to the public. In the event that the office determines that a regulation does not meet the standards set forth in Section 11349.1, it shall order the adopting agency to show cause why the regulation should not be repealed and shall proceed to seek repeal of the regulation as provided by this section in accordance with the following:

(a) In the event it determines that any of the regulations subject to the review do not meet the standards set forth in Section 11349.1, the office shall within 15 days of the determination order the adopting agency to show cause why the regulation should not be repealed. In issuing the order, the office shall specify in writing the reasons for its determination that the regulation does not meet the standards set forth in Section 11349.1. The reasons for its determination shall be made available to the public. The office shall also publish its order and the reasons therefor in the California Regulatory Notice Register. In the case of a regulation for which no, or inadequate, information relating to its necessity can be furnished by the adopting agency, the order shall specify the information which the office requires to make its determination.

(b) No later than 60 days following receipt of an order to show cause why a regulation should not be repealed, the agency shall respond in writing to the office. Upon written application by the agency, the office may extend the time for an additional 30 days.

(c) The office shall review and consider all information submitted by the agency in a timely response to the order to show cause why the regulation should not be repealed, and determine whether the regulation meets the standards set forth in Section 11349.1. The office shall make this determination within 60 days of receipt of an agency's response to the order to show cause. If the office does not make a determination within 60 days of receipt of an agency's response to the order to show cause, the regulation shall be deemed to meet the standards set forth in subdivision (a) of Section 11349.1. In making this determination, the office shall also review any written comments submitted to it by the public within 30 days of the publication of the order to show cause in the California Regulatory Notice Register. During the period of review and consideration, the information available to the office relating to each regulation for which the office has issued an order to show cause shall be made available to the public. The office shall notify the adopting agency within two working days of the receipt of information submitted by the public regarding a regulation for which an order to show cause has been issued. If the office determines that a regulation fails to meet the standards, it shall prepare a statement specifying the reasons for its determination. The statement shall be delivered to the adopting agency, the Legislature, and the Governor and shall be made available to the public and the courts. Thirty days after delivery of the statement required by this subdivision the office shall prepare an order of repeal of the regulation and shall transmit it to the Secretary of State for filing.

(d) The Governor, within 30 days after the office has delivered the statement specifying the reasons for its decision to repeal, as required by subdivision (c), may overrule the decision of the office ordering the repeal of a regulation. The regulation shall then remain in full force and effect. Notice of the Governor's action and the reasons therefor shall be published in the California Regulatory Notice Register.

The Governor shall transmit to the rules committee of each house of the Legislature a statement of reasons for overruling the decision of the office, plus any other information that may be requested by either of the rules committees.

(e) In the event that the office orders the repeal of a regulation, it shall publish the order and the reasons therefor in the California Regulatory Notice Register.

HISTORY:

Added Stats 1994 ch 1039 § 43 (AB 2531).

§ 11349.8. Repeal of regulation for which statutory authority is repealed, ineffective or inoperative

(a) If the office is notified of, or on its own becomes aware of, an existing regulation in the California Code of Regulations for which the statutory authority has been repealed or becomes ineffective or inoperative by its own terms, the office shall order the adopting agency to show cause why the regulation should not be repealed for lack of statutory authority and shall notify the Legislature in writing of this order. In issuing the order, the office shall specify in writing the reasons for issuance of the order. "Agency," for purposes of this section and Section 11349.9, refers to the agency that adopted the regulation and, if applicable, the agency that is responsible for administering the regulation in issue.

(b) The agency may, within 30 days after receipt of the written notification, submit in writing to the office any citations, legal arguments, or other information opposing the repeal, including public comments during this period. This section shall not apply where the agency demonstrates in its response that any of the following conditions exists:

(1) The statute or section thereof is simultaneously repealed and substantially reenacted through a single piece of legislation, or where subsequent legislation evinces a specific legislative intent to reenact the substance of the statute or section. When a regulation cites more than one specific statute or section as reference or authority for the adoption of a regulation, and one or more of the statutes or sections are repealed or become ineffective or inoperative, then the only provisions of the regulation which remain in effect shall be those for which the remaining statutes or sections provide specific or general authority.

(2) The statute is temporarily repealed, or rendered ineffective or inoperative by a provision of law which is effective only for a limited period, in which case any regulation described in subdivision (a) is thereby also temporarily repealed, rendered ineffective, or inoperative during that limited period. Any regulation so affected shall have the same force and effect upon the expiration of the limited period during which the provision of law was effective as if that temporary provision had not been enacted.

(3) The statute or section of a statute being repealed, or becoming ineffective or inoperative by its own terms, is to remain in full force and effect as regards events occurring prior to the date of repeal or ineffectiveness, in which case any regulation adopted to implement or interpret that statute shall likewise be deemed to remain in full force and effect in regards to those same events.

(c) This section shall not be construed to deprive any person or public agency of any substantial right which would have existed prior to, or hereafter exists subsequent to, the effective date of this section.

(d) Thirty days after receipt of the agency's opposition material, or the close of the 30-day agency and public response period if no response is submitted, the office shall do one of the following:

(1) Inform the agency and the Legislature in writing that the office has withdrawn its order to show cause.

(2) Issue a written notice to the agency specifying the reasons for the repeal and its intent to file a Notice of Repeal of the invalid regulation with the Secretary of State. Within seven calendar days of the filing of the Notice of Repeal, the office shall provide the agency, the Governor, and the Legislature with a written decision detailing the reasons for the repeal and a copy of the Notice of Repeal, and publish the office's written decision in the California Regulatory Notice Register.

(e) The office shall order the removal of the repealed regulation from the California Code of Regulations within 30 days after filing the Notice of Repeal, if the agency has not appealed the office's decision, or upon receipt of notification of the Governor's decision upholding the office's decision, if an appeal has been filed pursuant to Section 11349.9.

HISTORY:

Added Stats 1989 ch 1170 § 1, as Gov C § 11349.10. Amended and renumbered by Stats 1994 ch 1039 § 44 (AB 2531).

§ 11349.9. Review of notice of repeal

(a) To initiate a review of the office's Notice of Repeal pursuant to Section

11349.8, the agency shall appeal the office's decision by filing a written Request for Review with the Governor's Legal Affairs Secretary within 10 days of receipt of the Notice of Repeal and written decision provided for by paragraph (2) of subdivision (d) of Section 11349.8. The Request for Review shall include a complete statement as to why the agency believes the decision is incorrect and should be overruled. Along with the Request for Review, the agency shall submit all of the following:

(1) The office's written opinion detailing the reasons for repeal required by paragraph (2) of subdivision (d) of Section 11349.8.

(2) Copies of all statements and other documents that were submitted to the office.

(b) A copy of the agency's Request for Review shall be delivered to the office on the same day it is delivered to the Governor's office. The office shall file its written response to the agency's request with the Governor's Legal Affairs Secretary within 10 days, and deliver a copy of its response to the agency on the same day it is delivered to the Governor's office.

(c) The Governor's office shall provide the requesting agency and the office with a written decision within 15 days of receipt of the response by the office to the agency's Request for Review. Upon receipt of the decision, the office shall publish in the California Regulatory Notice Register the agency' s Request for Review, the office's response thereto, and the decision of the Governor's office.

(d) The time requirements set by subdivisions (a) and (b) may be shortened by the Governor's office for good cause.

(e) In the event the Governor overrules the decision of the office, the office shall immediately transmit the regulation to the Secretary of State for filing.

(f) Upon overruling the decision of the office, the Governor shall transmit to the rules committees of both houses of the Legislature a statement of the reasons for overruling the decision of the office.

HISTORY:

Added Stats 1989 ch 1170 § 2 as Gov C § 11349.11. Amended and renumbered by Stats 1994 ch 1039 § 45 (AB 2531); Amended Stats 1995 ch 938 § 15.7 (SB 523), operative January 1, 1996.

ARTICLE 8

JUDICIAL REVIEW

Section

11350. Judicial declaration regarding validity of regulation; Grounds for invalidity.
11350.3. Judicial declaration as to validity of disapproved or repealed regulation.

HISTORY: Added Stats 1979 ch 567 § 1, operative July 1, 1980, as Article 7. Renumbered by Stats 1994 ch 1039 § 46 (AB 2531), effective January 1, 1995. Former Article 8, entitled "Exemptions," consisting of §§ 11445, 11446, was added Stats 1979 ch 567 § 1, operative July 1, 1980, and repealed Stats 2015 ch 303 § 189, effective January 1, 2016.

§ 11350. Judicial declaration regarding validity of regulation; Grounds for invalidity

(a) Any interested person may obtain a judicial declaration as to the validity of any regulation or order of repeal by bringing an action for declaratory relief in the superior court in accordance with the Code of Civil Procedure. The right to judicial determination shall not be affected by the failure either to petition or to seek reconsideration of a petition filed pursuant to Section 11340.7 before the agency promulgating the regulation or order of repeal. The regulation or order of repeal may be declared to be invalid for a substantial failure to comply with this chapter, or, in the case of an emergency regulation or order of repeal, upon the ground that the facts recited in the finding of emergency prepared pursuant to subdivision (b) of Section 11346.1 do not constitute an emergency within the provisions of Section 11346.1.

(b) In addition to any other ground that may exist, a regulation or order of repeal may be declared invalid if either of the following exists:

(1) The agency's determination that the regulation is reasonably necessary to effectuate the purpose of the statute, court decision, or other provision of law that is being implemented, interpreted, or made specific by the regulation is not supported by substantial evidence.

(2) The agency declaration pursuant to paragraph (8) of subdivision (a) of Section 11346.5 is in conflict with substantial evidence in the record.

(c) The approval of a regulation or order of repeal by the office or the Governor's overruling of a decision of the office disapproving a regulation or order of repeal shall not be considered by a court in any action for declaratory relief brought with respect to a regulation or order of repeal.

(d) In a proceeding under this section, a court may only consider the following evidence:

(1) The rulemaking file prepared under Section 11347.3.

(2) The finding of emergency prepared pursuant to subdivision (b) of Section 11346.1.

(3) An item that is required to be included in the rulemaking file but is not included in the rulemaking file, for the sole purpose of proving its omission.

(4) Any evidence relevant to whether a regulation used by an agency is required to be adopted under this chapter.

HISTORY:

Added Stats 1979 ch 567 § 1, operative July 1, 1980. Amended Stats 1981 ch 592 § 1, ch 865 § 37; Stats 1982 ch 86 § 9, effective March 1, 1982, ch 1573 § 10; Stats 1991 ch 794 § 6 (AB 2061); Stats 1994 ch 1039 § 47 (AB 2531); Stats 1995 ch 938 § 15.8 (SB 523), operative January 1, 1996; Stats 2000 ch 1060 § 35 (AB 1822); Stats 2006 ch 713 § 5 (AB 1302), effective January 1, 2007.

§ 11350.3. Judicial declaration as to validity of disapproved or repealed regulation

Any interested person may obtain a judicial declaration as to the validity of a regulation or order of repeal which the office has disapproved pursuant to Section 11349.3, or 11349.6, or of a regulation that has been ordered repealed pursuant to Section 11349.7 by bringing an action for declaratory relief in the superior court in accordance with the Code of Civil Procedure. The court may declare the regulation valid if it determines that the regulation meets the standards set forth in Section 11349.1 and that the agency has complied with this chapter. If the court so determines, it may order the office to immediately file the regulation with the Secretary of State.

HISTORY:

Added Stats 1982 ch 1544 § 2, ch 1573 § 11. Amended Stats 1987 ch 1375 § 23.5; Stats 1994 ch 1039 § 48 (AB 2531); Stats 2000 ch 1060 § 36 (AB 1822).

ARTICLE 9
SPECIAL PROCEDURES

Section
11351. Applicability of specified provisions to Public Utilities Commission and Workers' Compensation Appeals Board.
11352. Applicability of chapter.
11353. Application of chapter to water quality control policy, plans, or guidelines.
11354. Effect of certain sections on court determination of applicability of chapter.
11354.1. Application of chapter to certain policies, plans and guidelines of San Francisco Bay Conservation and Development Commission.
11356. Applicability of articles to building standards.
11357. Instructions for determining impact of proposed action on local or state agencies or on school districts.
11359. Regulations relating to fire and panic safety.
11361. Applicability of chapter; Adoption or revision of regulations, guidelines, or criteria.

HISTORY: Heading added to precede Gov C § 11351 by Stats 1994 ch 1039 § 49.

§ 11351. Applicability of specified provisions to Public Utilities Commission and Workers' Compensation Appeals Board

(a) Except as provided in subdivision (b), Article 5 (commencing with Section 11346), Article 6 (commencing with Section 11349), Article 7 (commencing with Section 11349.7), and Article 8 (commencing with Section 11350) shall not apply to the Public Utilities Commission or the Workers' Compensation Appeals Board, and Article 3 (commencing with Section 11343) and Article 4 (commencing with Section 11344) shall apply only to the rules of procedure of these state agencies.

(b) The Public Utilities Commission and the Workers' Compensation Appeals Board shall comply with paragraph (5) of subdivision (a) of Section 11346.4 with respect to regulations that are required to be filed with the Secretary of State pursuant to Section 11343.

(c) Article 8 (commencing with Section 11350) shall not apply to the Division of Workers' Compensation.

HISTORY:

Added Stats 1979 ch 567 § 1, operative July 1, 1980, as Gov C § 11445. Amended and renumbered by Stats 1980 ch 204 § 6, effective June 20, 1980; Amended Stats 1982 ch 86 § 10, effective March 1, 1982; Stats 1983 ch 797 § 26; Stats 1987 ch 1375 § 24; Stats 1994 ch 1039 § 50 (AB 2531); Stats 1996 ch 14 § 1 (AB 1859).

§ 11352. Applicability of chapter

The following actions are not subject to this chapter:

(a) The issuance, denial, or waiver of any water quality certification as authorized under Section 13160 of the Water Code.

(b) The issuance, denial, or revocation of waste discharge requirements and permits pursuant to Sections 13263 and 13377 of the Water Code and waivers issued pursuant to Section 13269 of the Water Code.

(c) The development, issuance, and use of the guidance document pursuant to Section 13383.7 of the Water Code.

(d) The issuance of an order pursuant to Section 116400 of the Health and Safety Code.

(e) The issuance of a notification level, response level, or definition of a confirmed detection under Section 116455 of the Health and Safety Code.

(f) The issuance of an order or directive requiring the submittal of technical reports pursuant to Section 116530 of the Health and Safety Code.

HISTORY:

Added Stats 1992 ch 1112 § 1 (AB 3359). Amended Stats 2007 ch 610 § 1.5 (AB 739), effective January 1, 2008; Stats 2021 ch 187 § 1 (SB 776), effective January 1, 2022.

§ 11353. Application of chapter to water quality control policy, plans, or guidelines

(a) Except as provided in subdivision (b), this chapter does not apply to the adoption or revision of state policy for water quality control and the adoption or revision of water quality control plans and guidelines pursuant to Division 7 (commencing with Section 13000) of the Water Code.

(b)(1) Any policy, plan, or guideline, or any revision thereof, that the State Water Resources Control Board has adopted or that a court determines is subject to this part, after June 1, 1992, shall be submitted to the office.

(2) The State Water Resources Control Board shall include in its submittal to the office all of the following:

(A) A clear and concise summary of any regulatory provisions adopted or approved as part of that action, for publication in the California Code of Regulations.

(B) The administrative record for the proceeding. Proposed additions to a policy, plan, or guideline shall be indicated by underlined text and proposed deletions shall be indicated by strike-through text in documents submitted as part of the administrative record for the proceeding.

(C) A summary of the necessity for the regulatory provision.

(D) A certification by the chief legal officer of the State Water Resources Control Board that the action was taken in compliance with all applicable procedural requirements of Division 7 (commencing with Section 13000) of the Water Code.

(3) Paragraph (2) does not limit the authority of the office to review any regulatory provision which is part of the policy, plan, or guideline submitted by the State Water Resources Control Board.

(4) The office shall review the regulatory provisions to determine compliance with the standards of necessity, authority, clarity, consistency, reference, and nonduplication set forth in subdivision (a) of Section 11349.1. The office shall also review the responses to public comments prepared by the State Water Resources Control Board or the appropriate regional water quality control board to determine compliance with the public participation requirements of the Federal Water Pollution Control Act (33 U.S.C. Sec. 1251 et seq.). The office shall restrict its review to the regulatory provisions and the administrative record of the proceeding. Sections 11349.3, 11349.4, 11349.5, and 11350.3 shall apply to the review by the office to the extent that those sections are consistent with this section.

(5) The policy, plan, guideline, or revision shall not become effective unless and until the regulatory provisions are approved by the office in accordance with subdivision (a) of Section 11349.3.

(6) Upon approval of the regulatory provisions, the office shall transmit to the Secretary of State for filing the clear and concise summary of the regulatory provisions submitted by the State Water Resources Control Board.

(7) Any proceedings before the State Water Resources Control Board or a California regional water quality control board to take any action subject to this subdivision shall be conducted in accordance with the procedural requirements of Division 7 (commencing with Section 13000) of the Water Code, together with any applicable requirements of the Federal Water Pollution Control Act (33 U.S.C. Sec. 1251 et seq.), and the requirements of this chapter, other than the requirement for review by the office in accordance with this subdivision, shall not apply.

(8) This subdivision shall not provide a basis for review by the office under this subdivision or Article 6 (commencing with Section 11349) of any such policy, plan, or guideline adopted or revised prior to June 1, 1992.

(c) Subdivision (a) does not apply to a provision of any policy, plan, guideline, or revision, as applied to any person who, as of June 1, 1992, was a party to a civil action challenging that provision on the grounds that it has not been adopted as a regulation pursuant to this chapter.

(d) Copies of the policies, plans, and guidelines to which subdivision (a) applies shall be maintained at central locations for inspection by the public. The State Water Resources Control Board shall maintain, at its headquarters in Sacramento, a current copy of each policy, plan, or guideline in effect. Each regional water quality control board shall maintain at its headquarters a current copy of each policy, plan, or guideline in effect in its respective region. Any revision of a policy, plan, or guideline shall be made available for inspection by the public within 30 days of its effective date.

HISTORY:
Added Stats 1992 ch 1112 § 2 (AB 3359). Amended Stats 2000 ch 1060 § 37 (AB 1822).

§ 11354. Effect of certain sections on court determination of applicability of chapter

Sections 11352 and 11353 do not affect any court's determination, relating to the applicability of this chapter to any provision of a policy, plan, or guideline, in a civil action which was pending on June 1, 1992, and on that date included a challenge to a provision of a policy, plan, or guideline on the grounds that it has not been adopted in accordance with this chapter.

HISTORY:
Added Stats 1992 ch 1112 § 2 (AB 3359).

§ 11354.1. Application of chapter to certain policies, plans and guidelines of San Francisco Bay Conservation and Development Commission

(a) For purposes of this section, "commission" means the San Francisco Bay Conservation and Development Commission.

(b) This chapter does not apply to any policy, plan, or guideline adopted by the commission prior to January 1, 1996, pursuant to Chapter 5 (commencing with Section 66650) of Title 7.2 of this code or Division 19 (commencing with Section 29000) of the Public Resources Code.

(c) The issuance or denial by the commission of any permit pursuant to subdivision (a) of Section 66632, and the issuance or denial by, or appeal to, the commission of any permit pursuant to Chapter 6 (commencing with Section 29500) of Division 19 of the Public Resources Code, are not subject to this chapter.

(d)(1) Any amendments or other changes to the San Francisco Bay Plan or to a special area plan pursuant to Chapter 5 (commencing with Section 66650) of Title 7.2, adopted by the commission on or after January 1, 1996, and any amendments or other changes to the Suisun Marsh Protection Plan, as defined in Section 29113 of the Public Resources Code, or in the Suisun Marsh local protection program, as defined in Section 29111 of the Public Resources Code, adopted by the commission on and after January 1, 1996, shall be submitted to the office but are not subject to this chapter except as provided in this subdivision.

(2) The commission shall include in its submittal to the office pursuant to paragraph (1) both of the following documents:

(A) A clear and concise summary of any regulatory provision adopted or approved by the commission as part of the proposed change for publication in the California Code of Regulations.

(B) The administrative record for the proceeding, and a list of the documents relied upon in making the change. Proposed additions to the plans shall be indicated by underlined text, and proposed deletions shall be indicated by strike-through text in documents submitted as part of the administrative record for the proceeding.

(3) The office shall review the regulatory provisions to determine compliance with the standards of necessity, authority, clarity, consistency, reference, and nonduplication set forth in subdivision (a) of Section 11349.1. The office shall also review the responses to public comments prepared by the commission to determine compliance with the public participation requirements of Sections 11000 to 11007, inclusive, of Title 14 of the California Code of Regulations, and to ensure that the commission considers all relevant matters presented to it before adopting, amending, or repealing any regulatory provision, and that the commission explains the reasons for not modifying a proposed plan change to accommodate an objection or recommendation. The office shall restrict its review to the regulatory provisions and the administrative record of the proceeding. Sections 11349.3, 11349.4, 11349.5, and 11350.3 shall apply to the review by the office to the extent that those sections are consistent with this section.

(4) In reviewing proposed changes to the commission's plans for the criteria specified in subdivision (a) of Section 11349.1, the office shall consider the clarity of the proposed plan change in the context of the commission's existing plans.

(5) The proposed plan or program change subject to this subdivision shall not become effective unless and until the regulatory provisions are approved by the office in accordance with subdivision (a) of Section 11349.3.

(6) Upon approval of the regulatory provisions, the office shall transmit to the Secretary of State for filing the clear and concise summary of the regulatory provisions submitted by the commission.

(e) Except as provided in subdivisions (b), (c), and (d), the adoption of any regulation by the commission shall be subject to this chapter in all respects.

HISTORY:

Added Stats 1995 ch 951 § 1 (AB 1102). Amended Stats 1996 ch 124 § 35 (AB 3470); Stats 2002 ch 389 § 7 (AB 1857).

§ 11356. Applicability of articles to building standards

(a) Article 6 (commencing with Section 11349) is not applicable to a building standard.

(b) Article 5 (commencing with Section 11346) is applicable to those building standards, except that the office shall not disapprove those building standards nor refuse to publish any notice of proposed building standards if either has been approved by, and submitted to, the office by the California Building Standards Commission pursuant to Section 18935 of the Health and Safety Code.

HISTORY:

Added Stats 1979 ch 1152 § 13.5, operative July 1, 1980, as Gov C § 11446. Renumbered by Stats 1980 ch 676 § 106. Amended Stats 1984 ch 677 § 1; Stats 1987 ch 1375 § 25; Stats 1988 ch 1194 § 1.5, operative January 1, 1989; Stats 2000 ch 1060 § 38 (AB 1822).

§ 11357. Instructions for determining impact of proposed action on local or state agencies or on school districts

(a) The Department of Finance shall adopt and update, as necessary, instructions for inclusion in the State Administrative Manual prescribing the methods that an agency subject to this chapter shall use in making the determinations and the estimates of fiscal or economic impact required by Sections 11346.2, 11346.3, and 11346.5. The instructions shall include, but need not be limited to, the following:

(1) Guidelines governing the types of data or assumptions, or both, that may be used, and the methods that shall be used, to calculate the estimate of the cost or savings to public agencies mandated by the regulation for which the estimate is being prepared.

(2) The types of direct or indirect costs and savings that should be taken into account in preparing the estimate.

(3) The criteria that shall be used in determining whether the cost of a regulation must be funded by the state pursuant to Section 6 of Article XIII B of the California Constitution and Part 7 (commencing with Section 17500) of Division 4.

(4) The format the agency preparing the estimate shall follow in summarizing and reporting its estimate of the cost or savings to state and local agencies, school districts, and in federal funding of state programs that will result from the regulation and its estimate of the economic impact that will result from the regulation.

(b) An action by the Department of Finance to adopt and update, as necessary, instructions to any state or local agency for the preparation, development, or administration of the state budget, or instructions to a state agency on the preparation of an economic impact estimate or assessment of a proposed regulation, including any instructions included in the State Administrative Manual, shall be exempt from this chapter.

(c) The Department of Finance may review an estimate prepared pursuant to this section for content including, but not limited to, the data and assumptions used in its preparation.

HISTORY:

Added Stats 1994 ch 1039 § 51 (AB 2531). Amended Stats 2014 ch 779 § 3 (AB 1711), effective January 1, 2015.

§ 11359. Regulations relating to fire and panic safety

(a) Except as provided in subdivision (b), on and after January 1, 1982, no new regulation, or the amendment or repeal of any regulation, which regulation is intended to promote fire and panic safety or provide fire protection and prevention, including fire suppression systems, equipment, or alarm regulation, is valid or effective unless it is submitted by, or approved in writing by, the State Fire Marshal before transmittal to the Secretary of State or the Office of Administrative Law.

(b) Approval of the State Fire Marshal is not required if the regulation is expressly required to be at least as effective as federal standards published in the Federal Register pursuant to Section 6 of the Occupational Safety and Health Act of 1970 (P.L. 91–596) within the time period specified by federal law and as provided in subdivision (b) of Section 142.4 of the Labor Code, and as approved by the Occupational Safety and Health Administration of the United States Department of Labor as meeting the requirements of subdivision (a) of Section 142.3 of the Labor Code, unless the regulation is determined by the State Fire Marshal to be less effective in promoting fire and panic safety than regulations adopted by the State Fire Marshal.

HISTORY:

Added Stats 1981 ch 1177 § 1 as Gov C § 11342.3. Renumbered by Stats 1994 ch 1039 § 10 (AB 2531).

§ 11361. Applicability of chapter; Adoption or revision of regulations, guidelines, or criteria

This chapter does not apply to the adoption or revision of regulations, guidelines, or criteria to implement the Safe Neighborhood Parks, Clean Water, Clean Air, and Coastal Protection Bond Act of 2000 (the Villaraigosa-Keeley Act) (Chapter 1.692 (commencing with Section 5096.300) of Division 5 of the Public Resources Code), the California Clean Water, Clean Air, Safe Neighborhood Parks, and Coastal Protection Act of 2002 (Chapter 1.696 (commencing with Section 5096.600) of Division 5 of the Public Resources Code), or the Water Security, Clean Drinking Water, Coastal and Beach Protection Act of 2002 (Division 26.5 (commencing with Section 79500) of the Water Code). The adoption or revision of regulations, guidelines, or criteria, if necessary to implement those respective acts, shall instead be accomplished by means of a public process reasonably calculated to give those persons interested in their adoption or revision an opportunity to be heard.

HISTORY:

Added Stats 2000 ch 87 § 5 (SB 1679), effective July 5, 2000. Amended Stats 2003 ch 240 § 2 (AB 1747), effective August 13, 2003.

ARTICLE 10
CALIFORNIA TAXPAYERS' RIGHT TO SELF-GOVERNANCE AND PARTICIPATION [REPEALED]

HISTORY: Added Stats 2005 ch 686 § 3, repealed January 1, 2012, by the terms of former Gov C § 11365.

CHAPTER 4
OFFICE OF ADMINISTRATIVE HEARINGS

Article
1. General Provisions.
2. Medical Quality Hearing Panel.
3. State Agency Reports and Forms Appeals.

HISTORY: Added Stats 1947 ch 1425 § 1. Chapter heading amended Stats 1961 ch 2048 § 1; Stats 1971 ch 1303 § 1.

ARTICLE 1
GENERAL PROVISIONS

Section
11370. Chapters constituting Administrative Procedure Act.
11370.1. "Director".
11370.2. Office of Administrative Hearings in Department of General Services; Director.
11370.3. Appointment and assignment of administrative law judges and other personnel.
11370.4. Determination and collection of costs.
11370.5. Recommendations on administrative adjudication.

HISTORY: Added Stats 1995 ch 938 § 16 (SB 523), operative July 1, 1997. Former Article 1, entitled "General," consisting of §§ 11370–11373, was added Stats 1947 ch 1425 § 1 and heading repealed Stats 2015 ch 303 § 190, effective January 1, 2016. Former Article 1, entitled "General," consisting of §§ 11380–11385, was added Stats 1945 ch 111 § 3, and amended and renumbered Article 2, entitled "Filing and Publication," by Stats 1947 ch 1425 § 2.

§ 11370. Chapters constituting Administrative Procedure Act

Chapter 3.5 (commencing with Section 11340), Chapter 4 (commencing with Section 11370), Chapter 4.5 (commencing with Section 11400), and Chapter 5 (commencing with Section 11500) constitute, and may be cited as, the Administrative Procedure Act.

HISTORY:
Added Stats 1947 ch 1425 § 1. Amended Stats 1961 ch 2048 § 2; Stats 1981 ch 714 § 176, operative until July 1, 1997; Stats 1995 ch 938 § 16.5 (SB 523), operative July 1, 1997.

§ 11370.1. "Director"

As used in the Administrative Procedure Act "director" means the executive officer of the Office of Administrative Hearings.

HISTORY:
Added Stats 1961 ch 2048 § 3. Amended Stats 1971 ch 1303 § 2.

§ 11370.2. Office of Administrative Hearings in Department of General Services; Director

(a) There is in the Department of General Services the Office of Administrative Hearings which is under the direction and control of an executive officer who shall be known as the director.

(b) The director shall have the same qualifications as administrative law judges, and shall be appointed by the Governor subject to the confirmation of the Senate.

(c) Any and all references in any law to the Office of Administrative Procedure shall be deemed to be the Office of Administrative Hearings.

HISTORY:
Added Stats 1961 ch 2048 § 4. Amended Stats 1963 ch 1786 § 13, operative October 1, 1963; Stats 1971 ch 1303 § 3; Stats 1985 ch 324 § 13.

§ 11370.3. Appointment and assignment of administrative law judges and other personnel

The director shall appoint and maintain a staff of full-time, and may appoint pro tempore part-time, administrative law judges qualified under Section 11502 which is sufficient to fill the needs of the various state agencies. The director shall also appoint any other technical and clerical personnel as may be required to perform the duties of the office. The director shall assign an administrative law judge for any proceeding arising under Chapter 5 (commencing with Section 11500) and, upon request from any agency, may assign an administrative law judge to conduct other administrative proceedings not arising under that chapter and shall assign hearing reporters as required. Any administrative law judge or other employee so assigned shall be deemed an employee of the office and not of the agency to which he or she is assigned. When not engaged in hearing cases, administrative law judges may be assigned by the director to perform other duties vested in or required of the office, including those provided for in Section 11370.5.

HISTORY:
Added Stats 1961 ch 2048 § 5. Amended Stats 1971 ch 1303 § 3.5; Stats 1979 ch 199 § 2; Stats 1984 ch 1005 § 2; Stats § 1985 ch 324 § 14; Stats 1995 ch 938 § 17 (SB 523), operative July 1, 1997.

§ 11370.4. Determination and collection of costs

The total cost to the state of maintaining and operating the Office of Administrative Hearings shall be determined by, and collected by the Department of General Services in advance or upon such other basis as it may determine from the state or other public agencies for which services are provided by the office.

HISTORY:
Added Stats 1961 ch 2048 § 6. Amended Stats 1963 ch 1553 § 1; Stats 1965 ch 462 § 1; Stats 1971 ch 1303 § 4.

§ 11370.5. Recommendations on administrative adjudication

(a) The office is authorized and directed to study the subject of administrative adjudication in all its aspects; to submit its suggestions to the various agencies in the interests of fairness, uniformity and the expedition of business; and to report its recommendations to the Governor and Legislature. All departments, agencies, officers, and employees of the state shall give the office ready access to their records and full information and reasonable assistance in any matter of research requiring recourse to them or to data within their knowledge or control. Nothing in this section authorizes an agency to provide access to records required by statute to be kept confidential.

(b) The office may adopt rules and regulations to carry out the functions and duties of the office under the Administrative Procedure Act. The regulations are subject to Chapter 3.5 (commencing with Section 11340).

HISTORY:

Added Stats 1961 ch 2048 § 7. Amended Stats 1995 ch 938 § 18 (SB 523), operative July 1, 1997; Stats 2002 ch 370 § 3 (AB 2283).

ARTICLE 2

MEDICAL QUALITY HEARING PANEL

Section
11371. Members of panel; Published decisions; Experts.
11372. Conduct of hearing by administrative law judge.
11373. Conduct of proceedings under Administrative Procedure Act.
11373.3. Facilities and support personnel for review committee panel.

HISTORY: Heading added Stats 1995 ch 938 § 19, operative July 1, 1997.

§ 11371. Members of panel; Published decisions; Experts

(a) There is within the Office of Administrative Hearings a Medical Quality Hearing Panel, consisting of no fewer than five full-time administrative law judges. The administrative law judges shall have medical training as recommended by the Division of Medical Quality of the Medical Board of California and approved by the Director of the Office of Administrative Hearings.

(b) The director shall determine the qualifications of panel members, supervise their training, and coordinate the publication of a reporter of decisions pursuant to this section. The panel shall include only those persons specifically qualified and shall at no time constitute more than 25 percent of the total number of administrative law judges within the Office of Administrative Hearings. If the members of the panel do not have a full workload, they may be assigned work by the Director of the Office of Administrative Hearings. When the medically related case workload exceeds the capacity of the members of the panel, additional judges shall be requested to be added to the panels as appropriate. When this workload overflow occurs on a temporary basis, the Director of the Office of Administrative Hearings shall supply judges from the Office of Administrative Hearings to adjudicate the cases.

(c) The administrative law judges of the panel shall have panels of experts available. The panels of experts shall be appointed by the Director of the Office of Administrative Hearings, with the advice of the Medical Board of California. These panels of experts may be called as witnesses by the administrative law judges of the panel to testify on the record about any matter relevant to a proceeding and subject to cross-examination by all parties, and Section 11430.30 does not apply in a proceeding under this section. The administrative law judge may award reasonable expert witness fees to any person or persons serving on a panel of experts, which shall be paid from the Contingent Fund of the Medical Board of California upon appropriation by the Legislature.

HISTORY:
Added Stats 1993 ch 1267 § 51 (SB 916). Amended Stats 1994 ch 1206 § 27 (SB 1775); Stats 1995 ch 938 § 19.5 (SB 523), operative July 1, 1997; Stats 1998 ch 878 § 56 (SB 2239), operative until January 1, 2003; Stats 2002 ch 1085 § 31 (SB 1950); Stats 2005 ch 674 § 21 (SB 231), effective January 1, 2006.

§ 11372. Conduct of hearing by administrative law judge

(a) Except as provided in subdivision (b), all adjudicative hearings and proceedings relating to the discipline or reinstatement of licensees of the Medical Board of California, including licensees of affiliated health agencies within the jurisdiction of the Medical Board of California, that are heard pursuant to the Administrative Procedure Act, shall be conducted by an administrative law judge as designated in Section 11371, sitting alone if the case is so assigned by the agency filing the charging pleading.

(b) Proceedings relating to interim orders shall be heard in accordance with Section 11529.

HISTORY:
Added Stats 1990 ch 1597 § 32 (SB 2375). Amended Stats 1993 ch 1267 § 52 (SB 916); Stats 2007 ch 588 § 89 (SB 1048), effective January 1, 2008.

§ 11373. Conduct of proceedings under Administrative Procedure Act

All adjudicative hearings and proceedings conducted by an administrative law judge as designated in Section 11371 shall be conducted under the terms and conditions set forth in the Administrative Procedure Act, except as provided in the Medical Practice Act (Chapter 5 (commencing with Section 2000) of Division 2 of the Business and Professions Code).

HISTORY:
Added Stats 1990 ch 1597 § 33 (SB 2375). Amended Stats 1993 ch 1267 § 53 (SB 916).

§ 11373.3. Facilities and support personnel for review committee panel

The Office of Administrative Hearings shall provide facilities and support personnel for the review committee panel and shall assess the Medical Board of California for facilities and personnel, where used to adjudicate cases involving the Medical Board of California.

HISTORY:
Added Stats 1990 ch 1597 § 34 (SB 2375). Amended Stats 1991 ch 1091 § 44 (AB 1487).

ARTICLE 3

STATE AGENCY REPORTS AND FORMS APPEALS

Section
11380. Appeal filed by business.

HISTORY: Heading added Stats 1995 ch 938 § 20, operative July 1, 1997.

§ 11380. Appeal filed by business

(a)(1) The office shall hear and render a decision on any appeal filed by a business, pursuant to subdivision (c) of Section 14775, in the event the business contests the certification by a state agency head that reporting requirements meet established criteria and shall not be eliminated.

(2) Before a business may file an appeal with the office pursuant to subdivision (c) of Section 14775, the business shall file a challenge to a form or report required by a state agency with that state agency. Within 60 days of filing the challenge with a state agency, the state agency shall either eliminate the form or report or provide written justification for its continued use.

(3) A business may appeal a state agency's written justification for the continued use of a form or report with the office.

(4) If a state agency fails to respond within 60 days of the filing of a challenge pursuant to paragraph (2), the business shall have an immediate right to file an appeal with the office.

(b) No later than January 1, 1996, the office shall adopt procedures governing the filing, hearing, and disposition of appeals. The procedures shall include, but shall not be limited to, provisions that assure that appeals are heard and decisions rendered by the office in a fair, impartial, and timely fashion.

(c) The office may charge appellants a reasonable fee to pay for costs it incurs in complying with this section.

HISTORY:

Added Stats 1995 ch 938 § 20 (SB 523), operative July 1, 1997.

CHAPTER 4.5

ADMINISTRATIVE ADJUDICATION: GENERAL PROVISIONS

Article

1. Preliminary Provisions.
2. Definitions.
3. Application of Chapter.
4. Governing Procedure.
5. Alternative Dispute Resolution.
6. Administrative Adjudication Bill of Rights.
7. Ex Parte Communications.
8. Language Assistance.
9. General Procedural Provisions.
10. Informal Hearing.
11. Subpoenas.
12. Enforcement of Orders and Sanctions.
13. Emergency Decision.
14. Declaratory Decision.
15. Conversion of Proceeding.
16. Administrative Adjudication Code of Ethics.

HISTORY: Heading added Stats 1995 ch 938 § 21, operative July 1, 1997.

ARTICLE 1
PRELIMINARY PROVISIONS

Section
11400. Administrative Procedure Act; References to superseded provisions.
11400.10. Operative date of chapter; Applicability.
11400.20. Adoption of interim or permanent regulations.

§ 11400. Administrative Procedure Act; References to superseded provisions

(a) This chapter and Chapter 5 (commencing with Section 11500) constitute the administrative adjudication provisions of the Administrative Procedure Act.

(b) A reference in any other statute or in a rule of court, executive order, or regulation, to a provision formerly found in Chapter 5 (commencing with Section 11500) that is superseded by a provision of this chapter, means the applicable provision of this chapter.

HISTORY:
Added Stats 1995 ch 938 § 21 (SB 523), operative July 1, 1997.

§ 11400.10. Operative date of chapter; Applicability

(a) This chapter is operative on July 1, 1997.

(b) This chapter is applicable to an adjudicative proceeding commenced on or after July 1, 1997.

(c) This chapter is not applicable to an adjudicative proceeding commenced before July 1, 1997, except an adjudicative proceeding conducted on a remand from a court or another agency on or after July 1, 1997.

HISTORY:
Added Stats 1995 ch 938 § 21 (SB 523), operative July 1, 1997.

§ 11400.20. Adoption of interim or permanent regulations

(a) Before, on, or after July 1, 1997, an agency may adopt interim or permanent regulations to govern an adjudicative proceeding under this chapter or Chapter 5 (commencing with Section 11500). Nothing in this section authorizes an agency to adopt regulations to govern an adjudicative proceeding required to be conducted by an administrative law judge employed by the Office of Administrative Hearings, except to the extent the regulations are otherwise authorized by statute.

(b) Except as provided in Section 11351:

(1) Interim regulations need not comply with Article 5 (commencing with Section 11346) or Article 6 (commencing with Section 11349) of Chapter 3.5, but are governed by Chapter 3.5 (commencing with Section 11340) in all other respects.

(2) Interim regulations expire on December 31, 1998, unless earlier terminated or replaced by or readopted as permanent regulations under

paragraph (3). If on December 31, 1998, an agency has completed proceedings to replace or readopt interim regulations and has submitted permanent regulations for review by the Office of Administrative Law, but permanent regulations have not yet been filed with the Secretary of State, the interim regulations are extended until the date permanent regulations are filed with the Secretary of State or March 31, 1999, whichever is earlier.

(3) Permanent regulations are subject to all the provisions of Chapter 3.5 (commencing with Section 11340), except that if by December 31, 1998, an agency has submitted the regulations for review by the Office of Administrative Law, the regulations are not subject to review for necessity under Section 11349.1 or 11350.

HISTORY:

Added Stats 1995 ch 938 § 21 (SB 523), operative July 1, 1997. Amended Stats 1996 ch 390 § 5 (SB 794), effective August 19, 1996, operative July 1, 1997.

ARTICLE 2

DEFINITIONS

Section

11405.10. Definitions governing construction of chapter.
11405.20. "Adjudicative proceeding".
11405.30. "Agency".
11405.40. "Agency head".
11405.50. "Decision".
11405.60. "Party".
11405.70. "Person".
11405.80. "Presiding officer".

§ 11405.10. Definitions governing construction of chapter

Unless the provision or context requires otherwise, the definitions in this article govern the construction of this chapter.

HISTORY:

Added Stats 1995 ch 938 § 21 (SB 523), operative July 1, 1997.

§ 11405.20. "Adjudicative proceeding"

"Adjudicative proceeding" means an evidentiary hearing for determination of facts pursuant to which an agency formulates and issues a decision.

HISTORY:

Added Stats 1995 ch 938 § 21 (SB 523), operative July 1, 1997.

§ 11405.30. "Agency"

"Agency" means a board, bureau, commission, department, division, office, officer, or other administrative unit, including the agency head, and one or more members of the agency head or agency employees or other persons directly or indirectly purporting to act on behalf of or under the authority of the agency head. To the extent it purports to exercise authority pursuant to this chapter, an administrative unit otherwise qualifying as an agency shall be treated as a separate agency even if the unit is located within or subordinate to another agency.

HISTORY:
Added Stats 1995 ch 938 § 21 (SB 523), operative July 1, 1997.

§ 11405.40. "Agency head"

"Agency head" means a person or body in which the ultimate legal authority of an agency is vested, and includes a person or body to which the power to act is delegated pursuant to authority to delegate the agency's power to hear and decide.

HISTORY:
Added Stats 1995 ch 938 § 21 (SB 523), operative July 1, 1997.

§ 11405.50. "Decision"

(a) "Decision" means an agency action of specific application that determines a legal right, duty, privilege, immunity, or other legal interest of a particular person.

(b) Nothing in this section limits any of the following:

(1) The precedential effect of a decision under Section 11425.60.

(2) The authority of an agency to make a declaratory decision pursuant to Article 14 (commencing with Section 11465.10).

HISTORY:
Added Stats 1995 ch 938 § 21 (SB 523), operative July 1, 1997.

§ 11405.60. "Party"

"Party" includes the agency that is taking action, the person to which the agency action is directed, and any other person named as a party or allowed to appear or intervene in the proceeding. If the agency that is taking action and the agency that is conducting the adjudicative proceeding are separate agencies, the agency that is taking action is a party and the agency that is conducting the adjudicative proceeding is not a party.

HISTORY:
Added Stats 1995 ch 938 § 21 (SB 523), operative July 1, 1997.

§ 11405.70. "Person"

"Person" includes an individual, partnership, corporation, governmental subdivision or unit of a governmental subdivision, or public or private organization or entity of any character.

HISTORY:
Added Stats 1995 ch 938 § 21 (SB 523), operative July 1, 1997.

§ 11405.80. "Presiding officer"

"Presiding officer" means the agency head, member of the agency head, administrative law judge, hearing officer, or other person who presides in an adjudicative proceeding.

HISTORY:
Added Stats 1995 ch 938 § 21 (SB 523), operative July 1, 1997.

ARTICLE 3
APPLICATION OF CHAPTER

Section
11410.10. Decision requiring evidentiary hearing.
11410.20. Applicability to agencies.
11410.30. Applicability to local agencies.
11410.40. Adoption of chapter by exempt agency.
11410.50. Applicability to specified proceedings.
11410.60. Quasi-public entity.

§ 11410.10. Decision requiring evidentiary hearing

This chapter applies to a decision by an agency if, under the federal or state Constitution or a federal or state statute, an evidentiary hearing for determination of facts is required for formulation and issuance of the decision.

HISTORY:
Added Stats 1995 ch 938 § 21 (SB 523), operative July 1, 1997.

§ 11410.20. Applicability to agencies

Except as otherwise expressly provided by statute:

(a) This chapter applies to all agencies of the state.

(b) This chapter does not apply to the Legislature, the courts or judicial branch, or the Governor or office of the Governor.

HISTORY:
Added Stats 1995 ch 938 § 21 (SB 523), operative July 1, 1997.

§ 11410.30. Applicability to local agencies

(a) As used in this section, "local agency" means a county, city, district, public authority, public agency, or other political subdivision or public corporation in the state other than the state.

(b) This chapter does not apply to a local agency except to the extent the provisions are made applicable by statute.

(c) This chapter applies to an agency created or appointed by joint or concerted action of the state and one or more local agencies.

HISTORY:
Added Stats 1995 ch 938 § 21 (SB 523), operative July 1, 1997.

§ 11410.40. Adoption of chapter by exempt agency

Notwithstanding any other provision of this article, by regulation, ordinance, or other appropriate action, an agency may adopt this chapter or any of its provisions for the formulation and issuance of a decision, even though the agency or decision is exempt from application of this chapter.

HISTORY:
Added Stats 1995 ch 938 § 21 (SB 523), operative July 1, 1997.

APA

§ 11410.50. Applicability to specified proceedings

This chapter applies to an adjudicative proceeding required to be conducted under Chapter 5 (commencing with Section 11500) unless the statutes relating to the proceeding provide otherwise.

HISTORY:

Added Stats 1995 ch 938 § 21 (SB 523), operative July 1, 1997.

§ 11410.60. Quasi-public entity

(a) As used in this section, "quasi-public entity" means an entity, other than a governmental agency, whether characterized by statute as a public corporation, public instrumentality, or otherwise, that is expressly created by statute for the purpose of administration of a state function.

(b) This chapter applies to an adjudicative proceeding conducted by a quasi-public entity if all of the following conditions are satisfied:

(1) A statute vests the power of decision in the quasi-public entity.

(2) A statute, the United States Constitution, or the California Constitution, requires an evidentiary hearing for determination of facts for formulation and issuance of the decision. Nothing in this section is intended to create an evidentiary hearing requirement that is not otherwise statutorily or constitutionally imposed.

(3) The decision is not otherwise subject to administrative review in an adjudicative proceeding to which this chapter applies.

(c) For the purpose of application of this chapter to a decision by a quasi-public entity:

(1) "Agency," as defined in Section 11405.30, also includes the quasi-public entity.

(2) "Regulation" includes a rule promulgated by the quasi-public entity.

(3) Article 8 (commencing with Section 11435.05), requiring language assistance in an adjudicative proceeding, applies to a quasi-public entity to the same extent as a state agency under Section 11018.

(d) This section shall be strictly construed to effectuate the intent of the Legislature to apply this chapter only to a decision by a quasi-public entity that is expressly created by statute for the purpose of administration of a state function.

(e) This section shall not apply to a decision made on authority of an approved plan of operations of a quasi-public entity that is subject to the regulation or supervision of the Insurance Commissioner.

HISTORY:

Added Stats 1997 ch 220 § 9 (SB 68), effective August 4, 1997.

ARTICLE 4

GOVERNING PROCEDURE

Section

11415.10. Determination of procedure.
11415.20. Statute to prevail over provision of chapter.
11415.30. Actions by Governor to avoid loss or delay of federal funds.

Section
11415.40. Waiver of right conferred by provisions.
11415.50. Procedure for decision for which adjudicative proceeding not required.
11415.60. Decision by settlement.

§ 11415.10. Determination of procedure

(a) The governing procedure by which an agency conducts an adjudicative proceeding is determined by the statutes and regulations applicable to that proceeding. If no other governing procedure is provided by statute or regulation, an agency may conduct an adjudicative proceeding under the administrative adjudication provisions of the Administrative Procedure Act.

(b) This chapter supplements the governing procedure by which an agency conducts an adjudicative proceeding.

HISTORY:

Added Stats 1995 ch 938 § 21 (SB 523), operative July 1, 1997.

§ 11415.20. Statute to prevail over provision of chapter

A state statute or a federal statute or regulation applicable to a particular agency or decision prevails over a conflicting or inconsistent provision of this chapter.

HISTORY:

Added Stats 1995 ch 938 § 21 (SB 523), operative July 1, 1997.

§ 11415.30. Actions by Governor to avoid loss or delay of federal funds

(a) To the extent necessary to avoid a loss or delay of funds or services from the federal government that would otherwise be available to the state, the Governor may do any of the following by executive order:

(1) Suspend, in whole or in part, any administrative adjudication provision of the Administrative Procedure Act.

(2) Adopt a rule of procedure that will avoid the loss or delay.

(b) The Governor shall rescind an executive order issued under this section as soon as it is no longer necessary to prevent the loss or delay of funds or services from the federal government.

(c) If an administrative adjudication provision is suspended or rule of procedure is adopted pursuant to this section, the Governor shall promptly report the suspension or adoption to the Legislature. The report shall include recommendations concerning any legislation that may be necessary to conform the provision to federal law.

HISTORY:

Added Stats 1995 ch 938 § 21 (SB 523), operative July 1, 1997.

§ 11415.40. Waiver of right conferred by provisions

Except to the extent prohibited by another statute or regulation, a person may waive a right conferred on the person by the administrative adjudication provisions of the Administrative Procedure Act.

HISTORY:

Added Stats 1995 ch 938 § 21 (SB 523), operative July 1, 1997.

§ 11415.50. Procedure for decision for which adjudicative proceeding not required

(a) An agency may provide any appropriate procedure for a decision for which an adjudicative proceeding is not required.

(b) An adjudicative proceeding is not required for informal factfinding or an informal investigatory hearing, or a decision to initiate or not to initiate an investigation, prosecution, or other proceeding before the agency, another agency, or a court, whether in response to an application for an agency decision or otherwise.

HISTORY:

Added Stats 1995 ch 938 § 21 (SB 523), operative July 1, 1997.

§ 11415.60. Decision by settlement

(a) An agency may formulate and issue a decision by settlement, pursuant to an agreement of the parties, without conducting an adjudicative proceeding. Subject to subdivision (c), the settlement may be on any terms the parties determine are appropriate. Notwithstanding any other provision of law, no evidence of an offer of compromise or settlement made in settlement negotiations is admissible in an adjudicative proceeding or civil action, whether as affirmative evidence, by way of impeachment, or for any other purpose, and no evidence of conduct or statements made in settlement negotiations is admissible to prove liability for any loss or damage except to the extent provided in Section 1152 of the Evidence Code. Nothing in this subdivision makes inadmissible any public document created by a public agency.

(b) A settlement may be made before or after issuance of an agency pleading, except that in an adjudicative proceeding to determine whether an occupational license should be revoked, suspended, limited, or conditioned, a settlement may not be made before issuance of the agency pleading. A settlement may be made before, during, or after the hearing.

(c) A settlement is subject to any necessary agency approval. An agency head may delegate the power to approve a settlement. The terms of a settlement may not be contrary to statute or regulation, except that the settlement may include sanctions the agency would otherwise lack power to impose.

HISTORY:

Added Stats 1995 ch 938 § 21 (SB 523), operative July 1, 1997. Amended Stats 1996 ch 390 § 7 (SB 794), effective August 19, 1996, operative July 1, 1997.

ARTICLE 5
ALTERNATIVE DISPUTE RESOLUTION

Section

11420.10. Mediation or arbitration.
11420.20. Model regulations for alternative dispute resolution.
11420.30. Protection of communications.

§ 11420.10. Mediation or arbitration

(a) An agency, with the consent of all the parties, may refer a dispute that is the subject of an adjudicative proceeding for resolution by any of the following means:

(1) Mediation by a neutral mediator.

(2) Binding arbitration by a neutral arbitrator. An award in a binding arbitration is subject to judicial review in the manner provided in Chapter 4 (commencing with Section 1285) of Title 9 of Part 3 of the Code of Civil Procedure.

(3) Nonbinding arbitration by a neutral arbitrator. The arbitrator's decision in a nonbinding arbitration is final unless within 30 days after the arbitrator delivers the award to the agency head a party requests that the agency conduct a de novo adjudicative proceeding. If the decision in the de novo proceeding is not more favorable to the party electing the de novo proceeding, the party shall pay the costs and fees specified in Section 1141.21 of the Code of Civil Procedure insofar as applicable in the adjudicative proceeding.

(b) If another statute requires mediation or arbitration in an adjudicative proceeding, that statute prevails over this section.

(c) This section does not apply in an adjudicative proceeding to the extent an agency by regulation provides that this section is not applicable in a proceeding of the agency.

HISTORY:

Added Stats 1995 ch 938 § 21 (SB 523), operative July 1, 1997.

§ 11420.20. Model regulations for alternative dispute resolution

(a) The Office of Administrative Hearings shall adopt and promulgate model regulations for alternative dispute resolution under this article. The model regulations govern alternative dispute resolution by an agency under this article, except to the extent the agency by regulation provides inconsistent rules or provides that the model regulations are not applicable in a proceeding of the agency.

(b) The model regulations shall include provisions for selection and compensation of a mediator or arbitrator, qualifications of a mediator or arbitrator, and confidentiality of the mediation or arbitration proceeding.

HISTORY:

Added Stats 1995 ch 938 § 21 (SB 523), operative July 1, 1997.

§ 11420.30. Protection of communications

Notwithstanding any other provision of law, a communication made in alternative dispute resolution under this article is protected to the following extent:

(a) Anything said, any admission made, and any document prepared in the course of, or pursuant to, mediation under this article is a confidential communication, and a party to the mediation has a privilege to refuse to disclose and to prevent another from disclosing the communication, whether in an adjudicative proceeding, civil action, or other proceeding. This subdivision does not limit the admissibility of evidence if all parties to the proceedings consent.

(b) No reference to nonbinding arbitration proceedings, a decision of the arbitrator that is rejected by a party's request for a de novo adjudicative proceeding, the evidence produced, or any other aspect of the arbitration may be made in an adjudicative proceeding or civil action, whether as affirmative evidence, by way of impeachment, or for any other purpose.

(c) No mediator or arbitrator is competent to testify in a subsequent administrative or civil proceeding as to any statement, conduct, decision, or order occurring at, or in conjunction with, the alternative dispute resolution.

(d) Evidence otherwise admissible outside of alternative dispute resolution under this article is not inadmissible or protected from disclosure solely by reason of its introduction or use in alternative dispute resolution under this article.

HISTORY:

Added Stats 1995 ch 938 § 21 (SB 523), operative July 1, 1997.

ARTICLE 6

ADMINISTRATIVE ADJUDICATION BILL OF RIGHTS

Section

11425.10. Required procedures and rights of persons affected.
11425.20. Hearings open to public; Order for closure.
11425.30. Specified persons not to serve as presiding officer.
11425.40. Disqualification of presiding officer.
11425.50. Decision to be in writing; Statement of factual and legal basis.
11425.60. Decisions relied on as precedents; Index of precedent decisions.

§ 11425.10. Required procedures and rights of persons affected

(a) The governing procedure by which an agency conducts an adjudicative proceeding is subject to all of the following requirements:

(1) The agency shall give the person to which the agency action is directed notice and an opportunity to be heard, including the opportunity to present and rebut evidence.

(2) The agency shall make available to the person to which the agency action is directed a copy of the governing procedure, including a statement whether Chapter 5 (commencing with Section 11500) is applicable to the proceeding.

(3) The hearing shall be open to public observation as provided in Section 11425.20.

(4) The adjudicative function shall be separated from the investigative, prosecutorial, and advocacy functions within the agency as provided in Section 11425.30.

(5) The presiding officer is subject to disqualification for bias, prejudice, or interest as provided in Section 11425.40.

(6) The decision shall be in writing, be based on the record, and include a statement of the factual and legal basis of the decision as provided in Section 11425.50.

(7) A decision may not be relied on as precedent unless the agency designates and indexes the decision as precedent as provided in Section 11425.60.

(8) Ex parte communications shall be restricted as provided in Article 7 (commencing with Section 11430.10).

(9) Language assistance shall be made available as provided in Article 8 (commencing with Section 11435.05) by an agency described in Section 11018 or 11435.15.

(b) The requirements of this section apply to the governing procedure by which an agency conducts an adjudicative proceeding without further action by the agency, and prevail over a conflicting or inconsistent provision of the governing procedure, subject to Section 11415.20. The governing procedure by which an agency conducts an adjudicative proceeding may include provisions equivalent to, or more protective of the rights of the person to which the agency action is directed than, the requirements of this section.

HISTORY:

Added Stats 1995 ch 938 § 21 (SB 523), operative July 1, 1997.

§ 11425.20. Hearings open to public; Order for closure

(a) A hearing shall be open to public observation. This subdivision shall not limit the authority of the presiding officer to order closure of a hearing or make other protective orders to the extent necessary or proper for any of the following purposes:

(1) To satisfy the United States Constitution, the California Constitution, federal or state statute, or other law, including, but not limited to, laws protecting privileged, confidential, or other protected information.

(2) To ensure a fair hearing in the circumstances of the particular case.

(3) To conduct the hearing, including the manner of examining witnesses, in a way that is appropriate to protect a minor witness or a witness with a developmental disability, as defined in Section 4512 of the Welfare and Institutions Code, from intimidation or other harm, taking into account the rights of all persons.

(b) To the extent a hearing is conducted by telephone, television, or other electronic means, and is not closed as otherwise required by law, the requirement that the meeting is open to public observation pursuant to subdivision (a) is satisfied if members of the public have an opportunity to do both of the following:

(1) At reasonable times, hear or inspect the agency's record, and inspect any transcript obtained by the agency.

(2) Be physically or virtually present at the place where the presiding officer is conducting the hearing. For purposes of this section, the term "present" can be satisfied either by providing a designated location from which members of the public can observe the meeting via a live audio or a video feed of the hearing made available to the public on the internet or by teleconference.

(c) This section does not apply to a prehearing conference, settlement conference, or proceedings for alternative dispute resolution other than binding arbitration.

HISTORY:

Added Stats 1995 ch 938 § 21 (SB 523), operative July 1, 1997. Amended Stats 2021 ch 401 § 11 (AB 1578), effective January 1, 2022.

§ 11425.30. Specified persons not to serve as presiding officer

(a) A person may not serve as presiding officer in an adjudicative proceeding in any of the following circumstances:

(1) The person has served as investigator, prosecutor, or advocate in the proceeding or its preadjudicative stage.

(2) The person is subject to the authority, direction, or discretion of a person who has served as investigator, prosecutor, or advocate in the proceeding or its preadjudicative stage.

(b) Notwithstanding subdivision (a):

(1) A person may serve as presiding officer at successive stages of an adjudicative proceeding.

(2) A person who has participated only as a decisionmaker or as an advisor to a decisionmaker in a determination of probable cause or other equivalent preliminary determination in an adjudicative proceeding or its preadjudicative stage may serve as presiding officer in the proceeding.

(c) The provisions of this section governing separation of functions as to the presiding officer also govern separation of functions as to the agency head or other person or body to which the power to hear or decide in the proceeding is delegated.

HISTORY:

Added Stats 1995 ch 938 § 21 (SB 523), operative July 1, 1997.

§ 11425.40. Disqualification of presiding officer

(a) The presiding officer is subject to disqualification for bias, prejudice, or interest in the proceeding.

(b) It is not alone or in itself grounds for disqualification, without further evidence of bias, prejudice, or interest, that the presiding officer:

(1) Is or is not a member of a racial, ethnic, religious, sexual, or similar group and the proceeding involves the rights of that group.

(2) Has experience, technical competence, or specialized knowledge of, or has in any capacity expressed a view on, a legal, factual, or policy issue presented in the proceeding.

(3) Has as a lawyer or public official participated in the drafting of laws or regulations or in the effort to pass or defeat laws or regulations, the meaning, effect, or application of which is in issue in the proceeding.

(c) The provisions of this section governing disqualification of the presiding officer also govern disqualification of the agency head or other person or body to which the power to hear or decide in the proceeding is delegated.

(d) An agency that conducts an adjudicative proceeding may provide by regulation for peremptory challenge of the presiding officer.

HISTORY:

Added Stats 1995 ch 938 § 21 (SB 523), operative July 1, 1997.

§ 11425.50. Decision to be in writing; Statement of factual and legal basis

(a) The decision shall be in writing and shall include a statement of the factual and legal basis for the decision.

(b) The statement of the factual basis for the decision may be in the language of, or by reference to, the pleadings. If the statement is no more than mere repetition or paraphrase of the relevant statute or regulation, the statement shall be accompanied by a concise and explicit statement of the underlying facts of record that support the decision. If the factual basis for the decision includes a determination based substantially on the credibility of a witness, the statement shall identify any specific evidence of the observed demeanor, manner, or attitude of the witness that supports the determination, and on judicial review the court shall give great weight to the determination to the extent the determination identifies the observed demeanor, manner, or attitude of the witness that supports it.

(c) The statement of the factual basis for the decision shall be based exclusively on the evidence of record in the proceeding and on matters officially noticed in the proceeding. The presiding officer's experience, technical competence, and specialized knowledge may be used in evaluating evidence.

(d) Nothing in this section limits the information that may be contained in the decision, including a summary of evidence relied on.

(e) A penalty may not be based on a guideline, criterion, bulletin, manual, instruction, order, standard of general application or other rule subject to Chapter 3.5 (commencing with Section 11340) unless it has been adopted as a regulation pursuant to Chapter 3.5 (commencing with Section 11340).

HISTORY:

Added Stats 1995 ch 938 § 21 (SB 523), operative July 1, 1997.

§ 11425.60. Decisions relied on as precedents; Index of precedent decisions

(a) A decision may not be expressly relied on as precedent unless it is designated as a precedent decision by the agency.

(b) An agency may designate as a precedent decision a decision or part of a decision that contains a significant legal or policy determination of general application that is likely to recur. Designation of a decision or part of a decision as a precedent decision is not rulemaking and need not be done under Chapter 3.5 (commencing with Section 11340). An agency's designation of a decision or part of a decision, or failure to designate a decision or part of a decision, as a precedent decision is not subject to judicial review.

(c) An agency shall maintain an index of significant legal and policy determinations made in precedent decisions. The index shall be updated not less frequently than annually, unless no precedent decision has been designated since the last preceding update. The index shall be made available to the public by subscription, and its availability shall be publicized annually in the California Regulatory Notice Register.

(d) This section applies to decisions issued on or after July 1, 1997. Nothing in this section precludes an agency from designating and indexing as a precedent decision a decision issued before July 1, 1997.

HISTORY:

Added Stats 1995 ch 938 § 21 (SB 523), operative July 1, 1997. Amended Stats 1996 ch 390 § 8 (SB 794), effective August 19, 1996, operative July 1, 1997.

ARTICLE 7
EX PARTE COMMUNICATIONS

Section

11430.10. Ex parte communications.
11430.20. Permissible ex parte communications.
11430.30. Permissible ex parte communication from agency that is party.
11430.40. Disclosure of communication received while proceeding is pending.
11430.50. Communication in violation of provisions.
11430.60. Prohibited communication as grounds to disqualify presiding officer.
11430.70. Agency head delegated to hear or decide proceeding.
11430.80. Communication between presiding officer and agency head delegated to hear proceeding.

§ 11430.10. Ex parte communications

(a) While the proceeding is pending there shall be no communication, direct or indirect, regarding any issue in the proceeding, to the presiding officer from an employee or representative of an agency that is a party or from an interested person outside the agency, without notice and opportunity for all parties to participate in the communication.

(b) Nothing in this section precludes a communication, including a communication from an employee or representative of an agency that is a party, made on the record at the hearing.

(c) For the purpose of this section, a proceeding is pending from the issuance of the agency's pleading, or from an application for an agency decision, whichever is earlier.

HISTORY:

Added Stats 1995 ch 938 § 21 (SB 523), operative July 1, 1997.

§ 11430.20. Permissible ex parte communications

A communication otherwise prohibited by Section 11430.10 is permissible in any of the following circumstances:

(a) The communication is required for disposition of an ex parte matter specifically authorized by statute.

(b) The communication concerns a matter of procedure or practice, including a request for a continuance, that is not in controversy.

HISTORY:

Added Stats 1995 ch 938 § 21 (SB 523), operative July 1, 1997.

§ 11430.30. Permissible ex parte communication from agency that is party

A communication otherwise prohibited by Section 11430.10 from an employee or representative of an agency that is a party to the presiding officer is permissible in any of the following circumstances:

(a) The communication is for the purpose of assistance and advice to the presiding officer from a person who has not served as investigator, prosecutor, or advocate in the proceeding or its preadjudicative stage. An assistant or advisor may evaluate the evidence in the record but shall not furnish, augment, diminish, or modify the evidence in the record.

(b) The communication is for the purpose of advising the presiding officer concerning a settlement proposal advocated by the advisor.

(c) The communication is for the purpose of advising the presiding officer concerning any of the following matters in an adjudicative proceeding that is nonprosecutorial in character:

(1) The advice involves a technical issue in the proceeding and the advice is necessary for, and is not otherwise reasonably available to, the presiding officer, provided the content of the advice is disclosed on the record and all parties are given an opportunity to address it in the manner provided in Section 11430.50.

(2) The advice involves an issue in a proceeding of the San Francisco Bay Conservation and Development Commission, California Tahoe Regional Planning Agency, Delta Protection Commission, Water Resources Control Board, or a regional water quality control board.

HISTORY:

Added Stats 1995 ch 938 § 21 (SB 523), operative July 1, 1997.

§ 11430.40. Disclosure of communication received while proceeding is pending

If, while the proceeding is pending but before serving as presiding officer, a person receives a communication of a type that would be in violation of this article if received while serving as presiding officer, the person, promptly after starting to serve, shall disclose the content of the communication on the record and give all parties an opportunity to address it in the manner provided in Section 11430.50.

HISTORY:

Added Stats 1995 ch 938 § 21 (SB 523), operative July 1, 1997.

§ 11430.50. Communication in violation of provisions

(a) If a presiding officer receives a communication in violation of this article, the presiding officer shall make all of the following a part of the record in the proceeding:

(1) If the communication is written, the writing and any written response of the presiding officer to the communication.

(2) If the communication is oral, a memorandum stating the substance of the communication, any response made by the presiding officer, and the identity of each person from whom the presiding officer received the communication.

(b) The presiding officer shall notify all parties that a communication described in this section has been made a part of the record.

(c) If a party requests an opportunity to address the communication within 10 days after receipt of notice of the communication:

(1) The party shall be allowed to comment on the communication.

(2) The presiding officer has discretion to allow the party to present evidence concerning the subject of the communication, including discretion to reopen a hearing that has been concluded.

HISTORY:

Added Stats 1995 ch 938 § 21 (SB 523), operative July 1, 1997.

§ 11430.60. Prohibited communication as grounds to disqualify presiding officer

Receipt by the presiding officer of a communication in violation of this article may be grounds for disqualification of the presiding officer. If the presiding officer is disqualified, the portion of the record pertaining to the ex parte communication may be sealed by protective order of the disqualified presiding officer.

HISTORY:
Added Stats 1995 ch 938 § 21 (SB 523), operative July 1, 1997.

§ 11430.70. Agency head delegated to hear or decide proceeding

(a) Subject to subdivision (b) and (c), the provisions of this article governing ex parte communications to the presiding officer also govern ex parte communications in an adjudicative proceeding to the agency head or other person or body to which the power to hear or decide in the proceeding is delegated.

(b) An ex parte communication to the agency head or other person or body to which the power to hear or decide in the proceeding is delegated is permissible in an individualized ratemaking proceeding if the content of the communication is disclosed on the record and all parties are given an opportunity to address it in the manner provided in Section 11430.50.

(c) An ex parte communication to the agency head or other person or body to which the power to hear or decide in the proceeding is delegated is permissible in an individualized determination of an application for site certification pursuant to Chapter 6 (commencing with Section 25500) of Division 15 of the Public Resources Code, that is before the State Energy Resources Conservation and Development Commission, if the communication is made by an employee of another state agency and is made for the purpose of enabling the presiding officer to effectively manage the proceeding.

HISTORY:
Added Stats 1995 ch 938 § 21 (SB 523), operative July 1, 1997. Amended Stats 2009–2010 8th Ex Sess ch 9 § 4 (SB 34XXXXXXXX), effective March 22, 2010.

§ 11430.80. Communication between presiding officer and agency head delegated to hear proceeding

(a) There shall be no communication, direct or indirect, while a proceeding is pending regarding the merits of any issue in the proceeding, between the presiding officer and the agency head or other person or body to which the power to hear or decide in the proceeding is delegated.

(b) This section does not apply where the agency head or other person or body to which the power to hear or decide in the proceeding is delegated serves as both presiding officer and agency head, or where the presiding officer does not issue a decision in the proceeding.

HISTORY:
Added Stats 1995 ch 938 § 21 (SB 523), operative July 1, 1997.

ARTICLE 8
LANGUAGE ASSISTANCE

Section
11435.05. "Language assistance".

Section
11435.10. Interpretation for deaf or hard-of-hearing persons.
11435.15. Provision of language assistance by state agencies.
11435.20. Hearing or medical examination to be conducted in English.
11435.25. Cost of providing interpreter.
11435.30. Publication of list of certified interpreters.
11435.35. Publication of list of certified medical examination interpreters.
11435.40. Designation of languages for certification.
11435.45. Application fees to take interpreter examinations.
11435.50. Removal of person from list of certified interpreters.
11435.55. Qualification and use of noncertified interpreters.
11435.60. Party to be advised of right to interpreter.
11435.65. Rules of confidentiality applicable to interpreters.

§ 11435.05. "Language assistance"

As used in this article, "language assistance" means oral interpretation or written translation into English of a language other than English or of English into another language for a party or witness who cannot speak or understand English or who can do so only with difficulty.

HISTORY:
Added Stats 1995 ch 938 § 21 (SB 523), operative July 1, 1997.

§ 11435.10. Interpretation for deaf or hard-of-hearing persons

Nothing in this article limits the application or effect of Section 754 of the Evidence Code to interpretation for a deaf or hard-of-hearing party or witness in an adjudicative proceeding.

HISTORY:
Added Stats 1995 ch 938 § 21 (SB 523), operative July 1, 1997.

§ 11435.15. Provision of language assistance by state agencies

(a) The following state agencies shall provide language assistance in adjudicative proceedings to the extent provided in this article:

(1) Agricultural Labor Relations Board.
(2) State Department of Alcohol and Drug Programs.
(3) State Athletic Commission.
(4) California Unemployment Insurance Appeals Board.
(5) Board of Parole Hearings.
(6) State Board of Barbering and Cosmetology.
(7) State Department of Developmental Services.
(8) Public Employment Relations Board.
(9) Franchise Tax Board.
(10) State Department of Health Care Services.
(11) Department of Housing and Community Development.
(12) Department of Industrial Relations.
(13) State Department of State Hospitals.
(14) Department of Motor Vehicles.
(15) Notary Public Section, Office of the Secretary of State.
(16) Public Utilities Commission.
(17) Office of Statewide Health Planning and Development.
(18) State Department of Social Services.

(19) Workers' Compensation Appeals Board.
(20) Division of Juvenile Justice.
(21) Division of Juvenile Parole Operations.
(22) Department of Insurance.
(23) State Personnel Board.
(24) California Board of Podiatric Medicine.
(25) Board of Psychology.

(b) Nothing in this section prevents an agency other than an agency listed in subdivision (a) from electing to adopt any of the procedures in this article, provided that any selection of an interpreter is subject to Section 11435.30.

(c) Nothing in this section prohibits an agency from providing an interpreter during a proceeding to which this chapter does not apply, including an informal factfinding or informal investigatory hearing.

(d) This article applies to an agency listed in subdivision (a) notwithstanding a general provision that this chapter does not apply to some or all of an agency's adjudicative proceedings.

HISTORY:

Added Stats 1995 ch 938 § 21 (SB 523), operative July 1, 1997. Amended Stats 1996 ch 390 § 5, effective August 19, 1996, operative July 1, 1997; Stats 2012 ch 440 § 11 (AB 1488), effective September 22, 2012; Stats 2013 ch 76 § 82 (AB 383), effective January 1, 2014.

§ 11435.20. Hearing or medical examination to be conducted in English

(a) The hearing, or any medical examination conducted for the purpose of determining compensation or monetary award, shall be conducted in English.

(b) If a party or the party's witness does not proficiently speak or understand English and before commencement of the hearing or medical examination requests language assistance, an agency subject to the language assistance requirement of this article shall provide the party or witness an interpreter.

HISTORY:

Added Stats 1995 ch 938 § 21 (SB 523), operative July 1, 1997.

§ 11435.25. Cost of providing interpreter

(a) The cost of providing an interpreter under this article shall be paid by the agency having jurisdiction over the matter if the presiding officer so directs, otherwise by the party at whose request the interpreter is provided.

(b) The presiding officer's decision to direct payment shall be based upon an equitable consideration of all the circumstances in each case, such as the ability of the party in need of the interpreter to pay.

(c) Notwithstanding any other provision of this section, in a hearing before the Workers' Compensation Appeals Board or the Division of Workers' Compensation relating to workers' compensation claims, the payment of the costs of providing an interpreter shall be governed by the rules and regulations promulgated by the Workers' Compensation Appeals Board or the Administrative Director of the Division of Workers' Compensation, as appropriate.

HISTORY:

Added Stats 1995 ch 938 § 21 (SB 523), operative July 1, 1997.

§ 11435.30. Publication of list of certified interpreters

(a) The State Personnel Board shall establish, maintain, administer, and publish annually an updated list of certified administrative hearing interpreters it has determined meet the minimum standards in interpreting skills and linguistic abilities in languages designated pursuant to Section 11435.40. Any interpreter so listed may be examined by each employing agency to determine the interpreter's knowledge of the employing agency's technical program terminology and procedures.

(b) Court interpreters certified pursuant to Section 68562, and interpreters listed on the State Personnel Board's recommended lists of court and administrative hearing interpreters prior to July 1, 1993, shall be deemed certified for purposes of this section.

(c)(1) In addition to the certification procedure provided pursuant to subdivision (a), the Administrative Director of the Division of Workers' Compensation may establish, maintain, administer, and publish annually an updated list of certified administrative hearing interpreters who, based on testing by an independent organization designated by the administrative director, have been determined to meet the minimum standards in interpreting skills and linguistic abilities in languages designated pursuant to Section 11435.40, for purposes of administrative hearings conducted pursuant to proceedings of the Workers' Compensation Appeals Board. The independent testing organization shall have no financial interest in the training of interpreters or in the employment of interpreters for administrative hearings.

(2)(A) A fee, as determined by the administrative director, shall be collected from each interpreter seeking certification. The fee shall not exceed the reasonable regulatory costs of administering the testing and certification program and of publishing the list of certified administrative hearing interpreters on the Division of Workers' Compensation' Internet Web site.

(B) The Legislature finds and declares that the services described in this section are of such a special and unique nature that they may be contracted out pursuant to paragraph (3) of subdivision (b) of Section 19130. The Legislature further finds and declares that the services described in this section are a new state function pursuant to paragraph (2) of subdivision (b) of Section 19130.

HISTORY:

Added Stats 1995 ch 938 § 21 (SB 523), operative July 1, 1997. Amended Stats 2012 ch 363 § 2 (SB 863), effective January 1, 2013.

§ 11435.35. Publication of list of certified medical examination interpreters

(a) The State Personnel Board shall establish, maintain, administer, and publish annually, an updated list of certified medical examination interpreters it has determined meet the minimum standards in interpreting skills and linguistic abilities in languages designated pursuant to Section 11435.40.

(b) Court interpreters certified pursuant to Section 68562 and administrative hearing interpreters certified pursuant to Section 11435.30 shall be deemed certified for purposes of this section.

(c)(1) In addition to the certification procedure provided pursuant to subdivision (a), the Administrative Director of the Division of workers' Compensation may establish, maintain, administer, and publish annually an updated list of certified medical examination interpreters who, based on testing by an independent organization designated by the administrative director, have been determined to meet the minimum standards in interpreting skills and linguistic abilities in languages designated pursuant to Section 11435.40, for purposes of medical examinations conducted pursuant to proceedings of the workers' Compensation Appeals Board, and medical examinations conducted pursuant to Division 4 (commencing with Section 3200) of the Labor Code. The independent testing organization shall have no financial interest in the training of interpreters or in the employment of interpreters for medical examinations.

(2)(A) A fee, as determined by the administrative director, shall be collected from each interpreter seeking certification. The fee shall not exceed the reasonable regulatory costs of administering the testing and certification program and of publishing the list of certified medical examination interpreters on the Division of Workers' Compensation's Internet Web site.

(B) The Legislature finds and declares that the services described in this section are of such a special and unique nature that they may be contracted out pursuant to paragraph (3) of subdivision (b) of Section 19130. The Legislature further finds and declares that the services described in this section are a new state function pursuant to paragraph (2) of subdivision (b) of Section 19130.

HISTORY:

Added Stats 1995 ch 938 § 21 (SB 523), operative July 1, 1997. Amended Stats 2012 ch 363 § 3 (SB 863), effective January 1, 2013. Stats 2013 ch 287 § 1 (SB 375), effective January 1, 2014.

§ 11435.40. Designation of languages for certification

(a) The Department of Human Resources shall designate the languages for which certification shall be established under Sections 11435.30 and 11435.35. The languages designated shall include, but not be limited to, Spanish, Tagalog, Arabic, Cantonese, Japanese, Korean, Portuguese, and Vietnamese until the Department of Human Resources finds that there is an insufficient need for interpreting assistance in these languages.

(b) The language designations shall be based on the following:

(1) The language needs of non-English-speaking persons appearing before the administrative agencies, as determined by consultation with the agencies.

(2) The cost of developing a language examination.

(3) The availability of experts needed to develop a language examination.

(4) Other information the department deems relevant.

HISTORY:

Added Stats 1995 ch 938 § 21 (SB 523), operative July 1, 1997. Amended Stats 2012 ch 360 § 6 (SB 1309), effective January 1, 2013.

§ 11435.45. Application fees to take interpreter examinations

(a) The Department of Human Resources shall establish and charge fees for applications to take interpreter examinations and for renewal of certifications.

The purpose of these fees is to cover the annual projected costs of carrying out this article. The fees may be adjusted each fiscal year by a percent that is equal to or less than the percent change in the California Necessities Index prepared by the Commission on State Finance.

(b) Each certified administrative hearing interpreter and each certified medical examination interpreter shall pay a fee, due on July 1 of each year, for the renewal of the certification. Court interpreters certified under Section 68562 shall not pay any fees required by this section.

(c) If the amount of money collected in fees is not sufficient to cover the costs of carrying out this article, the department shall charge and be reimbursed a pro rata share of the additional costs by the state agencies that conduct administrative hearings.

HISTORY:

Added Stats 1995 ch 938 § 21 (SB 523), operative July 1, 1997. Amended Stats 2012 ch 360 § 7 (SB 1309), effective January 1, 2013.

§ 11435.50. Removal of person from list of certified interpreters

The Department of Human Resources may remove the name of a person from the list of certified interpreters if any of the following conditions occurs:

(a) The person is deceased.

(b) The person notifies the department that the person is unavailable for work.

(c) The person does not submit a renewal fee as required by Section 11435.45.

HISTORY:

Added Stats 1995 ch 938 § 21 (SB 523), operative July 1, 1997. Amended Stats 2012 ch 360 § 8 (SB 1309), effective January 1, 2013.

§ 11435.55. Qualification and use of noncertified interpreters

(a) An interpreter used in a hearing shall be certified pursuant to Section 11435.30. However, if an interpreter certified pursuant to Section 11435.30 cannot be present at the hearing, the hearing agency shall have discretionary authority to provisionally qualify and use another interpreter.

(b) An interpreter used in a medical examination shall be certified pursuant to Section 11435.35. However, if an interpreter certified pursuant to Section 11435.35 cannot be present at the medical examination, the physician provisionally may use another interpreter if that fact is noted in the record of the medical evaluation.

HISTORY:

Added Stats 1995 ch 938 § 21 (SB 523), operative July 1, 1997.

§ 11435.60. Party to be advised of right to interpreter

Every agency subject to the language assistance requirement of this article shall advise each party of the right to an interpreter at the same time that each party is advised of the hearing date or medical examination. Each party in need of an interpreter shall also be encouraged to give timely notice to the agency conducting the hearing or medical examination so that appropriate arrangements can be made.

HISTORY:
Added Stats 1995 ch 938 § 21 (SB 523), operative July 1, 1997.

§ 11435.65. Rules of confidentiality applicable to interpreters

(a) The rules of confidentiality of the agency, if any, that apply in an adjudicative proceeding shall apply to any interpreter in the hearing or medical examination, whether or not the rules so state.

(b) The interpreter shall not have had any involvement in the issues of the case prior to the hearing.

HISTORY:
Added Stats 1995 ch 938 § 21 (SB 523), operative July 1, 1997.

ARTICLE 9

GENERAL PROCEDURAL PROVISIONS

Section
11440.10. Review of decision.
11440.20. Service of writing or electronic document; Notice.
11440.30. Conduct of hearing by telephone, television, or other electronic means.
11440.40. Proceedings involving sexual offenses; Limitations on evidence.
11440.45. Benevolent gestures as admission of liability; Limitations on evidence.
11440.50. Intervention; Grant of motion; Conditions.
11440.60. Indication of person paying for written communication.

§ 11440.10. Review of decision

(a) The agency head may do any of the following with respect to a decision of the presiding officer or the agency:

(1) Determine to review some but not all issues, or not to exercise any review.

(2) Delegate its review authority to one or more persons.

(3) Authorize review by one or more persons, subject to further review by the agency head.

(b) By regulation an agency may mandate review, or may preclude or limit review, of a decision of the presiding officer or the agency.

HISTORY:
Added Stats 1995 ch 938 § 21 (SB 523), operative July 1, 1997.

§ 11440.20. Service of writing or electronic document; Notice

Service of a writing or electronic document on, or giving of a notice to, a person in a procedure provided in this chapter is subject to the following provisions:

(a) The writing, electronic document, or notice shall be delivered personally or sent by mail, electronic, or other means to the person at the person's last known address or, if the person is a party with an attorney or other authorized representative of record in the proceeding, to the party's attorney or other authorized representative. If a party is required by statute or regulation to maintain an address with an agency, the party's last known address is the address maintained with the agency.

(b) Unless a provision specifies the form of mail, service or notice by mail may be by first-class mail, registered mail, or certified mail, by mail delivery service, by facsimile transmission if complete and without error, or by other electronic means as provided by regulation, in the discretion of the sender.

HISTORY:

Added Stats 1995 ch 938 § 21 (SB 523), operative July 1, 1997. Amended Stats 2021 ch 401 § 12 (AB 1578), effective January 1, 2022.

§ 11440.30. Conduct of hearing by telephone, television, or other electronic means

(a) The presiding officer may conduct all or part of a hearing by telephone, television, or other electronic means if each participant in the hearing has an opportunity to participate in and to hear the entire proceeding while it is taking place and to observe exhibits.

(b)(1) Except as provided in paragraph (2), the presiding officer may not conduct all of a hearing by telephone, television, or other electronic means if a party objects.

(2) If a party objects pursuant to paragraph (1) to a hearing being conducted by electronic means, the presiding officer shall consider the objections and may, in the presiding officer's discretion, structure the hearing to address the party's specific objections and may require the presiding officer, parties, and witnesses, or a subset of parties and witnesses based on the specific objections, to be present in a physical location during all or part of the hearing.

(c) Subdivision (b) is not a limitation on the presiding officer transmitting the hearing by telephone, television, or other electronic means or receiving comments via electronic means from participants who are not parties or witnesses.

HISTORY:

Added Stats 1995 ch 938 § 21 (SB 523), operative July 1, 1997. Amended Stats 2021 ch 401 § 13 (AB 1578), effective January 1, 2022.

§ 11440.40. Proceedings involving sexual offenses; Limitations on evidence

(a) In any proceeding under subdivision (h) or (i) of Section 12940, or Section 19572 or 19702, alleging conduct that constitutes sexual harassment, sexual assault, or sexual battery, evidence of specific instances of a complainant's sexual conduct with individuals other than the alleged perpetrator is subject to all of the following limitations:

(1) The evidence is not discoverable unless it is to be offered at a hearing to attack the credibility of the complainant as provided for under subdivision (b). This paragraph is intended only to limit the scope of discovery; it is not intended to affect the methods of discovery allowed by statute.

(2) The evidence is not admissible at the hearing unless offered to attack the credibility of the complainant as provided for under subdivision (b). Reputation or opinion evidence regarding the sexual behavior of the complainant is not admissible for any purpose.

(b) Evidence of specific instances of a complainant's sexual conduct with individuals other than the alleged perpetrator is presumed inadmissible absent an offer of proof establishing its relevance and reliability and that its probative value is not substantially outweighed by the probability that its admission will create substantial danger of undue prejudice or confuse the issue.

(c) As used in this section "complainant" means a person claiming to have been subjected to conduct that constitutes sexual harassment, sexual assault, or sexual battery.

HISTORY:

Added Stats 1995 ch 938 § 21 (SB 523), operative July 1, 1997.

§ 11440.45. Benevolent gestures as admission of liability; Limitations on evidence

(a) In any proceedings pursuant to this chapter or Chapter 5 (commencing with Section 11500), the portion of statements, writings, or benevolent gestures expressing sympathy or a general sense of benevolence relating to the pain, suffering, or death of a person involved in an accident and made to that person or to the family of that person shall be inadmissible as evidence of an admission of liability. A statement of fault, however, which is part of, or in addition to, any of the above shall not be inadmissible pursuant to this section.

(b) For purposes of this section:

(1) "Accident" means an occurrence resulting in injury or death to one or more persons which is not the result of willful action by a party.

(2) "Benevolent gestures" means actions which convey a sense of compassion or commiseration emanating from humane impulses.

(3) "Family" means the spouse, parent, grandparent, stepmother, stepfather, child, grandchild, brother, sister, half brother, half sister, adopted children of parent, or spouse's parents of an injured party.

HISTORY:

Added Stats 2002 ch 92 § 1 (AB 2723).

§ 11440.50. Intervention; Grant of motion; Conditions

(a) This section applies in adjudicative proceedings of an agency if the agency by regulation provides that this section is applicable in the proceedings.

(b) The presiding officer shall grant a motion for intervention if all of the following conditions are satisfied:

(1) The motion is submitted in writing, with copies served on all parties named in the agency's pleading.

(2) The motion is made as early as practicable in advance of the hearing. If there is a prehearing conference, the motion shall be made in advance of the prehearing conference and shall be resolved at the prehearing conference.

(3) The motion states facts demonstrating that the applicant' s legal rights, duties, privileges, or immunities will be substantially affected by the proceeding or that the applicant qualifies as an intervenor under a statute or regulation.

(4) The presiding officer determines that the interests of justice and the orderly and prompt conduct of the proceeding will not be impaired by allowing the intervention.

(c) If an applicant qualifies for intervention, the presiding officer may impose conditions on the intervenor's participation in the proceeding, either at the time that intervention is granted or at a subsequent time. Conditions may include the following:

(1) Limiting the intervenor's participation to designated issues in which the intervenor has a particular interest demonstrated by the motion.

(2) Limiting or excluding the use of discovery, cross-examination, and other procedures involving the intervenor so as to promote the orderly and prompt conduct of the proceeding.

(3) Requiring two or more intervenors to combine their presentations of evidence and argument, cross-examination, discovery, and other participation in the proceeding.

(4) Limiting or excluding the intervenor's participation in settlement negotiations.

(d) As early as practicable in advance of the hearing the presiding officer shall issue an order granting or denying the motion for intervention, specifying any conditions, and briefly stating the reasons for the order. The presiding officer may modify the order at any time, stating the reasons for the modification. The presiding officer shall promptly give notice of an order granting, denying, or modifying intervention to the applicant and to all parties.

(e) Whether the interests of justice and the orderly and prompt conduct of the proceedings will be impaired by allowing intervention is a determination to be made in the sole discretion, and based on the knowledge and judgment at that time, of the presiding officer. The determination is not subject to administrative or judicial review.

(f) Nothing in this section precludes an agency from adopting a regulation that permits participation by a person short of intervention as a party, subject to Article 7 (commencing with Section 11430.10) of Chapter 4.5.

HISTORY:

Added Stats 1995 ch 938 § 21 (SB 523), operative July 1, 1997.

§ 11440.60. Indication of person paying for written communication

(a) For purposes of this section, the following terms have the following meaning:

(1) "Quasi-judicial proceeding" means any of the following:

(A) A proceeding to determine the rights or duties of a person under existing laws, regulations, or policies.

(B) A proceeding involving the issuance, amendment, or revocation of a permit or license.

(C) A proceeding to enforce compliance with existing law or to impose sanctions for violations of existing law.

(D) A proceeding at which action is taken involving the purchase or sale of property, goods, or services by an agency.

(E) A proceeding at which an action is taken awarding a grant or a contract.

(2) "Written communication" means any report, study, survey, analysis, letter, or any other written document.

(b) Any person submitting a written communication, which is specifically generated for the purpose of being presented at the agency hearing to which it is being communicated, to a state agency in a quasi-judicial proceeding that is directly paid for by anyone other than the person who submitted the written communication shall clearly indicate any person who paid to produce the written communication.

(c) A state agency may refuse or ignore a written communication submitted by an attorney or any other authorized representative on behalf of a client in a quasi-judicial proceeding, unless the written communication clearly indicates the client on whose behalf the communication is submitted to the state agency.

HISTORY:
Added Stats 1997 ch 192 § 1 (SB 504).

ARTICLE 10

INFORMAL HEARING

Section
11445.10. Legislative findings and declarations.
11445.20. Circumstances permitting use of informal hearing procedure.
11445.30. Notice of informal procedure.
11445.40. Application of procedures otherwise required.
11445.50. Denial of use of informal procedure; Conversion to formal hearing; Cross-examination.
11445.60. Identity of witnesses or other sources.

§ 11445.10. Legislative findings and declarations

(a) Subject to the limitations in this article, an agency may conduct an adjudicative proceeding under the informal hearing procedure provided in this article.

(b) The Legislature finds and declares the following:

(1) The informal hearing procedure is intended to satisfy due process and public policy requirements in a manner that is simpler and more expeditious than hearing procedures otherwise required by statute, for use in appropriate circumstances.

(2) The informal hearing procedure provides a forum in the nature of a conference in which a party has an opportunity to be heard by the presiding officer.

(3) The informal hearing procedure provides a forum that may accommodate a hearing where by regulation or statute a member of the public may participate without appearing or intervening as a party.

HISTORY:
Added Stats 1995 ch 938 § 21 (SB 523), operative July 1, 1997.

§ 11445.20. Circumstances permitting use of informal hearing procedure

Subject to Section 11445.30, an agency may use an informal hearing procedure in any of the following proceedings, if in the circumstances its use does not violate another statute or the federal or state Constitution:

(a) A proceeding where there is no disputed issue of material fact.

(b) A proceeding where there is a disputed issue of material fact, if the matter is limited to any of the following:

(1) A monetary amount of not more than one thousand dollars ($1,000).

(2) A disciplinary sanction against a student that does not involve expulsion from an academic institution or suspension for more than 10 days.

(3) A disciplinary sanction against an employee that does not involve discharge from employment, demotion, or suspension for more than 5 days.

(4) A disciplinary sanction against a licensee that does not involve an actual revocation of a license or an actual suspension of a license for more than five days. Nothing in this section precludes an agency from imposing a stayed revocation or a stayed suspension of a license in an informal hearing.

(c) A proceeding where, by regulation, the agency has authorized use of an informal hearing.

(d) A proceeding where an evidentiary hearing for determination of facts is not required by statute but where the agency determines the federal or state Constitution may require a hearing.

HISTORY:

Added Stats 1995 ch 938 § 21 (SB 523), operative July 1, 1997.

§ 11445.30. Notice of informal procedure

(a) The notice of hearing shall state the agency's selection of the informal hearing procedure.

(b) Any objection of a party to use of the informal hearing procedure shall be made in the party's pleading.

(c) An objection to use of the informal hearing procedure shall be resolved by the presiding officer before the hearing on the basis of the pleadings and any written submissions in support of the pleadings. An objection to use of the informal hearing procedure in a disciplinary proceeding involving an occupational license shall be resolved in favor of the licensee.

HISTORY:

Added Stats 1995 ch 938 § 21 (SB 523), operative July 1, 1997.

§ 11445.40. Application of procedures otherwise required

(a) Except as provided in this article, the hearing procedures otherwise required by statute for an adjudicative proceeding apply to an informal hearing.

(b) In an informal hearing the presiding officer shall regulate the course of the proceeding. The presiding officer shall permit the parties and may permit others to offer written or oral comments on the issues. The presiding officer may limit the use of witnesses, testimony, evidence, and argument, and may limit or eliminate the use of pleadings, intervention, discovery, prehearing conferences, and rebuttal.

HISTORY:

Added Stats 1995 ch 938 § 21 (SB 523), operative July 1, 1997.

§ 11445.50. Denial of use of informal procedure; Conversion to formal hearing; Cross-examination

(a) The presiding officer may deny use of the informal hearing procedure, or may convert an informal hearing to a formal hearing after an informal hearing is commenced, if it appears to the presiding officer that cross-examination is necessary for proper determination of the matter and that the delay, burden, or complication due to allowing cross-examination in the informal hearing will be more than minimal.

(b) An agency, by regulation, may specify categories of cases in which cross-examination is deemed not necessary for proper determination of the matter under the informal hearing procedure. The presiding officer may allow cross-examination of witnesses in an informal hearing notwithstanding an agency regulation if it appears to the presiding officer that in the circumstances cross-examination is necessary for proper determination of the matter.

(c) The actions of the presiding officer under this section are not subject to judicial review.

HISTORY:

Added Stats 1995 ch 938 § 21 (SB 523), operative July 1, 1997.

§ 11445.60. Identity of witnesses or other sources

(a) If the presiding officer has reason to believe that material facts are in dispute, the presiding officer may require a party to state the identity of the witnesses or other sources through which the party would propose to present proof if the proceeding were converted to a formal or other applicable hearing procedure. If disclosure of a fact, allegation, or source is privileged or expressly prohibited by a regulation, statute, or the federal or state Constitution, the presiding officer may require the party to indicate that confidential facts, allegations, or sources are involved, but not to disclose the confidential facts, allegations, or sources.

(b) If a party has reason to believe that essential facts must be obtained in order to permit an adequate presentation of the case, the party may inform the presiding officer regarding the general nature of the facts and the sources from which the party would propose to obtain the facts if the proceeding were converted to a formal or other applicable hearing procedure.

HISTORY:

Added Stats 1995 ch 938 § 21 (SB 523), operative July 1, 1997.

ARTICLE 11
SUBPOENAS

Section

11450.05. Application of article.
11450.10. Issuance for attendance or production of documents.
11450.20. Persons who may issue subpoenas; Service.
11450.30. Objection to subpoena; Motion for protective order; Motion to quash.
11450.40. Witness's mileage and fees.
11450.50. Written notice to witness to attend; Service.

§ 11450.05. Application of article

(a) This article applies in an adjudicative proceeding required to be conducted under Chapter 5 (commencing with Section 11500).

(b) An agency may use the subpoena procedure provided in this article in an adjudicative proceeding not required to be conducted under Chapter 5 (commencing with Section 11500), in which case all the provisions of this article apply including, but not limited to, issuance of a subpoena at the request of a party or by the attorney of record for a party under Section 11450.20.

HISTORY:

Added Stats 1995 ch 938 § 21 (SB 523), operative July 1, 1997.

§ 11450.10. Issuance for attendance or production of documents

(a) Subpoenas and subpoenas duces tecum may be issued for attendance at a hearing and for production of documents at any reasonable time and place or at a hearing.

(b) The custodian of documents that are the subject of a subpoena duces tecum may satisfy the subpoena by delivery of the documents or a copy of the documents, or by making the documents available for inspection or copying, together with an affidavit in compliance with Section 1561 of the Evidence Code.

HISTORY:

Added Stats 1995 ch 938 § 21 (SB 523), operative July 1, 1997.

§ 11450.20. Persons who may issue subpoenas; Service

(a) Subpoenas and subpoenas duces tecum shall be issued by the agency or presiding officer at the request of a party, or by the attorney of record for a party, in accordance with Sections 1985 to 1985.4, inclusive, of the Code of Civil Procedure.

(b) The process extends to all parts of the state and shall be served in accordance with Sections 1987 and 1988 of the Code of Civil Procedure. A subpoena or subpoena duces tecum may also be delivered by certified mail return receipt requested or by messenger. Service by messenger shall be effected when the witness acknowledges receipt of the subpoena to the sender, by telephone, by mail, or in person, and identifies himself or herself either by reference to date of birth and driver's license number or Department of Motor Vehicles identification number, or the sender may verify receipt of the subpoena by obtaining other identifying information from the recipient. The sender shall make a written notation of the acknowledgment. A subpoena issued and acknowledged pursuant to this section has the same force and effect as a subpoena personally served. Failure to comply with a subpoena issued and acknowledged pursuant to this section may be punished as a contempt and the subpoena may so state. A party requesting a continuance based upon the failure of a witness to appear at the time and place required for the appearance or testimony pursuant to a subpoena, shall prove that the party has complied with this section. The continuance shall only be granted for a period of time that would allow personal service of the subpoena and in no event longer than that allowed by law.

(c) No witness is obliged to attend unless the witness is a resident of the state at the time of service.

HISTORY:
Added Stats 1995 ch 938 § 21 (SB 523), operative July 1, 1997.

§ 11450.30. Objection to subpoena; Motion for protective order; Motion to quash

(a) A person served with a subpoena or a subpoena duces tecum may object to its terms by a motion for a protective order, including a motion to quash.

(b) The objection shall be resolved by the presiding officer on terms and conditions that the presiding officer declares. The presiding officer may make another order that is appropriate to protect the parties or the witness from unreasonable or oppressive demands, including violations of the right to privacy.

(c) A subpoena or a subpoena duces tecum issued by the agency on its own motion may be quashed by the agency.

HISTORY:
Added Stats 1995 ch 938 § 21 (SB 523), operative July 1, 1997.

§ 11450.40. Witness's mileage and fees

A witness appearing pursuant to a subpoena or a subpoena duces tecum, other than a party, shall receive for the appearance the following mileage and fees, to be paid by the party at whose request the witness is subpoenaed:

(a) The same mileage allowed by law to a witness in a civil case.

(b) The same fees allowed by law to a witness in a civil case. This subdivision does not apply to an officer or employee of the state or a political subdivision of the state.

HISTORY:
Added Stats 1995 ch 938 § 21 (SB 523), operative July 1, 1997.

§ 11450.50. Written notice to witness to attend; Service

(a) In the case of the production of a party to the record of a proceeding or of a person for whose benefit a proceeding is prosecuted or defended, the service of a subpoena on the witness is not required if written notice requesting the witness to attend, with the time and place of the hearing, is served on the attorney of the party or person.

(b) Service of written notice to attend under this section shall be made in the manner and is subject to the conditions provided in Section 1987 of the Code of Civil Procedure for service of written notice to attend in a civil action or proceeding.

HISTORY:
Added Stats 1995 ch 938 § 21 (SB 523), operative July 1, 1997.

ARTICLE 12
ENFORCEMENT OF ORDERS AND SANCTIONS

Section
11455.10. Grounds for contempt sanction.

Section
11455.20. Certification of facts to justify contempt sanction; Other procedure.
11455.30. Bad faith actions; Order to pay expenses including attorney's fees.

§ 11455.10. Grounds for contempt sanction

A person is subject to the contempt sanction for any of the following in an adjudicative proceeding before an agency:

(a) Disobedience of or resistance to a lawful order.

(b) Refusal to take the oath or affirmation as a witness or thereafter refusal to be examined.

(c) Obstruction or interruption of the due course of the proceeding during a hearing or near the place of the hearing by any of the following:

(1) Disorderly, contemptuous, or insolent behavior toward the presiding officer while conducting the proceeding.

(2) Breach of the peace, boisterous conduct, or violent disturbance.

(3) Other unlawful interference with the process or proceedings of the agency.

(d) Violation of the prohibition of ex parte communications under Article 7 (commencing with Section 11430.10).

(e) Failure or refusal, without substantial justification, to comply with a deposition order, discovery request, subpoena, or other order of the presiding officer, or moving, without substantial justification, to compel discovery.

HISTORY:
Added Stats 1995 ch 938 § 21 (SB 523), operative July 1, 1997.

§ 11455.20. Certification of facts to justify contempt sanction; Other procedure

(a) The presiding officer or agency head may certify the facts that justify the contempt sanction against a person to the superior court in and for the county where the proceeding is conducted. The court shall thereupon issue an order directing the person to appear before the court at a specified time and place, and then and there to show cause why the person should not be punished for contempt. The order and a copy of the certified statement shall be served on the person. Upon service of the order and a copy of the certified statement, the court has jurisdiction of the matter.

(b) The same proceedings shall be had, the same penalties may be imposed, and the person charged may purge the contempt in the same way, as in the case of a person who has committed a contempt in the trial of a civil action before a superior court.

HISTORY:
Added Stats 1995 ch 938 § 21 (SB 523), operative July 1, 1997.

§ 11455.30. Bad faith actions; Order to pay expenses including attorney's fees

(a) The presiding officer may order a party, the party's attorney or other authorized representative, or both, to pay reasonable expenses, including attorney's fees, incurred by another party as a result of bad faith actions or tactics that are frivolous or solely intended to cause unnecessary delay as defined in Section 128.5 of the Code of Civil Procedure.

(b) The order, or denial of an order, is subject to judicial review in the same manner as a decision in the proceeding. The order is enforceable in the same manner as a money judgment or by the contempt sanction.

HISTORY:
Added Stats 1995 ch 938 § 21 (SB 523), operative July 1, 1997.

ARTICLE 13
EMERGENCY DECISION

Section
11460.10. Conduct of proceeding under emergency procedure.
11460.20. Emergency decision.
11460.30. Conditions for issuance of emergency decision.
11460.40. Notice and hearing prior to decision.
11460.50. Statement of factual and legal basis and reasons for emergency decision.
11460.60. Formal or informal proceeding after issuance of emergency decision.
11460.70. Agency record.
11460.80. Judicial review of decision.

§ 11460.10. Conduct of proceeding under emergency procedure

Subject to the limitations in this article, an agency may conduct an adjudicative proceeding under the emergency decision procedure provided in this article.

HISTORY:
Added Stats 1995 ch 938 § 21 (SB 523), operative July 1, 1997.

§ 11460.20. Emergency decision

(a) An agency may issue an emergency decision for temporary, interim relief under this article if the agency has adopted a regulation that provides that the agency may use the procedure provided in this article.

(b) The regulation shall elaborate the application of the provisions of this article to an emergency decision by the agency, including all of the following:

(1) Define the specific circumstances in which an emergency decision may be issued under this article.

(2) State the nature of the temporary, interim relief that the agency may order.

(3) Prescribe the procedures that will be available before and after issuance of an emergency decision under this article. The procedures may be more protective of the person to which the agency action is directed than those provided in this article.

(c) This article does not apply to an emergency decision, including a cease and desist order or an interim or temporary suspension order, issued pursuant to other express statutory authority.

HISTORY:
Added Stats 1995 ch 938 § 21 (SB 523), operative July 1, 1997.

§ 11460.30. Conditions for issuance of emergency decision

(a) An agency may only issue an emergency decision under this article in a situation involving an immediate danger to the public health, safety, or welfare that requires immediate agency action.

(b) An agency may only take action under this article that is necessary to prevent or avoid the immediate danger to the public health, safety, or welfare that justifies issuance of an emergency decision.

(c) An emergency decision issued under this article is limited to temporary, interim relief. The temporary, interim relief is subject to judicial review under Section 11460.80, and the underlying issue giving rise to the temporary, interim relief is subject to an adjudicative proceeding pursuant to Section 11460.60.

HISTORY:

Added Stats 1995 ch 938 § 21 (SB 523), operative July 1, 1997.

§ 11460.40. Notice and hearing prior to decision

(a) Before issuing an emergency decision under this article, the agency shall, if practicable, give the person to which the agency action is directed notice and an opportunity to be heard.

(b) Notice and hearing under this section may be oral or written, including notice and hearing by telephone, facsimile transmission, or other electronic means, as the circumstances permit. The hearing may be conducted in the same manner as an informal hearing.

HISTORY:

Added Stats 1995 ch 938 § 21 (SB 523), operative July 1, 1997.

§ 11460.50. Statement of factual and legal basis and reasons for emergency decision

(a) The agency shall issue an emergency decision, including a brief explanation of the factual and legal basis and reasons for the emergency decision, to justify the determination of an immediate danger and the agency's emergency decision to take the specific action.

(b) The agency shall give notice to the extent practicable to the person to which the agency action is directed. The emergency decision is effective when issued or as provided in the decision.

HISTORY:

Added Stats 1995 ch 938 § 21 (SB 523), operative July 1, 1997.

§ 11460.60. Formal or informal proceeding after issuance of emergency decision

(a) After issuing an emergency decision under this article for temporary, interim relief, the agency shall conduct an adjudicative proceeding under a formal, informal, or other applicable hearing procedure to resolve the underlying issues giving rise to the temporary, interim relief.

(b) The agency shall commence an adjudicative proceeding under another procedure within 10 days after issuing an emergency decision under this article, notwithstanding the pendency of proceedings for judicial review of the emergency decision.

HISTORY:
Added Stats 1995 ch 938 § 21 (SB 523), operative July 1, 1997.

§ 11460.70. Agency record

The agency record consists of any documents concerning the matter that were considered or prepared by the agency. The agency shall maintain these documents as its official record.

HISTORY:
Added Stats 1995 ch 938 § 21 (SB 523), operative July 1, 1997.

§ 11460.80. Judicial review of decision

(a) On issuance of an emergency decision under this article, the person to which the agency action is directed may obtain judicial review of the decision in the manner provided in this section without exhaustion of administrative remedies.

(b) Judicial review under this section shall be pursuant to Section 1094.5 of the Code of Civil Procedure, subject to the following provisions:

(1) The hearing shall be on the earliest day that the business of the court will admit of, but not later than 15 days after service of the petition on the agency.

(2) Where it is claimed that the findings are not supported by the evidence, abuse of discretion is established if the court determines that the findings are not supported by substantial evidence in the light of the whole record.

(3) A party, on written request to another party, before the proceedings for review and within 10 days after issuance of the emergency decision, is entitled to appropriate discovery.

(4) The relief that may be ordered on judicial review is limited to a stay of the emergency decision.

HISTORY:
Added Stats 1995 ch 938 § 21 (SB 523), operative July 1, 1997.

ARTICLE 14
DECLARATORY DECISION

Section
11465.10. Conduct of proceeding under declaratory decision procedure.
11465.20. Application; Issuance of decision.
11465.30. Notice of application for decision.
11465.40. Applicable hearing procedure.
11465.50. Actions of agency after receipt of application.
11465.60. Contents of decision; Status and binding effect of decision.
11465.70. Model regulations.

§ 11465.10. Conduct of proceeding under declaratory decision procedure

Subject to the limitations in this article, an agency may conduct an adjudicative proceeding under the declaratory decision procedure provided in this article.

HISTORY:
Added Stats 1995 ch 938 § 21 (SB 523), operative July 1, 1997.

§ 11465.20. Application; Issuance of decision

(a) A person may apply to an agency for a declaratory decision as to the applicability to specified circumstances of a statute, regulation, or decision within the primary jurisdiction of the agency.

(b) The agency in its discretion may issue a declaratory decision in response to the application. The agency shall not issue a declaratory decision if any of the following applies:

(1) Issuance of the decision would be contrary to a regulation adopted under this article.

(2) The decision would substantially prejudice the rights of a person who would be a necessary party and who does not consent in writing to the determination of the matter by a declaratory decision proceeding.

(3) The decision involves a matter that is the subject of pending administrative or judicial proceedings.

(c) An application for a declaratory decision is not required for exhaustion of the applicant's administrative remedies for purposes of judicial review.

HISTORY:
Added Stats 1995 ch 938 § 21 (SB 523), operative July 1, 1997.

§ 11465.30. Notice of application for decision

Within 30 days after receipt of an application for a declaratory decision, an agency shall give notice of the application to all persons to which notice of an adjudicative proceeding is otherwise required, and may give notice to any other person.

HISTORY:
Added Stats 1995 ch 938 § 21 (SB 523), operative July 1, 1997.

§ 11465.40. Applicable hearing procedure

The provisions of a formal, informal, or other applicable hearing procedure do not apply to an agency proceeding for a declaratory decision except to the extent provided in this article or to the extent the agency so provides by regulation or order.

HISTORY:
Added Stats 1995 ch 938 § 21 (SB 523), operative July 1, 1997.

§ 11465.50. Actions of agency after receipt of application

(a) Within 60 days after receipt of an application for a declaratory decision, an agency shall do one of the following, in writing:

(1) Issue a decision declaring the applicability of the statute, regulation, or decision in question to the specified circumstances.

(2) Set the matter for specified proceedings.

(3) Agree to issue a declaratory decision by a specified time.

(4) Decline to issue a declaratory decision, stating in writing the reasons for its action. Agency action under this paragraph is not subject to judicial review.

(b) A copy of the agency's action under subdivision (a) shall be served promptly on the applicant and any other party.

(c) If an agency has not taken action under subdivision (a) within 60 days after receipt of an application for a declaratory decision, the agency is considered to have declined to issue a declaratory decision on the matter.

HISTORY:

Added Stats 1995 ch 938 § 21 (SB 523), operative July 1, 1997.

§ 11465.60. Contents of decision; Status and binding effect of decision

(a) A declaratory decision shall contain the names of all parties to the proceeding, the particular facts on which it is based, and the reasons for its conclusion.

(b) A declaratory decision has the same status and binding effect as any other decision issued by the agency in an adjudicative proceeding.

HISTORY:

Added Stats 1995 ch 938 § 21 (SB 523), operative July 1, 1997.

§ 11465.70. Model regulations

(a) The Office of Administrative Hearings shall adopt and promulgate model regulations under this article that are consistent with the public interest and with the general policy of this article to facilitate and encourage agency issuance of reliable advice. The model regulations shall provide for all of the following:

(1) A description of the classes of circumstances in which an agency will not issue a declaratory decision.

(2) The form, contents, and filing of an application for a declaratory decision.

(3) The procedural rights of a person in relation to an application.

(4) The disposition of an application.

(b) The regulations adopted by the Office of Administrative Hearings under this article apply in an adjudicative proceeding unless an agency adopts its own regulations to govern declaratory decisions of the agency.

(c) This article does not apply in an adjudicative proceeding to the extent an agency by regulation provides inconsistent rules or provides that this article is not applicable in a proceeding of the agency.

HISTORY:

Added Stats 1995 ch 938 § 21 (SB 523), operative July 1, 1997.

ARTICLE 15

CONVERSION OF PROCEEDING

Section

11470.10. Conversion into another type of proceeding.
11470.20. Appointment of successor to preside over new proceeding.
11470.30. Record of original proceeding.
11470.40. Duties of presiding officer of new proceeding.

Section
11470.50. Adoption of regulations to govern conversion.

§ 11470.10. Conversion into another type of proceeding

(a) Subject to any applicable regulation adopted under Section 11470.50, at any point in an agency proceeding the presiding officer or other agency official responsible for the proceeding:

(1) May convert the proceeding to another type of agency proceeding provided for by statute if the conversion is appropriate, is in the public interest, and does not substantially prejudice the rights of a party.

(2) Shall convert the proceeding to another type of agency proceeding provided for by statute, if required by regulation or statute.

(b) A proceeding of one type may be converted to a proceeding of another type only on notice to all parties to the original proceeding.

HISTORY:

Added Stats 1995 ch 938 § 21 (SB 523), operative July 1, 1997.

§ 11470.20. Appointment of successor to preside over new proceeding

If the presiding officer or other agency official responsible for the original proceeding would not have authority over the new proceeding to which it is to be converted, the agency head shall appoint a successor to preside over or be responsible for the new proceeding.

HISTORY:

Added Stats 1995 ch 938 § 21 (SB 523), operative July 1, 1997.

§ 11470.30. Record of original proceeding

To the extent practicable and consistent with the rights of parties and the requirements of this article relating to the new proceeding, the record of the original agency proceeding shall be used in the new agency proceeding.

HISTORY:

Added Stats 1995 ch 938 § 21 (SB 523), operative July 1, 1997.

§ 11470.40. Duties of presiding officer of new proceeding

After a proceeding is converted from one type to another, the presiding officer or other agency official responsible for the new proceeding shall do all of the following:

(a) Give additional notice to parties or other persons necessary to satisfy the statutory requirements relating to the new proceeding.

(b) Dispose of the matters involved without further proceedings if sufficient proceedings have already been held to satisfy the statutory requirements relating to the new proceeding.

(c) Conduct or cause to be conducted any additional proceedings necessary to satisfy the statutory requirements relating to the new proceeding, and allow the parties a reasonable time to prepare for the new proceeding.

HISTORY:

Added Stats 1995 ch 938 § 21 (SB 523), operative July 1, 1997.

§ 11470.50. Adoption of regulations to govern conversion

An agency may adopt regulations to govern the conversion of one type of proceeding to another. The regulations may include an enumeration of the factors to be considered in determining whether and under what circumstances one type of proceeding will be converted to another.

HISTORY:

Added Stats 1995 ch 938 § 21 (SB 523), operative July 1, 1997.

ARTICLE 16

ADMINISTRATIVE ADJUDICATION CODE OF ETHICS

Section

11475. Name of rules.
11475.10. Application.
11475.20. Law governing conduct.
11475.30. Definitions.
11475.40. Inapplicable provisions of Code of Judicial Ethics.
11475.50. Violations.
11475.60. Compliance requirements.
11475.70. Construction and intent.

HISTORY: Added Stats 1998 ch 95 § 1.

§ 11475. Name of rules

The rules imposed by this article may be referred to as the Administrative Adjudication Code of Ethics.

HISTORY:

Added Stats 1998 ch 95 § 1 (AB 2164).

§ 11475.10. Application

(a) This article applies to the following persons:

(1) An administrative law judge. As used in this subdivision, "administrative law judge" means an incumbent of that position, as defined by the State Personnel Board, for each class specification for Administrative Law Judge.

(2) A presiding officer to which this article is made applicable by statute or regulation.

(b) This article shall apply notwithstanding any general statutory provision that this chapter does not apply to some or all of a state agency's adjudicative proceedings.

HISTORY:

Added Stats 1998 ch 95 § 1 (AB 2164).

§ 11475.20. Law governing conduct

Except as otherwise provided in this article, the Code of Judicial Ethics adopted by the Supreme Court pursuant to subdivision (m) of Section 18 of

Article VI of the California Constitution for the conduct of judges governs the hearing and nonhearing conduct of an administrative law judge or other presiding officer to which this article applies.

HISTORY:
Added Stats 1998 ch 95 § 1 (AB 2164).

§ 11475.30. Definitions

For the purpose of this article, the following terms used in the Code of Judicial Ethics have the meanings provided in this section:

(a) "Appeal" means administrative review.

(b) "Court" means the agency conducting an adjudicative proceeding.

(c) "Judge" means administrative law judge or other presiding officer to which this article applies. Related terms, including "judicial," "judiciary," and "justice," mean comparable concepts in administrative adjudication.

(d) "Law" includes regulation and precedent decision.

HISTORY:
Added Stats 1998 ch 95 § 1 (AB 2164).

§ 11475.40. Inapplicable provisions of Code of Judicial Ethics

The following provisions of the Code of Judicial Ethics do not apply under this article:

(a) Canon 3B(7), to the extent it relates to ex parte communications.

(b) Canon 3B(10).

(c) Canon 3D(3).

(d) Canon 4C.

(e) Canons 4E(1), 4F, and 4G.

(f) Canons 5A–5D. However, the introductory paragraph of Canon 5 applies to persons subject to this article notwithstanding Chapter 9.5 (commencing with Section 3201) of Division 4 of Title 1, relating to political activities of public employees.

(g) Canon 6.

HISTORY:
Added Stats 1998 ch 95 § 1 (AB 2164).

§ 11475.50. Violations

A violation of an applicable provision of the Code of Judicial Ethics, or a violation of the restrictions and prohibitions on accepting honoraria, gifts, or travel that otherwise apply to elected state officers pursuant to Chapter 9.5 (commencing with Section 89500) of Title 9, by an administrative law judge or other presiding officer to which this article applies is cause for discipline by the employing agency pursuant to Section 19572.

HISTORY:
Added Stats 1998 ch 95 § 1 (AB 2164).

§ 11475.60. Compliance requirements

(a) Except as provided in subdivision (b), a person to whom this article applies shall comply immediately with all applicable provisions of the Code of Judicial Ethics.

(b) A person to whom this article applies shall comply with Canon 4D(2) of the Code of Judicial Ethics as soon as reasonably possible and shall do so in any event within a period of one year after the article becomes applicable.

HISTORY:
Added Stats 1998 ch 95 § 1 (AB 2164).

§ 11475.70. Construction and intent

Nothing in this article shall be construed or is intended to limit or affect the rights of an administrative law judge or other presiding officer under Chapter 10.3 (commencing with Section 3512) of Division 4 of Title 1.

HISTORY:
Added Stats 1998 ch 95 § 1 (AB 2164).

CHAPTER 5

ADMINISTRATIVE ADJUDICATION: FORMAL HEARING

Section

11500. Definitions.
11501. Application of chapter to agency.
11502. Administrative law judges.
11503. Accusation or District Statement of Reduction in Force.
11504. Statement of issues.
11504.5. Applicability of references to accusations to statements of issues.
11505. Service of accusation or District Statement of Reduction in Force and accompanying papers; Notice of defense or notice of participation; Request for hearing.
11506. Filing of notice of defense or notice of participation; Contents; Right to hearing on the merits.
11507. Amended or supplemental accusation or District Statement of Reduction in Force; Objections.
11507.3. Consolidated proceedings; Separate hearings.
11507.5. Exclusivity of discovery provisions.
11507.7. Motion to compel discovery; Order.
11508. Time and place of hearing.
11509. Notice of hearing.
11511. Depositions.
11511.5. Prehearing conference; Conduct by telephone or other electronic means; Conversion to ADR or informal hearing; Prehearing order.
11511.7. Settlement conference.
11512. Administrative law judge to preside over hearing; Disqualification; Reporting of proceedings.
11513. Evidence.
11514. Affidavits.
11515. Official notice.
11516. Amendment of accusation or District Statement of Reduction in Force after submission.
11517. Contested cases.
11518. Copies of decision to parties.
11518.5. Application to correct mistake or error in decision; Modification; Service of correction.
11519. Effective date of decision; Stay of execution; Notice of suspension or revocation; Restitution; Actual knowledge as condition of enforcement.
11519.1. Order of restitution for financial loss or damages.
11520. Defaults and uncontested cases.
11521. Reconsideration.
11522. Reinstatement of license or reduction of penalty.
11523. Judicial review.
11524. Continuances; Requirement of good cause; Judicial review of denial.
11526. Voting by mail.

Section
11527. Charge against funds of agency.
11528. Oaths.
11529. Interim orders.

HISTORY: Added Stats 1945 ch 867 § 1. Heading amended Stats 1947 ch 1425 § 14; Stats 1995 ch 938 § 22, operative July 1, 1997.

§ 11500. Definitions

In this chapter unless the context or subject matter otherwise requires:

(a) "Agency" includes the state boards, commissions, and officers to which this chapter is made applicable by law, except that wherever the word "agency" alone is used the power to act may be delegated by the agency, and wherever the words "agency itself" are used the power to act shall not be delegated unless the statutes relating to the particular agency authorize the delegation of the agency's power to hear and decide.

(b) "Party" includes the agency, the respondent, and any person, other than an officer or an employee of the agency in his or her official capacity, who has been allowed to appear or participate in the proceeding.

(c) "Respondent" means any person against whom an accusation or District Statement of Reduction in Force is filed pursuant to Section 11503 or against whom a statement of issues is filed pursuant to Section 11504.

(d) "Administrative law judge" means an individual qualified under Section 11502.

(e) "Agency member" means any person who is a member of any agency to which this chapter is applicable and includes any person who himself or herself constitutes an agency.

HISTORY:

Added Stats 1945 ch 867 § 1. Amended Stats 1947 ch 491 § 1, Stats 1977 ch 1057 § 1, operative July 1, 1978; Stats 1985 ch 324 § 15; Stats 1995 ch 938 § 23 (SB 523), operative July 1, 1997; Stats 2013 ch 90 § 2 (SB 546), effective January 1, 2014.

§ 11501. Application of chapter to agency

(a) This chapter applies to any agency as determined by the statutes relating to that agency.

(b) This chapter applies to an adjudicative proceeding of an agency created on or after July 1, 1997, unless the statutes relating to the proceeding provide otherwise.

(c) Chapter 4.5 (commencing with Section 11400) applies to an adjudicative proceeding required to be conducted under this chapter, unless the statutes relating to the proceeding provide otherwise.

HISTORY:

Added Stats 1995 ch 938 § 24.5 (SB 523), operative July 1, 1997.

§ 11502. Administrative law judges

(a) All hearings of state agencies required to be conducted under this chapter shall be conducted by administrative law judges on the staff of the Office of Administrative Hearings. This subdivision applies to a hearing required to be conducted under this chapter that is conducted under the informal hearing or emergency decision procedure provided in Chapter 4.5 (commencing with Section 11400).

(b) The Director of the Office of Administrative Hearings has power to appoint a staff of administrative law judges for the office as provided in Section 11370.3. Each administrative law judge shall have been admitted to practice law in this state for at least five years immediately preceding his or her appointment and shall possess any additional qualifications established by the State Personnel Board for the particular class of position involved.

HISTORY:

Added Stats 1945 ch 867 § 1. Amended Stats 1961 ch 2048 § 10; Stats 1971 ch 1303 § 7; Stats 1985 ch 324 § 16; Stats 1995 ch 938 § 26 (SB 523), operative July 1, 1997.

§ 11503. Accusation or District Statement of Reduction in Force

(a) A hearing to determine whether a right, authority, license, or privilege should be revoked, suspended, limited, or conditioned shall be initiated by filing an accusation or District Statement of Reduction in Force. The accusation or District Statement of Reduction in Force shall be a written statement of charges that shall set forth in ordinary and concise language the acts or omissions with which the respondent is charged, to the end that the respondent will be able to prepare their defense. It shall specify the statutes and rules that the respondent is alleged to have violated, but shall not consist merely of charges phrased in the language of those statutes and rules. The accusation or District Statement of Reduction in Force shall be verified unless made by a public officer acting in their official capacity or by an employee of the agency before which the proceeding is to be held. The verification may be on information and belief.

(b) In a hearing involving a reduction in force that is conducted pursuant to Section 44949, 45117, or 88017 of the Education Code, the hearing shall be initiated by filing a "District Statement of Reduction in Force." For purposes of this chapter, a "District Statement of Reduction in Force" shall have the same meaning as an "accusation." Respondent's responsive pleading shall be entitled "Notice of Participation in Reduction in Force Hearing."

HISTORY:

Added Stats 1945 ch 867 § 1. Amended Stats 1947 ch 491 § 3; Stats 2013 ch 90 § 3 (SB 546), effective January 1, 2014; Stats 2021 ch 655 § 4 (AB 438), effective January 1, 2022.

§ 11504. Statement of issues

A hearing to determine whether a right, authority, license, or privilege should be granted, issued, or renewed shall be initiated by filing a statement of issues. The statement of issues shall be a written statement specifying the statutes and rules with which the respondent must show compliance by producing proof at the hearing and, in addition, any particular matters that have come to the attention of the initiating party and that would authorize a denial of the agency action sought. The statement of issues shall be verified unless made by a public officer acting in his or her official capacity or by an employee of the agency before which the proceeding is to be held. The verification may be on information and belief. The statement of issues shall be served in the same manner as an accusation, except that, if the hearing is held at the request of the respondent, Sections 11505 and 11506 shall not apply and the statement of issues together with the notice of hearing shall be delivered or mailed to the parties as provided in Section 11509. Unless a statement to respondent is served pursuant to Section 11505, a copy of Sections 11507.5, 11507.6, and 11507.7, and the name and address of the person to whom requests permitted by Section 11505 may be made, shall be served with the statement of issues.

HISTORY:

Added Stats 1945 ch 867 § 1. Amended Stats 1947 ch 491 § 4; Stats 1968 ch 808 § 1; Stats 1996 ch 124 § 36 (AB 3470); Stats 1997 ch 17 § 50 (SB 947).

§ 11504.5. Applicability of references to accusations to statements of issues

In the following sections of this chapter, all references to accusations shall be deemed to be applicable to statements of issues except in those cases mentioned in subdivision (a) of Section 11505 and Section 11506 where compliance is not required.

HISTORY:

Added Stats 1963 ch 856 § 1.

§ 11505. Service of accusation or District Statement of Reduction in Force and accompanying papers; Notice of defense or notice of participation; Request for hearing

(a) Upon the filing of the accusation or District Statement of Reduction in Force the agency shall serve a copy thereof on the respondent as provided in subdivision (c). The agency may include with the accusation or District Statement of Reduction in Force any information that it deems appropriate, but it shall include a postcard or other form entitled Notice of Defense, or, as applicable, Notice of Participation, that, when signed by or on behalf of the respondent and returned to the agency, will acknowledge service of the accusation or District Statement of Reduction in Force and constitute a notice of defense, or, as applicable, notice of participation, under Section 11506. The copy of the accusation or District Statement of Reduction in Force shall include or be accompanied by (1) a statement that respondent may request a hearing by filing a notice of defense, or, as applicable, notice of participation, as provided in Section 11506 within 15 days after service upon the respondent of the accusation or District Statement of Reduction in Force, and that failure to do so will constitute a waiver of the respondent's right to a hearing, and (2) copies of Sections 11507.5, 11507.6, and 11507.7.

(b) The statement to respondent shall be substantially in the following form:

Unless a written request for a hearing signed by or on behalf of the person named as respondent in the accompanying accusation or District Statement of Reduction in Force is delivered or mailed to the agency within 15 days after the accusation or District Statement of Reduction in Force was personally served on you or mailed to you, (here insert name of agency) may proceed upon the accusation or District Statement of Reduction in Force without a hearing. The request for a hearing may be made by delivering or mailing the enclosed form entitled Notice of Defense, or, as applicable, Notice of Participation, or by delivering or mailing a notice of defense, or, as applicable, notice of participation, as provided by Section 11506 of the Government Code to: (here insert name and address of agency). You may, but need not, be represented by counsel at any or all stages of these proceedings.

If you desire the names and addresses of witnesses or an opportunity to inspect and copy the items mentioned in Section 11507.6 of the Government Code in the possession, custody, or control of the agency, you may contact: (here insert name and address of appropriate person).

The hearing may be postponed for good cause. If you have good cause, you are obliged to notify the agency or, if an administrative law judge has been assigned to the hearing, the Office of Administrative Hearings, within 10 working days after you discover the good cause. Failure to give notice within 10 days will deprive you of a postponement.

(c) The accusation or District Statement of Reduction in Force and all accompanying information may be sent to the respondent by any means selected by the agency, but no order adversely affecting the rights of the respondent shall be made by the agency in any case unless the respondent has been served personally or by registered mail as provided herein, or has filed a notice of defense, or, as applicable, notice of participation, or otherwise appeared. Service may be proved in the manner authorized in civil actions. Service by registered mail shall be effective if a statute or agency rule requires the respondent to file the respondent's address with the agency and to notify the agency of any change, and if a registered letter containing the accusation or District Statement of Reduction in Force and accompanying material is mailed, addressed to the respondent at the latest address on file with the agency.

(d) For purposes of this chapter, for hearings involving a reduction in force that are conducted pursuant to Section 44949, 45117, or 88017 of the Education Code, a "Notice of Participation" shall have the same meaning as a "Notice of Defense."

HISTORY:

Added Stats 1945 ch 867 § 1. Amended Stats 1968 ch 808 § 2; Stats 1970 ch 828 § 1; Stats 1979 ch 199 § 3; Stats 1995 ch 938 § 28 (SB 523), operative July 1, 1997; Stats 2013 ch 90 § 4 (SB 546), effective January 1, 2014; Stats 2021 ch 655 § 5 (AB 438), effective January 1, 2022.

§ 11506. Filing of notice of defense or notice of participation; Contents; Right to hearing on the merits

(a) Within 15 days after service of the accusation or District Statement of Reduction in Force the respondent may file with the agency a notice of defense, or, as applicable, notice of participation, in which the respondent may:

(1) Request a hearing.

(2) Object to the accusation or District Statement of Reduction in Force upon the ground that it does not state acts or omissions upon which the agency may proceed.

(3) Object to the form of the accusation or District Statement of Reduction in Force on the ground that it is so indefinite or uncertain that the respondent cannot identify the transaction or prepare a defense.

(4) Admit the accusation or District Statement of Reduction in Force in whole or in part.

(5) Present new matter by way of defense.

(6) Object to the accusation or District Statement of Reduction in Force upon the ground that, under the circumstances, compliance with the requirements of a regulation would result in a material violation of another regulation enacted by another department affecting substantive rights.

(b) Within the time specified the respondent may file one or more notices of defense, or, as applicable, notices of participation, upon any or all of these grounds but all of these notices shall be filed within that period unless the agency in its discretion authorizes the filing of a later notice.

(c) The respondent shall be entitled to a hearing on the merits if the respondent files a notice of defense or notice of participation, and the notice shall be deemed a specific denial of all parts of the accusation or District Statement of Reduction in Force not expressly admitted. Failure to file a notice of defense or notice of participation shall constitute a waiver of respondent's right to a hearing, but the agency in its discretion may nevertheless grant a hearing. Unless objection is taken as provided in paragraph (3) of subdivision (a), all objections to the form of the accusation or District Statement of Reduction in Force shall be deemed waived.

(d) The notice of defense or notice of participation shall be in writing signed by or on behalf of the respondent and shall state the respondent's mailing address. It need not be verified or follow any particular form.

(e) As used in this section, "file," "files," "filed," or "filing" means "delivered or mailed" to the agency as provided in Section 11505.

HISTORY:

Added Stats 1945 ch 867 § 1. Amended Stats 1963 ch 931 § 1; Stats 1982 ch 606 § 1; Stats 1986 ch 951 § 20; Stats 1995 ch 938 § 29 (SB 523), operative July 1, 1997; Stats 2013 ch 90 § 5 (SB 546), effective January 1, 2014.

§ 11507. Amended or supplemental accusation or District Statement of Reduction in Force; Objections

At any time before the matter is submitted for decision, the agency may file, or permit the filing of, an amended or supplemental accusation or District Statement of Reduction in Force. All parties shall be notified of the filing. If the amended or supplemental accusation or District Statement of Reduction in Force presents new charges, the agency shall afford the respondent a reasonable opportunity to prepare his or her defense to the new charges, but he or she shall not be entitled to file a further pleading unless the agency in its discretion so orders. Any new charges shall be deemed controverted, and any objections to the amended or supplemental accusation or District Statement of Reduction in Force may be made orally and shall be noted in the record.

HISTORY:

Added Stats 1945 ch 867 § 1. Amended Stats 2013 ch 90 § 6 (SB 546), effective January 1, 2014; Stats 2014 ch 71 § 69 (SB 1304), effective January 1, 2015.

§ 11507.3. Consolidated proceedings; Separate hearings

(a) When proceedings that involve a common question of law or fact are pending, the administrative law judge on the judge's own motion or on motion of a party may order a joint hearing of any or all the matters at issue in the proceedings. The administrative law judge may order all the proceedings consolidated and may make orders concerning the procedure that may tend to avoid unnecessary costs or delay.

(b) The administrative law judge on the judge's own motion or on motion of a party, in furtherance of convenience or to avoid prejudice or when separate hearings will be conducive to expedition and economy, may order a separate hearing of any issue, including an issue raised in the notice of defense or notice of participation, or of any number of issues.

HISTORY:

Added Stats 1995 ch 938 § 30 (SB 523), operative July 1, 1997. Amended Stats 2013 ch 90 § 7 (SB 546), effective January 1, 2014.

§ 11507.5. Exclusivity of discovery provisions

The provisions of Section 11507.6 provide the exclusive right to and method of discovery as to any proceeding governed by this chapter.

HISTORY:

Added Stats 1968 ch 808 § 3.

§ 11507.7. Motion to compel discovery; Order

(a) Any party claiming the party's request for discovery pursuant to Section 11507.6 has not been complied with may serve and file with the administrative law judge a motion to compel discovery, naming as respondent the party refusing or failing to comply with Section 11507.6. The motion shall state facts showing the respondent party failed or refused to comply with Section 11507.6, a description of the matters sought to be discovered, the reason or reasons why the matter is discoverable under that section, that a reasonable and good faith attempt to contact the respondent for an informal resolution of the issue has been made, and the ground or grounds of respondent's refusal so far as known to the moving party.

(b) The motion shall be served upon respondent party and filed within 15 days after the respondent party first evidenced failure or refusal to comply with Section 11507.6 or within 30 days after request was made and the party has failed to reply to the request, or within another time provided by stipulation, whichever period is longer.

(c) The hearing on the motion to compel discovery shall be held within 15 days after the motion is made, or a later time that the administrative law judge may on the judge's own motion for good cause determine. The respondent party shall have the right to serve and file a written answer or other response to the motion before or at the time of the hearing.

(d) Where the matter sought to be discovered is under the custody or control of the respondent party and the respondent party asserts that the matter is not a discoverable matter under the provisions of Section 11507.6, or is privileged against disclosure under those provisions, the administrative law judge may order lodged with it matters provided in subdivision (b) of Section 915 of the Evidence Code and examine the matters in accordance with its provisions.

(e) The administrative law judge shall decide the case on the matters examined in camera, the papers filed by the parties, and such oral argument and additional evidence as the administrative law judge may allow.

(f) Unless otherwise stipulated by the parties, the administrative law judge shall no later than 15 days after the hearing make its order denying or granting the motion. The order shall be in writing setting forth the matters the moving party is entitled to discover under Section 11507.6. A copy of the order shall forthwith be served by mail by the administrative law judge upon the parties. Where the order grants the motion in whole or in part, the order shall not become effective until 10 days after the date the order is served. Where the order denies relief to the moving party, the order shall be effective on the date it is served.

HISTORY:

Added Stats 1968 ch 808 § 5. Amended Stats 1971 ch 1303 § 8; Stats 1980 ch 548 § 2; Stats 1995 ch 938 § 32 (SB 523), operative July 1, 1997.

§ 11508. Time and place of hearing

(a) The agency shall consult the office, and subject to the availability of its staff, shall determine the time and place of the hearing. The hearing shall be held at a hearing facility maintained by the office in Sacramento, Oakland, Los Angeles, or San Diego and shall be held at the facility that is closest to the location where the transaction occurred or the respondent resides.

(b) Notwithstanding subdivision (a), the hearing may be held at any of the following places:

(1) A place selected by the agency that is closer to the location where the transaction occurred or the respondent resides.

(2) A place within the state selected by agreement of the parties.

(3) Virtually by telephone, videoconference, or other electronic means.

(c) The respondent may move for, and the administrative law judge has discretion to grant or deny, a change in the place of the hearing. A motion for a change in the place of the hearing shall be made within 10 days after service of the notice of hearing on the respondent.

(d) Unless good cause is identified in writing by the administrative law judge, hearings shall be held in a facility maintained by the office.

HISTORY:

Added Stats 1945 ch 867 § 1. Amended Stats 1963 ch 710 § 1; Stats 1967 ch 17 § 39; Stats 1987 ch 50 § 1; Stats 1995 ch 938 § 33 (SB 523), operative July 1, 1997; Stats 2005 ch 674 § 22 (SB 231), effective January 1, 2006; Stats 2021 ch 401 § 15 (AB 1578), effective January 1, 2022.

§ 11509. Notice of hearing

The agency shall deliver or mail a notice of hearing to all parties at least 10 days prior to the hearing. The hearing shall not be prior to the expiration of the time within which the respondent is entitled to file a notice of defense, or, as applicable, notice of participation.

The notice to respondent shall be substantially in the following form but may include other information:

You are hereby notified that a hearing will be held before [here insert name of agency] at [here insert place of hearing] on the ____ day of ____, 20____, at the hour of ____, upon the charges made in the accusation or District Statement of Reduction in Force served upon you. If you object to the place of hearing, you must notify the presiding officer within 10 days after this notice is served on you. Failure to notify the presiding officer within 10 days will deprive you of a change in the place of the hearing. You may be present at the hearing. You have the right to be represented by an attorney at your own expense. You are not entitled to the appointment of an attorney to represent you at public expense. You are entitled to represent yourself without legal counsel. You may present any relevant evidence, and will be given full opportunity to cross-examine all witnesses testifying against you. You are entitled to the issuance of subpoenas to compel the attendance of witnesses and the production of books, documents or other things by applying to [here insert appropriate office of agency].

HISTORY:

Added Stats 1945 ch 867 § 1. Amended Stats 1988 ch 362 § 2; Stats 1995 ch 938 § 34 (SB 523), operative July 1, 1997; Stats 2013 ch 90 § 8 (SB 546), effective January 1, 2014.

§ 11511. Depositions

On verified petition of any party, an administrative law judge or, if an administrative law judge has not been appointed, an agency may order that the testimony of any material witness residing within or without the state be taken by deposition in the manner prescribed by law for depositions in civil actions under Title 4 (commencing with Section 2016.010) of Part 4 of the Code of Civil Procedure. The petition shall set forth the nature of the pending proceeding; the name and address of the witness whose testimony is desired; a showing of the materiality of the testimony; a showing that the witness will be unable or cannot be compelled to attend; and shall request an order requiring the witness to appear and testify before an officer named in the petition for that purpose. The petitioner shall serve notice of hearing and a copy of the petition on the other parties at least 10 days before the hearing. Where the witness resides outside the state and where the administrative law judge or agency has ordered the taking of the testimony by deposition, the agency shall obtain an order of court to that effect by filing a petition therefor in the superior court in Sacramento County. The proceedings thereon shall be in accordance with the provisions of Section 11189.

HISTORY:

Added Stats 1945 ch 867 § 1. Amended Stats 1995 ch 938 § 36 (SB 523), operative July 1, 1997; Stats 1998 ch 931 § 182 (SB 2139), effective September 28, 1998; Stats 2004 ch 182 § 42 (AB 3081), operative July 1, 2005.

§ 11511.5. Prehearing conference; Conduct by telephone or other electronic means; Conversion to ADR or informal hearing; Prehearing order

(a) On motion of a party or by order of an administrative law judge, the administrative law judge may conduct a prehearing conference. The administrative law judge shall set the time and place for the prehearing conference, and shall give reasonable written notice to all parties.

(b) The prehearing conference may deal with one or more of the following matters:

(1) Exploration of settlement possibilities.
(2) Preparation of stipulations.
(3) Clarification of issues.
(4) Rulings on identity and limitation of the number of witnesses.

(5) Objections to proffers of evidence.

(6) Order of presentation of evidence and cross-examination.

(7) Rulings regarding issuance of subpoenas and protective orders.

(8) Schedules for the submission of written briefs and schedules for the commencement and conduct of the hearing.

(9) Exchange of witness lists and of exhibits or documents to be offered in evidence at the hearing.

(10) Motions for intervention.

(11) Exploration of the possibility of using alternative dispute resolution provided in Article 5 (commencing with Section 11420.10) of, or the informal hearing procedure provided in Article 10 (commencing with Section 11445.10) of, Chapter 4.5, and objections to use of the informal hearing procedure. Use of alternative dispute resolution or of the informal hearing procedure is subject to subdivision (d).

(12) Any other matters as shall promote the orderly and prompt conduct of the hearing.

(c) The administrative law judge may conduct all or part of the prehearing conference by telephone, television, or other electronic means if each participant in the conference has an opportunity to participate in and to hear the entire proceeding while it is taking place.

(d) With the consent of the parties, the prehearing conference may be converted immediately into alternative dispute resolution or an informal hearing. With the consent of the parties, the proceeding may be converted into alternative dispute resolution to be conducted at another time. With the consent of the agency, the proceeding may be converted into an informal hearing to be conducted at another time subject to the right of a party to object to use of the informal hearing procedure as provided in Section 11445.30.

(e) The administrative law judge shall issue a prehearing order incorporating the matters determined at the prehearing conference. The administrative law judge may direct one or more of the parties to prepare a prehearing order.

HISTORY:

Added Stats 1986 ch 899 § 1. Amended Stats 1995 ch 938 § 37 (SB 523), operative July 1, 1997.

§ 11511.7. Settlement conference

(a) The administrative law judge may order the parties to attend and participate in a settlement conference. The administrative law judge shall set the time and place for the settlement conference, and shall give reasonable written notice to all parties.

(b) The administrative law judge at the settlement conference shall not preside as administrative law judge at the hearing unless otherwise stipulated by the parties. The administrative law judge may conduct all or part of the settlement conference by telephone, television, or other electronic means if each participant in the conference has an opportunity to participate in and to hear the entire proceeding while it is taking place.

HISTORY:

Added Stats 1995 ch 938 § 38 (SB 523), operative July 1, 1997.

§ 11512. Administrative law judge to preside over hearing; Disqualification; Reporting of proceedings

(a) Every hearing in a contested case shall be presided over by an administrative law judge. The agency itself shall determine whether the administrative law judge is to hear the case alone or whether the agency itself is to hear the case with the administrative law judge.

(b) When the agency itself hears the case, the administrative law judge shall preside at the hearing, rule on the admission and exclusion of evidence, and advise the agency on matters of law; the agency itself shall exercise all other powers relating to the conduct of the hearing but may delegate any or all of them to the administrative law judge. When the administrative law judge alone hears a case, the judge shall exercise all powers relating to the conduct of the hearing. A ruling of the administrative law judge admitting or excluding evidence is subject to review in the same manner and to the same extent as the administrative law judge's proposed decision in the proceeding.

(c) An administrative law judge or agency member shall voluntarily disqualify themselves and withdraw from any case in which there are grounds for disqualification, including disqualification under Section 11425.40. The parties may waive the disqualification by a writing that recites the grounds for disqualification. A waiver is effective only when signed by all parties, accepted by the administrative law judge or agency member, and included in the record. Any party may request the disqualification of any administrative law judge or agency member by filing an affidavit, prior to the taking of evidence at a hearing, stating with particularity the grounds upon which it is claimed that the administrative law judge or agency member is disqualified. Where the request concerns an agency member, the issue shall be determined by the other members of the agency. Where the request concerns the administrative law judge, the issue shall be determined by the agency itself if the agency itself hears the case with the administrative law judge, otherwise the issue shall be determined by the administrative law judge. No agency member shall withdraw voluntarily or be subject to disqualification if their disqualification would prevent the existence of a quorum qualified to act in the particular case, except that a substitute qualified to act may be appointed by the appointing authority.

(d) The proceedings at the hearing shall be reported by a stenographic reporter. However, upon the consent of all the parties, or if a stenographic reporter is unavailable and upon finding of good cause by the administrative law judge, the proceedings may be recorded electronically.

(e) Whenever, after the agency itself has commenced to hear the case with an administrative law judge presiding, a quorum no longer exists, the administrative law judge who is presiding shall complete the hearing as if sitting alone and shall render a proposed decision in accordance with subdivision (b) of Section 11517.

HISTORY:

Added Stats 1945 ch 867 § 1. Amended Stats 1973 ch 231 § 1; Stats 1983 ch 635 § 1; Stats 1985 ch 324 § 19; Stats 1995 ch 938 § 39 (SB 523), operative July 1, 1997; Stats 2022 ch 48 § 23 (SB 189), effective June 30, 2022.

§ 11513. Evidence

(a) Oral evidence shall be taken only on oath or affirmation.

(b) Each party shall have these rights: to call and examine witnesses, to introduce exhibits; to cross-examine opposing witnesses on any matter relevant to the issues even though that matter was not covered in the direct examination; to impeach any witness regardless of which party first called him or her to testify; and to rebut the evidence against him or her. If respondent does not testify in his or her own behalf he or she may be called and examined as if under cross-examination.

(c) The hearing need not be conducted according to technical rules relating to evidence and witnesses, except as hereinafter provided. Any relevant evidence shall be admitted if it is the sort of evidence on which responsible persons are accustomed to rely in the conduct of serious affairs, regardless of the existence of any common law or statutory rule which might make improper the admission of the evidence over objection in civil actions.

(d) Hearsay evidence may be used for the purpose of supplementing or explaining other evidence but over timely objection shall not be sufficient in itself to support a finding unless it would be admissible over objection in civil actions. An objection is timely if made before submission of the case or on reconsideration.

(e) The rules of privilege shall be effective to the extent that they are otherwise required by statute to be recognized at the hearing.

(f) The presiding officer has discretion to exclude evidence if its probative value is substantially outweighed by the probability that its admission will necessitate undue consumption of time.

HISTORY:

Added Stats 1992 ch 1302 § 9 (AB 3107), effective September 30, 1992, operative July 1, 1995. Amended Stats 1995 ch 938 § 40 (SB 523), operative July 1, 1997.

§ 11514. Affidavits

(a) At any time 10 or more days prior to a hearing or a continued hearing, any party may mail or deliver to the opposing party a copy of any affidavit which he proposes to introduce in evidence, together with a notice as provided in subdivision (b). Unless the opposing party, within seven days after such mailing or delivery, mails or delivers to the proponent a request to cross-examine an affiant, his right to cross-examine such affiant is waived and the affidavit, if introduced in evidence, shall be given the same effect as if the affiant had testified orally. If an opportunity to cross-examine an affiant is not afforded after request therefor is made as herein provided, the affidavit may be introduced in evidence, but shall be given only the same effect as other hearsay evidence.

(b) The notice referred to in subdivision (a) shall be substantially in the following form:

The accompanying affidavit of (here insert name of affiant) will be introduced as evidence at the hearing in (here insert title of proceeding). (Here insert name of affiant) will not be called to testify orally and you will not be entitled to question him unless you notify (here insert name of proponent or his attorney) at (here insert address) that you wish to cross-examine him. To be effective your request must be mailed or delivered to (here insert name of proponent or his attorney) on or before (here insert a date seven days after the date of mailing or delivering the affidavit to the opposing party).

HISTORY:

Added Stats 1947 ch 491 § 6.

§ 11515. Official notice

In reaching a decision official notice may be taken, either before or after submission of the case for decision, of any generally accepted technical or scientific matter within the agency's special field, and of any fact which may be judicially noticed by the courts of this State. Parties present at the hearing shall be informed of the matters to be noticed, and those matters shall be noted in the record, referred to therein, or appended thereto. Any such party shall be given a reasonable opportunity on request to refute the officially noticed matters by evidence or by written or oral presentation of authority, the manner of such refutation to be determined by the agency.

HISTORY:
Added Stats 1945 ch 867 § 1.

§ 11516. Amendment of accusation or District Statement of Reduction in Force after submission

The agency may order amendment of the accusation or District Statement of Reduction in Force after submission of the case for decision. Each party shall be given notice of the intended amendment and opportunity to show that he or she will be prejudiced thereby unless the case is reopened to permit the introduction of additional evidence on his or her behalf. If such prejudice is shown, the agency shall reopen the case to permit the introduction of additional evidence.

HISTORY:
Added Stats 1945 ch 867 § 1. Amended Stats 2013 ch 90 § 9 (SB 546), effective January 1, 2014.

§ 11517. Contested cases

(a) A contested case may be originally heard by the agency itself and subdivision (b) shall apply. Alternatively, at the discretion of the agency, an administrative law judge may originally hear the case alone and subdivision (c) shall apply.

(b) If a contested case is originally heard before an agency itself, all of the following provisions apply:

(1) An administrative law judge shall be present during the consideration of the case and, if requested, shall assist and advise the agency in the conduct of the hearing.

(2) No member of the agency who did not hear the evidence shall vote on the decision.

(3) The agency shall issue its decision within 100 days of submission of the case.

(c)(1) If a contested case is originally heard by an administrative law judge alone, he or she shall prepare within 30 days after the case is submitted to him or her a proposed decision in a form that may be adopted by the agency as the final decision in the case. Failure of the administrative law judge to deliver a proposed decision within the time required does not prejudice the rights of the agency in the case. Thirty days after the receipt by the agency of the proposed decision, a copy of the proposed decision shall be filed by the agency as a public record and a copy shall be served by the agency on each party and his or her attorney. The filing and service is not an adoption of a proposed decision by the agency.

(2) Within 100 days of receipt by the agency of the administrative law judge's proposed decision, the agency may act as prescribed in subparagraphs (A) to (E), inclusive. If the agency fails to act as prescribed in subparagraphs (A) to (E), inclusive, within 100 days of receipt of the proposed decision, the proposed decision shall be deemed adopted by the agency. The agency may do any of the following:

(A) Adopt the proposed decision in its entirety.

(B) Reduce or otherwise mitigate the proposed penalty and adopt the balance of the proposed decision.

(C) Make technical or other minor changes in the proposed decision and adopt it as the decision. Action by the agency under this paragraph is limited to a clarifying change or a change of a similar nature that does not affect the factual or legal basis of the proposed decision.

(D) Reject the proposed decision and refer the case to the same administrative law judge if reasonably available, otherwise to another administrative law judge, to take additional evidence. If the case is referred to an administrative law judge pursuant to this subparagraph, he or she shall prepare a revised proposed decision, as provided in paragraph (1), based upon the additional evidence and the transcript and other papers that are part of the record of the prior hearing. A copy of the revised proposed decision shall be furnished to each party and his or her attorney as prescribed in this subdivision.

(E) Reject the proposed decision, and decide the case upon the record, including the transcript, or upon an agreed statement of the parties, with or without taking additional evidence. By stipulation of the parties, the agency may decide the case upon the record without including the transcript. If the agency acts pursuant to this subparagraph, all of the following provisions apply:

(i) A copy of the record shall be made available to the parties. The agency may require payment of fees covering direct costs of making the copy.

(ii) The agency itself shall not decide any case provided for in this subdivision without affording the parties the opportunity to present either oral or written argument before the agency itself. If additional oral evidence is introduced before the agency itself, no agency member may vote unless the member heard the additional oral evidence.

(iii) The authority of the agency itself to decide the case under this subdivision includes authority to decide some but not all issues in the case.

(iv) If the agency elects to proceed under this subparagraph, the agency shall issue its final decision not later than 100 days after rejection of the proposed decision. If the agency elects to proceed under this subparagraph, and has ordered a transcript of the proceedings before the administrative law judge, the agency shall issue its final decision not later than 100 days after receipt of the transcript. If the agency finds that a further delay is required by special circumstance, it shall issue an order delaying the decision for no more than 30 days and specifying the reasons therefor. The order shall be subject to judicial review pursuant to Section 11523.

(d) The decision of the agency shall be filed immediately by the agency as a public record and a copy shall be served by the agency on each party and his or her attorney.

HISTORY:

Added Stats 1999 ch 339 § 2 (AB 1692).

§ 11518. Copies of decision to parties

Copies of the decision shall be delivered to the parties personally or sent to them by registered mail.

HISTORY:

Added Stats 1945 ch 867 § 1. Amended Stats 1947 ch 491 § 7; Stats 1995 ch 938 § 43 (SB 523), operative July 1, 1997.

§ 11518.5. Application to correct mistake or error in decision; Modification; Service of correction

(a) Within 15 days after service of a copy of the decision on a party, but not later than the effective date of the decision, the party may apply to the agency for correction of a mistake or clerical error in the decision, stating the specific ground on which the application is made. Notice of the application shall be given to the other parties to the proceeding. The application is not a prerequisite for seeking judicial review.

(b) The agency may refer the application to the administrative law judge who formulated the proposed decision or may delegate its authority under this section to one or more persons.

(c) The agency may deny the application, grant the application and modify the decision, or grant the application and set the matter for further proceedings. The application is considered denied if the agency does not dispose of it within 15 days after it is made or a longer time that the agency provides by regulation.

(d) Nothing in this section precludes the agency, on its own motion or on motion of the administrative law judge, from modifying the decision to correct a mistake or clerical error. A modification under this subdivision shall be made within 15 days after issuance of the decision.

(e) The agency shall, within 15 days after correction of a mistake or clerical error in the decision, serve a copy of the correction on each party on which a copy of the decision was previously served.

HISTORY:

Added Stats 1995 ch 938 § 44 (SB 523), operative July 1, 1997.

§ 11519. Effective date of decision; Stay of execution; Notice of suspension or revocation; Restitution; Actual knowledge as condition of enforcement

(a) The decision shall become effective 30 days after it is delivered or mailed to respondent unless: a reconsideration is ordered within that time, or the agency itself orders that the decision shall become effective sooner, or a stay of execution is granted.

(b) A stay of execution may be included in the decision or if not included therein may be granted by the agency at any time before the decision becomes effective. The stay of execution provided herein may be accompanied by an express condition that respondent comply with specified terms of probation; provided, however, that the terms of probation shall be just and reasonable in the light of the findings and decision.

(c) If respondent was required to register with any public officer, a notification of any suspension or revocation shall be sent to the officer after the decision has become effective.

(d) As used in subdivision (b), specified terms of probation may include an order of restitution. Where restitution is ordered and paid pursuant to the provisions of this subdivision, the amount paid shall be credited to any subsequent judgment in a civil action.

(e) The person to which the agency action is directed may not be required to comply with a decision unless the person has been served with the decision in the manner provided in Section 11505 or has actual knowledge of the decision.

(f) A nonparty may not be required to comply with a decision unless the agency has made the decision available for public inspection and copying or the nonparty has actual knowledge of the decision.

(g) This section does not preclude an agency from taking immediate action to protect the public interest in accordance with Article 13 (commencing with Section 11460.10) of Chapter 4.5.

HISTORY:

Added Stats 1945 ch 867 § 1. Amended Stats 1949 ch 314 § 2; Stats 1976 ch 476 § 1; Stats 1977 ch 680 § 1; Stats 1995 ch 938 § 45 (SB 523), operative July 1, 1997.

§ 11519.1. Order of restitution for financial loss or damages

(a) A decision rendered against a licensee under Article 1 (commencing with Section 11700) of Chapter 4 of Division 5 of the Vehicle Code may include an order of restitution for any financial loss or damage found to have been suffered by a person in the case.

(b) The failure to make the restitution in accordance with the terms of the decision is separate grounds for the Department of Motor Vehicles to refuse to issue a license under Article 1 (commencing with Section 11700) of Chapter 4 of Division 5 of the Vehicle Code, and constitutes a violation of the terms of any applicable probationary order in the decision.

(c) Nothing in this section is intended to limit or restrict actions, remedies, or procedures otherwise available to an aggrieved party pursuant to any other provision of law.

HISTORY:

Added Stats 2007 ch 93 § 1 (SB 525), effective January 1, 2008.

§ 11520. Defaults and uncontested cases

(a) If the respondent either fails to file a notice of defense, or, as applicable, notice of participation, or to appear at the hearing, the agency may take action based upon the respondent's express admissions or upon other evidence and affidavits may be used as evidence without any notice to respondent; and where the burden of proof is on the respondent to establish that the respondent is entitled to the agency action sought, the agency may act without taking evidence.

(b) Notwithstanding the default of the respondent, the agency or the administrative law judge, before a proposed decision is issued, has discretion to grant a hearing on reasonable notice to the parties. If the agency and administrative law judge make conflicting orders under this subdivision, the agency's order takes precedence. The administrative law judge may order the respondent, or the respondent's attorney or other authorized representative, or both, to pay reasonable expenses, including attorney's fees, incurred by another party as a result of the respondent's failure to appear at the hearing.

(c) Within seven days after service on the respondent of a decision based on the respondent's default, the respondent may serve a written motion requesting that the decision be vacated and stating the grounds relied on. The agency in its discretion may vacate the decision and grant a hearing on a showing of good cause. As used in this subdivision, good cause includes, but is not limited to, any of the following:

(1) Failure of the person to receive notice served pursuant to Section 11505.

(2) Mistake, inadvertence, surprise, or excusable neglect.

HISTORY:

Added Stats 1945 ch 867 § 1. Amended Stats 1947 ch 491 § 8; Stats 1963 ch 931 § 2; Stats 1995 ch 938 § 46 (SB 523), operative July 1, 1997; Stats 2013 ch 90 § 10 (SB 546), effective January 1, 2014.

§ 11521. Reconsideration

(a) The agency itself may order a reconsideration of all or part of the case on its own motion or on petition of any party. The agency shall notify a petitioner of the time limits for petitioning for reconsideration. The power to order a reconsideration shall expire 30 days after the delivery or mailing of a decision to a respondent, or on the date set by the agency itself as the effective date of the decision if that date occurs prior to the expiration of the 30-day period or at the termination of a stay of not to exceed 30 days which the agency may grant for the purpose of filing an application for reconsideration. If additional time is needed to evaluate a petition for reconsideration filed prior to the expiration of any of the applicable periods, an agency may grant a stay of that expiration for no more than 10 days, solely for the purpose of considering the petition. If no action is taken on a petition within the time allowed for ordering reconsideration, the petition shall be deemed denied.

(b) The case may be reconsidered by the agency itself on all the pertinent parts of the record and such additional evidence and argument as may be permitted, or may be assigned to an administrative law judge. A reconsideration assigned to an administrative law judge shall be subject to the procedure provided in Section 11517. If oral evidence is introduced before the agency itself, no agency member may vote unless he or she heard the evidence.

HISTORY:

Added Stats 1945 ch 867 § 1. Amended Stats 1953 ch 964 § 1; Stats 1985 ch 324 § 22; Stats 1987 ch 305 § 1; Stats 2004 ch 865 § 34 (SB 1914).

§ 11522. Reinstatement of license or reduction of penalty

A person whose license has been revoked or suspended may petition the agency for reinstatement or reduction of penalty after a period of not less than one year has elapsed from the effective date of the decision or from the date of the denial of a similar petition. The agency shall give notice to the Attorney General of the filing of the petition and the Attorney General and the petitioner shall be afforded an opportunity to present either oral or written argument before the agency itself. The agency itself shall decide the petition, and the decision shall include the reasons therefor, and any terms and conditions that the agency reasonably deems appropriate to impose as a condition of reinstatement. This section shall not apply if the statutes dealing with the particular agency contain different provisions for reinstatement or reduction of penalty.

HISTORY:

Added Stats 1945 ch 867 § 1. Amended Stats 1985 ch 587 § 4.

§ 11523. Judicial review

Judicial review may be had by filing a petition for a writ of mandate in accordance with the provisions of the Code of Civil Procedure, subject, however, to the statutes relating to the particular agency. Except as otherwise provided in this section, the petition shall be filed within 30 days after the last day on which reconsideration can be ordered. The right to petition shall not be affected by the failure to seek reconsideration before the agency. On request of the petitioner for a record of the proceedings, the complete record of the proceedings, or the parts thereof as are designated by the petitioner in the request, shall be prepared by the Office of Administrative Hearings or the agency and shall be delivered to the petitioner, within 30 days after the request, which time shall be extended for good cause shown, upon the payment of the cost for the preparation of the transcript, the cost for preparation of other portions of the record and for certification thereof. The complete record includes the pleadings, all notices and orders issued by the agency, any proposed decision by an administrative law judge, the final decision, a transcript of all proceedings, the exhibits admitted or rejected, the written evidence and any other papers in the case. If the petitioner, within 10 days after the last day on which reconsideration can be ordered, requests the agency to prepare all or any part of the record, the time within which a petition may be filed shall be extended until 30 days after its delivery to him or her. The agency may file with the court the original of any document in the record in lieu of a copy thereof. If the petitioner prevails in overturning the administrative decision following judicial review, the agency shall reimburse the petitioner for all costs of transcript preparation, compilation of the record, and certification.

HISTORY:

Added Stats 1945 ch 867 § 1. Amended Stats 1947 ch 491 § 9; Stats 1953 ch 962 § 1; Stats 1955 ch 246 § 1; Stats 1965 ch 1458 § 10; Stats 1971 ch 984 § 1; Stats 1985 ch 324 § 23, Stats 1985 ch 973 § 1; Stats 1986 ch 597 § 3; Stats 1994 ch 1206 § 29 (SB 1775); Stats 1995 ch 938 § 47 (SB 523), operative July 1, 1997; Stats 2005 ch 674 § 23 (SB 231), effective January 1, 2006.

§ 11524. Continuances; Requirement of good cause; Judicial review of denial

(a) The agency may grant continuances. When an administrative law judge of the Office of Administrative Hearings has been assigned to the hearing, no continuance may be granted except by him or her or by the presiding judge of the appropriate regional office of the Office of Administrative Hearings, for good cause shown.

(b) When seeking a continuance, a party shall apply for the continuance within 10 working days following the time the party discovered or reasonably should have discovered the event or occurrence which establishes the good cause for the continuance. A continuance may be granted for good cause after the 10 working days have lapsed if the party seeking the continuance is not responsible for and has made a good faith effort to prevent the condition or event establishing the good cause.

(c) In the event that an application for a continuance by a party is denied by an administrative law judge of the Office of Administrative Hearings, and the party seeks judicial review thereof, the party shall, within 10 working days of the denial, make application for appropriate judicial relief in the superior court or be barred from judicial review thereof as a matter of jurisdiction. A party applying for judicial relief from the denial shall give notice to the agency and other parties. Notwithstanding Section 1010 of the Code of Civil Procedure, the notice may be either oral at the time of the denial of application for a continuance or written at the same time application is made in court for judicial relief. This subdivision does not apply to the Department of Alcoholic Beverage Control.

HISTORY:
Added Stats 1945 ch 867 § 1. Amended Stats 1953 ch 962 § 2; Stats 1963 ch 842 § 1; Stats 1971 ch 1303 § 9; Stats 1979 ch 199 § 5; Stats 1985 ch 324 § 24; Stats 1995 ch 938 § 48 (SB 523), operative July 1, 1997.

§ 11526. Voting by mail

The members of an agency qualified to vote on any question may vote by mail or another appropriate method.

HISTORY:
Added Stats 1945 ch 867 § 1. Amended Stats 1995 ch 938 § 50 (SB 523), operative July 1, 1997.

§ 11527. Charge against funds of agency

Any sums authorized to be expended under this chapter by any agency shall be a legal charge against the funds of the agency.

HISTORY:
Added Stats 1945 ch 867 § 1.

§ 11528. Oaths

In any proceedings under this chapter any agency, agency member, secretary of an agency, hearing reporter, or administrative law judge has power to administer oaths and affirmations and to certify to official acts.

HISTORY:
Added Stats 1945 ch 867 § 1. Amended Stats 1969 ch 191 § 1; Stats 1985 ch 324 § 25.

§ 11529. Interim orders

(a) The administrative law judge of the Medical Quality Hearing Panel established pursuant to Section 11371 may issue an interim order suspending a license, imposing drug testing, continuing education, supervision of procedures, limitations on the authority to prescribe, furnish, administer, or dispense controlled substances, or other license restrictions. Interim orders may be issued only if the affidavits in support of the petition show that the licensee has engaged in, or is about to engage in, acts or omissions constituting a violation of the Medical Practice Act or the appropriate practice act governing each allied health profession, or is unable to practice safely due to a mental or physical condition, and that permitting the licensee to continue to engage in the profession for which the license was issued will endanger the public health, safety, or welfare. The failure to comply with an order issued pursuant to Section 820 of the Business and Professions Code may constitute grounds to issue an interim suspension order under this section.

(b) All orders authorized by this section shall be issued only after a hearing conducted pursuant to subdivision (d), unless it appears from the facts shown by affidavit that serious injury would result to the public before the matter can be heard on notice. Except as provided in subdivision (c), the licensee shall receive at least 15 days' prior notice of the hearing, which notice shall include affidavits and all other information in support of the order.

(c) If an interim order is issued without notice, the administrative law judge who issued the order without notice shall cause the licensee to be notified of the order, including affidavits and all other information in support of the order by a 24-hour delivery service. That notice shall also include the date of the hearing on the order, which shall be conducted in accordance with the requirement of subdivision (d), not later than 20 days from the date of issuance. The order shall be dissolved unless the requirements of subdivision (a) are satisfied.

(d) For the purposes of the hearing conducted pursuant to this section, the licentiate shall, at a minimum, have the following rights:

(1) To be represented by counsel.

(2) To have a record made of the proceedings, copies of which may be obtained by the licentiate upon payment of any reasonable charges associated with the record.

(3) To present written evidence in the form of relevant declarations, affidavits, and documents.

The discretion of the administrative law judge to permit testimony at the hearing conducted pursuant to this section shall be identical to the discretion of a superior court judge to permit testimony at a hearing conducted pursuant to Section 527 of the Code of Civil Procedure.

(4) To present oral argument.

(e) Consistent with the burden and standards of proof applicable to a preliminary injunction entered under Section 527 of the Code of Civil Procedure, the administrative law judge shall grant the interim order if, in the exercise of discretion, the administrative law judge concludes that:

(1) There is a reasonable probability that the petitioner will prevail in the underlying action.

(2) The likelihood of injury to the public in not issuing the order outweighs the likelihood of injury to the licensee in issuing the order.

(f) In all cases in which an interim order is issued, and an accusation or petition to revoke probation is not filed and served pursuant to Sections 11503 and 11505 within 30 days of the date on which the parties to the hearing on the interim order have submitted the matter, the order shall be dissolved.

Upon service of the accusation or petition to revoke probation the licensee shall have, in addition to the rights granted by this section, all of the rights and privileges available as specified in this chapter. If the licensee requests a hearing on the accusation, the board shall provide the licensee with a hearing within 30 days of the request, unless the licensee stipulates to a later hearing, and a decision within 15 days of the date the decision is received from the administrative law judge, or the board shall nullify the interim order previously issued, unless good cause can be shown by the Division of Medical Quality for a delay.

(g) If an interim order is issued, a written decision shall be prepared within 15 days of the hearing, by the administrative law judge, including findings of fact and a conclusion articulating the connection between the evidence produced at the hearing and the decision reached.

(h) Notwithstanding the fact that interim orders issued pursuant to this section are not issued after a hearing as otherwise required by this chapter, interim orders so issued shall be subject to judicial review pursuant to Section 1094.5 of the Code of Civil Procedure. The relief that may be ordered shall be limited to a stay of the interim order. Interim orders issued pursuant to this section are final interim orders and, if not dissolved pursuant to subdivision (c) or (f), may only be challenged administratively at the hearing on the accusation.

(i) The interim order provided for by this section shall be:

(1) In addition to, and not a limitation on, the authority to seek injunctive relief provided for in the Business and Professions Code.

(2) A limitation on the emergency decision procedure provided in Article 13 (commencing with Section 11460.10) of Chapter 4.5.

HISTORY:

Added Stats 1990 ch 1597 § 35 (SB 2375). Amended Stats 1993 ch 1267 § 54 (SB 916); Stats 1995 ch 938 § 51 (SB 523), operative July 1, 1997; Stats 1998 ch 878 § 57 (SB 2239); Stats 2013 ch 399 § 3 (SB 670), effective January 1, 2014, ch 515 § 29.5 (SB 304), effective January 1, 2014; Stats 2017 ch 775 § 110 (SB 798), effective January 1, 2018.

APA

EXTRACTED FROM
CALIFORNIA CODE OF REGULATIONS

TITLE 1
GENERAL PROVISIONS

Division
2. Office of Administrative Hearings

DIVISION 2
OFFICE OF ADMINISTRATIVE HEARINGS

Chapter
1. General APA Hearing Procedures

CHAPTER 1
GENERAL APA HEARING PROCEDURES

Chapter
1000. Purpose.
1002. Definitions.
1004. Construction of Regulations.
1006. Format and Filing of Papers.
1008. Service; Proof of Service.
1012. Ex Parte Petitions and Applications for Temporary or Interim Orders.
1014. Pleadings; Notice of Defense; Withdrawal of Notice of Defense.
1015. Notice of Representation and Withdrawal of Counsel or Other Representative.
1016. Consolidated Proceedings; Separate Hearings.
1018. Agency Request for Hearing; Required Documents.
1019. Request for Security.
1020. Motion for Continuance of Hearing.
1022. Motions.
1024. Subpoenas; Motion for a Protective Order.
1026. Prehearing Conferences.
1027. Informal Hearings.
1028. Settlement Conferences; Settlements.
1030. Conduct of Hearing; Protective Orders.
1032. Interpreters and Accommodation.
1034. Peremptory Challenge.
1038. Ordering the Record.
1040. Monetary Sanctions.
1042. Cost Recovery.
1044. Request for Expenses After Default.
1046. Amicus Briefs.
1048. Technical and Minor Changes to Proposed and Final Decisions.
1050. Remand or Reconsideration.

§ 1000. Purpose.

These regulations specify the procedures for the conduct of matters before the Office of Administrative Hearings. Parties should also refer to the Administrative Procedure Act (Government Code sections 11370 through

11529) and/or other laws which apply to their Case. When a statute is in conflict or inconsistent with these regulations, the statute shall take precedence.

Authority cited: Section 11370.5(b), Government Code. Reference: Sections 11370-11529, Government Code.

History

1. New section filed 6-30-97 as an interim regulation pursuant to Government Code section 11400.20; operative 7-1-97 (Register 97, No. 27). Interim regulations expire on 12-31-98 unless earlier repealed or amended.

2. Amendment of subsection (a) filed 8-27-97 as an interim regulation pursuant to Government Code section 11400.20; operative 8-27-97 (Register 97, No. 35). Interim regulations expire on 12-31-98 unless earlier amended or repealed.

3. Interim regulation, including repealer of subsection (a) designator, amendment of text, repealer of subsection (b) and amendment of Note, filed 5-19-98 as a permanent regulation pursuant to Government Code section 11400.20; operative 5-30-98 pursuant to Government Code section 11343.4(d) (Register 98, No. 21).

4. Amendment of division heading and chapter heading filed 7-1-2003; operative 7-1-2003 pursuant to Government Code section 11343.4 (Register 2003, No. 27).

5. Amendment filed 10-13-2004; operative 12-1-2004 (Register 2004, No. 42).

§ 1002. Definitions.

(a) As used in these regulations, the following definitions apply:

(1) "ALJ" means an administrative law judge of the Office of Administrative Hearings.

(2) "Case" means the administrative action referred by an agency to OAH.

(3) "Day" means a calendar day, unless otherwise specified.

(4) "Declaration" means a statement under penalty of perjury that complies with Code of Civil Procedure section 2015.5.

(5) "Hearing" means the adjudicative hearing on the merits of the Case.

(6) "Motions" shall include all motions or applications for orders.

(7) "OAH" means the Office of Administrative Hearings. Unless otherwise specified, "OAH" means the appropriate regional office to which the Case is assigned.

(8) "Presiding Judge" means the Presiding Judge of the regional office of the Office of Administrative Hearings or his or her designee.

(9) "Serve" or "Service" of papers means delivery of the document by the means specified in Regulation 1008 and as required by law.

(b) These definitions are supplementary to those found in Government Code section 11500 and other applicable laws and regulations.

Authority cited: Section 11370.5(b), Government Code. Reference: Section 11500, Government Code; and Section 2015.5, Code of Civil Procedure.

History

1. New section filed 6-30-97 as an interim regulation pursuant to Government Code section 11400.20; operative 7-1-97 (Register 97, No. 27). Interim regulations expire on 12-31-98 unless earlier repealed or amended.

2. Interim regulation, including amendment of section and Note, filed 5-19-98 as a permanent regulation pursuant to Government Code section 11400.20; operative 5-30-98 pursuant to Government Code section 11343.4(d) (Register 98, No. 21).

3. Amendment filed 10-13-2004; operative 12-1-2004 (Register 2004, No. 42).

§ 1004. Construction of Regulations.

(a) As used in these regulations, words in the singular shall include the plural and words in the plural shall include the singular, unless the context otherwise requires.

(b) Statutory references are to the Government Code unless otherwise specified.

(c) In these regulations, whenever a time is stated within which an act is to be done, the time is computed by excluding the first Day and including the last Day. If the last Day is any day OAH is closed for business, that Day is also excluded.

(d) Time limits set forth in these regulations are not jurisdictional.

Authority cited: Section 11370.5(b), Government Code. Reference: Section 11370.5(b), Government Code.

History

1. New section filed 6-30-97 as an interim regulation pursuant to Government Code section 11400.20; operative 7-1-97 (Register 97, No. 27). Interim regulations expire on 12-31-98 unless earlier repealed or amended.

2. Interim regulation, including amendment of section heading, subsection (d) and Note, filed 5-19-98 as a permanent regulation pursuant to Government Code section 11400.20; operative 5-30-98 pursuant to Government Code section 11343.4(d) (Register 98, No. 21).

3. Repealer of subsection (a), subsection relettering and amendment of newly designated subsection (c) filed 10-13-2004; operative 12-1-2004 (Register 2004, No. 42).

§ 1006. Format and Filing of Papers.

(a) After a Case has been assigned to a regional office of OAH for Hearing, all papers filed pursuant to any provision of law, regulation, or ALJ order shall be filed at that regional office within applicable time limits.

(b) The first page of each paper filed should include the following:

(1) The name, address, and telephone number of the person filing the paper, including the State Bar number if the person filing the paper is an attorney;

(2) A caption setting forth the title of the Case, including the names of the agency and the respondent;

(3) The agency case number;

(4) The OAH Case number, if assigned;

(5) A brief title describing the paper filed;

(6) The dates of the Hearing and any future prehearing or settlement conferences, if known.

(c) Papers should be filed on 8 1/2" x 11" stock paper of customary weight and quality, with two normal-sized holes punched at the top (centered 2 1/2 inches apart, and 5/8 inch from the top of the paper).

(d) Papers should be typed or computer-printed. Type should be at least pica (10 characters per inch) or 12 point print. The color of the type should be blue-black or black.

(e) In addition to a paper copy, the ALJ may direct a party to submit pleadings or other papers on computer compatible diskette or by other electronic means if the party is able to do so.

(f) A party may obtain proof of the filing of a paper by submitting either an extra copy of the paper or the first page only, with a self-addressed, return envelope, postage prepaid. The clerk will return the copy marked with the date of filing.

(g) Papers may be filed with OAH by facsimile transmission. Unless required by the ALJ, the original paper need not be filed with OAH if the party obtains telephonic or other confirmation from OAH that a complete and legible copy of the papers was received.

(h) Papers delivered by the U.S. Postal Service are filed on the date received by OAH. Papers hand delivered to OAH and complete papers received by OAH by facsimile transmission during regular business hours (8 a.m. to 5 p.m.) will be filed on the date received. Papers received after regular business hours are deemed filed on the next regular business day.

Authority cited: Section 11370.5(b), Government Code. Reference: Sections 11507.3, 11507.7, 11508(c), 11511, 11511.5, 11512(c) and 11524, Government Code.

History

1. New section filed 6-30-97 as an interim regulation pursuant to Government Code section 11400.20; operative 7-1-97 (Register 97, No. 27). Interim regulations expire on 12-31-98 unless earlier repealed or amended.

2. Interim regulation, including amendment of subsections (a), (b)(4), (e) and (h), filed 5-19-98 as a permanent regulation pursuant to Government Code section 11400.20; operative 5-30-98 pursuant to Government Code section 11343.4(d) (Register 98, No. 21).

3. Amendment filed 10-13-2004; operative 12-1-2004 (Register 2004, No. 42).

§ 1008. Service; Proof of Service.

(a) Proof of Service of papers shall be a Declaration stating the title of the paper Served or filed, the name and address of the person making the Service, and that he or she is over the age of 18 years and not a party to the matter.

(b) Service may be made by leaving the paper at the residence or business of the person named to be Served, with a person not less than 18 years of age. Where Service is made in this manner, the proof of Service shall also state the date and place of delivery and the name of the person to whom the papers were handed. Where the person making the Service is unable to obtain the name of the person to whom the papers were handed, the person making the Service may substitute a physical description for the name.

(c) Where Service is made by mail, the proof of Service shall show the date and place of deposit in the mail, the name and address of the person Served as shown on the mailing envelope and that the envelope was sealed and deposited in the mail with the postage fully prepaid.

(d) Where Service is by facsimile the proof of Service shall state the method of Service upon each party, the date and time sent and the facsimile number to which the document was sent.

(e) The proof of Service shall be signed by the person making it and contain the following statement above the signature:

"I declare under penalty of perjury under the laws of the State of California that the foregoing is true and correct, and this Declaration was executed at ____(city, state)____ on ____(date)____."

The name of the declarant shall be typed and signed below this statement.

(f) A proof of Service made in accordance with Code of Civil Procedure section 1013a complies with this Regulation.

Authority cited: Section 11370.5(b), Government Code. Reference: Section 11440.20, Government Code; and Section 1013a, Code of Civil Procedure.

History

1. New section filed 6-30-97 as an interim regulation pursuant to Government Code section 11400.20; operative 7-1-97 (Register 97, No. 27). Interim regulations expire on 12-31-98 unless earlier repealed or amended.

2. Interim regulation, including amendment of subsections (a)-(e), filed 5-19-98 as a permanent regulation pursuant to Government Code section 11400.20; operative 5-30-98 pursuant to Government Code section 11343.4(d) (Register 98, No. 21).

3. Amendment filed 10-13-2004; operative 12-1-2004 (Register 2004, No. 42).

§ 1012. *Ex Parte* Petitions and Applications for Temporary or Interim Orders.

(a) This regulation applies to any *ex parte* petition or application an agency files with OAH for temporary relief or interim orders specifically authorized by statute or regulation.

(b) Absent a showing of good cause, parties shall be given at least 24 hours notice of the specific relief sought and the date, time, and place of the *ex parte* proceeding. Notice may be given by telephone or facsimile transmission.

(c) At the time of the *ex parte* appearance the petitioner or applicant shall submit a written Declaration stating the manner in which the notice was given.

(d) If prior notice was not given, the petitioner or applicant shall submit a written Declaration stating the facts showing cause why the notice under subdivision (b) could not be given or should not be required.

(e) *ex parte* petitions and applications shall be in writing and comply with Regulation 1006. The petition or application shall state the statutory authority for the temporary relief and include a proposed order.

(f) Except as provided in Regulation 1022(b), Regulation 1022 does not apply to *ex parte* petitions and applications filed under this regulation.

Authority cited: Section 11370.5(b), Government Code. Reference: Section 494, Business and Professions Code; Sections 1550.5 and 1558, Health and Safety Code; and Section 11529, Government Code.

History

1. New section filed 6-30-97 as an interim regulation pursuant to Government Code section 11400.20; operative 7-1-97 (Register 97, No. 27). Interim regulations expire on 12-31-98 unless earlier repealed or amended.

2. Interim regulation, including amendment of subsections (c) and (d), filed 5-19-98 as a permanent regulation pursuant to Government Code section 11400.20; operative 5-30-98 pursuant to Government Code section 11343.4(d) (Register 98, No. 21).

3. Amendment of section heading and section filed 10-13-2004; operative 12-1-2004 (Register 2004, No. 42).

§ 1014. Pleadings; Notice of Defense; Withdrawal of Notice of Defense.

(a) When a party amends a pleading, the party shall Serve on all other parties and promptly file with OAH a complete, new pleading incorporating the amendments. The new pleading shall be titled a "First Amended" pleading, and subsequent amended pleadings shall be titled consecutively. If the amendments are made during the Hearing, the party shall use highlighting or any other effective method to identify the changes made to the pleading. The ALJ may allow exceptions for minor amendments during Hearing.

(b) OAH prefers amended to supplemental pleadings. However, if a party issues a supplemental pleading, the party shall Serve on all other parties and promptly file with OAH the supplemental pleading which shall be titled a "First Supplemental" pleading. Subsequent supplemental pleadings shall be titled consecutively.

(c) A party who withdraws a notice of defense, a request for Hearing, or an asserted special defense shall immediately notify OAH and all other parties.

(d) When a party withdraws a notice of defense or a request for Hearing, the agency shall promptly notify OAH of the agency's decision either to proceed with the Hearing as a default or request that the scheduled Hearing be taken off calendar as a result of the party's withdrawal of the notice of defense or request for Hearing. If the agency's request to take the Hearing off calendar is made before the scheduled Hearing, the agency shall file the request in writing and include the name of the party who has withdrawn the notice of defense or request for Hearing.

Authority cited: Section 11370.5(b), Government Code. Reference: Sections 11505, 11506 and 11507, Government Code.

History

1. New section filed 6-30-97 as an interim regulation pursuant to Government Code section 11400.20; operative 7-1-97 (Register 97, No. 27). Interim regulations expire on 12-31-98 unless earlier repealed or amended.

2. Interim regulation filed 5-19-98 as a permanent regulation pursuant to Government Code section 11400.20; operative 5-30-98 pursuant to Government Code section 11343.4(d) (Register 98, No. 21).

3. Amendment of section heading and section filed 10-13-2004; operative 12-1-2004 (Register 2004, No. 42).

§ 1015. Notice of Representation and Withdrawal of Counsel or Other Representative.

(a) Any counsel or other representative who has assumed representation of a party after the agency has referred a Case to OAH shall give written notice to OAH and all other parties of his or her name, address, telephone and fax number (if any) and the name of the represented party, within a reasonable time after assuming representation.

(b) Any counsel or other representative may withdraw as counsel or representative of record by giving written notice to OAH and all parties of the withdrawal. The written notice shall include the last known address of the formerly represented party.

(c) Upon withdrawal by counsel or other representative:

(1) OAH retains jurisdiction over the Case.

(2) The formerly represented party bears the burden of keeping OAH and all other parties informed of a current address for purposes of Service. If notice of address is not given, any party may Serve the formerly represented party at the last known address and the current address of record with the agency, if a statute or regulation requires the party to maintain an address with the agency and to notify the agency of any change of address.

(3) The formerly represented party is responsible for preparation and representation throughout the remainder of the Case, unless and until such party retains new counsel or other representative.

(d) Withdrawal or change of counsel or other representative does not alone constitute grounds for continuance of any previously scheduled proceeding in the Case.

Authority cited: Section 11370.5(b), Government Code. Reference: Sections 11505, 11506 and 11524, Government Code.

History

1. New section filed 10-13-2004; operative 12-1-2004 (Register 2004, No. 42).

§ 1016. Consolidated Proceedings; Separate Hearings.

(a) A party who brings a Motion for consolidated proceedings or separate Hearings pursuant to section 11507.3 shall comply with Regulation 1022.

(b) Before an ALJ orders consolidated proceedings or separate Hearings pursuant to section 11507.3, the ALJ shall provide notice; to all parties and allow a reasonable time for the parties to file with OAH and Serve on all other parties any written opposition. Failure to file a timely opposition shall constitute a waiver of objection to an order of consolidation or severance.

(c) The parties may stipulate to consolidated proceedings or separate Hearings. In the event a stipulation is reached, the moving party shall file a written stipulation with OAH, signed by all parties, and with a signature line for the ALJ to order the consolidation. The ALJ has sole discretion to decide whether proceedings shall be consolidated or separated.

(d) If OAH consolidates Cases for Hearing, the ALJ shall prepare a separate proposed decision for each agency pleading that was consolidated, unless the agency requests or agrees otherwise.

Authority cited: Section 11370.5(b), Government Code. Reference: Section 11507.3, Government Code.

History

1. New section filed 6-30-97 as an interim regulation pursuant to Government Code section 11400.20; operative 7-1-97 (Register 97, No. 27). Interim regulations expire on 12-31-98 unless earlier repealed or amended.

2. Interim regulation filed 5-19-98 as a permanent regulation pursuant to Government Code section 11400.20; operative 5-30-98 pursuant to Government Code section 11343.4(d) (Register 98, No. 21).

3. Amendment filed 10-13-2004; operative 12-1-2004 (Register 2004, No. 42).

§ 1018. Agency Request for Hearing; Required Documents.

(a) An agency's request to OAH to set a Hearing date shall be in writing and contain the following information:

(1) The title of the Case including the identities of the agency and respondent(s);

(2) The agency case number and, if known, the OAH number assigned to the Case;

(3) The names, addresses and phone numbers of all parties who must receive notice of the hearing and their representatives, if any;

(4) The time estimate for Hearing, taking into account the time for respondent's presentation of evidence;

(5) The dates the agency and its counsel are unavailable for Hearing over the next six months; and the unavailable dates of all other parties for Hearing, if known;

(6) Preferred Hearing dates, but only if the agency includes at least three alternative preferred Hearing dates and the agency confirms in the request either that all parties have agreed to the specific dates or that it has made reasonable efforts to confer with all other parties for mutually acceptable Hearing dates, and includes the reasonable efforts the agency has made;

(7) A reference to any statute or regulation (if other than section 11517(c)) which specifies the time within which the Hearing shall be held or the proposed decision issued; and

(8) The city or county in which the Hearing will be held, pursuant to section 11508.

(b) OAH may defer setting a matter for Hearing until the agency supplies all of the information set forth in subparagraph (a).

(c) The document used by the agency to request the Hearing date shall contain a space for OAH to insert the OAH number assigned to the Case, and the date(s), time and location set for the Hearing. OAH shall transmit this information simultaneously to the agency, respondent(s), and each respondent's representative as identified in the written request to set. The transmission of this information by OAH does not replace the notice of Hearing required by section 11509.

(d) The agency shall file the following documents with OAH at the time it files the written request to set a Hearing date or as soon thereafter as the documents become available:

(1) accusation, statement of issues, statement of charges, suspension order, or other initial pleading, with proof of Service on all parties;

(2) notice of defense executed by respondent(s);

(3) notice of Hearing, with proof of Service on all parties.

Authority cited: Section 11370.5(b), Government Code. Reference: Sections 11508 and 11509, Government Code.

History

1. New section filed 6-30-97 as an interim regulation pursuant to Government Code section 11400.20; operative 7-1-97 (Register 97, No. 27). Interim regulations expire on 12-31-98 unless earlier repealed or amended.

2. Interim regulation, including amendment of section heading and subsections (a)(2), (a)(6), (a)(7) and (b), filed 5-19-98 as a permanent regulation pursuant to Government Code section 11400.20; operative 5-30-98 pursuant to Government Code section 11343.4(d) (Register 98, No. 21).

3. Amendment of section heading and section filed 10-13-2004; operative 12-1-2004 (Register 2004, No. 42).

§ 1019. Request for Security.

(a) Any party or participant in a proceeding before OAH may request security for the proceeding. The request for security shall be made to the Presiding Judge as soon as the need for security is known.

(b) The Presiding Judge or the ALJ presiding over the proceeding may determine on his or her own initiative that security is required.

(c) To assure that appropriate safety measures are arranged, the person requesting security shall inform the Presiding Judge of the nature of the safety risk.

(d) If the request for security is made without sufficient time for OAH to obtain appropriate security, the Presiding Judge has discretion to continue the proceeding.

Authority cited: Section 11370.5(b), Government Code. Reference: *Zaheri v New Motor Vehicle Board* (1997) 55 Cal.App.4th 1305, 64 Cal.Rptr.2d 705.

History

1. New section filed 10-13-2004; operative 12-1-2004 (Register 2004, No. 42).

§ 1020. Motion for Continuance of Hearing.

(a) A Case filed with OAH is assigned to the Presiding Judge until reassigned to another ALJ.

(b) A Motion to continue a Hearing shall be in writing, directed to the Presiding Judge, and Served on all other parties.

(c) Before filing the Motion, the moving party shall make reasonable efforts to confer with all other parties to determine whether any party opposes the Motion and to obtain future dates when all parties are unavailable for Hearing over the next six months and at least three alternative preferred future Hearing dates.

(d) The Motion shall include all facts which support a showing of good cause to continue the Hearing, as well as:

(1) the Case name, and OAH Case number;

(2) the date, time and place of the Hearing;

(3) the address and daytime telephone number of the moving party;

(4) the name, address and telephone number of all other parties;

(5) a list of all previous Motions to continue the Hearing and the dispositions thereof;

(6) whether or not any party opposes the Motion;

(7) any future dates when the parties are unavailable for Hearing over the next six months and any preferred future Hearing dates obtained pursuant to paragraph (c);

(8) if the moving party has not included all of the information required pursuant to this paragraph (d), the reasons why it is not included;

(9) a reference to any legal or other requirement to set the Hearing within a certain period of time, and whether or not the parties have waived the requirement.

(e) If the Motion is not timely pursuant to section 11524(b) or other applicable law, the Motion shall include all facts justifying the lack of timeliness.

(f) The Motion may include a proposed order granting the continuance.

(g) Any party may request a written order from OAH reflecting the disposition of the Motion.

(h) Any party opposing the Motion shall file with OAH and Serve on all other parties a written opposition.

(i) The Presiding Judge may waive any requirement of this regulation, including but not limited to the requirement for a written Motion, written opposition, written order, and/or any notice to other parties.

(j) Regulation 1022 does not apply to Motions for continuance filed under this regulation.

Authority cited: Section 11370.5(b), Government Code. Reference: Section 11524, Government Code. *Arnett v Office of Administrative Hearings*, 49 Cal. App. 4th 332 (1996).

History

1. New section filed 6-30-97 as an interim regulation pursuant to Government Code section 11400.20; operative 7-1-97 (Register 97, No. 27). Interim regulations expire on 12-31-98 unless earlier repealed or amended.

2. Interim regulation, including amendment of section heading, section and Note, filed 5-19-98 as a permanent regulation pursuant to Government Code section 11400.20; operative 5-30-98 pursuant to Government Code section 11343.4(d) (Register 98, No. 21).

3. Repealer and new section filed 10-13-2004; operative 12-1-2004 (Register 2004, No. 42).

§ 1022. Motions.

(a) All Motions made prior to the Hearing shall be directed to the Presiding Judge. Thereafter, Motions shall be directed to the ALJ assigned to the Hearing.

(b) A Motion shall be made with written notice to all parties, unless the Motion is made during a Hearing while on the record. If a specific statute or regulation permits an *ex parte* petition or application, the moving party shall give all other parties 24-hour notice in accordance with Regulation 1012. Every written Motion shall be filed with an attached proof of Service showing that all parties have been Served with the Motion.

(c) If a prehearing conference has been scheduled, all Motions to be heard at the prehearing conference shall be filed in accordance with Regulation 1026(b), unless the Presiding Judge determines otherwise.

(d) Motions and any response thereto shall conform to the requirements of Regulation 1006. The Motion shall state in plain language the relief sought and the facts, circumstances, and legal authority that support the Motion.

(e) Except as otherwise provided by statute or regulation, or as ordered by the Presiding Judge, a Motion shall be filed and Served at least 15 Days before the date set for the commencement of the Hearing, and any response to the Motion shall be filed and Served no later than 3 Days before the date the Motion is scheduled to be heard.

(f) Except as otherwise provided by statute or regulation, or as ordered by the Presiding Judge, a Motion shall be decided without oral argument. A party may request oral argument at the time of filing the Motion or response.

(g) If the Presiding Judge orders oral argument, OAH shall set the date, time and place. The Presiding Judge may direct a party to Serve written notice on all other parties of the date, time, and place of the oral argument. Oral argument may be made in person or by telephone conference call, video conference, or any other electronic means, in compliance with section 11440.30 and Regulation 1030.

(h) The Presiding Judge has discretion to decide whether oral argument shall be stenographically reported on his or her own motion or upon the written request of any party which includes the reasons for the request.

(i) The ruling on any Motion shall be made by written order, unless the Motion and ruling are made during the course of a Hearing while on the record. The ALJ may direct the prevailing party to prepare the order, or dispense with the requirement of a written order.

(j) This regulation does not apply to a Motion to continue a Hearing pursuant to section 11524 and Regulation 1020. Requests for *ex parte* Petitions and Applications for Temporary or Interim Orders shall be made pursuant to the provisions of Regulation 1012, and do not constitute a Motion within the meaning of this regulation. A request for a settlement conference pursuant to Regulation 1028, a prehearing conference pursuant to Regulation 1026, or security pursuant to Regulation 1019 does not constitute a Motion within the meaning of this regulation.

Authority cited: Section 11370.5(b), Government Code. Reference: Sections 11440.30, 11507.3, 11507.7, 11508(c), 11511 and 11524, Government Code.

History

1. New section filed 6-30-97 as an interim regulation pursuant to Government Code section 11400.20; operative 7-1-97 (Register 97, No. 27). Interim regulations expire on 12-31-98 unless earlier repealed or amended.

2. Interim regulation, including new subsection (a), repealer of subsection (c), subsection relettering, and amendment of subsection (f), filed 5-19-98 as a permanent regulation pursuant to Government Code section 11400.20; operative 5-30-98 pursuant to Government Code section 11343.4(d) (Register 98, No. 21).

3. Repealer and new section filed 10-13-2004; operative 12-1-2004 (Register 2004, No. 42).

§ 1024. Subpoenas; Motion for a Protective Order.

(a) Subpoena forms are available from OAH. Subpoenas may also be issued pursuant to section 11450.20(a).

(b) A Motion pursuant to section 11450.30 for a protective order, including a Motion to quash, shall be made in compliance with Regulation 1022. The Motion shall be made within a reasonable period after receipt of the subpoena.

The person bringing the Motion shall Serve copies of the Motion on all parties and persons who are required by law to receive notice of the subpoena.

Authority cited: Section 11370.5(b), Government Code. Reference: Sections 1985-1985.4, Code of Civil Procedure; and Sections 11450.05, 11450.20, 11450.50 and 11450.30, Government Code.

History

1. New section filed 6-30-97 as an interim regulation pursuant to Government Code section 11400.20; operative 7-1-97 (Register 97, No. 27). Interim regulations expire on 12-31-98 unless earlier repealed or amended.

2. Interim regulation, including amendment of subsection (a) and Note, filed 5-19-98 as a permanent regulation pursuant to Government Code section 11400.20; operative 5-30-98 pursuant to Government Code section 11343.4(d) (Register 98, No. 21).

3. Amendment of section and Note filed 10-13-2004; operative 12-1-2004 (Register 2004, No. 42).

§ 1026. Prehearing Conferences.

(a) After a Case is assigned to OAH, any party may file with OAH and Serve on all parties a request for a prehearing conference. A request for a prehearing conference shall be directed to the Presiding Judge and state the reasons for the conference. If the request is granted, OAH shall set the date and time for the conference. Regulation 1022 does not apply to a request for a prehearing conference.

(b) Motions to be heard at the prehearing conference shall be filed with OAH no later than 15 Days before the prehearing conference and shall otherwise comply with Regulation 1022. Responses shall be filed with OAH no later than 3 business days prior to the prehearing conference. The ALJ may, in his or her discretion, allow oral Motions during the prehearing conference.

(c) A request to continue the date of the prehearing conference shall be directed to the Presiding Judge. After commencement of the prehearing conference, the assigned ALJ may continue it to any other convenient time prior to the Hearing date.

(d) At least 3 business days before a prehearing conference, each party shall file with OAH and Serve on all other parties a prehearing conference statement containing the following information:

(1) Identification of all operative pleadings by title and date signed;

(2) The party's current estimate of time necessary to try the Case;

(3) The name of each witness the party may call at the Hearing along with a brief statement of the subject matter of the witness's expected testimony;

(4) The identity of any witness whose testimony will be presented by affidavit pursuant to section 11514;

(5) The name and address of each expert witness the party intends to call at the Hearing along with a brief statement of the opinion the expert is expected to give and a copy of the expert's current resume;

(6) The need for an interpreter or special accommodation;

(7) A list of the documentary exhibits the party intends to present and a description of any physical or demonstrative evidence; and

(8) A concise statement of any legal issues or affirmative defenses that may affect the presentation of evidence or the disposition of the Case.

(e) Exhibits need not be premarked or filed with the prehearing conference statements unless requested by the ALJ. Exhibits shall be exchanged between the parties at least 3 business days before the prehearing conference. On agreement of the parties, exhibits already produced in discovery need not be exchanged.

(f) The prehearing conference may be held by telephone or other electronic means pursuant to section 11511.5(c).

(g) After the prehearing conference, the ALJ shall issue a prehearing conference order which incorporates the matters determined at the conference. This order may be issued orally if an accurate record is made. Agreements on the simplification of issues, amendments, stipulations, or other matters may be entered on the record or may be made the subject of a written order by the ALJ. If no matters were determined or dates set at the prehearing conference, a prehearing conference order is not required.

(h) Upon request of a party, the ALJ shall prepare a written prehearing conference order. The ALJ may direct a party to prepare a proposed prehearing conference order.

Authority cited: Section 11370.5(b), Government Code. Reference: Sections 11420.10, 11445.10, 11511.5 and 11514, Government Code.

History

1. New section filed 6-30-97 as an interim regulation pursuant to Government Code section 11400.20; operative 7-1-97 (Register 97, No. 27). Interim regulations expire on 12-31-98 unless earlier repealed or amended.

2. Interim regulation, including amendment of subsections (a), (b), (d), (d)(3), (d)(5), (d)(7) and (e), filed 5-19-98 as a permanent regulation pursuant to Government Code section 11400.20; operative 5-30-98 pursuant to Government Code section 11343.4(d) (Register 98, No. 21).

3. Amendment filed 10-13-2004; operative 12-1-2004 (Register 2004, No. 42).

§ 1027. Informal Hearings.

An agency may file a written request directed to the Presiding Judge to set a Case for an informal hearing. The request shall explain how the circumstances are appropriate for an informal hearing procedure, pursuant to section 11445.10 et seq. The Presiding Judge may order the Case to proceed as an informal hearing. If the Case proceeds by informal hearing, the Presiding Judge or assigned ALJ shall advise the parties of the procedures to be applied pursuant to section 11445.40.

Authority cited: Section 11370.5(b), Government Code. Reference: Sections 11445.10-11445.60 and 11470.10, Government Code.

History

1. New section filed 5-19-98; operative 5-30-98 pursuant to Government Code section 11343.4(d) (Register 98, No. 21).

2. Repealer and new section filed 10-13-2004; operative 12-1-2004 (Register 2004, No. 42).

§ 1028. Settlement Conferences; Settlements.

(a) After a Case is assigned to OAH, any party may file with OAH and Serve on all parties a request for a settlement conference. A request for a settlement conference shall be directed to the Presiding Judge. If the request is granted, OAH shall set the date and time for the conference. Regulation 1022 does not apply to a request for a settlement conference.

(b) Each respondent and his or her representative and an agency counsel or other representative, if the agency is not represented by counsel, shall appear in person at all settlement conferences. Each party or representative who attends the settlement conference shall be fully familiar with the facts and issues in the Case and shall have authority, or be able to obtain authority immediately by telephone, to negotiate settlement terms subject to the approval by the agency head. An agency representative who is familiar with the case, and has authority to approve settlement terms subject to the approval by the agency head, must be available to participate in the settlement conference in person or by telephone, subject to section 11511.7.

(c) The Presiding Judge may excuse the attendance or participation of a party or representative upon a showing of good cause. A request to be excused shall be made not less than 3 business days before the date of the conference.

(d) A Request to continue the settlement conference shall be addressed to the Presiding Judge.

(e) The settlement conference ALJ may structure the conference to meet the needs of the particular dispute. A telephonic settlement conference may be arranged pursuant to section 11511.7(b).

(f) A party may file a written settlement conference statement with OAH that describes the factual and legal issues and the status of any previous settlement discussions in the Case. The statement may be Served on all other parties or it may be marked "confidential" and submitted only to the Presiding Judge or the settlement conference ALJ. The statement should be submitted at least 3 business days before the conference. The Presiding Judge or settlement conference ALJ may require a party to file a settlement conference statement.

(g) A party should bring any pertinent documents and a draft of any settlement proposal on disk or in writing to the settlement conference.

(h) The settlement conference statement, other settlement materials, and settlement discussions shall not be disclosed to the Hearing ALJ and are deemed confidential unless the parties agree otherwise.

(i) Any settlement shall be included in a written stipulation, settlement agreement or consent order, or an oral agreement placed on the record.

(j) The parties shall promptly notify the OAH calendar clerk of any resolution that terminates a Case before OAH. OAH will vacate all Hearing dates upon receipt of a written request and notice of final resolution of the Case from the agency. A copy shall be Served on all other parties. Notice of final resolution of a Case consists of written confirmation from the agency that all parties have signed a final written agreement resolving the Case (subject to approval by the agency head) or that the agency has taken any unilateral actions legally required to withdraw, dismiss, or otherwise resolve the Case. A copy of the signed settlement, stipulation, agency order or any other paperwork terminating a matter before OAH, or, at the discretion of the agency, the first page and signature pages thereof, shall be filed with OAH.

Authority cited: Section 11370.5(b), Government Code. Reference: Sections 11415.60 and 11511.7, Government Code.

History

1. New section filed 6-30-97 as an interim regulation pursuant to Government Code section 11400.20; operative 7-1-97 (Register 97, No. 27). Interim regulations expire on 12-31-98 unless earlier repealed or amended.

2. Interim regulation, including amendment of subsections (e), (j) and (r), filed 5-19-98 as a permanent regulation pursuant to Government Code section 11400.20; operative 5-30-98 pursuant to Government Code section 11343.4(d) (Register 98, No. 21).

3. Repealer and new section filed 10-13-2004; operative 12-1-2004 (Register 2004, No. 42).

§ 1030. Conduct of Hearing; Protective Orders.

(a) A party seeking an order for closure or other protective order for all or part of a Hearing, including a request to seal the record, pursuant to section 11425.20 shall file a Motion stating in plain language the relief sought and the facts, circumstances, and legal authority that support the Motion.

(b) A party seeking to have all or part of a Hearing conducted by electronic means pursuant to section 11440.30 shall file a Motion stating in plain language the relief sought and the facts, circumstances, and legal authority that support the Motion.

(c) An ALJ, in his or her discretion, and with due consideration for the effect on witnesses, the Hearing process, and existing protective orders, may grant a request by a party or interested person to film, photograph, or record the Hearing. A record made pursuant to this section shall not be part of the official record.

(d) If a party's Motion or request under subsections (a), (b), or (c) of this Regulation is granted, the ALJ may direct the moving party to make the necessary arrangements and pay the related costs.

(e) The ALJ may:

(1) Exclude persons whose actions impede the orderly conduct of the Hearing;

(2) Restrict attendance because of the physical limitations of the Hearing facility; or

(3) Take other action to promote due process or the orderly conduct of the Hearing.

Authority cited: Section 11370.5(b), Government Code. Reference: Sections 11425.20, 11440.30 and 11455.10, Government Code.

History

1. New section filed 6-30-97 as an interim regulation pursuant to Government Code section 11400.20; operative 7-1-97 (Register 97, No. 27). Interim regulations expire on 12-31-98 unless earlier repealed or amended.

2. Interim regulation filed 5-19-98 as a permanent regulation pursuant to Government Code section 11400.20; operative 5-30-98 pursuant to Government Code section 11343.4(d) (Register 98, No. 21).

3. Repealer and new section heading and section and amendment of Note filed 10-13-2004; operative 12-1-2004 (Register 2004, No. 42).

§ 1032. Interpreters and Accommodation.

(a) A party shall give timely notice to OAH and the agency when that party or the party's representative or witness needs any of the following accommodations during a proceeding before OAH:

(1) Language assistance, including sign language.

(2) Accommodation for a disability.

(3) Electronic amplification for hearing impairment.

(4) Any other special accommodation.

(b) Unless otherwise provided by contract, the agency shall provide the appropriate language assistance.

(c) An interpreter at a Hearing or other proceeding shall be sworn by oath or affirmation to perform his or her duties truthfully. The oath or affirmation shall be in substantially the following form:

"Do you swear or affirm that, to the best of your skill and judgment, you will make a true interpretation of the questions asked and the answers given and that you will make a true translation of any documents which require translation?"

(d) A party may ask the ALJ assigned to the Hearing to direct payment for the cost of interpreter services pursuant to section 11435.25.

Authority cited: Section 11370.5(b), Government Code. Reference: Section 751, Evidence Code; and Sections 11435.05, 11435.10, 11435.55 and 11435.65, Government Code.

History

1. New section filed 6-30-97 as an interim regulation pursuant to Government Code section 11400.20; operative 7-1-97 (Register 97, No. 27). Interim regulations expire on 12-31-98 unless earlier repealed or amended.

2. Interim regulation, including amendment of Note, filed 5-19-98 as a permanent regulation pursuant to Government Code section 11400.20; operative 5-30-98 pursuant to Government Code section 11343.4(d) (Register 98, No. 21).

3. Repealer and new section and amendment of Note filed 10-13-2004; operative 12-1-2004 (Register 2004, No. 42).

§ 1034. Peremptory Challenge.

(a) Pursuant to section 11425.40(d), a party is entitled to one peremptory challenge (disqualification without cause) of an ALJ assigned to an OAH Hearing. A peremptory challenge is not allowed in proceedings involving petitions or applications for temporary relief or interim order or in a proceeding on reconsideration or remand; and shall not apply to panel members of a Commission on Professional Competence, other than the ALJ, in proceedings under Education Code section 44944. In no event will a peremptory challenge be allowed if it is made after the Hearing has commenced.

(b) A peremptory challenge shall be:

(1) Directed to the Presiding Judge;

(2) Filed by a party, attorney or authorized representative;

(3) Made in writing or orally on the record in substantially the following form:

"I am a party to [CASENAME] and am exercising my right to a peremptory challenge regarding ALJ [NAME], pursuant to Regulation 1034 and Government Code section 11425.40(d)";

(4) Served on all parties if made in writing; and

(5) Filed in compliance with the time requirements of subsections (c), (d), and (e) herein.

(c) If, at the time of a scheduled prehearing conference, an ALJ has been assigned to the Hearing, any challenge to the assigned ALJ shall be made no later than commencement of that prehearing conference.

(d) Except as provided in (c), if the Hearing is to be held at an OAH regional office, the peremptory challenge of the assigned ALJ shall be made no later than 2 business days before the Hearing.

(e) Except as provided in (c), if the Hearing is to be held at a site other than an OAH regional office, the peremptory challenge of the assigned ALJ shall be made by noon on Friday prior to the week in which the Hearing is to commence.

(f) A party may contact OAH to determine the name of the ALJ assigned to the Hearing.

(g) A Hearing shall not be continued by reason of a peremptory challenge unless a continuance is required for the convenience of OAH. If continued, the Hearing shall be rescheduled to the first convenient date for OAH.

(h) Nothing in this regulation shall affect or limit the provisions of a challenge for cause under sections 11425.40, 11430.60 and 11512(c) or any other applicable provisions of law.

Authority cited: Section 11370.5(b), Government Code. Reference: Sections 11425.40, 11430.60 and 11512(c), Government Code.

History

1. New section filed 6-30-97 as an interim regulation pursuant to Government Code section 11400.20; operative 7-1-97 (Register 97, No. 27). Interim regulations expire on 12-31-98 unless earlier repealed or amended.

2. Interim regulation, including amendment of subsections (c), (f), (g) and (i), filed 5-19-98 as a permanent regulation pursuant to Government Code section 11400.20; operative 5-30-98 pursuant to Government Code section 11343.4(d) (Register 98, No. 21).

3. Repealer and new section filed 10-13-2004; operative 12-1-2004 (Register 2004, No. 42).

§ 1038. Ordering the Record.

(a) Any person may request a copy of all or a portion of the record, subject to any protective orders or provisions of law prohibiting disclosure. The complete record includes the pleadings, all notices and orders issued by the agency, any proposed decision by an ALJ, the final decision, a transcript of all proceedings, all exhibits whether admitted or rejected, the written evidence and any other papers in the Case, except as provided by law.

(b) Except as provided in (f), no portion of the record will be prepared until the requesting person has paid a deposit equal to the estimated cost of preparation. The deposit will be applied to the actual cost and any excess will be returned to the person who submitted it. The record will not be released until the person ordering the record has paid any balance due for the actual cost of preparing the record.

(c) If OAH has contracted for the stenographic reporting or tape recording of the proceeding, a person may contact the OAH transcript clerk to order and pay for preparation of all or a portion of the transcript in the Case. If the agency for whom OAH has conducted the proceeding has contracted for the stenographic reporting or tape recording, a person seeking to order all or a portion of the transcript or a copy of the tape must contact the agency directly.

(d) Any person may contact the OAH transcript clerks or the agency to order and pay for copying of any other portions of the record in a Case, except as provided in (c).

(e) If the official record of the Hearing or other proceeding was made by audio tape, copies of the audio tape(s) are available upon written request to the OAH transcript clerk and payment of the costs of duplication, except as provided in (c). Copies of audio tapes and transcripts made from the copies are not part of the official record.

(f) A party seeking a waiver of fees and costs to prepare the record for the purpose of judicial review under Code of Civil Procedure section 1094.5 who has been declared *in forma pauperis* (Government Code section 68511.3) shall submit a valid order issued by the Superior Court.

Authority cited: Section 11370.5(b), Government Code. Reference: Section 1094.5, Code of Civil Procedure; Sections 11512, 11523 and 69950, Government Code; and Section 985, California Rules of Court.

History

1. New section filed 6-30-97 as an interim regulation pursuant to Government Code section 11400.20; operative 7-1-97 (Register 97, No. 27). Interim regulations expire on 12-31-98 unless earlier repealed or amended.

2. Interim regulation, including amendment of subsection (h), filed 5-19-98 as a permanent regulation pursuant to Government Code section 11400.20; operative 5-30-98 pursuant to Government Code section 11343.4(d) (Register 98, No. 21).

3. Repealer and new section filed 7-1-2003; operative 7-1-2003 pursuant to Government Code section 11343.4 (Register 2003, No. 27).

4. Editorial correction adding text of new section and correcting History 3 (Register 2003, No. 33).

5. Amendment of section and Note filed 10-13-2004; operative 12-1-2004 (Register 2004, No. 42).
6. Change without regulatory effect amending subsection (b) and Note filed 12-29-2005 pursuant to section 100, title 1, California Code of Regulations (Register 2005, No. 52).

§ 1040. Monetary Sanctions.

(a) The ALJ may order a party, a party's representative or both, to pay reasonable expenses, including attorney's fees, incurred by another party as a result of bad faith actions or tactics that are frivolous or solely intended to cause unnecessary delay.

(1) "Actions or tactics" include, but are not limited to, the making or opposing of Motions or the failure to comply with a lawful order of the ALJ.

(2) "Frivolous" means

(A) totally and completely without merit or

(B) for the sole purpose of harassing an opposing party.

(b) The ALJ shall not impose sanctions without providing notice and an opportunity to be heard.

(c) The ALJ shall determine the reasonable expenses based upon testimony under oath or a Declaration setting forth specific expenses incurred as a result of the bad faith conduct. An order for sanctions may be made on the record or in writing, setting forth the factual findings on which the sanctions are based.

Authority cited: Section 11370.5(b), Government Code. Reference: Section 128.5, Code of Civil Procedure; and Section 11455.30, Government Code.

History

1. New section filed 6-30-97 as an interim regulation pursuant to Government Code section 11400.20; operative 7-1-97 (Register 97, No. 27). Interim regulations expire on 12-31-98 unless earlier repealed or amended.
2. Interim regulation, including amendment of subsections (c)(1) and (c)(2), filed 5-19-98 as a permanent regulation pursuant to Government Code section 11400.20; operative 5-30-98 pursuant to Government Code section 11343.4(d) (Register 98, No. 21).
3. Amendment of section heading and section filed 10-13-2004; operative 12-1-2004 (Register 2004, No. 42).

§ 1042. Cost Recovery.

(a) An agency shall allege in its pleading any request for costs, citing the applicable cost recovery statute or regulation.

(b) Except as otherwise provided by law, proof of costs at the Hearing may be made by Declarations that contain specific and sufficient facts to support findings regarding actual costs incurred and the reasonableness of the costs, which shall be presented as follows:

(1) For services provided by a regular agency employee, the Declaration may be executed by the agency or its designee and shall describe the general tasks performed, the time spent on each task and the method of calculating the cost. For other costs, the bill, invoice or similar supporting document shall be attached to the Declaration.

(2) For services provided by persons who are not agency employees, the Declaration shall be executed by the person providing the service and describe the general tasks performed, the time spent on each task and the hourly rate or other compensation for the service. In lieu of this Declaration, the agency may attach to its Declaration copies of the time and billing records submitted by the service provider.

(3) When the agency presents an estimate of actual costs incurred, its Declaration shall explain the reason actual cost information is not available.

(4) The ALJ may permit a party to present testimony relevant to the amount and reasonableness of costs.

(c) The proposed decision shall include a factual finding and legal conclusion on the request for costs and shall state the reasons for denying a request or awarding less than the amount requested. Any award of costs shall be specified in the order.

Authority cited: Section 11370.5(b), Government Code. Reference: Sections 125.3(c), 3753.5(a), 4990.17 and 5107(b), Business and Professions Code; and Sections 11507.6 and 11520(b), Government Code.

History

1. New section filed 6-30-97 as an interim regulation pursuant to Government Code section 11400.20; operative 7-1-97 (Register 97, No. 27). Interim regulations expire on 12-31-98 unless earlier repealed or amended.

2. Interim regulation, including amendment of subsections (a), (b)(1)-(5) and (d), filed 5-19-98 as a permanent regulation pursuant to Government Code section 11400.20; operative 5-30-98 pursuant to Government Code section 11343.4(d) (Register 98, No. 21).

3. Repealer and new section heading and section filed 10-13-2004; operative 12-1-2004 (Register 2004, No. 42).

§ 1044. Request for Expenses After Default.

When a request is made for expenses pursuant to section 11520(b), the requesting party shall submit a Declaration setting forth, with specificity, the expenses incurred as a result of respondent's failure to appear.

Authority cited: Section 11370.5(b), Government Code. Reference: Section 11520(b), Government Code.

History

1. New section filed 6-30-97 as an interim regulation pursuant to Government Code section 11400.20; operative 7-1-97 (Register 97, No. 27). Interim regulations expire on 12-31-98 unless earlier repealed or amended.

2. Interim regulation, including amendment of section, filed 5-19-98 as a permanent regulation pursuant to Government Code section 11400.20; operative 5-30-98 pursuant to Government Code section 11343.4(d) (Register 98, No. 21).

3. Amendment filed 10-13-2004; operative 12-1-2004 (Register 2004, No. 42).

§ 1046. Amicus Briefs.

A non-party with an interest in the outcome of the Hearing may, by Motion, request permission to file an Amicus brief. The Motion shall show good cause for allowing the brief, giving consideration to the following factors:

(a) Due process of law;

(b) Whether matters in the Amicus brief will be helpful to the ALJ;

(c) The interests of the public and public policy; and

(d) The costs to the parties to reply to the Amicus brief.

Authority cited: Section 11370.5(b), Government Code. Reference: Sections 11500(b) and 11512(b), Government Code.

History

1. New section filed 6-30-97 as an interim regulation pursuant to Government Code section 11400.20; operative 7-1-97 (Register 97, No. 27). Interim regulations expire on 12-31-98 unless earlier repealed or amended.

2. Interim regulation filed 5-19-98 as a permanent regulation pursuant to Government Code section 11400.20; operative 5-30-98 pursuant to Government Code section 11343.4(d) (Register 98, No. 21).

3. Amendment of section heading and repealer and new section filed 10-13-2004; operative 12-1-2004 (Register 2004, No. 42).

§ 1048. Technical and Minor Changes to Proposed and Final Decisions.

(a) The agency may make an application to OAH to correct a mistake or clerical error, or make minor or technical changes, in a proposed decision by filing a written request addressed to the Presiding Judge.

(1) The application must be signed on behalf of the agency that is seeking the correction(s) and identify the correction(s) being sought and the reasons therefor. The application shall be served on all other parties, together with a copy of the proposed decision. A copy of the proof of service shall be filed with the application.

(2) A party shall have a period of 10 days from the date the application is served to file written opposition. The opposition shall be served on all parties and filed with OAH, with a copy of the proof of service.

(3) If opposition is filed, the Presiding Judge may permit oral argument or decide the matter on the papers alone. If the Presiding Judge permits oral argument, at least 5 days notice of the time and place for oral argument shall be given. The Presiding Judge shall decide the matter no later than 5 days after it is submitted.

(4) If the application is granted, the Presiding Judge shall prepare, and cause to be served on all parties, a notice and order of correction and/or a corrected proposed decision, which shall identify the correction(s) made.

(5) If the application is denied, the Presiding Judge shall cause notice of the denial to be served on all parties.

(6) The Presiding Judge will designate the same ALJ who prepared the proposed decision in the case to review and decide the application for correction. If the same ALJ is not reasonably available, the Presiding Judge may designate another ALJ.

(b) Any party other than the agency shall file an application with the agency to correct a mistake or clerical error, or make minor or technical changes, in a proposed decision. Subject to section 11517(c)(2)(C), the agency may decide the application itself or refer it to the Presiding Judge to decide. If the application is referred to the Presiding Judge, the provisions of paragraph (a)(1)-(6) shall apply.

(c) An ALJ who prepares a proposed decision may, on his or her own motion, correct any mistakes or clerical errors or make minor or technical changes in the proposed decision. The ALJ must cause to be served on all parties, a notice and order of correction and/or a corrected proposed decision, each of which shall identify the correction(s) made. Before making any correction under this paragraph, an ALJ may, in his or her discretion, provide notice to all parties and an opportunity to be heard.

(d) Section 11517(c)(2)(C) authorizes the agency to make technical or other minor changes to a proposed decision and adopt it as the decision in the Case. The agency may obtain an electronic copy of the proposed decision for this purpose upon written request addressed to the Presiding Judge of the OAH office that issued the proposed decision. When OAH provides an electronic copy of the proposed decision to the agency, it does not constitute OAH's approval of any changes the agency proposes. The agency shall send a copy of the proposed decision, as corrected, to OAH.

(e) OAH may correct a clerical error or mistake, or make technical or minor changes, in a proposed decision if all of the parties agree to the correction. The stipulation pursuant to the agreement must be in writing, signed by all parties, and clearly identify the change(s) or correction(s) to be made in the proposed decision. The stipulation must be filed with the Presiding Judge. If the stipulation is accepted, the Presiding Judge shall prepare, and cause to be served on all parties, a notice and order of correction and/or a corrected proposed decision, each of which shall identify the correction(s) made. If the stipulation is rejected, the Presiding Judge shall cause notice thereof to be served on all parties.

(f) No change or correction to a proposed decision shall be effective if the agency rejects or adopts the existing proposed decision without the change or correction.

(g) Government Code section 11518.5 governs corrections of mistakes or clerical errors in agency decisions issued after adjudicative proceedings that are subject to the formal hearing provisions of the Administrative Procedure Act in Title 2, Division 3, Part 1, Chapter 5, commencing with Government Code section 11500.

(h) Decisions issued by an ALJ in proceedings that are not subject to the formal hearing provisions of the Administrative Procedure Act (Title 2, Division 3, Part 1, Chapter 5, commencing with Government Code section 11500) may be corrected in accordance with the procedures provided in paragraphs (a), (b), and (e).

(i) In no event may any correction made pursuant to this policy statement result in reconsideration, or change the factual or legal basis, of a proposed or final decision.

(j) All documents filed or issued with a request to correct a proposed or final decision shall become a part of the record in the Case.

Authority cited: Section 11370.5(b), Government Code. Reference: Sections 11517(c) and 11518.5, Government Code.

History

1. New section filed 10-13-2004; operative 12-1-2004 (Register 2004, No. 42).

§ 1050. Remand or Reconsideration.

(a) An agency referral of a Case to OAH for rehearing or reconsideration pursuant to sections 11517(c)(2)(D) or 11521(b) shall be filed in the OAH regional office that issued the proposed decision. The referral shall be in writing, directed to the Presiding Judge, and shall contain the following:

(1) Information as required in Regulation 1018, except for Hearing dates if no Hearing is requested;

(2) The name of the ALJ who prepared the proposed decision;

(3) A copy of any agency order or decision for rehearing or reconsideration and the proof of Service of the order or decision on all parties; and

(4) The evidence or issues to be considered on rehearing or reconsideration.

(b) The agency shall lodge the record in the Case, including the transcript, exhibits, and other papers that are part of the record, with OAH promptly after the agency has received it. If the agency has not lodged the complete record at least 15 days before the scheduled Hearing in the Case, it shall provide written notice thereof to OAH and all other parties.

Authority cited: Section 11370.5(b), Government Code. Reference: Sections 11517(c)(2)(D) and 11521(b), Government Code.

History

1. New section filed 10-13-2004; operative 12-1-2004 (Register 2004, No. 42).